Springer Japan KK

M. Endoh · M. Morad
H. Scholz · T. Iijima (Eds.)

Molecular and Cellular Mechanisms of Cardiovascular Regulation

With 201 Figures

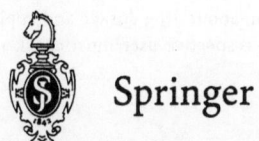 Springer

MASAO ENDOH, M.D., PH.D.
Professor, Department of Pharmacology, Yamagata University School of Medicine,
2-2-2 Iida-nishi, Yamagata 990-23, Japan

MARTIN MORAD, PH.D.
Professor of Pharmacology and Medicine, Georgetown University Medical Center,
3900 Reservoir Rd., NW, Washington, D.C. 20007, USA

HASSO SCHOLZ, M.D.
Professor, Universitäts-Krankenhaus Eppendorf, Pharmakologisches Institut,
Martinistrasse 52, D-20246 Hamburg, Germany

TOSHIHIKO IIJIMA, M.D., PH.D.
Professor, Department of Pharmacology, Akita University School of Medicine,
1-1-1 Hondoh, Akita 010, Japan

ISBN 978-4-431-65954-9   ISBN 978-4-431-65952-5 (eBook)
DOI 10.1007/978-4-431-65952-5

Printed on acid-free paper

© Springer Japan 1996
Originally published by Springer-Verlag Tokyo Berlin Heidelberg New York in 1996

Typesetting: Best-set Typesetter Ltd., Hong Kong

Preface

This volume contains selected papers presented at the Sendai International Symposium on Molecular and Cellular Mechanisms of Cardiovascular Regulation held from May 10–12, 1995, to honor the contributions of Professor Norio Taira, Chairman of the Department of Pharmacology (1972–1995), Tohoku University School of Medicine, Sendai, Japan.

The Department of Pharmacology at Sendai has a long tradition of significant contribution to the development of drug therapy for cardiovascular diseases. The late Professor Koroku Hashimoto, the predecessor of Professor Norio Taira, first suggested the mode of action of calcium antagonists and their potential usefulness in therapy of ischemic heart disease and hypertension at an early stage of their development.

The need for greater understanding of the pathophysiology of cardiovascular diseases is more critical now than ever before because modern advances in basic and clinical sciences have prolonged the average life expectancy. Using a wide range of molecular and electrophysiological techniques, major advances are occurring frequently in the field of cardiovascular physiology and pharmacology. Such multifaceted approaches are preferred because human cardiovascular diseases are complex, requiring multiple interventions and an in-depth understanding of molecular mechanisms underlying the disease.

The first section of this book focuses on molecular mechanisms of ion channel regulation. Eight of ten chapters in this section are devoted to the recent advances in molecular characterization and regulation of various types of potassium channels in cardiac, vascular, and neuronal tissues. A discussion of the structure and function of sodium and calcium channels is also included.

The second section of the book deals with molecular mechanisms regulating vascular smooth muscle. Individual chapters in this section discuss the regulation of vascular tone by various interventions, including membrane receptors, calcium channels, and membrane potential. Two of the eight chapters treat the mode of action of phosphodiesterase III inhibitors and the possible role of compartmentalization of intracellular calcium in smooth muscle cells.

The third and by far the largest section of the book concentrates on a wide range of topics dealing with regulatory mechanisms of cardiac excitation–contraction coupling, including the L-type calcium channel, calcium release and uptake mechanisms in the cardiac sarcoplasmic reticulum, intracellular calcium signaling and its receptor-mediated modulation, cardiac NO pathways, calcium sensitivity of contractile proteins, and cardiac energetics.

The fourth and last section is devoted to pathophysiological modulation and suppression or reversal of pathophysiological changes, including beta receptor downregulation in heart failure, mechanisms of cardiac hypertrophy and its pharmacological modulation, alpha adrenergic activity in ischemic heart diseases, and the present state of treatment of congestive heart failure.

It is hoped that this volume will provide graduate students in biomedical and pharmaceutical sciences and scientists in cardiovascular sciences and clinical cardiology with an opportunity to integrate molecular and cellular knowledge into physiologic and pathophysiologic components that regulate the cardiovascular system. In dedicating this text to Professor Taira, we point with pride to the fact that such a wide array of talented scientists have come together to share their valuable information and experimental data.

The Editors

Contents

Part 2. Mechanisms of Vascular Regulation

Part 3. Mechanisms of Cardiac Regulation

Part 4. Pathophysiological Modulation of Regulatory Mechanisms

List of Contributors

ABE, FUJIO   (p 195)
Department of Pharmacology, Yamagata University School of Medicine, Yamagata 990-23, Japan

ARAKI, JUNICHI   (p 373)
Department of Physiology II, Okayama University Medical School, Okayama 700, Japan

BALLIGAND, JEAN-LUC   (p 353)
Cardiovascular Division, Department of Medicine, Brigham and Women's Hospital and Harvard Medical School, Boston, MA 02115, USA

BRODDE, OTTO-ERICH   (p 393)
Institute of Pharmacology and Toxicology, Martin-Luther-University of Halle-Wittenberg, D-06097 Halle (Saale), Germany

CATTERALL, WILLIAM A.   (p 15)
Department of Pharmacology, University of Washington, Seattle, WA 98195, USA

CAVERO, ICILIO   (p 69)
Rhône-Poulenc Rorer, Pharmaceutical Research Vitry-Alfortville Research Center, 94403 Vitry-sur-Seine, France

DAVIES, MICHAEL P.   (p 33)
Department of Physiology, University of Rochester Medical Center, Rochester, NY 14624, USA

DESSY, CHANTAL   (p 125)
Laboratoire de Pharmacologie, Université Catholique de Louvain, B-1200 Brussels, Belgium

DJELLAS, YASMINE   (p 69)
Department of Pharmacology, University of Illinois, Medical Center, 835 South Wolcott Avenue, Chicago, IL 60612-7343, USA

EDWARDS, GILLIAN   (p 93)
School of Biological Sciences, University of Manchester, Manchester M13 9PT, UK

ENDOH, MASAO   (pp 195, 327)
Department of Pharmacology, Yamagata University School of Medicine, Yamagata
990-23, Japan

ESCHENHAGEN, THOMAS   (p 317)
Pharmakologisches Institut, Universitäts-Krankenhaus Eppendorf, Universität
Hamburg, D-20246 Hamburg, Germany

FAN, JING   (p 221)
Department of Pharmacology, Georgetown University School of Medicine, Washington, DC 20007, USA, and Mt. Desert Island Biological Laboratory, Salisbury Cove, ME
04672, USA

FERON, OLIVIER   (p 125)
Laboratoire de Pharmacologie, Université Catholique de Louvain, B-1200 Brussels,
Belgium

FREEMAN, LISA C.   (p 33)
Department of Physiology, University of Rochester Medical Center, Rochester, NY
14624, USA

FURUKAWA, TETSUSHI   (p 83)
Department of Autonomic Physiology, Medical Research Institute, Tokyo Medical
and Dental University, 1-5-45 Yushima, Bunkyo-ku, Tokyo 113, Japan

GODFRAIND, THÉOPHILE   (p 125)
Laboratoire de Pharmacologie, Université Catholique de Louvain, B-1200 Brussels,
Belgium

GOLLOT-ROBERT, VÉRONIQUE   (p 69)
Rhône-Poulenc Rorer, Pharmaceutical Research Vitry-Alfortville Research Center,
94403 Vitry-sur-Seine, France

GROSS, WENDY L.   (p 353)
Department of Anesthesiology, Brigham and Women's Hospital and Harvard Medical
School, Boston, MA 02115, USA

GROSSMAN, JESSICA   (p 269)
Harvard-Thorndike Laboratories, Beth Israel Hospital, Harvard Medical School,
Boston, MA 02159, USA

HAMPTON, THOMAS   (p 269)
Harvard-Thorndike Laboratories, Beth Israel Hospital, Harvard Medical School,
Boston, MA 02159, USA

HAN, XINQIANG   (p 353)
Cardiovascular Division, Department of Medicine, Brigham and Women's Hospital
and Harvard Medical School, Boston, MA 02115, USA

HARADA, KATSUHIKO   (p 47)
Department of Pharmacology, Akita University School of Medicine, 1-1-1 Hondoh,
Akita 010, Japan

HARADA, KEN-ICHI   (p 195)
Department of Veterinary Pharmacology, Graduate School of Agriculture and Life
Sciences, University of Tokyo, Bunkyo-ku, Tokyo 113, Japan

HECQUET, CLAUDIE   (p 69)
Department of Pharmacology, University of Illinois, Medical Center, 835 South Wolcott Avenue, Chicago, IL 60612-7343, USA

HIDAKA, HIROYOSHI   (p 169)
Department of Pharmacology, Nagoya University School of Medicine, Showa-ku, Nagoya 466, Japan

HIRAOKA, MASAYASU   (p 83)
Department of Cardiovascular Diseases, Medical Research Institute, Tokyo Medical and Dental University, 1-5-45 Yushima, Bunkyo-ku, Tokyo 113, Japan

HOFMANN, FRANZ   (p 231)
Institute of Pharmacology and Toxicology, Technische Universität München, D-80802 München, Germany

HONGYU, LI   (p 243)
Department of Physiology, Juntendo University, School of Medicine, Hongo, Bunkyo-ku, Tokyo 113, Japan

HORI, MASATOSHI   (p 195)
Department of Veterinary Pharmacology, Graduate School of Agriculture and Life Sciences, University of Tokyo, Bunkyo-ku, Tokyo 113, Japan

HORI, MASATSUGU   (p 417)
First Department of Medicine, Osaka University, School of Medicine, Suita, Osaka 565, Japan

IIJIMA, TOSHIHIKO   (p 47)
Department of Pharmacology, Akita University, School of Medicine, 1-1-1 Hondoh, Akita 010, Japan

IMAGAWA, JUN-ICHI   (p 47)
Department of Pharmacology, Akita University School of Medicine, 1-1-1 Hondoh, Akita 010, Japan

ISENBERG, GERRIT   (p 149)
Department of Physiology, Martin-Luther-University of Halle-Wittenberg, D-06097 Halle (Saale), Germany

ISHII, KUNIAKI   (p 3)
Department of Pharmacology, Tohoku University School of Medicine, Aoba-ku, Sendai 980, Japan

KAMADA, TAKENOBU   (p 417)
First Department of Medicine, Osaka University, School of Medicine, Suita, Osaka 565, Japan

KARAKI, HIDEAKI   (p 195)
Department of Veterinary Pharmacology, Graduate School of Agriculture and Life Sciences, University of Tokyo, Bunkyo-ku, Tokyo 113, Japan

KASS, ROBERT S.   (p 33)
Department of Physiology, University of Rochester Medical Center, Rochester, NY 14624, USA

KAYE, DAVID M.   (p 353)
Cardiovascular Division, Department of Medicine, Brigham and Women's Hospital and Harvard Medical School, Boston, MA 02115, USA

KELLY, RALPH A.   (p 353)
Cardiovascular Division, Department of Medicine, Brigham and Women's Hospital and Harvard Medical School, Boston, MA 02115, USA

KIMURA, JUNKO   (p 327)
Department of Pharmacology, Fukushima Medical College, Fukushima 960-12, Japan

KIMURA, YUKIO   (p 169)
Tokushima Research Institute, Otsuka Pharmaceutical Co., Ltd., Kawauchi-chou, Tokushima 771-01, Japan

KITAJIMA, SATOSHI   (p 195)
Department of Veterinary Pharmacology, Graduate School of Agriculture and Life Sciences, University of Tokyo, Bunkyo-ku, Tokyo 113, Japan

KITAKAZE, MASAFUMI   (p 417)
First Department of Medicine, Osaka University, School of Medicine, Suita, Osaka 565, Japan

KLUGBAUER, NORBERT   (p 231)
Institute of Pharmacology and Toxicology, Technische Universität München, D-80802 München, Germany

KOMUKAI, KIMIAKI   (p 281)
Department of Physiology, Jikei University of School of Medicine, Minato-ku, Tokyo 105, Japan

KOMURO, ISSEI   (p 409)
Third Department of Medicine, University of Tokyo School of Medicine, Bunkyo-ku, Tokyo 113, Japan

KONDO, CHIKAKO   (p 59)
Department of Pharmacology II, Faculty of Medicine, Osaka University, Suita, Osaka 565, Japan

KURACHI, YOSHIHISA   (p 59)
Department of Pharmacology II, Faculty of Medicine, Osaka University, Suita, Osaka 565, Japan

KURIHARA, SATOSHI   (p 281)
Department of Physiology, Jikei University of School of Medicine, Minato-ku, Tokyo 105, Japan

LACINOVÁ, LUBICA   (p 231)
Institute of Pharmacology and Toxicology, Technische Universität München, D-80802 München, Germany

LAKATTA, EDWARD G.   (p 291)
Laboratory of Cardiovascular Science, Gerontology Research Center, National Institute on Aging, National Institutes of Health, Baltimore, MD 21224, USA

LINDE, CLAUDIA   (p 111)
Department of Pharmacology, University of Tübingen, D-72074 Tübingen, Germany

LÖFFLER, CORNELIA   (p 111)
Department of Pharmacology, University of Tübingen, D-72074 Tübingen, Germany

MATSUBARA, HIROMI   (p 373)
Department of Physiology II, Okayama University Medical School, Okayama 700, Japan

MATSUI, SIGEO   (p 433)
Department of Cardiovascular Medicine, Kyoto University, Sakyo-ku, Kyoto 606, Japan

MATSUMORI, AKIRA   (p 433)
Department of Cardiovascular Medicine, Kyoto University, Sakyo-ku, Kyoto 606, Japan

MESTRE, MICHEL   (p 69)
Rhône-Poulenc Rorer, Pharmaceutical Research Vitry-Alfortville Research Center, 94403 Vitry-sur-Seine, France

METZGER, FRIEDRICH   (p 111)
Department of Pharmacology, University of Tübingen, D-72074 Tübingen, Germany

MITSUI-SAITO, MINORI   (p 195)
Department of Veterinary Pharmacology, Graduate School of Agriculture and Life Sciences, University of Tokyo, Bunkyo-ku, Tokyo 113, Japan

MORAD, MARTIN   (p 221)
Department of Pharmacology, Georgetown University School of Medicine, Washington, DC 20007, USA, and Mt. Desert Island Biological Laboratory, Salisbury Cove, ME 04672, USA

MOREL, NICOLE   (p 125)
Laboratoire de Pharmacologie, Université Catholique de Louvain, B-1200 Brussels, Belgium

MORGAN, JAMES   (p 269)
Harvard-Thorndike Laboratories, Beth Israel Hospital, Harvard Medical School, Boston, MA 02159, USA

MORISHIGE, KEN-ICHIROU   (p 59)
Department of Obstetrics and Gynecology, Faculty of Medicine, Osaka University, Suita, Osaka 565, Japan

MORITA, HIDEYUKI   (p 327)
Department of Pharmacology, Yamagata University School of Medicine, Yamagata 990-23, Japan

NAGAI, RYOZO   (p 409)
Third Department of Medicine, University of Tokyo School of Medicine, Bunkyo-ku, Tokyo 113, Japan

NAKAMURA, TAKESHI   (p 243)
Laboratory of Cellular Neurobiology, School of Life Science, Tokyo University of Pharmacy and Life Science, Tokyo 192-03, Japan

NEUMANN, JOACHIM   (p 317)
Pharmakologisches Institut, Universitäts-Krankenhaus Eppendorf, Universität Hamburg, D-20246 Hamburg, Germany

OCHI, RIKUO   (p 243)
Department of Physiology, Juntendo University, School of Medicine, Hongo, Bunkyo-ku, Tokyo 113, Japan

OKAMURA, TOMIO   (p 211)
Department of Pharmacology, Shiga University of Medical Sciences, Seta, Ohtsu 520-21, Japan

OZAKI, HIROSHI   (p 195)
Department of Veterinary Pharmacology, Graduate School of Agriculture and Life Sciences, University of Tokyo, Bunkyo-ku, Tokyo 113, Japan

QIU, ZHIHUA   (p 269)
Harvard-Thorndike Laboratories, Beth Israel Hospital, Harvard Medical School, Boston, MA 02159, USA

QUAST, ULRICH   (p 111)
Department of Pharmacology, University of Tübingen, D-72074 Tübingen, Germany

SALOMONE, SALVATORE   (p 125)
Laboratoire de Pharmacologie, Université Catholique de Louvain, B-1200 Brussels, Belgium

SASAYAMA, SHIGETAKE   (p 433)
Department of Cardiovascular Medicine, Kyoto University, Sakyo-ku, Kyoto 606, Japan

SATO, KOICHI   (p 195)
Department of Veterinary Pharmacology, Graduate School of Agriculture and Life Sciences, University of Tokyo, Bunkyo-ku, Tokyo 113, Japan

SAWANOBORI, TOHRU   (p 83)
Department of Cardiovascular Diseases, Medical Research Institute, Tokyo Medical and Dental University, 1-5-45 Yushima, Bunkyo-ku, Tokyo 113, Japan

SCHEUER, TODD   (p 15)
Department of Pharmacology, University of Washington, Seattle, WA 98195, USA

SCHOLZ, HASSO   (p 317)
Pharmakologisches Institut, Universitäts-Krankenhaus Eppendorf, Universität Hamburg, D-20246 Hamburg, Germany

SCHUSTER, ANGELA   (p 231)
Institute of Pharmacology and Toxicology, Technische Universität München, D-80802 München, Germany

SCHWARTZ, ARNOLD (p 27)
Institute of Molecular Pharmacology and Biophysics, University of Cincinnati College of Medicine, Cincinnati, OH 45267-0828, USA

SEISENBERGER, CLAUDIA   (p 231)
Institute of Pharmacology and Toxicology, Technische Universität München, D-80802 München, Germany

SHIOI, TETSUO   (p 433)
Department of Cardiovascular Medicine, Kyoto University, Sakyo-ku, Kyoto 606, Japan

SHIOJIMA, ICHIRO   (p 409)
Third Department of Medicine, University of Tokyo School of Medicine, Bunkyo-ku, Tokyo 113, Japan

SHUBA, YAROSLAV   (p 221)
Department of Pharmacology, Georgetown University School of Medicine, Washington, DC 20007, USA, and Mt. Desert Island Biological Laboratory, Salisbury Cove, ME 04672, USA

SIMMONS, WILLIAM W.   (p 353)
Cardiovascular Division, Department of Medicine, Brigham and Women's Hospital and Harvard Medical School, Boston, MA 02115, USA

SMITH, THOMAS W.   (p 353)
Cardiovascular Division, Department of Medicine, Brigham and Women's Hospital and Harvard Medical School, Boston, MA 02115, USA

SOLARO, R. JOHN   (p 363)
Department of Physiology and Biophysics, College of Medicine (M/C 901), University of Illinois-Chicago, Chicago, IL 60612-7342, USA

STEIN, BIRGITT   (p 317)
Pharmakologisches Institut, Universitäts-Krankenhaus Eppendorf, Universität Hamburg, D-20246 Hamburg, Germany

SUGA, HIROYUKI   (p 373)
Department of Physiology II, Okayama University Medical School, Okayama 700, Japan

TADA, MICHIHIKO   (p 255)
Department of Medicine and Pathophysiology, Osaka University, School of Medicine, Suita, Osaka 565, Japan

TAIRA, NORIO   (p 3)
Department of Pharmacology, Tohoku University School of Medicine, Aoba-ku, Sendai 980, Japan

TAKAHASHI, NAOHIKO   (p 59)
Department of Pharmacology II, Faculty of Medicine, Osaka University, Suita, Osaka 565, Japan

TAKAKI, MIYAKO   (p 373)
Department of Physiology II, Okayama University Medical School, Okayama 700, Japan

TODA, NOBORU   (p 211)
Department of Pharmacology, Shiga University of Medical Sciences, Seta, Ohtsu 520-21, Japan

TOYOFUKU, TOSHIHIKO   (p 255)
Department of Medicine and Pathophysiology, Osaka University, School of Medicine, Suita, Osaka 565, Japan

WANG, JIANXUN   (p 269)
Harvard-Thorndike Laboratories, Beth Israel Hospital, Harvard Medical School, Boston, MA 02159, USA

WELLING, ANDREA   (p 231)
Institute of Pharmacology and Toxicology, Technische Universität München, D-80802 München, Germany

WESTON, ARTHUR H.   (p 93)
School of Biological Sciences, University of Manchester, Manchester M13 9PT, UK

XIAO, RUI-PING   (p 291)
Laboratory of Cardiovascular Science, Gerontology Research Center, National Institute on Aging, National Institutes of Health, Baltimore, MD 21224, USA

YAMADA, MITSUHIKO   (p 59)
Department of Pharmacology II, Faculty of Medicine, Osaka University, Suita, Osaka 565, Japan

YAMADA, TAKEHIKO   (p 433)
Department of Cardiovascular Medicine, Kyoto University, Sakyo-ku, Kyoto 606, Japan

YAMANE, TEIICHI   (p 83)
Department of Cardiovascular Diseases, Medical Research Institute, Tokyo Medical and Dental University, 1-5-45 Yushima, Bunkyo-ku, Tokyo 113, Japan

YAMAZAKI, TSUTOMU   (p 409)
Third Department of Medicine, University of Tokyo School of Medicine, Bunkyo-ku, Tokyo 113, Japan

YANAGISAWA, TERUYUKI   (p 183)
Department of Pharmacology, Tohoku University School of Medicine, Aoba-ku, Sendai 980, Japan

YAZAKI, YOSHIO   (p 409)
Third Department of Medicine, University of Tokyo School of Medicine, Bunkyo-ku, Tokyo 113, Japan

Part 1

Molecular Mechanisms of Ion-Channel Regulation

Artificial Modulation of
Potassium Channels

Norio Taira and Kuniaki Ishii

Summary. The inactivation mechanism of the *Drosophila Shaker* K+ channel is explained by a ball-and-chain model. The initial 20 amino acids in the amino-terminus and the following region (about 60 amino acids) have been identified as the ball and chain, respectively. In a mammalian counterpart of the *Shaker* K+ channel, rat Kv1.4, the structural elements responsible for rapid inactivation were investigated. The inactivation mechanisms of the Kv1.4 channel could be explained by a ball-and-chain model; however, the structures involved in the mechanisms seem to be more complicated than those of the *Shaker* K+ channel. Besides the inactivation ball, the composition of the acceptor sites exerts great influence on rapid inactivation. Receptor-mediated modulation of cloned K+ channels, rat Kv1.2 and Kv1.4, were also investigated. The currents flowing through both channels [$I_{(Kv1.2)}$ and $I_{(Kv1.4)}$] were suppressed by stimulation of the coexpressed receptor, which is coupled to phosphatidylinositol turnover. Although the two pathways, activation of protein kinase C (PKC) and increase in intracellular Ca^{2+}, were involved in current suppression in both channels, the contribution of each pathway was not of the same extent in each channel. For example, PKC seemed to contribute more to the suppression of $I_{(Kv1.2)}$ than $I_{(Kv1.4)}$.

Key words. K+ channel—PKC—Ca^{2+}—Inactivation—Ball-and-chain model

Introduction

Ion channels are integral membrane proteins that regulate the movement of ions across the cell membrane and thereby play fundamental roles in excitability of the cells [1]. Almost all ion channels are hetero-oligomeric proteins having a pore-forming subunit and other auxiliary subunits. For example, the voltage-dependent Na+ channel of the brain consists of one pore-forming α-subunit and two other subunits (β_1 and β_2), and the voltage-dependent Ca^{2+} channel of skeletal muscle consists of one pore-forming α_1-subunit and four other subunits (β, γ, α_2, and δ) [2]. In addition to a pore-forming subunit (α-subunit), β-subunits of the voltage-dependent K+ channel have been cloned [3–5], but its precise subunit composition still remains to be elucidated. Among voltage-dependent ion channels, K+ channels form the most diversified

Department of Pharmacology, Tohoku University School of Medicine, Aoba-ku, Sendai 980, Japan

3

class of ion channels in terms of both physiological characteristics and molecular structures.

On a structural basis, they are classified at present into three major groups as follows: (1) outwardly rectifying K+ channels with six transmembrane segments [6–8], (2) inwardly rectifying K+ channels with two transmembrane segments [9,10], and (3) slowly activating, outwardly rectifying K+ channel with one transmembrane segment [11–13]. In contrast, no such structural diversity is found in voltage-dependent Na+ and Ca2+ channels cloned so far. The pore-forming subunit of the Na+ or Ca2+ channel contains four homologous domains, each of which resembles one α-subunit of the voltage-dependent K+ channel with six transmembrane segments. Therefore, the protein encoded by the K+ channel gene of group 1 (six transmembranes) is about one-fourth the size of the protein encoded by the Na+ or Ca2+ channel gene, and the pore-forming subunits of the K+ channel are thought to assemble as homo- or heterotetramers. The K+ channel proteins of other groups are even smaller. This smaller size makes the K+ channel more amenable to genetic manipulation, and many important structural elements involved in the fundamental function of voltage-dependent ion channels, such as the inactivation gate and channel pore, have been identified through mutagenesis experiments of the K+ channel [14–20].

Since the cloning of the *Drosophila Shaker* gene, many mammalian voltage-dependent K+ channels have been cloned from the neuron, heart, lymphocyte, and so on. In the heart, the K+ channels are thought to be involved in maintaining the resting membrane potential and determining action potential duration, and to be targets for some kinds of antiarrhythmic drugs.

We have cloned two voltage-dependent K+ channels with six transmembrane segments from rat heart [21,22] and one from rabbit heart [23]. We have also cloned an inwardly rectifying K+ channel with two transmembrane segments from rabbit heart [24]. The K+ channels that we cloned from rat heart were Kv1.2 and Kv1.4, according to the currently used nomenclature: Kv1.2 is a delayed rectifier type and Kv1.4 is a transient outward type K+ channel. Our studies on inactivation mechanisms and receptor-mediated modulation of K+ channels cloned from rat heart are reviewed next.

Inactivation Mechanisms of Rat Transient Type K+ Channel

The transient-type K+ channel encoded by the *Drosophila Shaker* locus and also its mammalian counterpart Kv1.4 inactivate within a few milliseconds like voltage-dependent Na+ channels. For inactivation mechanisms of Na+ channels, a ball-and-chain model was proposed by Armstrong and Bezanilla [25]. A ball composed of protein is tethered by a chain to the cytoplasmic side of the channel. On the opening of the channel, an acceptor for the ball becomes exposed and the ball binds it to occlude the channel pore. About a decade later, Aldrich and co-workers [14,15] showed that this ball-and-chain model was suitable for explaining the inactivation mechanism of the transient type K+ channel. They used the *Shaker* K+ channel and experimentally demonstrated the existence of an inactivation ball at the amino-terminus and a chain following the ball. Later it was suggested that the region between the fourth and fifth transmembrane segment (S4–S5 loop) of the *Shaker* K+ channel forms part of an acceptor for the inactivation ball [26].

Inactivation Ball

In the *Shaker* K⁺ channel, the initial 20 amino acids in the amino-terminus have been identified as the inactivation ball, which is composed of the first 11 hydrophobic amino acids and the following hydrophilic amino acids containing four positive and two negative charges. The region following the ball and preceding the assembly domain [27] has been identified as the chain tethering the ball [14,15]. In the mammalian transient-type K⁺ channel, however, the ball-and-chain structure had not been identified. Tseng and co-workers [28] first tackled this problem making a number of deletion mutants in the amino-terminus of rat Kv1.4. They have not identified a chain structure in rat Kv1.4, as has been proposed for the *Shaker* K⁺ channel. However, as to a ball structure, they found that deletion of the amino-terminal hydrophobic domain (the first 25 amino acids) abolished the inactivation and that deletion of the following hydrophilic region containing five positive and two negative charges greatly attenuated the inactivation. They have suggested that the amino-terminus of rat Kv1.4 may be similar to that of the *Shaker* K⁺ channel in having a ball composed of hydrophobic and hydrophilic regions and that the inactivation mechanism of rat Kv1.4 is similar to that of the *Shaker* K⁺ channel.

We have also made a number of deletions in the amino-terminus of rat Kv1.4 and tackled the problem concerning ball-and-chain structures in a mammalian transient-type K⁺ channel. Detailed analysis of the mutants has not been completed yet. However, the data obtained so far suggest that there may exist a potential inactivation ball besides the amino-terminal hydrophobic region, which has been proposed to be an essential component of inactivation ball by Tseng and co-workers. Thus, although the inactivation mechanisms in rat Kv1.4 could be explained by a ball-and-chain model, the structural elements involved in ball and chain may be more complicated in rat Kv1.4 than in the *Shaker* K⁺ channel. This question has not been settled yet.

Acceptor for Inactivation Ball

When the amino acid sequence of Kv1.4 (a transient type) is compared with that of Kv1.2 (a delayed rectifier type), the most striking difference is found in the amino-terminal region. Kv1.4 has a much longer amino-terminal region, which is supposed to contain an inactivation ball. Therefore, we constructed a chimera channel in which the amino-terminal region of Kv1.4 (the residues 1–183) preceding the channel assembly domain was ligated to Kv1.2 at the corresponding site to test whether the amino-terminal region of Kv1.4 can cause inactivation in Kv1.2. When expressed in *Xenopus* oocytes, the chimera channel rapidly inactivated, indicating that the Kv1.4 ball binds to the potential acceptor site of Kv1.2 and occludes the channel pore. The time constant for inactivation of the chimera channel was about 40 ms, and that of Kv1.4 was about 70 ms at test potential of +20 mV. The current decay was even faster in the chimera channel than in the Kv1.4 channel. As K⁺ channels are generally thought to assemble as tetramers, the chimera channel has four sets of inactivation ball-and-acceptor sites like the wild-type Kv1.4 channel. Because the inactivation ball of the chimera channel is the same as that of Kv1.4, the difference in time constant for inactivation between the chimera and Kv1.4 channel is probably the result of the difference of the acceptor site.

MacKinnon et al. [29] have reported that the only a single inactivation gate is necessary to produce inactivation in the *Shaker* K+ channel and that the inactivation rate constant is dependent on the number of gates. However, it is still unknown how many acceptor sites there are and how each acceptor site is involved in inactivation. Therefore, we studied this matter. It has been suggested that coexpression of *Shaker*-related vertebrate homologues can form heteromultimeric K+ channels [30–32]. It has also been shown that two *Shaker* subfamily K+ channel subunits, Kv1.2 and Kv1.4, coassemble and actually form a heteromultimeric K+ channel in vivo in the rat brain [33]. In that case, the heteromultimeric K+ channel is likely to have two Kv1.4 inactivation balls and four acceptor sites (two from Kv1.4 and two from Kv1.2).

We made a tandem construct by linking the 5′ end of Kv1.2 cDNA to the 3′ end of Kv1.4 cDNA and examined how the currents flowing through the hybrid channel inactivate. We also made tandem constructs by similarly linking Kv1.4 and mutants of Kv1.2 instead of wild-type Kv1.2 [34]. The Kv1.2 mutants we used for tandem construction have a single amino acid change in the S4–S5 loop that is expected to form part of the acceptor site for the inactivation ball. Among the mutants, m1Kv1.2, in which the threonine residue at position 320 was substituted with alanine, generated similar current amplitudes to wild-type Kv1.2, but m2 or m5Kv1.2, in which the serine residue at position 324 was substituted with glycine or alanine, did not lead to the expression of functional channels. All the tandem constructs, however, were functional channels, although the amplitude of the currents flowing through them varied depending on the amino acid substitution made in Kv1.2.

Figure 1 shows the proposed membrane topology of the channels encoded by the tandem dimeric constructs and a sequence alignment of a portion of the S4–S5 loop of Kv1.2 and its mutants. The currents flowed by the dimeric constructs in which both subunits could form functional K+ channels by themselves (Kv1.4-Kv1.2 and Kv1.4-m1Kv1.2) showed similar amplitudes and characteristics to those shown with Kv1.4 alone, whereas the currents of the dimeric constructs in which nonfunctional Kv1.2 mutants were ligated to Kv1.4 (Kv1.4-m2Kv1.2 and Kv1.4-m5Kv1.2) were smaller and inactivated less than those of Kv1.4 (Fig. 2). On depolarization, the currents of the former hybrid channels activated rapidly and subsequently inactivated with an exponential time-course, although the currents generated by Kv1.4-m1Kv1.2 inactivated more slowly than those of the Kv1.4 homotetramer or Kv1.4-Kv1.2. The current decay of Kv1.4, Kv1.4-Kv1.2, and Kv1.4-m1Kv1.2 was best fitted to a single exponential function. Interestingly, the time constant for inactivation was not significantly different between Kv1.4 homotetramer and Kv1.4-Kv1.2, even though the number of inactivation balls of Kv1.4-Kv1.2 is considered to be half that of Kv1.4.

As mentioned earlier, MacKinnon et al. have reported that in the homomeric *Shaker* K+ channel the inactivation rate constant is dependent on the number of inactivation balls. If the inactivation process were determined only by the number of the balls, the hybrid channel Kv1.4-Kv1.2 would show much slower inactivation kinetics than Kv1.4, but it is not. Therefore, the foregoing observation could be explained by the difference in the composition of the acceptor site between the hybrid and homomeric K+ channel. There are two amino acid differences in the S4–S5 loop between Kv1.4 and Kv1.2, and these differences could result in an alteration of binding interaction of inactivation balls of the hybrid K+ channel and confer fast inactivation on the hybrid channel similar to that of homomeric Kv1.4 channel.

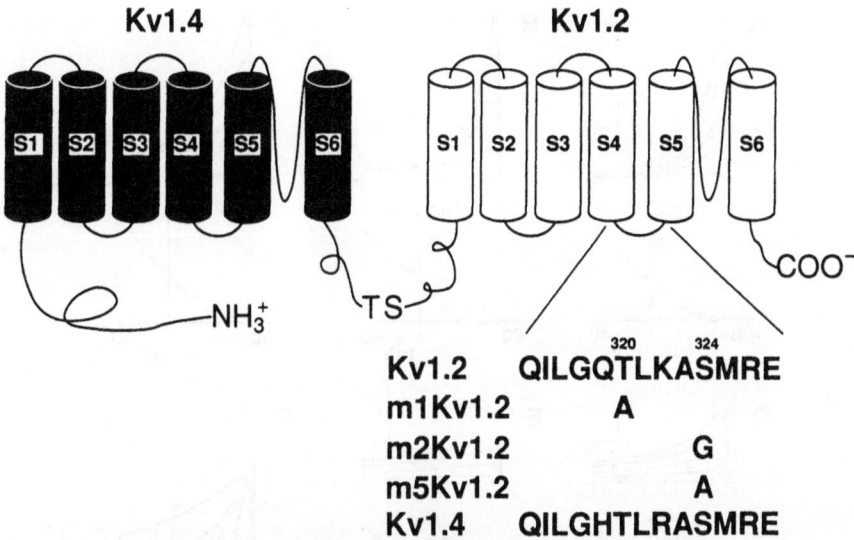

FIG. 1. Heterodimeric constructs generated by tandem linkage of *Kv1.4* and *Kv1.2* or its mutants. *Upper panel*: proposed membrane topology of tandem dimeric polypeptide encoded by the fusion genes. In these tandem dimers, the last residue of the first subunit (*Kv1.4*) polypeptide is connected by a linker of threonine (*T*) and serine (*S*) residues with the first residue of the second subunit (Kv1.2 or its mutants) polypeptide. *Lower panel*: sequence alignment of a portion of the S4–S5 loop of Kv1.2 and its mutants. The amino acid sequence of the cytoplasmic segment connecting S4 and S5 of Kv1.2 is shown as well as that of the corresponding part of Kv1.4. The positions of amino acid substitutions are indicated below the sequence of Kv1.2. Each mutant is named as *m1Kv1.2*, *m2Kv1.2*, and *m5Kv1.2*, respectively. (From [34], with permission)

When inactivation kinetics of the mutant hybrid channels was compared with that of the wild-type hybrid channel, Kv1.4-Kv1.2, the time constant for inactivation of the macroscopic current increased markedly on point mutation of the amino acid at the proposed acceptor site (S4–S5 loop) in the second subunit (Kv1.2). The time constant for inactivation of Kv1.4-m1Kv1.2 was about 110 ms for test pulses to +20 mV, and that of Kv1.4-Kv1.2 was about 79 ms. Further increases in the time constant for inactivation occurred in two other mutant hybrid channels (Kv1.4-m2Kv1.2 and Kv1.4-m5Kv1.2). Because the acceptor sites for the inactivation ball likely have some effects on recovery from inactivation, the rate of recovery was also examined. Rate of recovery from inactivation was significantly faster in the channels from tandem constructs than in the parent Kv1.4 channel. Therefore, we further estimated the microscopic inactivation rate constant (k_{inact}) from the values of inactivation time constant of macroscopic currents and time constant of recovery assuming that a channel recovers from inactivated state to open state and then deactivates.

The following equation is applied to calculate k_{inact}:

$$k_{inact} = 1/\tau_{inact} - 1/\tau_{rec}$$

The ratio of k_{inact} for Kv1.4-Kv1.2 to Kv1.4 is close to 1. This indicates that, as macroscopic inactivation, the microscopic inactivation rate constant of the wild-type hybrid channel, Kv1.4-Kv1.2, is not different from the homomeric Kv1.4 channel even though the number of the inactivation balls of the hybrid channel is half that of Kv1.4 channel.

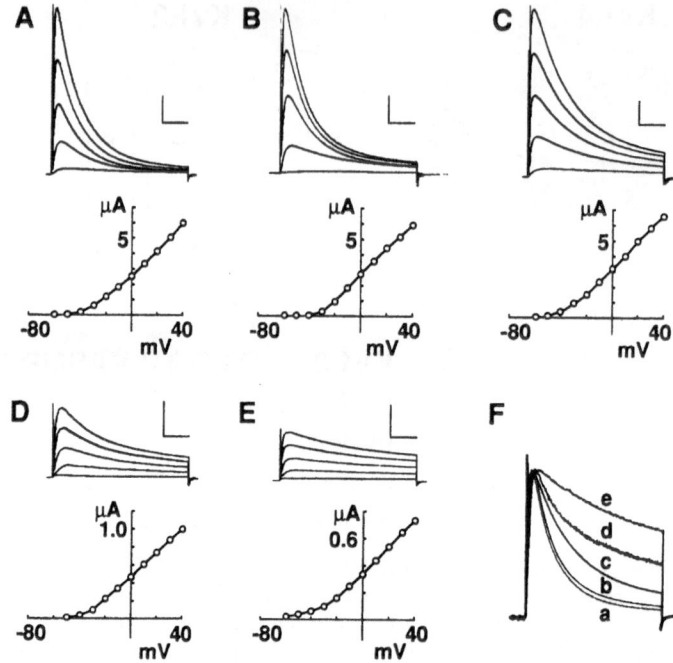

FIG. 2A–F. Macroscopic currents obtained by two-microelectrode voltage clamp from injected *Xenopus* oocytes. Currents shown in A, B, C, D, and E were obtained from the oocytes injected with cRNAs of Kv1.4, Kv1.4-Kv1.2, Kv1.4-m1Kv1.2, Kv1.4-m2Kv1.2, and Kv1.4-m5Kv1.2, respectively. Current traces elicited by steps to +40, +20, 0, −20, and −40 mV from a holding potential of −80 mV are shown in each panel. Calibration bars, 100 ms, and 1 μA (A–C) or 0.5 μA (D, E). The current-voltage relationships of the peak currents measured at each test potential plotted are presented under the current traces. Normalized macroscopic currents from *Xenopus* oocytes in A–E are also given in F. Currents evoked by a test potential to +20 mV from each clone are normalized and superimposed to illustrate the differences in their waveforms. Current traces in F are named as follows: a, (Kv1.4); b, (Kv1.4-Kv1.2); c, (Kv1.4-m1Kv1.2); d, (Kv1.4-m2Kv1.2); e, (Kv1.4-m5Kv1.2). Note that the differences of the time-courses of K⁺ current inactivation are evident between the homotetrameric Kv1.4 channel and the hybrid channels, which contain substitutions of single amino acids in the S4–S5 loop of the second subunit. (From [34], with permission)

In contrast, the ratios of k_{inact} for the mutant hybrid channels to the wild-type hybrid channel are much less than unity; the ratios of k_{inact} for Kv1.4-m1Kv1.2, Kv1.4-m2Kv1.2, and Kv1.4-m5Kv1.2 to the wild-type hybrid channel were approximately 0.7, 0.6, and 0.4, respectively. Thus, microscopic inactivation rate constants as well as the time constants for inactivation of macroscopic current were increased in the mutant hybrid channels.

The marked slowing of inactivation could be attributed to the differences in the characteristics and/or the number of the potential acceptor regions of the non-inactivating second subunit, because all the hybrid channels have the same two inactivation balls. Obviously, the second subunit participates in inactivation of the hybrid channels. From comparison of the inactivation kinetics of the wild-type and mutant hybrid channels, it is also obvious that the S4–S5 loop of the second subunit exerts great influence on the inactivation. Substitution of a single amino acid in that region of the second subunit might lead to a change in the structure and alter the accessibility of the inactivation balls to the acceptor sites.

Considering that m1Kv1.2 is functional but m2 and m5Kv1.2 are nonfunctional, the results obtained with the three mutant hybrid channels may have different meanings. The S4–S5 loop of m1Kv1.2 may serve as an acceptor site with different affinity for an inactivation ball (differences in characteristics), although the S4–S5 loop of m2 and m5Kv1.2 may not be able to work as an acceptor at all (differences in number).

Receptor-Mediated Modulation

It is well known that voltage-dependent ion channels can be modulated by receptor-mediated mechanisms, among which the best investigated is phosphorylation by protein kinase A or protein kinase C (PKC) [35]. Such modulation of ion channels can affect the activity of the cells in which they reside. In the heart, for example, stimulation of β-receptor enhances not only the slow inward (L-type) Ca^{2+} current that is responsible for the plateau phase of the action potential but also the delayed rectifier K⁺ current which is responsible for the repolarization of the action potential [36–38]. The enhancement of the Ca^{2+} current produces positive inotropy, and the enhancement of the K⁺ current causes shortening of action potential duration. It has also been reported that stimulation of α-receptor suppresses the transient outward K⁺ current [39–41]. Because of advances in molecular biological techniques, it became possible to study mechanisms of receptor-mediated modulation of cloned voltage-dependent ion channels by coexpressing cloned receptors and channels.

We have studied receptor-mediated modulation of the cloned rat cardiac K⁺ channels, Kv1.2 and Kv1.4 [21,22,42]. They were coexpressed with a subtype of endothelin receptor (ET_A) or a subtype of metabotropic glutamate receptor (mGluR5) in *Xenopus* oocytes. When Kv1.2 was coexpressed with ET_A or mGluR5, stimulation of either receptor resulted in suppression of the Kv1.2 current ($I_{(Kv1.2)}$). Similarly, when Kv1.4 was coexpressed with ET_A or mGluR5, stimulation of either receptor resulted in suppression of the Kv1.4 current ($I_{(Kv1.4)}$). Both $I_{(Kv1.2)}$ and $I_{(Kv1.4)}$ were suppressed in a similar time-course and to similar extent. Because both receptors are known to couple to phosphatidylinositol turnover, the involvement of activation of PKC and increase of intracellular Ca^{2+} concentration in current suppression was investigated. To inhibit PKC, staurosporine was applied, and to chelate intracellular Ca^{2+}, ethyleneglycoltetraacetic acid (EGTA) was injected into the cells.

Involvement of PKC

ET_A- or mGluR5-mediated suppression of $I_{(Kv1.2)}$ and $I_{(Kv1.4)}$ was inhibited by staurosporine and mimicked by PMA (4-beta-phorbol 12-myristate 13-acetate). An inactive analogue of PMA (α-PMA), however, had no effect on both currents. This suggests that PKC is involved in the receptor-mediated suppression. Interestingly, the suppression of $I_{(Kv1.2)}$ was attenuated more than that of $I_{(Kv1.4)}$ by staurosporine, although the suppression by stimulation of coexpressed receptor was to a similar extent in both currents (Fig. 3). Therefore, it seems likely that the contribution of PKC in receptor-mediated suppression is not the same between $I_{(Kv1.2)}$ and $I_{(Kv1.4)}$; that is, PKC contributes more to the suppression of $I_{(Kv1.2)}$ than $I_{(Kv1.4)}$.

The Kv1.2 channel has two putative phosphorylation sites for PKC in the S4–S5 loop (threonine at 320 and serine at 324), and the Kv1.4 channel has six putative phosphorylation sites, two in the S4–S5 loop (threonine at 471 and serine at 475), the same as Kv1.2, three in the amino-terminus (serine at 82, threonine at 90, and serine at 169) and one in the carboxyl-terminus (threonine at 639). To determine whether these sites are responsible for the suppression of the currents by activation of PKC, we made point mutations at these sites.

For Kv1.2, m1Kv1.2 in which threonine residue at position 320 was substituted with alanine generated similar current amplitudes to wild-type Kv1.2, whereas substitution of serine residue at 324 hampered the expression of the functional channel. Therefore, we substituted an arginine residue at 326 with gulutamine to destroy the consensus sequence for PKC phosphorylation (m9Kv1.2, which is a functional channel). We also made a mutant in which both threonine at 320 and arginine at 326 were substituted (m14Kv1.2). If these potential phosphorylation sites for PKC are responsible for current suppression, we could expect no effect of PKC activator on the current amplitudes of the mutants. However, the currents of all the functional mutants were suppressed by the PKC activator PMA, as was wild-type Kv1.2. Huang et al. [43] have reported that the m_1 muscarinic acetylcholine receptor suppressed the rat Kv1.2 current through a pathway involving phospholipase C activation and direct tyrosine phosphorylation of the channel, which is a quite novel mechanism. Taken together, direct phosphorylation of the Kv1.2 channel by PKC is unlikely to be involved in the suppression of the current.

For Kv1.4, we have made mutations at six potential phosphorylation sites for PKC. Mutations in the S4–S5 loop (threonine at 471 and serine at 475) resulted in loss of expression of the functional channel, but mutations at four other potential PKC sites did not interfere with channel expression. Although one of the mutants in which serine residue at 169 was substituted with alanine seemed to be less susceptible to PKC, we could not obtain conclusive evidence as to its direct involvement in current suppression by PKC. The currents of three other functional mutants were suppressed by a PKC activator similar to wild-type Kv1.4. Murray et al. [44] have reported that human Kv1.4 current was modulated by PKC activation and that the K^+ channel was directly phosphorylated by PKC. Taken together, it is possible that suppression of Kv1.4 current by PKC activation results in part from direct phosphorylation of the channel protein by PKC and in part from another, unknown mechanism.

Involvement of Ca^{2+}

Intracellular Ca^{2+} injection suppressed both $I_{(Kv1.2)}$ and $I_{(Kv1.4)}$ over a period of 30–60 min. Direct binding of Ca^{2+} to the channel is probably not responsible for the current suppression, because a transient rise in intracellular Ca^{2+} levels has been observed following injection of the oocyte with Ca^{2+}; the Ca^{2+} levels would return in a short time period. The involvement of intracellular Ca^{2+} in receptor-mediated suppression was investigated. Intracellular injection of EGTA attenuated ET_A- or mGluR5-mediated suppression of $I_{(Kv1.2)}$ and $I_{(Kv1.4)}$, but again to a different extent between the two currents. In contrast to staurosporine, intracellular injection of EGTA attenuated the receptor-mediated suppression of $I_{(Kv1.4)}$ more than that of $I_{(Kv1.2)}$ (see Fig. 3). Thus, the contribution of intracellular Ca^{2+} to receptor-mediated suppression is not the same between $I_{(Kv1.2)}$ and $I_{(Kv1.4)}$; that is, intracellular Ca^{2+} contributes more to the suppression of $I_{(Kv1.4)}$ than $I_{(Kv1.2)}$.

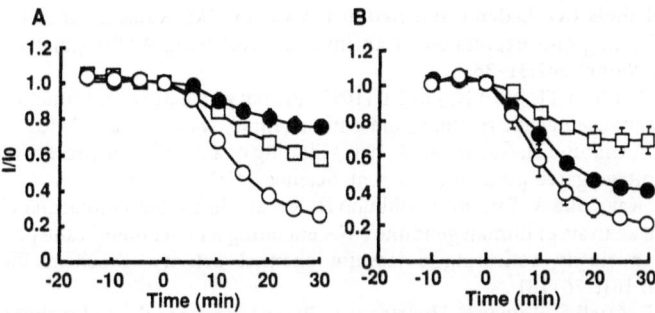

FIG. 3A,B. Time-course of endothelin receptor- (ET$_A$-) mediated suppression of I$_{(Kv1.2)}$ (A) and I$_{(Kv1.4)}$ (B) amplitudes in the absence (*open circles*) or presence (*solid circles*) of 1 μM staurosporine or in ethyleneglycoltetraacetic acid- (EGTA-) injected oocytes (*open squares*). Currents were elicited by depolarizations from −80 mV to +20 mV every 5 min and plotted as a value relative to the current at time zero when ET-1 (10 nM) was applied. Similar results were obtained with oocytes coexpressing mGluR5 and Kv1.2 or Kv1.4.

When the relative contribution of PKC and Ca^{2+} is compared in the receptor-mediated suppression of I$_{(Kv1.2)}$, PKC activation seems to contribute more to suppression than intracellular Ca^{2+}. On the other hand, in I$_{(Kv1.4)}$ intracellular Ca^{2+} seems to contribute more than PKC activation to current suppression. Attali et al. [45] reported that Kv1.3 current underwent suppression mediated by serotonine receptor, which is coupled to phosphatidylinositol turnover. The suppression of I$_{(Kv1.3)}$ seems to be equally inhibited by staurosporine and intracellular EGTA. Thus, even though all the cloned K+ channels mentioned earlier are suppressed by phospholipase C-mediated mechanisms, Ca^{2+} or PKC do not seem to contribute equally to suppression in each K+ channel clone.

References

1. Hille B (1992) Ionic channels of excitable membranes, 2nd edn. Sinauer, Sunderland, MA
2. Catterall WA (1988) Structure and function of voltage-sensitive ion channels. Science 242:50–61
3. Rettig J, Heinemann SH, Wunder F, Lorra C, Parcej DN, Dolly JO, Pongs O (1994) Inactivation properties of voltage-gated K+ channels altered by presence of β-subunit. Nature 369:289–294
4. Majumder K, De Biasi M, Wang Z, Wible BA (1995) Molecular cloning and functional expression of a novel potassium channel β-subunit from human atrium. FEBS Lett 361:13–16
5. Morales MJ, Castellino RC, Crews AL, Rasmusson RL, Strauss HC (1995) A novel β subunit increases rate of inactivation of specific voltage-gated potassium channel α subunits. J Biol Chem 270:6272–6277
6. Papazian DM, Schwarz TL, Tempel BL, Jan YN, Jan LY (1987) Cloning of genomic and complementary DNA from *Shaker*, a putative potassium channel gene from *Drosophila*. Science 237:749–753
7. Kamb A, Iverson LE, Tanouye MA (1987) Molecular characterization of *Shaker*, a *Drosophila* gene that encodes a potassium channel. Cell 50:405–413
8. Pongs O, Kecskemethy N, Müller R, Krah-Jentgens I, Baumann A, Kiltz HH, Canal I, Llamazares S, Ferrus A (1988) *Shaker* encodes a family of putative potassium channel proteins in the nervous system of *Drosophila*. EMBO J 7:1087–1096

9. Ho K, Nichols CG, Lederer WJ, Lytton J, Vassilev PM, Kanazirska MV, Hebert SC (1993) Cloning and expression of an inwardly rectifying ATP-regulated potassium channel. Nature 362:31–38

10. Kubo Y, Baldwin TJ, Jan YN, Jan LY (1993) Primary structure and functional expression of a mouse inward rectifier potassium channel. Nature 362:127–133

11. Takumi T, Ohkubo H, Nakanishi S (1988) Cloning of a membrane protein that induces a slow voltage-gated potassium current. Science 242:1042–1045

12. Murai T, Kakizuka A, Takumi T, Ohkubo H, Nakanishi S (1989) Molecular cloning and sequence analysis of human genomic DNA encoding a novel membrane protein which exhibits a slowly activating potassium channel activity. Biochem Biophys Res Commun 161:176–181

13. Honoré E, Attali B, Romey G, Heurteaux C, Ricard P, Lesage F, Lazdunski M, Barhanin J (1991) Cloning, expression, pharmacology and regulation of a delayed rectifier K⁺ channel in mouse heart. EMBO J 10:2805–2811

14. Hoshi T, Zagotta WN, Aldrich RW (1990) Biophysical and molecular mechanisms of *Shaker* potassium channel inactivation. Science 250:533–538

15. Zagotta WN, Hoshi T, Aldrich RW (1990) Restoration of inactivation in mutants of *Shaker* potassium channels by a peptide derived from ShB. Science 250:568–571

16. MacKinnon R, Miller C (1989) Mutant potassium channels with altered binding of charybdotoxin, a pore-blocking peptide inhibitor. Science 245:1382–1385

17. MacKinnon R, Heginbotham L, Abramson T (1990) Mapping the receptor site for charybdotoxin, a pore-blocking potassium channel inhibitor. Neuron 5:767–771

18. Yellen G, Jurman ME, Abramson T, MacKinnon R (1991) Mutations affecting internal TEA blockade identify the probable pore-forming region of a K⁺ channel. Science 251:939–942

19. Hartmann HA, Kirsch GE, Drewe JA, Taglialatela M, Joho RH, Brown AM (1991) Exchange of conduction pathways between two related K⁺ channels. Science 251:942–944

20. Jan LY, Jan YN (1992) Structural elements involved in specific K⁺ channel functions. Annu Rev Physiol 54:537–555

21. Ishii K, Nunoki K, Murakoshi H, Taira N (1992) Cloning and modulation by endothelin-1 of rat cardiac K channel. Biochem Biophys Res Commun 184:1484–1489

22. Okada H, Ishii K, Nunoki K, Abe T, Taira N (1992) Modulation of transient type K channel cloned from rat heart. Biochem Biophys Res Commun 189:430–436

23. Sasaki Y, Ishii K, Nunoki K, Yamagishi T, Taira N (1995) Voltage-dependent K⁺ channel (Kv1.5) cloned from rabbit heart and facilitation of inactivation of the delayed rectifier current by rat β subunit. FEBS Lett 372:20–24

24. Ishii K, Yamagishi T, Taira N (1994) Cloning and functional expression of a cardiac inward rectifier K⁺ channel. FEBS Lett 338:107–111

25. Armstrong CM, Bezanilla F (1977) Inactivation of the sodium channel II. Gating current experiments. J Gen Pysiol 70:567–590

26. Isacoff EY, Jan YN, Jan LY (1991) Putative receptor for the cytoplasmic inactivation gate in the *Shaker* K⁺ channel. Nature 353:86–90

27. Li M, Jan YN, Jan LY (1992) Specification of subunit assembly by the hydrophilic amino-terminal domain of the *Shaker* potassium channel. Science 257:1225–1230

28. Tseng-Crank J, Yao JA, Berman MF, Tseng GN (1993) Functional role of the NH₂-terminal cytoplasmic domain of a mammalian A-type K channel. J Gen Physiol 102:1057–1083

29. MacKinnon R, Aldrich RW, Lee AW (1993) Functional stoichiometry of *Shaker* potassium channel inactivation. Science 262:757–759

30. Christie MJ, North RA, Osborne PB, Douglass J, Adelman JP (1990) Heteropolymeric potassium channels expressed in *Xenopus* oocytes from cloned subunits. Neuron 2:405–411

31. Isacoff EY, Jan YN, Jan LY (1990) Evidence for the formation of heteromultimeric potassium channels in *Xenopus* oocytes. Nature 345:530–534

32. Ruppersberg JP, Schröter KH, Sakmann B, Stocker M, Sewing S, Pongs O (1990) Heteromultimeric channels formed by rat brain potassium-channel proteins. Nature 345:535–537

33. Sheng M, Liao YJ, Jan YN, Jan LY (1993) Presynaptic A-current based on heteromultimeric K$^+$ channels detected *in vivo*. Nature 365:72–75

34. Nunoki K, Ishii K, Okada H, Yamagishi T, Murakoshi H, Taira N (1994) Hybrid potassium channels by tandem linkage of inactivating and non-inactivating subunits. J Biol Chem 269:24138–24142

35. Levitan IB (1985) Phosphorylation of ion channels. J Membr Biol 87:177–190

36. Tsien RW, Giles WR, Greengard P (1972) Cyclic AMP mediates the effects of adrenaline on cardiac Purkinje fibres. Nature New Biol 240:181–183

37. Kameyama M, Hofmann F, Trautwein W (1985) On the mechanism of β-adrenergic regulation of the Ca channel in the guinea-pig heart. Pflügers Arch 405:285–293

38. Yazawa K, Kameyama M (1990) Mechanism of receptor-mediated modulation of the delayed outward potassium current in guinea-pig ventricular myocytes. J Physiol (Camb) 421:135–150

39. Apkon M, Nerbonne JM (1988) α_1-Adrenergic agonists selectively suppress voltage-dependent K$^+$ currents in rat ventricular myocytes. Proc Natl Acad Sci USA 85:8756–8760

40. Fedida D, Shimoni Y, Giles WR (1989) A novel effect of norepinephrine on cardiac cells is mediated by α_1-adrenoceptors. Am J Physiol 256:H1500–H1504

41. Tohse N, Nakaya H, Hattori Y, Endou M, Kanno M (1990) Inhibitory effect mediated by α_1-adrenoceptors on transient outward current in isolated rat ventricular cells. Eur J Physiol 415:575–581

42. Murakoshi H, Ishii K, Nunoki K, Taira N (1994) Receptor-mediated modulation of rat Kv1.2 in *Xenopus* oocytes. Eur J Pharmacol Mol Pharmacol Sect 268:451–454

43. Huang XY, Morielli AD, Peralta EG (1993) Tyrosine kinase-dependent suppression of a potassium channel by the G protein-coupled m$_1$ muscarinic acetylcholine receptor. Cell 75:1145–1156

44. Murray KT, Fahrig SA, Deal KK, Po SS, Hu NN, Snyders DJ, Tamkun MM, Bennett PB (1994) Modulation of an inactivating human cardiac K$^+$ channel by protein kinase C. Circ Res 75:999–1005

45. Attali B, Honoré E, Lesage F, Lazdunski M, Barhanin J (1992) Regulation of a major cloned voltage-gated K$^+$ channel from human T lymphocytes. FEBS Lett 303:229–232

Molecular Mechanisms of Sodium Channel Inactivation and Block by Local Anesthetics

TODD SCHEUER and WILLIAM A. CATTERALL

Summary. Voltage-dependent sodium channels initiate electrical activity in many excitable cells but inactivation terminates their activity within 2 ms of activation. Local anesthetics block sodium channels and stabilize the inactivated state. The rat brain Na^+ channel consists of a 260-kDa α-subunit, a 36-kDa β_1 subunit and a 33-kDa β_2 subunit. The α-subunit contains four homologous transmembrane domains (I–IV), each with six predicted α-helical transmembrane repeats (S1–S6). A conserved intracellular loop between homologous domains III and IV (L_{III-IV}) is required for inactivation and is proposed to form the inactivation gate. A hydrophobic cluster of amino acids, IFM, binds to a receptor in the pore and occludes it. Amino acids in transmembrane segment IVS6 are also required for inactivation. Overlapping amino acids in IVS6 are necessary for use- and voltage-dependent block by local anesthetics, indicating that IVS6 contains the binding site for these drugs and also forms part of the ion-conducting pore.

Key words. Sodium channel—Inactivation—Local anesthetics—Electrical excitability—Site-directed mutagenesis

Introduction

Voltage-dependent sodium channels are responsible for the upstroke of the action potential in most excitable cells including neurons, cardiac muscle, and skeletal muscle. Sodium currents activate in less than a millisecond in response to a depolarization and then inactivate almost completely within a few milliseconds. The sodium channel from rat brain consists of a large α-subunit (260 kDa) that is associated with smaller β_1 (36-kDa) and β_2 (33-kDa) subunits. The β_2-subunit is linked to the α-subunit by disulfide bonds. Sodium channel α-subunit cDNAs have been isolated from a variety of sources including rat brain, skeletal muscle, and cardiac muscle. Each cDNA encodes a protein consisting of four homologous domains (I–IV), each consisting of six predicted transmembrane α-helices (S1–S6). Each homologous domain has extensive homology to a single subunit of voltage-dependent K^+ channels, four of which are thought to form a functional channel. By analogy, the four homologous domains of the voltage-dependent sodium channels are thought to be arranged in a tetrad, surrounding a central, ion-conducting pore.

Department of Pharmacology, University of Washington, Seattle, WA 98195, USA

Using mutagenesis of specific amino acids, several functional regions of the channel have been identified. Residues contributing to the ion-conducting pore were first identified in potassium channels in the loop between transmembrane helices S5 and S6 [1]. The analogous loops in each homologous domain of the sodium channel contain residues that affect binding of tetrodotoxin [2], which is thought to act by "plugging" the extracellular mouth of the ion-conducting pore [3]. Also, ion-binding sites controlling permeability of the Na^+ channel have been identified in these regions of the channel [4]. Segment S4 of each homologous domain contains positively charged amino acids at every third position, and these are proposed to act as voltage sensors for opening the channel. Charge neutralization and reversal mutations reduce the voltage dependence of channel opening, consistent with some of these residues serving as gating charges [5]. Neutralization of positively charged amino acid residues reduces the steepness of activation consistent with these residues serving as gating charges. Recent work from our group has focused on two aspects of sodium channel structure and function, the molecular basis for sodium channel inactivation and the identification of amino acids critical for block of sodium channels by local anesthetics. These studies and the basis for them are reviewed next.

Molecular Mechanisms of Inactivation

Sodium channels activate and then inactivate within a few milliseconds. The rate of activation is strongly voltage dependent and is thought to derive its voltage dependence from intrinsic, voltage-dependent transitions in the sodium channel molecule. The fast inactivation process begins with a delay [6–8] and is thought to be less voltage dependent and to derive much of its voltage dependence from its coupling to the voltage-dependent activation process [7,9]. The structural basis underlying this process has been a major emphasis of our laboratory.

Pharmacological interventions that block the inactivation process give valuable clues to regions of the Na^+ channel molecule that participate in the inactivation process. Alpha-scorpion toxins such as the toxin from *Leiurus quinquestriatus* (LqTX) are charged peptide molecules that act from the extracellular surface of the membrane and slow the inactivation process. Binding of these toxins to the channel is highly voltage dependent, suggesting that the binding site for these molecules represents an extracellular site that undergoes voltage-dependent conformational changes that are required for channel inactivation [10]. Photolabeling of the brain sodium channel with a photoreactive scorpion toxin derivative resulted in labeling of α- and $β_1$-subunits [11]. However, actions of α-scorpion toxins are normal on channels resulting from expression of the α-subunit alone, indicating that the physiologically relevant sites are on that subunit [12,13]. The sites on the α-subunit that were photolabeled were identified by proteolytic digestion of the labeled protein followed by identification of the labeled fragment using site-directed antibodies [14]. This site is located on the extracellular loop connecting transmembrane segments S5 and S6. Site-directed antibodies recognizing this loop also inhibit LqTX binding. Likewise, similar antibodies recognizing the loop connecting segments S5 and S6 in the homologous domain IV also inhibit LqTX binding [15]. In the properly folded sodium channel, these loops must be near each other and contain or be close to the binding site for LqTX. These results indicate that regions near these locations on the sodium channel α-subunit are expected to undergo conformational changes leading to Na^+ channel inactivation.

Armstrong and colleagues initially demonstrated that intracellular perfusion of Na^+ channel-expressing cells with proteases removes the inactivation process [16]. Activation was virtually unaffected. A variety of other intracellularly acting chemical modifying agents can also remove inactivation (see [3] for review). Molecular interpretation of the inactivation process has also been strongly influenced by studies describing the behavior of intracellularly applied charged blocking compounds. Application of derivatives of tetraethylammonium to normally noninactivating squid axon potassium channels induced an inactivation-like process that required channel activation before the drug could reach its binding site [17]. Similar block of protease-treated, noninactivated sodium channels by pancuronium [18], N-methyl strychnine [19], and thiazin dyes [20] as well as other positively charged compounds has been described. Armstrong and coworkers [21] combined these findings with observations on the kinetics of sodium channel gating to propose what has come to be called the "ball-and-chain model" of inactivation. They suggested that the channel contained a physically distinct structure similar to a ball and chain on its intracellular surface. Channel activation in response to voltage makes a receptor available on the intracellular surface of the channel. The ball can then swing in and bind to the receptor, thus blocking the channel and "immobilizing" the voltage-dependent particle to which it is bound. This scheme has dominated the design and interpretation of experiments examining the molecular nature of fast Na^+ and K^+ channel inactivation.

As originally conceived, this scheme fits most completely with data from the *Shaker* potassium channel molecule. Hoshi et al. showed that the N-terminus of each potassium channel subunit is required for inactivation [22]. The extreme N-terminus is composed of a mixture of hydrophobic and hydrophilic amino acids and is most critical for inactivation. Truncating this portion of the channel results in a noninactivating channel. This ball is connected to the rest of the channel by a hydrophilic protein chain. Application of peptides corresponding to the truncated N-terminus to the intracellular surface of excised inside-out patches results in the reconstitution of the inactivation process [23]. This series of experiments corresponded to the original ball-and-chain proposal of Armstrong in a remarkable way.

Role of L_{III-IV} in Sodium Channel Inactivation

Sodium channels from a broad range of organisms have functionally similar inactivation processes. This suggests that portions of the channel involved in inactivation are likely to be structurally conserved. The short intracellular loop connecting homologous domains III and IV (L_{III-IV}) of the sodium channel is highly conserved among sodium channel α-subunits. A site-directed antibody recognizing this loop specifically blocked sodium channel inactivation without affecting activation of brain and muscle cells [24,25]. Other intracellularly directed antibodies left inactivation unaffected. Interestingly, the rate at which these antibodies removed inactivation after application depended on membrane potential. Effects were more rapid at negative potentials than at more depolarized potentials at which the channel was inactivated. These results suggested that this region of the molecule becomes hidden and inaccessible to antibodies when the channel inactivates. The involvement of L_{III-IV} in inactivation was also detected in experiments employing molecular biological techniques. Introducing a break in this region of the channel by dividing the channel in two in this loop and coexpressing the two halves in *Xenopus* oocytes yielded channels with defective inactivation [5]. Finally, two of a series of five large deletions in this loop virtually prevented inactivation [26]. The combination of these experimental approaches strongly implicated L_{III-IV} in the inactivation process and suggested that its overall structure was important for supporting normal sodium channel inactivation.

The sequence of amino acids in L_{III-IV} is characterized by multiple positively and negatively charged residues as well as a series of hydrophobic residues. The multiple charged residues are likely targets for the proteases that effectively remove inactivation. However, mutation of charged residues singly and in combination had only minor effects on inactivation [26,27]. Mutation of hydrophobic amino acids had far more dramatic effects. Mutation of a hydrophobic triplet of amino acids, isoleucine 1488, phenylalanine 1489, and methionine 1490, all to glutamine (IFM1488,1489,1490QQQ) produced a channel with minimal macroscopic inactivation [28]. However, after similar mutation of phenylalanine 1483 to glutamine, inactivation was unaffected. Individual mutation of phenylalanine 1489 to glutamine caused almost as strong a disruption of inactivation as the IFM combination. Individual mutations I1488Q and M1490Q caused much smaller changes in the inactivation behavior of the channel. To date, no other individual amino acid change in this region causes nearly as great a disruption of inactivation as that observed with F1489Q. Thus, phenylalanine 1489 appears to be the key amino acid residue controlling inactivation in this region.

The currents produced by mutant IFM1488,1489,1490QQQ were reminiscent of the removal of sodium channel inactivation observed after intracellular treatment with proteases [16]. However, the structure of L_{III-IV} is unlike the tethered ball of the ball-and-chain model [21]. Instead, L_{III-IV} is short (50 amino acids) and fixed at both ends with the critical IFM (hydrophobic amino acid cluster) motif lying approximately one-third of the distance from the N-terminal end of the loop. To accommodate this structure, it was proposed that L_{III-IV} forms a "hinged lid" analogous to the protein lids that fold over the active site of certain allosteric enzymes and control substrate access. Conserved glycine and proline residues found at either end of the loop would serve as molecular hinges. In this scheme, after channel activation, L_{III-IV} would fold over the intracellular mouth of the pore and bind, with phenylalanine 1489 forming a hydrophobic latch that holds the inactivation gate closed [28].

Two aspects of this scheme have been tested experimentally. First, the scheme predicts that phenylalanine 1489 is a critical part of a blocking particle that enters the intracellular mouth of the pore and blocks it during inactivation. Thus, the pore of the channel is predicted to contain a binding site for a blocking particle containing the IFM motif. Application of synthetic peptides corresponding to the IFM motif are expected to reconstitute inactivation in noninactivating sodium channels, much as synthetic peptides corresponding to the N-terminus of potassium channels can reconstitute potassium channel inactivation [23].

Large synthetic peptides corresponding to the native sequence were unsuccessful at reproducing sodium channel inactivation [13]. However, a short, five-residue peptide containing the IFM motif KIFMK successfully reconstituted inactivation in channels that had been made inactivation deficient, either by the mutation F1480Q or by treatment with α-scorpion toxin [13,29]. Just as mutation F1489Q blocked inactivation of the channel, a peptide with the sequence KIQMK produced no inactivation. Thus, a receptor exists in the pore of the channel that specifically binds the phenylalanine in the IFM motif [13,29].

This model has also been evaluated by examining the chemical properties of the amino acid at position 1489 that are required for effective inactivation. Phenylalanine 1489 was substituted with a range of different amino acids. Amino acids that were hydrophobic and aromatic in character caused minimal disruption of inactivation, but polar and charged amino acids almost completely blocked it [30]. These data indicate that phenylalanine 1489 makes a hydrophobic or π-electron interaction with its receptor.

Role of Transmembrane Segment IVS6 in Sodium Channel Inactivation

Relatively little information is available concerning the portions of the channel that might contribute to formation of the receptor for the inactivation gate. Local anesthetics [31,32] and other charged drugs [18,20,33,34] acting from the cytoplasmic surface of the channel mimic inactivation and immobilize gating charge movement of the channel, much as the inactivation gate does. Some local anesthetics act by stabilizing the inactivated state of channel [35–37]. Other intracellular blocking drugs [18,33,34], as well as the peptide KIFMK [13], prevent closure of the inactivation gate. Phenylalkylamines block calcium [38] and sodium channels [39,40] with characteristics that are reminiscent of sodium channel block by local anesthetics. Thus, a range of compounds appear to share the same or an overlapping binding site with the inactivation gate in the intracellular portion of the ion-conducting pore.

Photoreactive phenylalkylamines label the voltage-dependent skeletal muscle calcium channels. The site of labeling was localized to the intracellular portion of transmembrane segment IVS6, indicating that this segment is near the phenylalkylamine binding site of the L-type calcium channel. The homology between sodium and calcium channels suggested that this region might also be involved in drug binding in the sodium channel and also might contain the receptor for the inactivation gate. The involvement of IVS6 in sodium channel inactivation was also suggested by location in this segment of mutations causing hyperkalemic periodic paralysis, a disease characterized by incomplete sodium channel inactivation [41,42]. Thus, this region was chosen as a target for mutagenic analysis to locate residues participating in inactivation and local anesthetic binding [43–45].

To identify residues involved in inactivation, sodium channel constructs were created containing mutations of individual amino acids in this region to alanine. Alanine was chosen because it produces chemical differences without disrupting the helical structure of the region mutated [46]. Three amino acids in this region produced significant disruption of inactivation. Each produced a fraction of noninactivating current, although the strongest mutant of an individual amino acid, V1774A, produced an approximately 30% noninactivating current, far less than produced by F1489Q in L_{III-IV}. However, combination of two of these mutations in the same construct, F1764A and V1774A, produced a channel with no detectable inactivation [44]. The degree of inactivation disruption produced by FV1764,1774AA was that predicted if each of the component amino acids made independent contributions to the total effect.

A mutation that acts primarily by disrupting the binding of an inactivation particle to its receptor is expected to speed the rate at which it leaves the receptor once it is bound. To detect such behavior, single-channel recordings were obtained from each of the constructs affecting inactivation. The wild-type rat brain type IIA channel normally opened only once or twice for a total time of less than 1 ms and then inactivated and failed to reopen for the remainder of the depolarization. Inactivation was effectively absorbing. Single-channel recordings from the mutant constructs were characterized by multiple, individual openings during a depolarization, but openings were short and well separated from one another. The mean channel open time was minimally affected. Thus, in the mutant channels the inactivated state was much less stable once formed, behavior that is expected for a disrupted inactivation gate [44].

These mutant channels had the kinetic phenotype expected for a disrupted inactivation gate receptor. Several tests were designed to determine whether they interacted with phenylalanine 1489 in L_{III-IV}. First, block by the peptide KIFMK was examined. If the receptor for phenylalanine 1489 was one of the identified residues, KIFMK would not be expected to block that mutant effectively. However, KIFMK blocked the mutant FV1764,1774AA with normal affinity and kinetics, indicating that its receptor had not been disrupted [44].

Second, the interaction between phenylalanine 1489 and its receptor had been proposed to be hydrophobic or aromatic in nature [30]. Thus, if F1489 interacted with V1774 in the wild-type channel, making the amino acid at position 1774 less hydrophobic, then alanine would be expected to further disrupt inactivation. Substitution of the polar residues serine and asparagine for the native valine disrupted inactivation less effectively than the mutation to alanine. Thus, in contrast to results at position 1489, effects of mutations at 1774 are not correlated with the hydrophobicity of the substituted amino acid [44].

A third strategy was to combine mutations at position 1489 and positions 1764 or 1774 to examine whether their effects on inactivation were energetically independent. Thus, mutation F1489W was combined with mutation F1764A or V1774A. The sum of the changes in free energy caused by each of the individual mutations was equivalent to the change in free energy from the double mutation. This result indicated that these mutations had independent effects on the stability of the inactivated state and that residues at either position 1764 or 1774 were unlikely to pair with the residue at position 1489 [44].

Molecular Determinants of Block by Local Anesthetics

Local anesthetics block current through sodium channels more effectively when the membrane is depolarized or when the channel is repetitively activated. These use- and voltage-dependent properties are thought to result from differential drug binding to the depolarized channel. The dependence of drug binding on channel state can be explained using a model in which drugs have a higher affinity for the channel when it is open and inactivated than when it is at rest [35–37,47,48].

Most biophysical evidence concerning the location of the binding site for local anesthetics relies on the use of permanently charged derivatives of local anesthetics such as QX314. These drugs are inactive when applied to the extracellular surface of axonal sodium channels but produce an effective use-dependent block when added intracellularly [49,50]. They appear to bind to a site in the ion-conducting pore that is accessible from the intracellular surface of the channel. Finally, they can be trapped within the pore at negative potentials, presumably between an intracellular inactivation gate and the selectivity filter [50–53].

Charged phenylalkylamine binding to calcium channels behave much as QX314 does in blocking sodium channels [38]. Photolabeling with phenylalkylamines has identified segment IVS6 of the calcium channel as a possible phenylalkylamine-binding site [54]. Therefore, mutations in this region of the sodium channel were good candidates for having effects on local anesthetic binding. Because of the use- and voltage-dependent properties of local anesthetic block, experiments were designed to separate effects on resting hyperpolarized channels and depolarized and active channels.

Drug block of resting channels was measured during infrequent depolarizations from the holding potential or after strong hyperpolarizations to remove residual drug block present at the holding potential [45]. Under these conditions etidocaine bound to resting wild-type channels with an inhibition constant for the resting channel, K_r, of $325\,\mu M$. Three mutations, I1761A, V1766A, and N1769A, caused increased resting block. K_rs were approximately $100\,\mu M$ for I1761A and V1766A and $20\,\mu M$ for N1769A, a 15-fold increase in sensitivity to block or resting channels by etidocaine. One mutation, F1764A, caused a pronounced decrease in the sensitivity of the channel to resting block by etidocaine ($K_r = 1\,\mu M$).

Mutations that affected affinity of the drug for depolarized channels were detected by examining shifts in channel availability or inactivation curves. Local anesthetic drugs induce a dose-dependent negative shift in inactivation curves. This has been interpreted as being caused by the increased affinity of the drug for the inactivated as opposed to the resting conformation of the channel [35–37]. Mutant F1764A gave a decreased negative shift in the inactivation curve, suggesting that this drug had a decreased binding affinity for the inactivated state of the channel [45].

The binding affinity of the drug for depolarized and inactivated channels was determined directly by measuring drug block at −40 mV, a potential at which most of the channels were inactivated [45]. Using this approach, the dissociation constant for drug binding to inactivated channels, K_i, was $1\,\mu M$ for the wild-type channel. In contrast, the K_i for F1764A was $130\,\mu M$. Apparently, this mutation causes reduced affinity of the inactivated channel for local anesthetics.

Use-dependent block induced by trains of depolarizing pulses results from binding of the drug to the channel during each depolarization that does not unbind completely during the interval between pulses [50,51]. Several mutations in this region caused reductions in use-dependent block, the largest being caused by I1760A, F1764A, and Y1771A [45].

The mechanism by which use-dependent block was reduced differed between mutants. Both F1774A and Y1771A reduced the amount of drug that bound to the channel on depolarization, thus reducing use-dependent block. In contrast, for mutant I1760A, the number of channels blocked on depolarization was unaffected. Instead, these mutant channels recovered from drug block eightfold more rapidly between pulses than the wild-type channel. For mutant I1760A, this more rapid escape of drug from closed channels at negative potentials was responsible for the reduction in use-dependent block [45].

Tertiary amine local anesthetics are thought to arrive at blocking sites in the channel by both hydrophilic and hydrophobic pathways [36]. Quaternary amine local anesthetics do not pass readily through cell membranes and thus have been used as probes for identifying hydrophilic pathways for drug access to blocking sites. As discussed previously, these drugs only block from the intracellular surface of the channel. Intracellular application of the quaternary drug QX314 caused potent use-dependent block of wild-type brain sodium channels [45]. Recovery from this block was extremely slow (τ = 12 min), consistent with evidence from other preparations that the drug becomes trapped in the channel by closed activation and inactivation gates at negative potentials [50–53]. When tested on mutant channel I1760A, QX314 caused a use-dependent block that was nearly as potent as in the wild type. However, the drug escaped from the channel much more rapidly with a time constant of 0.8 min [45]. Mutation I1760A appeared to create a new pathway for drug escape from the channel or greatly facilitate passage through an existing pathway. The location of this residue near the predicted extracellular end of the channel suggested that it might create a pathway between the drug-binding site and the extracellular mouth of the pore by which drug molecules could escape from the channel. As predicted by this scheme and in contrast to the wild-type channel, extracellularly added QX314 blocks sodium currents by expression of I1760A. Thus, mutation of I1760 to A creates an extracellular pathway by which quaternary local anesthetics can both enter and leave their binding site [45].

The position of each of the three mutations having strong effects on use-dependent block by local anesthetics falls on approximately the same face of the predicted IVS6 α-helix. Mutants F1764A and Y1771A, which reduced depolarized channel affinity for local anesthetics, are separated by two helical turns and thus are about 11 Å apart. Effective local anesthetics are 10–15 Å in length [55] with charged and hydrophobic residues at either end [56–58]. Ragsdale et al. [45] proposed that these residues interact with either end of local anesthetic molecules by hydrophobic or π-electron interactions. I1760 was proposed to lie at a narrow point in the pore extracellular to the local anesthetic-binding site. Replacing the isoleucine residue with the smaller alanine created an extracellular access pathway by which extracellularly applied QX314 can enter and leave the pore.

Conclusion

Molecular approaches have, to date, defined three regions that are involved in sodium channel inactivation. An extracellular region defined by the binding site for α-scorpion toxin is located near the loops connecting transmembrane segments S5 and S6 of homologous domains I and IV. Loop L_{III-IV} has the properties expected of an inactivation gate, and phenylalanine 1489 stabilizes the inactivated state by binding via either hydrophobic or π-electron interactions. Transmembrane segment IVS6 also contains residues that are required for stabilizing the inactivated state, properties that are expected for an inactivation gate receptor. However, residues in this region do not appear to interact directly with F1489. Residues in transmembrane segment IVS6 also contribute to the binding site for local anesthetics. Two residues, F1764 and Y1771, are required for effective binding of local anesthetics to the depolarized state of the channel. A third residue, I1760, is located at a narrow point in the pore that normally prevents access of extracellularly applied quaternary local anesthetics to their binding site. Thus, mutations in IVS6 define a new region contributing to the sodium channel pore containing functionally important interaction sites for inactivation and for local anesthetic block.

References

1. Yellen G, Jurman ME, Abramson T, MacKinnon R (1991) Mutations affecting internal TEA blockade identify the probable pore-forming region of a K^+ channel. Science 251:939–942

2. Terlau H, Heinemann SH, Stuhmer W, Pusch M, Conti F, Imoto K, Numa S (1991) Mapping the site of block by tetrodotoxin and saxitoxin of sodium channel II. FEBS Lett 293:93–96

3. Hille B (1992) Ionic channels of excitable membranes. Sinauer Associates, Sunderland, MA

4. Backx PH, Yue DT, Lawrence JH, Marban E, Tomaselli GH (1992) Molecular localization of an ion-binding site within the pore of mammalian sodium channels. Science 257:248–251

5. Stuhmer W, Conti F, Suzuki H, Wang X, Noda M, Yahagi N, Kubo H, Numa S (1988) Structural parts involved in activation and inactivation of the sodium channel. Nature 339:597–603

6. Schauf CL, Goldman L (1972) Inactivation of the sodium current in *Myxicola* giant axons. J Gen Physiol 59:659–675

7. Armstrong CM, Bezanilla F (1977) Inactivation of the sodium channel. II. Gating current experiments. J Gen Physiol 70:567–590

8. Bean BP (1981) Sodium channel inactivation in the crayfish giant axon. Biophys J 35:595–614

9. Aldrich RW, Corey DP, Stevens CF (1983) A reinterpretation of mammalian sodium channel gating based on single channel recording. Nature 306:436–441

10. Catterall WA (1992) Cellular and molecular biology of voltage-gated sodium channels. Physiol Rev 72:S15–S48

11. Beneski D, Catterall WA (1980) Covalent labelling of protein components of the sodium channel with a photoactivatable derivative of scorpion toxin. Proc Natl Acad Sci USA 77:639–642

12. Scheuer T, Auld VJ, Boyd S, Offord J, Dunn R, Catterall WA (1990) Functional properties of rat brain sodium channels expressed in a somatic cell line. Science 247:854–858

13. Eaholtz G, Scheuer T, Catterall WA (1994) Restoration of inactivation and block of open sodium channels by an inactivation gate peptide. Neuron 12:1041–1072

14. Tejedor FJ, Catterall WA (1988) Site of covalent attachment of α-scorpion toxin derivatives in domain I of the sodium channel α subunit. Proc Natl Acad Sci USA 85:8742–8746

15. Thomsen WJ, Catterall WA (1989) Localization of the receptor site for α-scorpion toxins by antibody mapping: implications for sodium channel topology. Proc Natl Acad Sci USA 86:10161–10165

16. Armstrong CM, Bezanilla F, Rojas E (1973) Destruction of sodium conductance inactivation in squid giant axons perfused with pronase. J Gen Physiol 63:375–391

17. Armstrong CM (1971) Interaction of tetraethylammonium derivatives with the potassium channels of squid giant axons. J Gen Physiol 58:413–437

18. Yeh JZ, Narahashi T (1977) Kinetic analysis of pancuronium interaction with sodium channels in squid axon membranes. J Gen Physiol 69:293–323

19. Shapiro BI (1977) Effects of strychnine on the sodium conductance of the frog node of Ranvier. J Gen Physiol 69:915–926

20. Armstrong CM, Croop RS (1982) Simulation of Na channel inactivation by thiazin dyes. J Gen Physiol 80:641–662

21. Armstrong CM (1981) Sodium channels and gating currents. Physiol Rev 61:644–683

22. Hoshi T, Zagotta WN, Aldrich RW (1990) Biophysical and molecular mechanisms of *Shaker* potassium channel inactivation. Science 250:533–538

23. Zagotta WN, Hoshi T, Aldrich RW (1990) Restoration of inactivation in mutants of *Shaker* potassium channels by a peptide derived from ShB. Science 250:568–571

24. Vassilev PM, Scheuer T, Catterall WA (1988) Identification of an intracellular peptide segment involved in sodium channel inactivation. Science 241:1658–1661

25. Vassilev P, Scheuer T, Catterall WA (1989) Inhibition of inactivation of single sodium channels by a site-directed antibody. Proc Natl Acad Sci USA 86:8147–8151

26. Patton DE, West JW, Catterall WA, Goldin AL (1992) Amino acid residues required for fast Na$^+$-channel inactivation: charge neutralizations and deletions in the III-IV linker. Proc Natl Acad Sci USA 89:10905–10909

27. Moorman JR, Kirsch GE, Brown AM, Joho RH (1990) Changes in sodium channel gating produced by point mutations in a cytoplasmic linker. Science 250:688–691

28. West JW, Patton DE, Scheuer T, Wang Y, Goldin AL, Catterall WA (1992) A cluster of hydrophobic amino acid residues required for fast Na$^+$-channel inactivation. Proc Natl Acad Sci USA 89:10910–10914

29. Eaholtz G, Zagotta WA, Catterall WA (1995) Kinetic analysis of time-dependent open channel block by an inactivation gate peptide of non-inactivating type IIA sodium channels. Biophys J 68:A159

30. Scheuer T, West JW, Wang YL, Catterall WA (1993) Effects of amino acid hydrophobicity at position 1489 on sodium channel inactivation. Biophys J 64:A88

31. Cahalan MD (1978) Local anesthetic block of sodium channels in normal and pronase-treated squid giant axons. Biophys J 23:285–311

32. Cahalan MD, Almers W (1979) Interactions between quaternary lidocaine, the sodium channel gates and tetrodotoxin. Biophys J 27:39–56

33. Cahalan MD, Almers W (1979) Block of sodium conductance and gating current in squid giant axons poisoned with quaternary strychnine. Biophys J 27:57–74

34. Yeh JZ, Armstrong CM (1978) Immobilisation of gating charge by a substance that simulates inactivation. Nature 273:387–389

35. Hondeghem LM, Katzung BG (1977) Time- and voltage-dependent interactions of anti-arrhythmic drugs with cardiac sodium channels. Biochem Biophys Acta 427:373

36. Hille B (1977) Local anesthetics: hydrophilic and hydrophobic pathways for the drug-receptor reaction. J Gen Physiol 69:497–515

37. Bean BP, Cohen CJ, Tsien RW (1983) Lidocaine block of cardiac sodium channels. J Gen Physiol 81:613–642

38. McDonald TF, Pelzer S, Trautwein W, Pelzer DJ (1994) Regulation and modulation of calcium channels in cardiac, skeletal, and smooth muscle cells. Physiol Rev 74:365–506

39. Ragsdale DS, Scheuer T, Catterall WA (1991) Frequency and voltage-dependent inhibition of type IIA Na$^+$ channels, expressed in a mammalian cell line, by local anesthetic, antiarrhythmic, and anticonvulsant drugs. Mol Pharmacol 40:756–765

40. Ragsdale DS, Catterall WA, Scheuer T (1993) Biophysical characterization of Na channel block by the quarternary phenylalkylamine D890. Biophys J 64:A90

41. Rojas CV, Wang JZ, Schwartz LS, Hoffman EP, Powell BR, Brown RH Jr (1991) A Met-to-Val mutation in the skeletal muscle Na$^+$ channel alpha-subunit in hyperkalaemic periodic paralysis. Nature 354:387–389

42. Cannon SC, Strittmatter SM (1993) Functional expression of sodium channel mutations identified in families with periodic paralysis. Neuron 10:317–326

43. McPhee JC, Ragsdale DS, Scheuer T, Catterall WA (1994) A mutation in segment IVS6 disrupts fast inactivation of sodium channels. Proc Natl Acad Sci USA 91:12346–12350

44. McPhee JC, Ragsdale DS, Scheuer T, Catterall WA (1995) A critical role for transmembrane segment IVS6 of the sodium channel α subunit in fast inactivation. J Biol Chem 270:12025–12034

45. Ragsdale DS, McPhee JC, Scheuer T, Catterall WA (1994) Molecular determinants of state-dependent block of Na$^+$ channels by local anesthetics. Science 265:1724–1728

46. Blaber M, Zhang X-J, Matthews BW (1993) Stuctural basis of amino acid α helix propensity. Science 260:1637–1640

47. Butterworth JF, Strichartz GR (1990) Molecular mechanisms of local anesthesia: a review. Anesthesiology 72:711–734

48. Catterall WA (1987) Common modes of drug action on Na$^+$ channels: local anesthetics, antiarrhythmics and anticonvulsants. Trends Pharmacol Sci 8:57–65

49. Frazier DT, Narahashi T, Yamada M (1970) The site of action and active form of local anesthetics. II. Experiments with quaternary compounds. J Pharmacol Exp Ther 171:45–51

50. Strichartz GR (1973) The inhibition of sodium currents in myelinated nerve by quarternary derivatives of lidocaine. J Gen Physiol 62:37–57

51. Courtney KR (1975) Mechanism of frequency-dependent inhibition of sodium currents in frog myelinated nerve by the lidocaine derivative GEA968. J Pharmacol Exp Ther 195:225–236

52. Starmer CF, Yeh JZ, Tanguy J (1986) A quantitative description of QX222 blockade of sodium channels in squid axons. Biophys J 49:913–920

53. Yeh JZ, Tanguy J (1985) Na channel activation gate modulates slow recovery from use-dependent block by local anesthetics in squid giant axons. Biophys J 47:685–694

54. Striessnig J, Glossman H, Catterall WA (1991) Identification of a phenylalkylamine binding region within the alpha 1 subunit of skeletal muscle Ca^{2+} channels. Proc Natl Acad Sci USA 88:9203–9207

55. Courtney KR (1994) Why do some drugs preferentially block open sodium channels? J Mol Cell Cardiol 20:461–464

56. Sheldon RS, Hill RJ, Taouis M, Wilson LM (1991) Aminoalkyl structural requirements for interaction of lidocaine with the class I antiarrhythmic drug receptor on rat cardiac myocytes. Mol Pharmacol 39:609–614

57. Bokesch PM, Post C, Strichartz G (1986) Structure-activity relationship of lidocaine homologs producing tonic and frequency-dependent impulse blockade in nerve. J Pharmacol Exp Ther 237:773–781

58. Zamponi GW, French RJ (1993) Dissecting lidocaine action: diethylamide and phenol mimic separate modes of lidocaine block of sodium channels from heart and skeletal muscle. Biophys J 65:2335–2347

Molecular Properties of Calcium Channels: A Summary

ARNOLD SCHWARTZ

Summary. The voltage-dependent L-type calcium channel consists of four major subunits: α_1, α_2, β, and γ. The α_1 contains the pore and calcium channel modulator sites. The nature, regulation, and asymmetry of the pore and the putatitive binding sites of the drugs are being studied.

Key words. Calcium antagonist binding sites—Calcium channels—Pore

Introduction

Voltage-dependent Ca channels (VDCC) play a vital role in a variety of cellular functions [1]. On the basis of electrophysiological and pharmacological properties, at least six types of VDCCs—the L-, N-, P-, Q-, R-, and T-types—have been distinguished. In cardiac muscle, where Ca influx across the sarcolemma is essential for contraction, the dihydropyridine (DHP)-sensitive L-type VDCC represents the major entry pathway of extracellular Ca. VDCC are heterooligomeric protein complexes composed of α_1, α_2, and β subunits, and other tissue-specific associated proteins such as the γ subunit in the skeletal muscle (Fig. 1). It is now recognized that the pore, gating apparatus, and Ca channel modulator drug-binding sites are located in a large membrane-spanning subunit known as α_1, and that the other, so-called auxiliary subunits, α_2 and β, modulate the VDCC function by interacting with the α_1 protein. In our recent research efforts, we have focused on determining functional regions of the pore-forming subunit α_1.

DHP Binding Sites

The three major classes of Ca antagonists, dihydropyridines (DHP) (e.g., nifedipine), benzothiazepines (BTZ) (e.g., diltiazem), and phenylalkylamines (PAA) (e.g., verapamil), represent a clinically important set of molecules. From the experimental point of view, DHPs have been most extensively used as pharmacological "tools" to probe functional states of L-type VDCCs in relation to their structure. As a matter of fact, DHPs can distinguish two main subfamilies of the six distinct α_1 subunit genes

---

Institute of Molecular Pharmacology and Biophysics, University of Cincinnati College of Medicine, Cincinnati, OH 45267-0828, USA

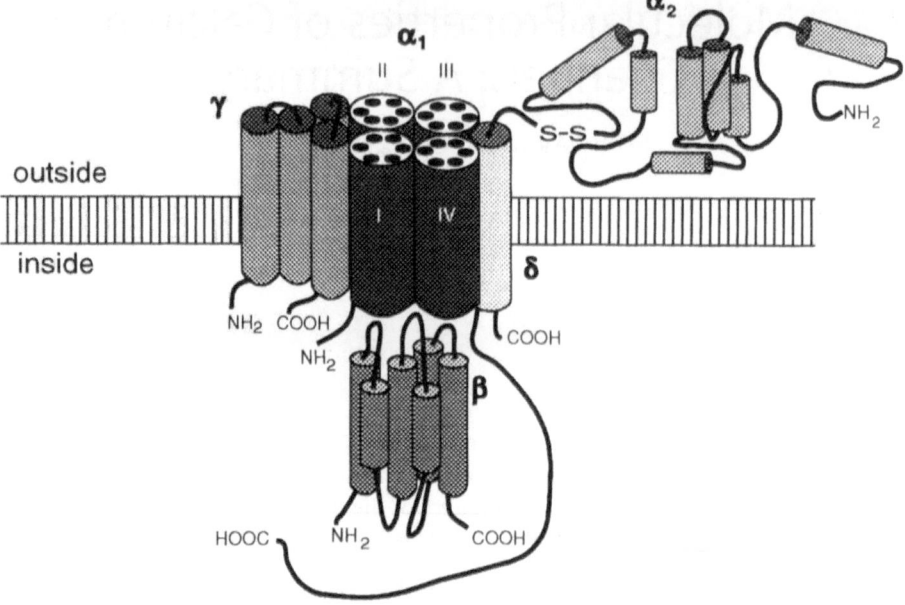

FIG. 1. Hypothetical structure of a high voltage activated (HVA) Ca channel complex showing subunit arrangement for the skeletal muscle HVA Ca channel. (Based on [1])

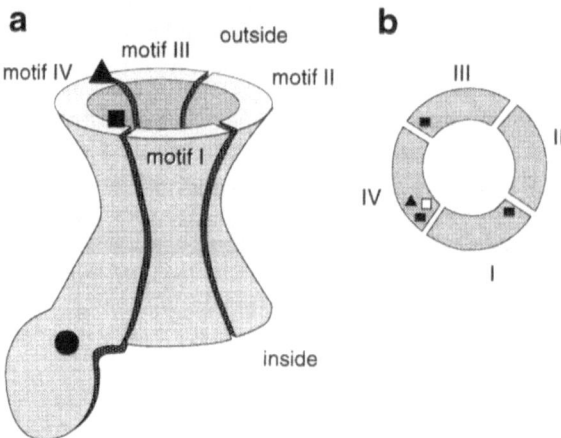

FIG. 2. a High-affinity binding sites for organic Ca channel blockers on the α_1 subunit. *Filled triangle*, benzothiazepines; *filled square*, dihydropyridines; *filled circle*, phenylalkylamines. b Photoaffinity labeling sites of dihydropyridines and benzothiazepines on the α_1 subunit. *Filled triangle*, azidobutyryl clentiazem; *filled squares*, azidopine; *open square*, isradipine. (Based on [1])

[2]: the L-type, and the neuronal non-L-type subfamilies originally classified on the basis of amino acid comparison. In addition, DHPs are the only group that includes both antagonists and agonists. Initially, mapping the binding sites of the three classes of Ca channel blockers on the skeletal muscle α_1 subunit involved photoreactive drug labeling and purification (Fig. 2). The region covalently labeled PAAs was localized on

a 42-amino-acid segment that encompasses part of the transmembrane segment S6 in the internal repeat IV and the adjacent short sequence in the intracellular tail of the α_1 subunit [3]. A photoreactive analog of diltiazem specifically labeled the S5–S6 extracellular connecting loop of motif IV [4]. An attempt to determine the DHP site using similar photoaffinity labeling methods assigning DHP binding to different regions (S5 to S6 in motifs I, III, and IV) [3,5] turned out to be more controversial than other drugs. This inconsistency appears to derive from at least three characteristic drawbacks of the photolabeling procedure [1]: (1) photoreactive groups on the side chain are at a distance of 10–15 Å from the core structure of the derivatives; (2) the availability of antibodies that can precipitate proteolytically digested short fragments of the α_1 subunit is limited; (3) the labeling pattern somewhat depends on whether the photolabeled sample was a purified or crude membrane preparation. To overcome these intrinsic problems of photoaffinity labeling, we employed a chimeric approach [6]. In a series of experiments, chimeric α_1 subunits engineered between cardiac α_{1C} and brain α_{1A} (BI α_1), that produce the DHP-sensitive L-type VDCC and DHP-insensitive Q-type VDCC, respectively, were constructed and expressed in *Xenopus* oocytes to test for sensitivity to blockade by DHPs. A chimera, in which a region from S3 to S6 of repeat IV of the cardiac L channel was replaced with the corresponding region of the BI DHP-insensitive channel, exhibited no DHP sensitivity. In another chimeric construct, which had the BI channel region from S5 to S6 of repeat IV, a markedly decreased sensitivity to DHP agonists was observed, but antagonist sensitivity was fully retained. However, a chimera in which parts of the repeat III-S5-S6 connecting loop and the S6 segment were replaced with the corresponding region from the BI channel retained sensitivity to both DHP antagonists and agonists. These studies clearly emphasize the critical involvement of the IV S5–S6 connecting loop and part of the segment S6 in the functional binding domain of DHPs. Taken together, using both photoaffinity labeling and chimeric techniques, the data to date suggest that DHPs and BTZs bind to a region in close proximity to the pore-lining region. Binding of the DHPs and BTZs may introduce "distortion" into the polypeptide that propagate into the pore structure, thereby reducing probability of the permeable "open conformation" or the L-type channel.

Pore Structure

Under physiological conditions, VDCCs must be highly selective in allowing Ca fluxes to the exclusion of other ions such as Na, K, and Mg, even though these ions are present at comparatively higher concentrations. Although several theoretical models have been proposed to explain this selective permeability, little direct information concerning its structural basis is available. However, evidence accumulated using voltage-gated Na and K channels, whose overall transmembrane topology is the same as VDCC α_1 subunits, strongly suggests a direct involvement of the loops between S5 and S6, termed "P loop" (previously called the SS1–SS2 region) (Fig. 3a), in the architecture of the channel pore. We therefore systematically replaced the negatively charged Glu (E) residues with Gln (Q), Ala, or Lys in the P loops of the four repeats of the cardiac L-type α_{1C} subunit by site-directed mutagenesis and the mutant channels were examined for divalent cation selectivity [7,8]. In the absence of divalent cations, the mutant channels carry large monovalent cation currents which are blocked by Ca in the order EIIIQ > EIIQ > EIVQ > EIQ. Blockade of Ba or Li currents by Cd also

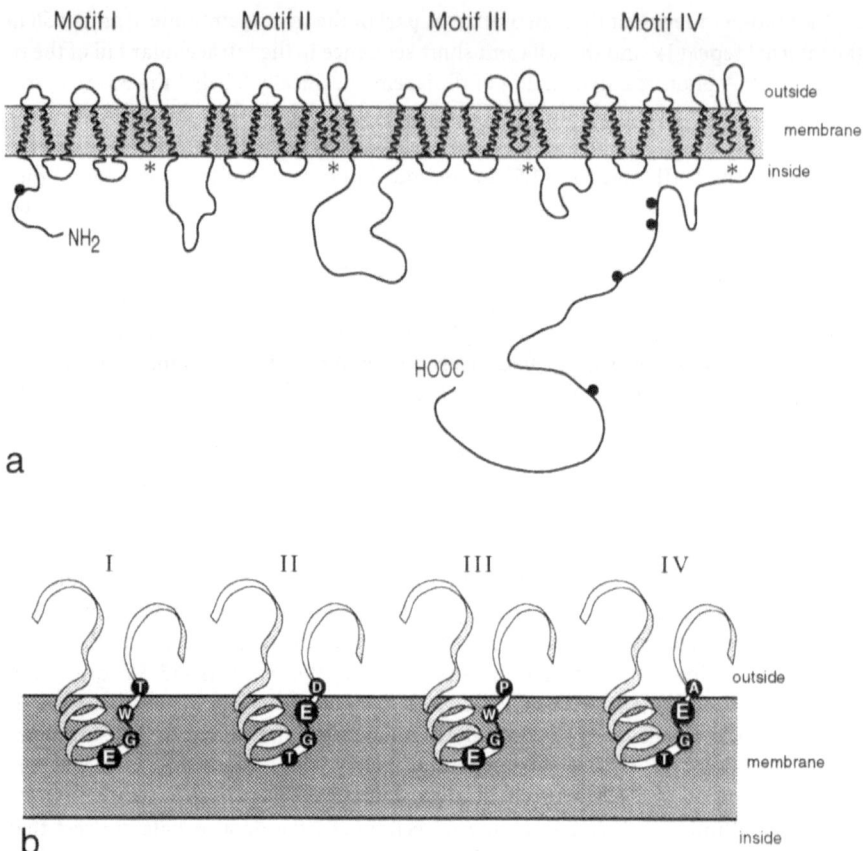

FIG. 3. **a** Proposed secondary structure of the α_1 subunit. The *asterisks* mark the SS1–SS2 segments that form P loops in each motif. The *open circles* indicate PKA phosphorylation sites. **b** Hypothetical bend structure of the Ca channel pore-lining region showing α-helix/bend arrangement of pore-lining regions for each motif. (Based on [1])

shows a non-equivalence of the Glu positions, in the order EIIIQ > EIQ > EIIQ > EIVQ. These results clearly show that Glu residues in the P loop of all four motifs collectively contribute to the high affinity of Ca. The interaction of Ca with Glu residues probably occurs in a cooperative manner, so that the binding of the first Ca with high affinity at the first site will be weakened by the association of the incoming second Ca at the binding site. A three-dimensional geometrical arrangement for the P loop, predicted from the data and theoretical calculations, suggests that the four Glu residues are arranged on two close but non-equivalent planes in a *trans* configuration to accept two Ca ions at the high-affinity site in the pore (Fig. 3b).

Carboxy-Terminal (C-Terminal) Region

Molecular cloning and genomic analysis of the human heart L-type α_{1C} subunit have revealed that structural variability in the C-terminal region is due to three message variants generated by alternative utilization of two C-terminal exons [9]. Quantitation of reverse transcriptase/polymerase chain reaction (RT/PCR) products showed significant variation in the distribution of these isoforms in distinct areas of the heart, aorta, and fibroblasts, which suggests physiological significance for the C-terminal variability. To determine functional differences among three variants, we compared the Ba currents produced by the isoforms in *Xenopus* oocytes. The kinetics and voltage dependence of the induced currents showed no significant differences. Furthermore, when the isoforms were coexpressed with three human β subunits, no α_1-specific functional divergence was observed. These data suggest that gating parameters of the Ca channel current are not determined by naturally occurring modifications in the C-terminal region of the α_1 subunit.

We also constructed a C-terminal deletion mutant where part of the C-terminal tail until amino acid residue 1673 was removed, and we transfected the mutant cDNA in human embryo kidney (HEK) cells to further explore functional significance of the C-terminal region [10]. The Ca channel current induced by the deletion mutant had a threefold higher current density in comparison to the wild type. The observed effect of the mutation mimicked the stimulatory effect of intracellular proteolytic treatment of the wild-type α_{1C} channel expressed alone or together with the α_2 and/or β_3 subunit in a manner similar to Ca current in native cardiac myocytes. Interestingly, the mutant Ca currents no longer responded to dialysis with trypsin. From these results we conclude that digestion of part of the C-terminal tail of the α_{1C} subunit is responsible for proteolytic stimulation of the cardiac Ca current, and that this structure may be part of the inactivation mechanism.

PKA (Protein Kinase A) Phosphorylation Sites

Modulation of L-type VDCC activity by cyclic adenosine monophosphate (cAMP)-dependent phosphorylation reaction is of key importance in sympathetic (adrenergic) stimulation of cardiac function. It is well established that the activation of protein kinase A (PKA) by elevated levels of intracellular cAMP, which activates the catalytic subunit of PKA, leads to an enhanced L-type Ca current in the native setting. The question whether basal function of the VDCC depends on phosphorylation is an area of considerable controversy. Using site-directed mutagenesis of the human heart α_{1C} subunit followed by transient expression in HEK 293 cells, we have studied the role of high-consensus cAMP-dependent phosphorylation (PKA) sites (Fig. 3a) on basal activity of the cardiac L-type VDCC [11]. Individual elimination of putative PKA sites by substituting Ser residues for Ala at the C- and N-terminus of the α_{1C} subunit resulted in Ca channel currents indistinguishable from the wild type. Even simultaneous replacements of two to five (full removal) high-consensus sites did not alter current density and kinetic parameters. From these results, it is possible to conclude that high-consensus cAMP-dependent phosphorylation sites are not required for basal activity of recombinant human L-type Ca channel.

Conclusions

Molecular studies of the Ca channel here revealed substantial diversity. The physiological significance of such diversity remains a topic of much interest and activity. During the last 5 years, a number of investigations in many laboratories have contributed to a contemporary "picture" of the Ca channel. The pore is comprised of amino acids, chiefly critical glutamates that are arranged in an asymmetric configuration. The Ca antagonist drugs clearly regulate the pore by binding to specific regions on the

α_1 subunit close to the pore. While phosphorylation must be important in the regulation of the Ca channel, identification of the site(s) of phosphorylation and the exact polypeptide(s) involved remain an enigma.

Acknowledgments. The original studies reported were supported by National Institues of Health grants (PO1 HL 22619, R37 HL 43231, PO1 HL 41496) and the Tanabe Seiyaku Fund for Molecular Pharmacology and Biophysics. I am extremely grateful to all of my students and associates for their contribution to the research. In particular, I should like to give special thanks to Dr. Yasuo Mori (assistant professor), who provided his expertise in summarizing our studies in this draft, and to Dr. Gabor Mikala (research associate), who assisted Dr. Mori with this manuscript.

References

1. Varadi G, Mori Y, Mikala G, Schwartz A (1995) Molecular determinants of Ca^{2+}-channel function and drug administration. Trends Pharmacol Sci 16:43–49
2. Mori Y (1994) Molecular biology of voltage-dependent calcium channels. In: Peracchia C (ed) Handbook of membrane channels. Academic, New York, pp 163–186
3. Catterall WA, Striessnig J (1992) Receptor sites for Ca^{2+} channel antagonists. Trends Pharmacol Sci 13:256–262
4. Watanabe T, Kalasz H, Yabana H, Kuniyasu A, Mershon J, Itagaki K, Vaghy PL, Naito K, Nakayama H, Schwartz A (1993) Azidobutyryl diltiazem a new photoactivatable diltiazem analog labels benzothiazepine binding site in the α_1 subunit of the skeletal muscle Ca channel. FEBS Lett 334:261–264
5. Kalasz H, Watanabe T, Yabana H, Itagaki K, Naito K, Nakayama H, Schwartz A, Vaghy PL (1993) Identification of 1,4-DHP binding domains within the primary structure of the α_1 subunit of the skeletal muscle L-type Ca channel. FEBS Lett 331:177–181
6. Tang S, Yatani A, Bahinski A, Mori Y, Schwartz A (1993) Molecular localization of regions in the L-type Ca channel critical for dihydropyridine action. Neuron 11:1013–1021
7. Tang S, Mikala G, Bahinski A, Yatani A, Varadi G, Schwartz A (1993) Molecular localization of ion selectivity sites within the pore of a human L-type cardiac Ca channel. J Biol Chem 268:13026–13029
8. Yang J, Ellinor PT, Sather WA, Zhang J-F, Tsien RW (1993) Molecular determinants of Ca-selectivity and ion permeation permeation in L-type Ca channels. Nature 366:158–161
9. Mikala G, Klöckner U, Eisfeld J, Iles DE, Schwartz A, Varadi G (1994) Molecular characteristics and functional expression of three COOH-terminal splice variants of human cardiac L-type Ca channel α_1 subunit (abstract). Circulation 90:I-37
10. Klöckner U, Mikala G, Varadi M, Varadi G, Schwartz A (1995) Involvement of the carboxyl-terminal region of the α_1 subunit in voltage-dependent inactivation of cardiac calcium channels. J Biol Chem 270:17306–17310
11. Mikala G, Klöckner U, Eisfeld J, Varadi M, Varadi G, Schwartz A (1995) cAMP-dependent phosphorylation sites are not required for activity of the recombinant cardiac L-type Ca channel. Biophys J 68:A349

Functional Differences Between Native and Recombinant Forms of Delayed Rectifier Potassium Channel Currents

ROBERT S. KASS, MICHAEL P. DAVIES, and LISA C. FREEMAN

Summary. Two components of delayed rectifier potassium channels are known to contribute repolarizing currents in cardiac tissue. One component is characterized by very slow activation kinetics and insensitivity to class III antiarrhythmic agents such as E4031. This component, referred to as I_{Ks}, has been linked to a gene that encodes a unique and small (130 amino acids) protein that has been shown to induce channel activity in heterologous expression systems remarkably similar to native I_{Ks}. In this chapter, several lines of experimental evidence are reviewed that strongly suggest that, despite the similarity between native and recombinant forms of minK or I_{Ks} channel activity, a sufficient number of differences have emerged that raise the possibility that the minK gene product, while contributing to the functioning I_{Ks} channel, is not sufficient to account for important functional channel properties. Thus these data suggest that the channel underlying I_{Ks} is likely to be heteromultimeric with subunit components that are yet to be identified.

Key words. Minimal K^+ channel protein—Delayed rectifier potassium current—Patch-clamp

Introduction

Potassium channels are membrane-spanning proteins that regulate potassium ion movement across the cell membrane. They are important in maintaining the electrical activity in most excitable cells because they control cellular resting potential and action potential duration. Based on cellular electrophysiology and pharmacology, at least seven cardiac K^+ channels have been identified [1]. The molecular genetic approach has revealed multiple subfamilies of K^+ channels cloned from the heart based on sequence homology with *Shaker* K^+ channels [2–6]. Expression cloning has recently been reported for inward rectifier K channels [7,8] as well as for an ATP-regulated K channel (K_{ATP}) [9]. The clones for these channel types show substantial homology with *Shaker* K^+ channels in the pore (H5 or P) region, but only limited similarities in other regions. Most notably, inward rectifier and K_{ATP} clones are much smaller than *Shaker* K^+ channel clones, and hydropathy plots suggest only two, instead of six, membrane-spanning regions.

Department of Physiology, University of Rochester Medical Center, Rochester, NY 14624, USA

Additionally, a gene encoding a distinct slowly activating, non-inactivating K$^+$ channel with a putatively unique minimal molecular structure has also been cloned from cardiac tissue [10]. The protein encoded by this message contains 129–130 amino acids and only one membrane-spanning domain, has no homology with other cloned voltage-gated K$^+$ channels, and is referred to either as Isk or minK. The functional properties of ionic current expressed in *Xenopus* oocytes injected with, or HEK 293 cells transfected with, minK message strongly resemble properties of the slowly activated delayed rectifier potassium current (I_{Ks}) that has been well characterized in mammalian cardiac preparations [11–13].

Cardiac delayed potassium currents were first shown to contribute to control of cardiac action potential duration by Noble and Tsien [14]. Although it is now known that multiple types of K$^+$ channels contribute to cardiac electrical activity [1], delayed rectifier channels remain of considerable interest as potential targets for class III antiarrhythmics because of the unique relationship between their activation kinetics and the time-course of the heart action potential plateau [15]. Pharmacological data [16,17] have confirmed the existence of at least two types of cardiac delayed rectifier currents in ventricular and atrial cells that can be distinguished by their kinetics and pharmacology: I_{Kr}, a rapidly activating and rectifying component that is blocked by the benzene sulfonamide antiarrhythmic drug E-4031 and by La^{+3}; and I_{Ks}, which is lanthanum- and E-4031 insensitive and does not inactivate [18]. I_{Ks}, but not I_{Kr}, is increased by protein kinase A (PKA), protein kinase C (PKC), and intracellular calcium in distinct temperature- and voltage-dependent manners [19–25].

In the ventricle, muscarinic stimulation does not affect I_{Ks} in the absence of prior PKA activation; it does antagonize its enhancement by isoproterenol or forskolin, but has no effect on cyclic adenosine monophosphate- (cAMP-) stimulated I_{Ks}, suggesting that the antagonism occurs at a step in the signaling pathway proximal to stimulation of PKA by cAMP [26,27]. Delayed potassium currents have been described in mammalian sinoatrial and atrioventricular nodes [28]. Rabbit sinoatrial nodal (SAN) cells are dominated by a delayed rectifier component similar to ventricular I_{Kr} [29], but in the guinea pig SAN, the major delayed rectifier component strongly resembles ventricular I_{Ks} in its voltage- and time-dependent properties [30]. However, regulation of guinea pig SAN I_{Ks} is distinct from that of I_{Ks} in the guinea pig ventricle: stimulation by PKA and PKC is not temperature dependent, and inhibition by muscarinic agonists does not require prior stimulation by β-adrenergic agonists [31]. Thus, expression of I_{Ks} may differ regionally in the heart.

The biophysical properties of I_{Ks} most closely resemble the properties of ionic currents induced by the minK gene. Like ventricular I_{Ks} [32], the currents induced by minK in heterologous expression systems are blocked by the antiarrhythmic drugs clofilium and NE 10064 [13,33,34] and are modulated by PKA, PKC, and calcium in a temperature-dependent manner [35]. Modulatory responses depend on species variants of the minK gene. *Xenopus* oocyte-expressed rat kidney minK currents (I_{minK}) are *decreased* by PKC activators, apparently by phosphorylation of the minK protein [36], but guinea pig minK currents are *enhanced* by PKC stimulation, consistent with modulation of native guinea pig I_{Ks} channels [37,38]. PKA stimulation enhances currents induced by the rat minK clone in *Xenopus* oocytes but likely not via phosphorylation of the minK protein [39,40]. Perhaps most important, single-channel currents have not been reported either for native I_{Ks} or currents in heterologous expression systems [41,42]. Instead, single-channel currents estimated by noise analysis have suggested high-density, very low conductance channels underlie I_{Ks} and recombinant currents. This small conductance distinguishes the channel protein(s) that underlie I_{Ks} from all other candidate K^+ channel clones. Further investigation of the unitary currents underlying I_{Ks} are clearly important in identifying the channel and associated subunits underlying this current.

Determination of the molecular structure(s) underlying I_{Ks} may have direct relevance to at least one form of an inherited cardiac disorder. The long QT syndrome (LQTS) is an inherited disease in which the ventricular repolarization period is unusually long and there is high risk for sudden death. The disease can exist in autosomal recessive and autosomal dominant forms and also can be "acquired," often as the result of therapeutic drug therapy [43]. Changes in sympathetic tone can exacerbate arrhythmias associated with LQTS [44], and thus LQTS is regarded as a unique example of noncoronary, neurally modulated sudden cardiac death. Genetic studies have already shown linkage to at least three different chromosomes [45–47], but the underlying mechanism(s) remain(s) unknown. Identification of a genetic fingerprint for LQTS would make possible presymptomatic diagnosis, and identification of the functional basis of the disorder has the promise of determining more specific pharmacological probes as well as unraveling the basis for the acquired form of the disorder. Because of its putative importance to regulation of the ventricular action potential and its marked sensitivity to sympathetic stimulation, I_{Ks} is one of several ion channel currents that could contribute to congenital and acquired forms of this disease.

Despite the attraction of associating the minK gene with the putative I_{Ks} channel and the indirect functional evidence just described, identification of the protein encoded by the minK gene as an ion channel is controversial. Takumi et al. [48] and Goldstein and Miller [33] provided evidence that the minK gene product is an ion channel by altering ion selectivity, open channel block by Cs^+ and tetraethylammonium (TEA), and channel gating by mutations of the minK gene. Hice et al. [49] have reported sequence-specific changes in biophysical properties of *Xenopus*-expressed I_{sK} that supported the view that the I_{sK} gene encodes an ion channel. However, Attali et al. [50] found that the type of channel activity expressed by *Xenopus* oocytes injected with minK cRNA was dependent on the [cRNA] injected: low concentrations induced K^+-selective currents and high concentrations Cl^--selective currents with properties very similar to currents encoded by the phospholemman gene [51,52]. Furthermore, truncation or deletion of specific regions of the minK gene caused selective expression of Cl^-- or K^+-selective channels.

Consequently, Attali et al. [50] have postulated that the minK gene does not encode a K^+-selective ion channel, but rather a regulator of endogenous ion channel proteins (either K^+- or Cl^--selective) that must exist in the membranes of *Xenopus* occytes (and, by implication, all other cells that express this current). Blumenthal and Kaczmarek [53] also found that the minK protein can exist in both functional and nonfunctional forms in *Xenopus* oocyte membranes [53], suggesting that the minK protein forms functional channels by association with an endogenous membrane subunit or cofactor [53], which would very well vary with expression cell type and be the protein suggested by the work of Attali et al. [50]. Expression of minK currents in mammalian HEK 293 cells in our laboratory has demonstrated that minK expression is not limited to *Xenopus* oocytes, but does not rule out the existence of similar endogenous channels in the HEK 293 cell membrane.

This chapter reviews recent functional evidence suggesting that the minK gene product is, in fact, insufficient to explain the functional properties of native I_{ks} channel activity.

Methods

Cells and Recording Conditions

The methodology used in the experiments described here have all been described in detail elsewhere and thus are only briefly summarized here. Isolation of SAN and ventricular cells from adult guinea pig hearts was carried out using procedures previously described [30,32]. HEK 293 cells were obtained either from American Type Cell Culture (Bethesda, MD, USA) or from Dr. Bruce Spillman (Cold Spring Harbor Laboratories, Cold Spring Harbor, NY, USA). HEK 293 cells were grown in modified essential medium (MEM) (Gibco, Grand Island, NY, USA) supplemented with 10% fetal bovine serum, penicillin, and glucamine, and transfected at an exponential stage of growth. Cells were then washed with phosphate-buffered saline (PBS) and returned to normal 10% fetal calf serum- (FCS-) enhanced MEM for an additional 24–48 h, after which they could be studied for expression of channel activity. Most experiments were carried out using patch-clamp procedures in whole-cell or perforated patch configurations [54,55]. Previously described intra- and extracellular recording solutions designed to isolate K^+ currents were used [32,56].

Noise Analysis

Current fluctuations from I_{Ks} were analyzed using techniques developed by Sigworth [57] for nonstationary signals. Macroscopic current (I) from identical, independent channels with one conducting state is determined by the current through a single channel (i) and the number of functional open channels (N_o):

$$I = i * N_o \tag{1}$$

N_o is a function of time in the nonstationary state case and includes contributions from gating behavior of the channel. It is equal to the total number of channels in the membrane, N, times the probability, $P(t)$, that a channel is open. The macroscopic current will fluctuate according to the number of channels open at any given time. The variance (<VAR>) of the macroscopic current is related to the parameters in Eq. 1 as follows:

$$\langle VAR \rangle = I * i - I^2 / N_o \tag{2}$$

According to Eq. 2, the variance of the macroscopic current is a parabolic function of the mean current with an initial slope equal to the single-channel current (i). If the number of channels is large or the probability of channel opening is small, then the relationship approaches a linear relationship between variance and single-channel current.

Results

Expression of minK-Encoded Activity in Mammalian Cells

Freeman and Kass [58] transiently transfected HEK 293 cells with a synthetic (rat) minK gene using a modified lipofection procedure and found that transfected, but not control or sham-transfected, cells expressed slowly activating, noninactivating currents that strongly resembled native guinea pig I_{ks} (Fig. 1). The currents share similar

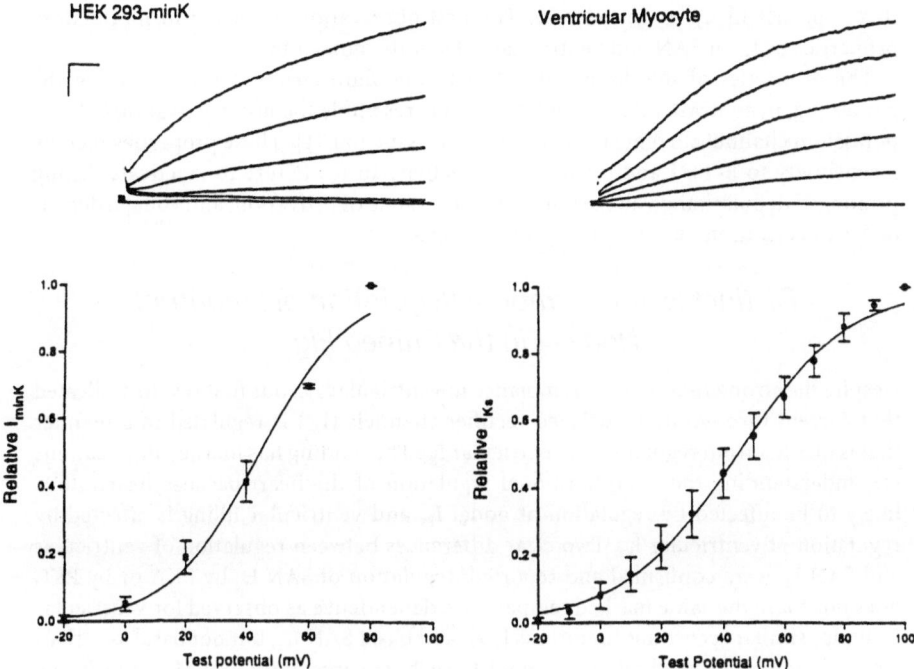

FIG. 1. Comparison of minK-expressed currents with native delayed rectifier potassium channels (I_{Ks}) measured in guinea pig ventricular myocytes. *Upper panel*: families of current traces in response to depolarizing voltage pulses. *Bottom panels*: isochronal activation curves from series of 2-s depolarizations

voltage-dependent activation, kinetics, and sensitivity to barium, LY97241, and the novel class III antiarrhythmic compound NE10064. These data thus provided evidence that expression of minK-mediated current in heterologous systems is not limited to *Xenopus* oocytes, but our results do not definitively prove that the protein encoded by the minK gene is in fact an ion channel. In addition to testing for expression of minK-mediated ionic currents in HEK 293 cells, a polyclonal antibody that had been raised against the predicted amino acid sequence of the rat minK protein was used to test for expression efficiency in our HEK 293 cells and also to determine whether the minK protein was present in guinea pig SAN and ventricular cells. Freeman and Kass [58] found that transfected, but not control or sham-transfected, cells stained positively for the minK antibody.

The transfection efficiency estimated by immunostaining was in good agreement with our estimates based on electrophysiology. Additionally, both guinea pig SAN and ventricular cells were stained positively by the minK antibody, providing strong evidence that the minK protein is present in these cells. Because the cells were not treated with detergent, it is likely that the minK protein is present in the sarcolemmal membrane. These results strongly suggest that the minK protein is present in cells that express I_{Ks}. However, these experiments cannot rule out the possibility that the minK gene product must associate with other membrane proteins (subunits) to confer complete functional properties to the expressed ionic currents. Since this work, several observations on both native and recombinant ionic channel activity suggest that this is in fact likely to be the case. The first observation is related to modulatory properties of I_{Ks} in SAN and ventricular cells of the guinea pig.

The properties of the dominant delayed potassium current in SAN cells of the guinea pig, in contrast with the rabbit, strongly resemble the noninactivating delayed potassium channel current (I_{Ks}) is ventricular tissue [30,31]. These properties include insensitivity to E-4031 and lanthanum, selectivity to K$^+$, failure to inactivate during prolonged depolarizing voltage pulses, voltage range of activation, and voltage dependence of activation and deactivation time constants.

Distinct Neurohormonal Regulation of Sinoatrial Node I_{Ks} in the Guinea Pig

Despite the strong functional resemblance to ventricular I_{Ks}, our first results indicated that current through nodal delayed rectifier channels (I_{Ks}) is regulated in a manner that is distinct from regulation of ventricular I_{Ks}. This finding has marked implications for understanding the neurohormonal regulation of the heart because heartrate is likely to be affected by regulation of nodal I_{Ks} and ventricular filling is affected by regulation of ventricular I_{Ks}. Two clear differences between regulation of ventricular and SAN I_{Ks} were confirmed and reported: regulation of SAN I_{Ks} by PKA or by PKC does not share the same marked temperature dependence as observed for ventricular I_{Ks} under similar recording conditions [19]; and basal SAN I_{Ks}, but not basal ventricular I_{Ks}, is inhibited by cholinergic agonists such as carbachol (100 nM), even in the absence of prior stimulation of the β-adrenergic pathway.

Further investigation of the modulation of SAN I_{Ks} by muscarinic agonists has revealed that this modulation is not via muscarinic receptors [59]. Using conventional whole-cell or perforated patch arrangements of the patch clamp, it was shown that cholinergic agonists, including the endogenous neurotransmitter acetylcholine, decrease the amplitude of I_{Ks} in guinea pig SAN cells via a nonmuscarinic, nonnicotinic, cAMP-independent mechanism (Fig. 2). Although we have not identified the precise nature of this signal transduction pathway, it is clearly different than those described for regulation of other nodal currents. Furthermore, these data indicated that differential regulation of I_{Ks} in guinea pig SAN and ventricle cannot be attributed to higher basal adenylate cyclase activity in SAN cells compared with cells of the ventricle. The inhibitory effect of carbachol on I_{Ks} was not additive with that of verapamil, a drug that is both an allosteric muscarinic antagonist and a potassium channel blocking agent. Freeman and Kass [59] suggested that cholinergic agonists may inhibit I_{Ks} in SAN cells via a direct interaction with the SAN I_{Ks} channel. This interaction may occur via expression of distinct channels or channel-associated subunits in the SAN compared with the ventricle of the guinea pig. Molecular cloning of the SAN I_{Ks} channel is needed to distinguish between these possibilities.

Nonstationary Noise Analysis: Estimation of Unitary Conductances

A second set of data based on estimation of single-channel properties of native and recombinant I_{Ks} channel activity have also begun to suggest that functional properties of channels expressed in heterologous systems such as the HEK 293 cells may differ from native channels. In previous work from this laboratory, it was demonstrated that it is possible to record I_{Ks} channel activity in cell-attached and excised patches of

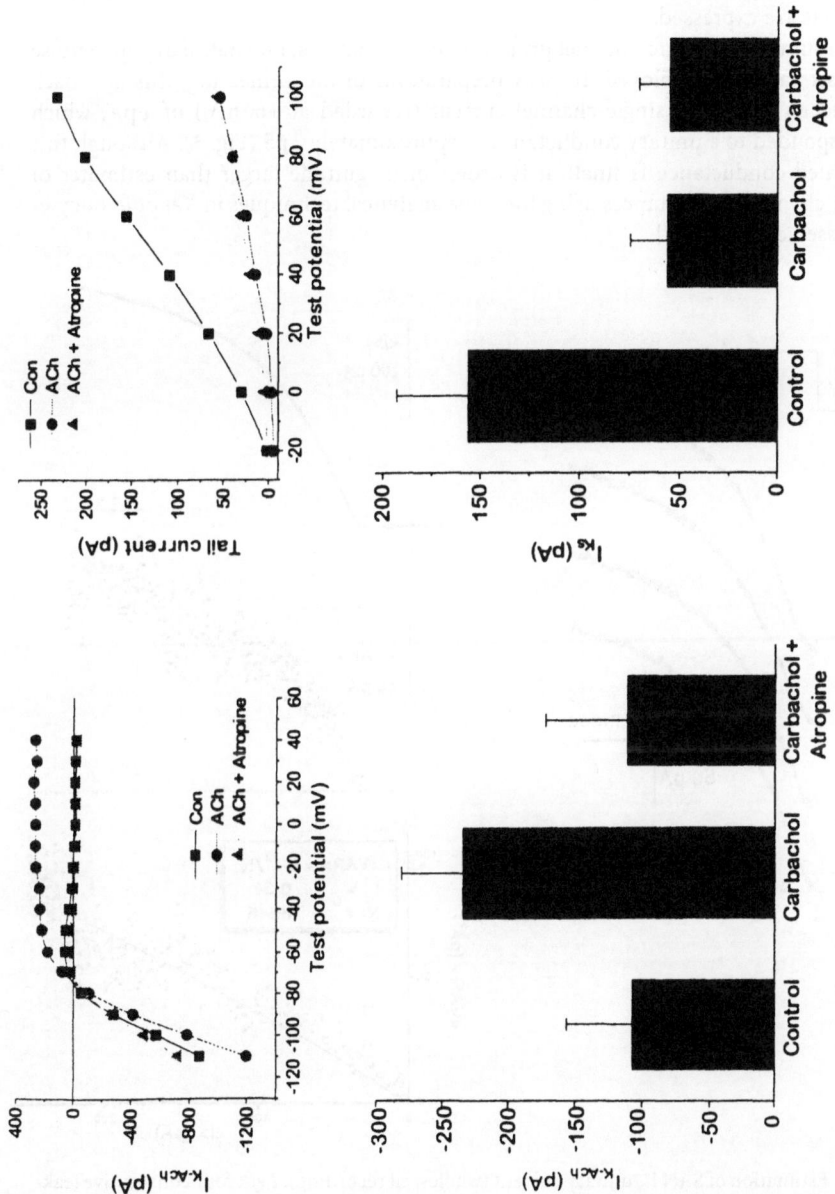

FIG. 2. Inhibiton of sinoatrial node (SAN) I_{Ks} is not antagonized by atropine (*right*) in cells in which stimulation of muscarinic K$^+$ current is antagonized (*left*)

guinea pig ventricular cell membranes [56], not as unitary channel events, but instead as macroscopic currents that strongly resemble whole-cell currents recorded under similar conditions. These results have now been confirmed in *Xenopus* oocytes injected with minK mRNA [42], indicating that this appears to be a general property of the channels that underlie I_{Ks} regardless of the cellular environment in which the channels are expressed.

To estimate the single-channel properties of I_{Ks} channels, nonstationary state noise analysis has been employed. In SAN preparations of the guinea pig, this approach yielded an estimated single-channel current (recorded at +60 mV) of 1 pA, which corresponded to a unitary conductance of approximately 2 pS (Fig. 3). Although this estimated conductance is small, it is orders of magnitude larger than estimates of single-channel conductances using the same analytical techniques in *Xenopus* oocyte-expressed currents [42].

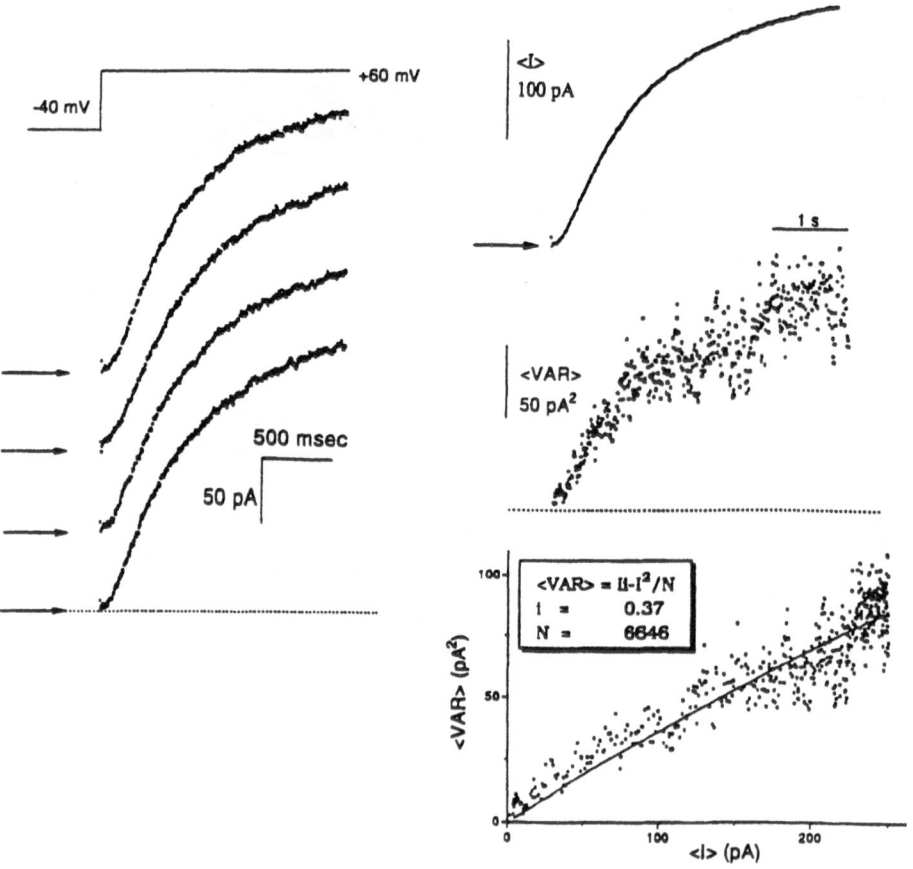

FIG. 3. Estimation of SAN I_{Ks} unitary current (whole-cell recording). *Left*: four consecutive leak-subtracted current traces recorded in response to successive depolarizations to + 60 mV aligned at the start of the depolarizations. *Arrows* indicate zero current level. *Right top*: ensemble average of 16 consecutive current records. *Right middle*: variance at each sample point computed for the same group of 16 records and plotted using the same time scale. *Right bottom*: scatter plot of variance (<VAR>) *vs* mean current (<I>). Continuous curve is best fit of <VAR> = iI – I²/N. Estimated unitary current, i = 0.37 pA; estimated total number of channels, N > 1000

Preliminary estimates have now been obtained for guinea pig SAN and ventricular I_{K_s} in whole-cell and membrane patch configurations as well as from whole-cell recordings in HEK 293-transfected cells. We have found that cells expressing smaller whole-cell currents are best suited for noise analysis because clear voltage-dependent increases in current noise can be resolved in these cases. Generally, ventricular cells of the guinea pig heart are not well suited for noise analysis because resolution of this noise is not clear. Examples of this problem are well documented in the literature [60]. In each case, nonstationary state noise analysis predicts very small (<1 pA) unitary currents and large channel numbers ($N > 1000$) for all cell types at voltages near +60 mV, and physiological K^+ gradients. However, as summarized in Fig. 4, our data to date suggest that there may be small but significant differences in single-channel properties of the channels underlying I_{K_s}-like currents that depend both on the cell type and on the configuration of the recording conditions. The data of Fig. 4 suggest (1) that guinea pig SAN and ventricular I_{K_s} unitary conductances are the same, but that (2) I_{mink} unitary conductance estimated in HEK cells is significantly larger than the estimates of guinea pig I_{K_s} unitary conductance. If, under the same recording conditions, unitary conductances estimated for I_{K_s} and I_{mink} channels were significantly different, this would strongly suggest that the assembled functional channels underlying these currents are not the same and thus provide indirect support for the view that the minK gene does not encode the entire functioning I_{K_s} channel.

Distinct Interactions of H+ with Native and Recombinant I_{K_s}

We have begun to measure the influence of hydrogen ions on I_{K_s} in guinea pig SAN and ventricle as well as transfected HEK 293 cells to determine whether native and recombinant channels share a similar pH sensitivity [61]. Figure 5 shows the result of a preliminary experiment on guinea pig ventricular I_{K_s} indicating that this current is

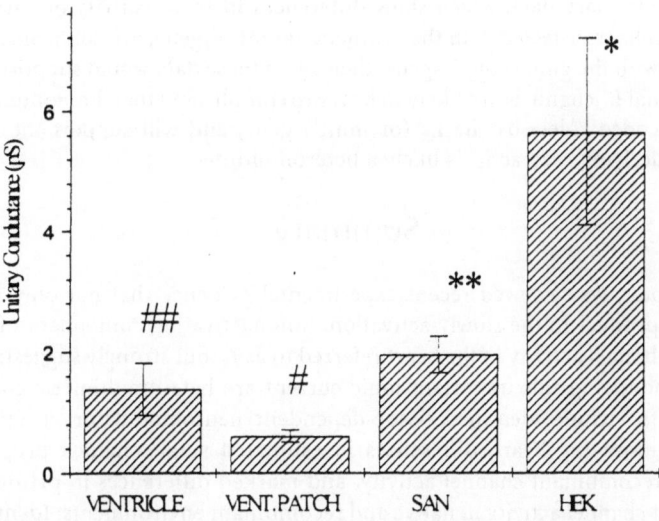

FIG. 4. Estimates of minK-induced unitary conductance are significantly greater than estimates of native channel unitary conductances in preliminary experiments (*, **; *, #, *, ##). *Vent.*, ventricular; *HEK*, HEK293 cells

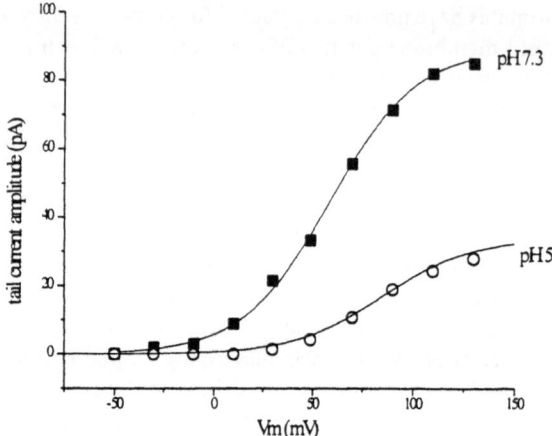

Fɪɢ. 5. External H⁺ shifts gating of, and blocks, guinea pig ventricular I_{Ks}. Two-second isoch-ronal activation curves measured at pH 7.4 (*squares*) and pH 5.0 (*circles*) solutions. Botzmann curve fitted through control data was shifted by + 36 mV and scaled down by a factor of 0.63 to fit the data obtained at pH 5.0

very sensitivity to external H⁺, and that both shifts in channel gating and voltage-dependent block of the channel are likely to underlie this interaction. These results are in contrast with results of Yamane et al. [62], who showed that expression of rat minK channel activity in *Xenopus* oocytes is inhibited by external H⁺, but not in a voltage-dependent manner and without accompanying gating shifts. Thus, if our preliminary results are confirmed they will be important not only for implications about regula-tion of the native channel by H⁺, but also for possible differences between native channel activity and activity measured in heterologous expression systems.

If our preliminary data, which show differences in H⁺ sensitivity of currents ex-pressed by cells transfected with the synthetic rat minK gene, are confirmed for cells transfected with the guinea pig I_{sK} gene, then again these data would support the view that functional I_{Ks} channels are likely to be more complicated than homomultimers of proteins encoded solely by the I_{sK} (or minK) gene, and will support the view the channel underlying cardiac I_{Ks} is likely a heteromultimer.

Summary

In this chapter, we reviewed recent experimental evidence that not only links the minK gene product to the slowly activation, noninactivating component of delayed potassium channel activity in the heart referred to as I_{Ks} but strongly suggests that the channels underlying this important ionic current are heteromultimeric complexes. These results include identified tissue-dependent neuromodulatory properties of I_{Ks} in the guinea pig heart, differences in estimated single-channel properties of native and recombinant channel activity, and marked differences in pH-dependent inhibition of channel activity in native and recombinant environments. Identification of minK-associated subunits would confirm the predictions of these functional experiments.

References

1. Kass RS, Freeman LC (1993) Potassium channels in the heart: cellular, molecular, and clinical implications. Trends Cardiovasc Med 3:149–159
2. Fedida D, Wible B, Wang Z, Fermini B, Faust F, Nattel S, Brown AM (1993) Identity of a novel delayed rectifier current from human heart with a cloned K channel current. Circ Res 73:210–216
3. Po S, Snyders DJ, Baker R, Tamkun MM, Bennett PB (1992) Functional expression of an inactivating potassium channel cloned from human heart. Circ Res 71:732–736
4. Po S, Roberds S, Snyders DJ, Tamkun MM, Bennett PB (1993) Heteromultimeric assembly of human potassium channels: molecular basis of a transient outward current? Circ Res 72:1326–1336
5. Snyders DJ, Fish FA, Roberds SL, Knoth KM, Tamkun MM, Bennett PB (1991) Stable exogenous expression of K^+ channels cloned from the mammalian cardiovascular system in mouse Ltk cells. Circulation 84:II-444
6. Roberds SL, Tamkun MM (1991) Cloning and tissue-specific expression of five voltage-gated potassium channel cDNAs expressed in rat heart, Proc Natl Acad Sci USA 88:1798–1802
7. Ho K, Nichols CG, Lederer J, Lytton J, Vassilev PM, Kanazirska MV, Heber SC (1993) Cloning and expression of an inwardly rectifying ATP-regulated potassium channel. Nature 362:31–38
8. Kubo Y, Baldwin TJ, Jan YN, Jan LY (1993) Primary structure and functional expression of a mouse inward recitfier potassium channel. Nature 362:127–132
9. Ashford ML, Bond CT, Blair TA, Adelman JP (1994) Cloning and functional expression of a rat heart KATP channel. Nature 370:456–459
10. Folander K, Smith JS, Antanavage J, Bennett C, Stein RB, Swanson R (1990) Cloning and expression of the delayed-rectifier IsK channel from neonatal rat heart and diethylstilbestrol-primed rat uterus. Proc Natl Acad Sci USA 87:2975–2979
11. Takumi T, Ohkubo H, Nakanishi S (1988) Cloning of a membrane protein that induces a slow voltage-gated potassium current. Science 242:1042–1045
12. Pragnell M, Snay KJ, Trimmer JS, MacLusky NJ, Naftolin F, Kaczmarek LK, Boyle M (1990) Estrogen induction of a small, putative K channel mRNA in rat uterus. Neuron 4:807–812
13. Honore E, Attali B, Romey G, Heurteaux C, Ricard P, Lesage F, Lazdunski M, Barhanin J (1991) Cloning, expression, pharmacology, and regulation of a delayed rectifier K channel in mouse heart. EMBO J 10:2805–2811
14. Noble D, Tsien RW (1969) Outward membrane currents activated in the plateau range of potentials in cardiac Purkinje fibres. J Physiol (Lond) 200:205–231
15. Colatsky TJ (1992) Potassium channel blockers: synthetic agents and their antiarrhythmic potential. In: Weston AH, Hamilton EC (eds) Potassium channel modulators. Blackwell, London, pp 304–340
16. Balser JR, Bennett PB, Roden DM (1990) Time-dependent outward current in guinea pig ventricular myocytes. Gating kinetics of the delayed rectifier. J Gen Physiol 96:835–863
17. Sanguinetti MC, Jurkiewicz NK (1991) Delayed rectifier outward K current is composed of two currents in guinea pig atrial cells. Am J Physiol 260:H393–H399
18. Sanguinetti MC, Jurkiewicz NK (1990) Two components of cardiac delayed rectifier K^+ current. Differential sensitivity to block by class III antiarrhythmic agents. J Gen Physiol 96:195–215
19. Walsh KB, Begenisich TB, Kass RS (1989) β-Adrenergic modulation of cardiac ion channels: differential temperature-sensitivity of potassium and calcium currents. J Gen Physiol 93:841–854
20. Walsh KB, Kass RS (1988) Regulation of a heart potassium channel by protein kinase A and C. Science 242:67–69

21. Walsh KB, Kass RS (1991) Distinct voltage-dependent regulation of a heart delayed IK by protein kinases A and C. Am J Physiol 261:C1081–C1090
22. Sanguinetti MC, Jurkiewicz NK, Scott A, Siegle PK (1993) Isoproterenol antagonizes prolongation of refractory period by the class III antiarrhythmic agent E-4031 in guina pig myocytes. Circ Res 68(1):77–84
23. Toshe N, Kameyama M, Sekiguchi K, Shearman ME, Kanno M (1990) Protein kinase C activation enhances the delayed rectifier potassium current in guinea pig heart cells. J Mol Cell Cardiol 22:725–734
24. Hartzell HC, Duchatelle-Gourdon I (1993) Regulation of the cardiac delayed rectifier K current by neurotransmitters and magnesium [review]. Cardiovasc Drugs Ther 7(suppl 3):547–554
25. Levesque PC, Clark CD, Zakarov SI, Rosenshtraukh LV, Hume JR (1993) Anion and cation modulation of the guinea-pig ventricular action potential during beta-adrenoceptor stimulation. Pfluegers Arch Eur J Physiol 424:54–62
26. Harvey RD, Hume JR (1989) Autonomic regulation of delayed rectifier K⁺ current in mammalian heart involves G proteins. Am J Physiol 257(26):H818–H823
27. Yazawa K, Kameyama M (1990) Mechanism of receptor-mediated modulation of the delayed outward potassium current in guinea-pig ventricular myocytes. J Physiol (Camb) 421:135–150
28. Irisawa H, Hagiwara N (1991) Ionic current in sinoatrial node cells. J Cardiovasc Electrophysiol 2:531–540
29. Shibasaki T (1987) Conductance and kinetics of delayed rectifier potassium channels in nodal cells of the rabbit heart. J Physiol (Lond) 387:227–250
30. Anumonwo JMB, Freeman LC, Kwok WM, Kass RS (1992) Delayed rectification in single cells isolated from guinea pig sino-atrial node. Am J Physiol 262:H921–H925
31. Freeman LC, Kass RS (1993) Delayed rectifier potassium channels in ventricle and sinoatrial node of the guinea pig: molecular and regulatory properties. Cardiovasc Drugs Ther 7:627–635
32. Arena JP, Kass RS (1988) Block of heart potassium channels by clofilium and its tertiary analogs: relationship between drug structure and type of channel blocked. Mol Pharmacol 34:60–66
33. Goldstein SAN, Miller C (1991) Site-specific mutations in a minimal voltage-dependent K⁺ channel alter ion selectivity and open-channel block. Neuron 7:403–408
34. Hausdorff SF, Goldstein SAN, Rushin EE, Miller C (1991) Functional characterization of a minimal K channel expressed from a synthetic gene. Biochemistry 30:3341–3346
35. Busch AE, Lang F (1993) Effects of calcium and temperature on minK channels expressed in Xenopus oocytes. FEBS Lett 334(2):221–224
36. Busch AE, Varnum MD, North RA, Adelman JP (1992) An amino acid mutation on a potassium channel that prevents inhibition by protein kinase C. Science 255:1705–1707
37. Varnum MD, Busch AE, Bond CT, Maylie J, Adelman JP (1993) The min K channel underlies the cardiac potassium current IKs and mediates species-specific responses to protein kinase C. Proc Natl Acad Sci USA 90:11528–11532
38. Zhang ZJ, Jurkiewicz NK, Folander K, Lazarides E, Salata JJ, Swanson R (1994) K⁺ currents expressed from the guinea pig cardiac IsK protein are enhanced by activators of protein kinase C. Proc Natl Acad Sci USA 91:1766–1770
39. Blumenthal EM, Kaczmarek LK (1992) Modulation by cAMP of a slowly activating potassium channel expressed by Xenopus oocytes. J Neurosci 12:290–296
40. Busch AE, Kavanaugh MP, Varnum MD, Adelman JP, North RA (1992) Regulation by second messengers of the slowly activating, voltage-dependent potassium current expressed in Xenopus oocytes. J Physiol (Lond) 450:491–502
41. Freeman LC, Kass RS (1994) Non-stationary fluctuation analysis of delayed K current in guinea pig sinoatrial node and transfected HEK 293 cells. Biophys J 66(2):A143
42. Yang Y, Sigworth FJ (1995) The conductance of Mink "channels" is very small. Biophys J 68:A22

43. Moss AJ, Robinson J (1992) Clinical features of the idiopathic long QT syntrome. Circulation 85(suppl I):I140–I144
44. Schwartz PJ, Locati EH, Napolitano C, Priori SG (1994) The long QT syndrome. In: Zipes DF, Jalife J (eds) Cardiac electrophysiology from cell to bedside. Saunders, Philadelphia, pp 788–811
45. Moss AJ, Robinson JL (1993) The long-QT syndrome: genetic considerations. Trends Cardiovasc Med 2:81–83
46. Benhorin J, Kalman YM, Medina A, Towbin J, Rave-Harel N, Dyer TD, Blangero J, MacCluer JW, Krem B (1993) Evidence of genetic heterogeneity in the long QT syndrome. Science 260:1960–1961
47. Jiang C, Atkinson D, Towbin JA, Splawski I, Lehmann MH, Li H, Timothy K, Taggart RT, Schwartz PJ, Vincent GM, Moss AM, Keating MT (1994) Two long AT syndrome loci map to chromosomes 3 and 7 with evidence for further heterogeneity. Nature Genet 8:141–147
48. Takumi T, Moriyoshi K, Aramori I, Ishii T, Oiki S, Okada Y, OhkuboH, Nakanishi S (1991) Alteration of channel activities and gating by mutations of slow ISK potassium channel. J Biol Chem 266:22192–22198
49. Hice RE, Folander K, Salata JJ, Smith JS, Sanguinetti MC, Swanson R (1994) Species variants of the IsK protein: differences in kinetics, voltage dependence, and La3+ block of the currents expressed in *Xenopus* oocytes. Pfleugers Arch Eur J Physiol 426:139–145
50. Attali B, Gullemare E, Lessage F, Honore E, Romey G, Lazdunski M, Barhanin J (1993) The protein IsK is a dual activator of K+ and Cl− channels. Nature 365:850–852
51. Kowdley GC, Ackerman SJ, John JE, Jones LR, Moorman JR (1994) Hyperpolarization-activated chloride currents in *Xenopus* oocytes. J Gen Physiol 103:217–230
52. Moorman JR, Palmer CJ, John JE, Durieux ME, Jones LR (1992) Phospholemman expression induces a hyperpolarization-activated chloride current in *Xenopus* oocytes. J Biol Chem 267:14551–14554
53. Blumenthal EM, Kaczmarek LK (1994) The minK potassium channel exists in functional and nonfunctional forms when expressed in the plasma membrane of *Xenopus* oocytes. J Neurosci 14:3097–3105
54. Hammill OP, Marty A, Neher E, Sakmann B, Sigworth FJ (1981) Improved patch-clamp techniques for high-resolution current recording from cells and cell-free membrane patches. Pfleugers Arch 391:85–100
55. Horn R, Marty A (1988) Muscarinic activation of ionic currents measured by a new whole-cell recording method. J Gen Physiol 92:145–159
56. Walsh KB, Arena JP, Kwok WM, Freeman L, Kass RS (1991) Delayed-rectifier potassium channel activity in isolated membrane patches of guinea pig ventricular myocytes. Am J Physiol 260:H1390–H1393
57. Sigworth F (1980) The variance of sodium current fluctuations at the node of Ranvier. J Physiol (Lond) 307:97–129
58. Freeman LC, Kass RS (1993) Expression of a minimal K channel protein in mammalian cells and immunolocalization in guinea pig heart. Circ Res 73:968–973
59. Freeman LC, and Kass RS (1995) Cholinergic inhibition of slow delayed rectifier K+ current (I_{Ks}) in guinea pig sino-atrial node is not mediated by muscarinc receptors. Mol Pharmacol 47:1248–1254
60. Toshe N (1990) Calcium-sensitive delayed rectifier potassium current in guinea pig ventricular cells. Am J Physiol 258:1200–H1207
61. Davies M, Kass RS (1995) Hydrogen ions shift gating of and block current through I_{Ks} channels in guinea pig ventricular cells but not I_{mink} in human embryonic kidney cells. Biophys J 68:A22
62. Yamane T, Furukawa T, Horikawa S, Hiraoka M (1993) External pH regulates the slowly activating potassium curent Isk expressed in *Xenopus* oocytes. FEBS lett 319:229–232

Modulation of Cardiac L-Type Calcium and Delayed Rectifier Potassium Current by β_1-Adrenoceptor and Adenylate Cyclase in Ventricular Myocytes of Guinea Pig Heart

Toshihiko Iijima, Jun-ichi Imagawa, and Katsuhiko Harada

Summary. This study was designed to investigate the differential modulation of the L-type calcium current (I_{Ca}) and the delayed rectifier potassium current (I_K) by β-adrenoceptor stimulation and by direct activation of adenylate cyclase in single ventricular cells of the guinea pig heart. Single ventricular cells were prepared by the collagenase dispersion procedure, and membrane currents were recorded with a patch electrode by use of the whole-cell voltage-clamp method. I_{Ca} was obtained by intra- and extra-cellular perfusion with the Cs^+ solutions that suppressed potassium currents. I_K was evaluated in Co^{2+}-Tyrode solution in which $0.9\,mM$ Co^{2+} was substituted for equimolar Ca^{2+} to abolish I_{Ca}. Isoproterenol, a nonselective β-adrenoceptor agonist, increased not only I_{Ca} but also I_K at the same threshold concentration ($1\,nM$). In contrast, the threshold concentration of T-1583, a selective β_1-adrenoceptor agonist, for increasing I_{Ca} ($1\,nM$) was distinctly lower than that for increasing I_K ($100\,nM$). The threshold concentration of NKH-477, a water-soluble forskolin analog for increasing I_K ($\sim 1\,nM$) was clearly less than that for increasing I_{Ca} ($10\,nM$). These results suggest that increases in I_{Ca} and I_K elicited by β_1-adrenoceptor and adenylate cyclase stimulation appear to be generated by different biophysical mechanisms.

Key words. L-Type calcium current—Delayed rectifier potassium current—T-1583—NKH-477—Guinea pig ventricular myocytes

Introduction

The molecular mechanism that mediates signals from drug receptors to L-type Ca^{2+} (I_{Ca}) and delayed rectifier K^+ (I_K) channels in the heart have recently been well analyzed in relation to β-adrenoceptors. These two kinds of ion channels are regulated by the cyclic adenosine monophosphate- (cAMP-) dependent protein kinase mediated through β-adrenoceptors. β-Adrenoceptor stimulation increases not only the slow inward current (I_{si}) [1] but also I_K [2,3] in several mammalian cardiac preparations. Although such mechanisms for the regulation of Ca^{2+} and K^+ channels have been supported by a number of studies [4,5], it still remains unclear whether both channel currents are equally and simultaneously increased by β-adrenoceptor stimulation through the same intracellular signal transduction pathway. Direct regulation of these

---

Department of Pharmacology, Akita University School of Medicine, 1-1-1 Hondoh, Akita 010, Japan

channels by stimulatory guanine nucleotide (Gs) proteins through membrane-delim-
ited pathways has been reported [6,7], but the physiological role has been questioned
[8] (Fig. 1).

A selective β_1-adrenoceptor agonist, T-1583 [9], has been reported to produce a
positive inotropic response with a smaller increase in cAMP content than that caused
by isoproterenol in isolated canine ventricular muscles [10]. The difference might be
produced by stimulation of β_2-adrenoceptors with isoproterenol, because canine ventricular muscles contain 85% β_1- and 15% β_2-adreoceptors [11]. However, the results
may also suggest that the nonselective and the selective β_1-adrenoceptor agonist
might differentially modulate the β-adrenoceptor–cAMP cascade and the ion channels [10]. On the other hand, forskolin directly activates adenylate cyclase and increases intracellular cAMP, but not through β-adrenoceptors [12,13]. NKH-477, a
water-soluble forskolin analog that has recently been synthesized, is a more potent
activator of adenylate cyclase than forskolin [14,15]. Precise concentration–response
relationships can be obtained with NKH-477 without concern for any nonpolar
solvent effects.

We have examined differences in the effects of a nonselective β-adrenoceptor
agonist, isoproterenol, a selective β_1-adrenoceptor agonist, T-1583, and a water-
soluble forskolin analog, NKH-477, on I_{Ca} and I_K in single ventricular cells from
the guinea pig heart using the whole-cell, voltage-clamp technique [16,17]. In this
chapter, we review these studies and discuss differential modulation of I_{Ca} and I_K by
β-adrenoceptor and adenylate cyclase.

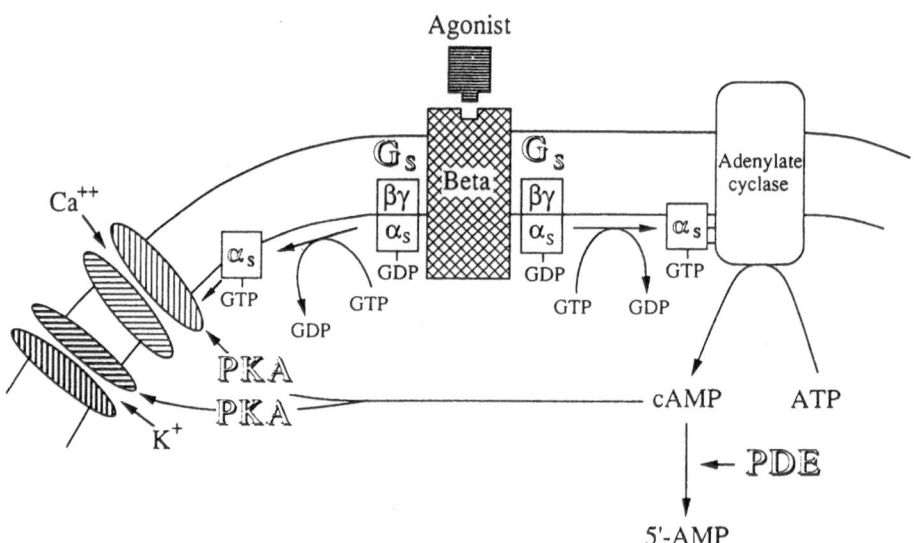

FIG. 1. Schematic representation of the signal transduction pathway from beta-(β-)
adrenoceptors to L-type Ca^{2+} and delayed rectifier K^+ channel. *5'-AMP*, 5'-adenosine monophosphate; *ATP*, adenosine triphosphate; *cAMP*, cyclic adenosine monophosphate; *GDP*, guanosine
diphosphate; *Gs*, stimulatory guanine nucleotide binding protein; *GTP*, guanosine triphosphate;
PDE, phosphodiesterase; *PKA*, cAMP-dependent protein kinase; α_S, and β and γ, subunits of
guanine nucleotide binding protein

Methods

Isolation of Ventricular Cells and Whole-Cell Recording

Single ventricular cells of the guinea pig heart were obtained by an enzymatic dissociation method, and the preparation of single cells was essentially the same as in previous reports [18,19]. The single-pipette, whole-cell recording technique was used to record membrane currents [20]. The electrode resistance ranged between 2 and 4 MΩ when filled with the pipette solutions. After formation of a gigaohm seal, the patch of membrane was disrupted by suction of −50 to −100 cm H_2O. It has been reported and discussed previously that I_{Ca} and I_K exhibit "rundown" associated with dialysis. To minimize the influence of the rundown, only one or two concentrations of drugs were tested in one preparation, and maximum responses were not elicited by high concentrations of drugs. The holding current, I_{Ca}, the current at the end of the test pulse, and the outward tail current were evaluated. The amplitude of I_{Ca} was measured as the difference between the peak of the inward current and the current at the end of the test pulse. Amplitude of the outward tail current, which has been thought to reflect I_K [21], was measured as the difference between the peak of the outward tail and the holding current.

Solutions and Drugs

Normal Tyrode solution for single-cell experiments contained (in mM): 136.9 NaCl, 5.4 KCl, 1.8 $CaCl_2$, 0.53 $MgCl_2$, 0.33 NaH_2PO_4, and 5.0 hydroxyethylpiperazine ethanesulfonic acid (HEPES), 5.5 glucose; the pH was adjusted to 7.4 with NaOH. Co^{2+}-Tyrode solution, in which Co^{2+} was applied by substituting 0.9 mM Co^{2+} for 0.9 mM Ca^{2+} in normal Tyrode solution, was prepared to abolish I_{Ca}. The Cs^+-Tyrode solution was prepared simply by substituting Cs^+ for K^+ in normal Tyrode solution. The storage solution contained (in mM): 10 taurine, 10 oxalic acid, 70 L-glutamic acid, 10 KH_2PO_4, 10 HEPES, 25 KCl, 11 glucose, and 0.5 ethyleneglycoltetraacetic acid (EGTA); pH was adjusted to pH 7.4 with KOH. The standard pipette solution contained (in mM): 110 potassium aspartate, 20 KCl, 2 $MgCl_2$, 4 ATP (dipotassium salt), 6 creatine phosphate (disodium salt), 5 HEPES, and 0.1 EGTA, adjusted to pH 7.0 with KOH. The Cs^+ pipette solution was prepared simply substituting Cs^+ for all K^+ except dipotassium-ATP in the standard pipette solution.

The drugs used in the experiments were (−)-isoproterenol hydrochloride (Merck AG, Darmstadt, Germany, and Sigma Chemical, St. Louis, MO, USA), α-(3,4,5-trimethoxyphenethylaminomethyl)-3,4-dihydroxybenzylalcohol hydrochloride (T-1583; a gift from Tanabe Seiyaku, Osaka, Japan), 6-(3-dimethylaminopropionyl) forskolin hydrochloride (NKH-477; a gift from Nippon Kayaku, Tokyo, Japan), and $CoCl_2$ (Wako, Osaka, Japan).

Data Analysis

The results are expressed as means ± SE. Student's paired or unpaired t-test was applied where appropriate; differences were considered significant if $P < .05$. Changes in amplitude of the currents were expressed as a percentage of the respective basal value. To evaluate the potency of the drugs, relatively linear ranges in the concentration–response curves were fitted by linear regressions. The value of the potency of the drug is given in the text with the confidence limits for .95 probability shown in parentheses.

Results

Effects of Isoproterenol and T-1583 on I_{Ca}

The effects of isoproterenol and T-1583 on I_{Ca} were examined under the condition in which potassium currents were abolished by Cs^+. The I_{Ca} was obtained in the cells that were dialyzed internally with the Cs^+ internal pipette solution through the patch electrode and were superfused with Cs^+-Tyrode solution. Under such circumstances (Cs/Cs condition), potassium currents were almost abolished within 4–6 min [22]. The cell was voltage clamped at −30 mV, and 300-ms depolarizing test pulses from −20 to +70 mV were applied every 10 s. I_{Ca} was maximum around 0 mV, and the apparent reversal potential was +60 to +70 mV in the Cs/Cs condition (data not shown).

In the Cs/Cs condition, isoproterenol and T-1583 increased I_{Ca} just as in the normal condition. The results obtained with isoproterenol (10 nM) and T-1583 (100 nM) are shown in Fig. 2(a–c). The increase in I_{Ca} was concentration dependent, and the slopes of the concentration-response curves, calculated by a linear regression for isoproterenol (1–100 nM) and T-1583 (10–1000 nM), were 55.3% and 51.0% per log unit dose, respectively (Fig. 3). The threshold concentrations of isoproterenol and T-

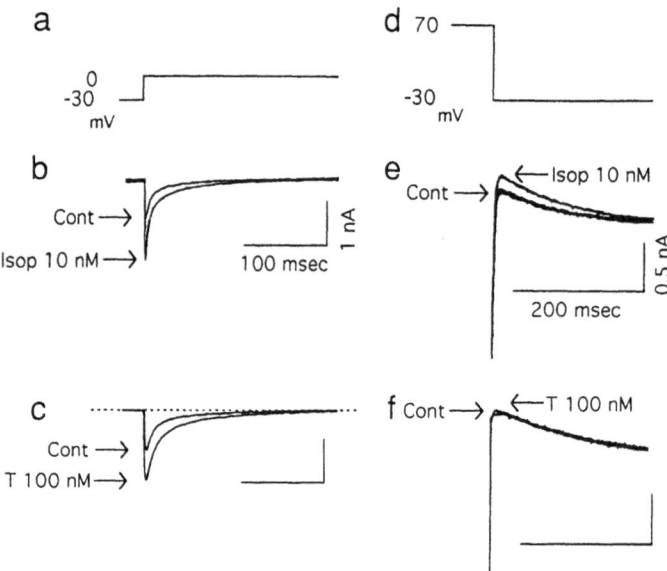

FIG. 2a–f. Effects of isoproterenol (*Isop*) and T-1583 (*T*) on I_{Ca} and the outward tail current. a, d Voltage-clamp protocols to evaluate I_{Ca} and the outward tail current, respectively. b, c Currents recorded during voltage pulses to 0 mV in the absence (*Cont*) and in the presence of 10 nM isoproterenol (b) or 100 nM T-1583 (c) in the Cs/Cs condition. e, f Currents recorded following 300-ms clamp pulses to +70 mV in the absence (*Cont*) and in the presence of 10 nM isoproterenol (e) or 100 nM T-1583 (f) in Co^{2+}-Tyrode solution. Currents were superimposed. *Dotted lines* show the zero current leve. (Modified from [16] with permission)

1583 were approximately 1 and 10 nM, respectively. To evaluate the potency of the drugs on the I_{Ca}, we calculated the concentration that produced a 75% increase in the amplitude of I_{Ca} ($EC_{75\%}I_{Ca}$). $EC_{75\%}I_{Ca}$ was 8.11 nM (confidence limit, 2.35–47.4 nM) for isoproterenol and 68.7 nM) confidence limit, 27.7–140 nM) for T-1583.

Effects of Isoproterenol and NKH-477 on I_{Ca}

The effects of isoproterenol and NKH-477 on I_{Ca} were examined under the condition in which K⁺ currents were abolished by Cs⁺. As shown in Fig. 4(a–c), isoproterenol and NKH-477 increased I_{Ca} just as in the normal condition. To obtain concentration-response relationships, I_{Ca} was eclicited by clamp pulses from −30 to 0 mV. The increase in I_{Ca} was concentration dependent, and slopes of the concentration-response curves calculted by a linear regression for isoproterenol (1–10 nM) and NKH-477 (30–300 nM) were 154% and 112%/log unit concentration, respectively (Fig. 5). The threshold concentrations for increasing I_{Ca} by isoproterenol and NKH-477 were ~0.3 and 10 nM, respectively. The maximal response for increasing I_{Ca}, however, was not evaluated in these experiments to avoid deterioration of the cells. To evaluate the potency of the drugs on I_{Ca}, we calculated the concentration that produced a 100% increase in the amplitude of I_{Ca} ($EC_{100\%}I_{Ca}$). $EC_{100\%}I_{Ca}$ was 2.97 nM (confidence limit, 0.28–31.3 nM) for isoproterenol and 143 nM (confidence limit, 29.0–710 nM) for NKH-477.

Effects of Isoproterenol and T-1583 on the Outward Tail Current

Effects of isoproterenol and T-1583 on I_K were examined in the absence of I_{Ca}. I_{Ca} was abolished by Co^{2+} (0.9 mM) substituted for 0.9 mM Ca^{2+} in normal Tyrode solution. Under this condition, the time-dependent outward and the outward tail current were

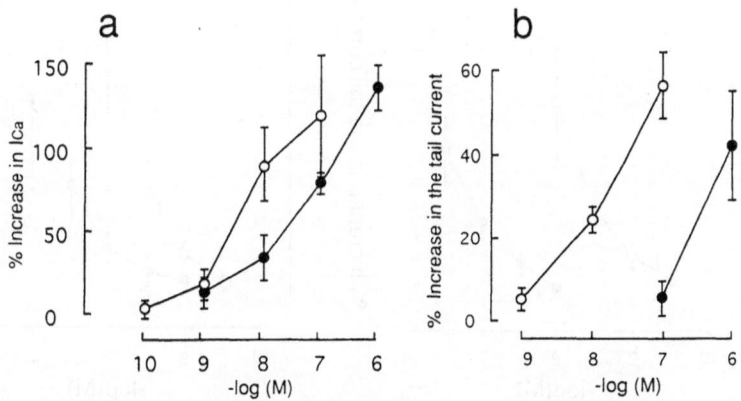

FIG. 3a,b. Concentration–response curves to isoproterenol (*open circles*) and T-1583 (*solid circles*) for increasing I_{Ca} (a) in the Cs/Cs condition and the outward tail current (b) in Co^{2+}–Tyrode solution. I_{Ca} was elicited by clamp pulses from −30 to 0 mV, and the outward tail current was elicited by clamp pulses from −30 to +70 mV. Values are expressed as percent increases from values before the application of the drug. Data points represent means ± SE of 2–9 cells. (Modified from [16] with permission)

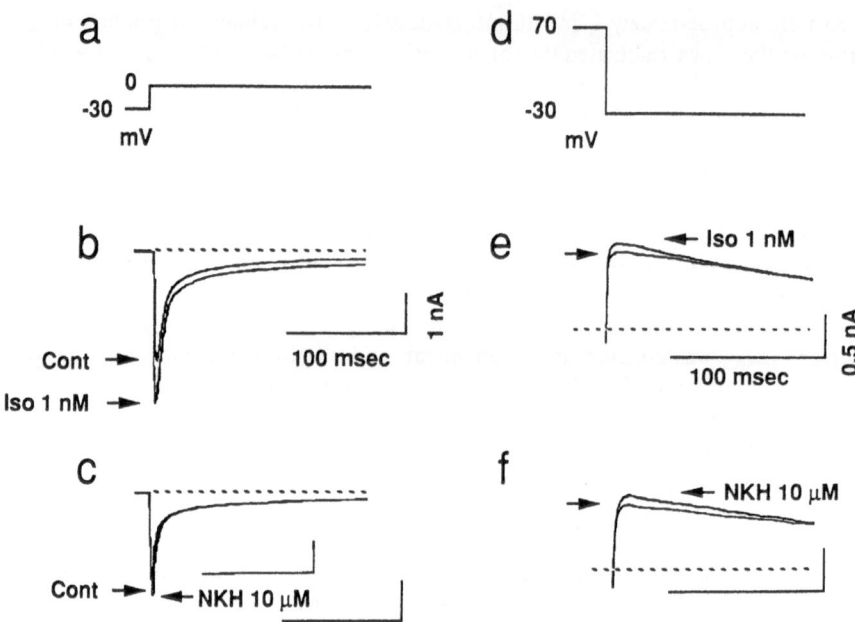

FIG. 4a–f. Effects of isoproterenol (*Iso*) and NKH-477 (*NKH*) on I_{Ca} and outward tail current. **a, d** Voltage-clamp protocols to evaluate I_{Ca} and outward tail current, respectively. **b, c** Currents recorded during voltage pulses to 0 mB in absence (*Cont*) and presence of 1 n*M* isoprepterenol (**b**) or 10 n*M* NKH-477 (**c**) in Cs/Cs condition. **e, f** Currents recorded after 300-ms clamp pulses to 70 mB in absence and presence of 1 n*M* isoproterenol (**e**) or 10 n*M* NKH-477. (**f**) in Co^{2+}-Tyrode solution. Currents were superimposed. *Dotted lines*, zero current levels. (Modified from [17] with permission)

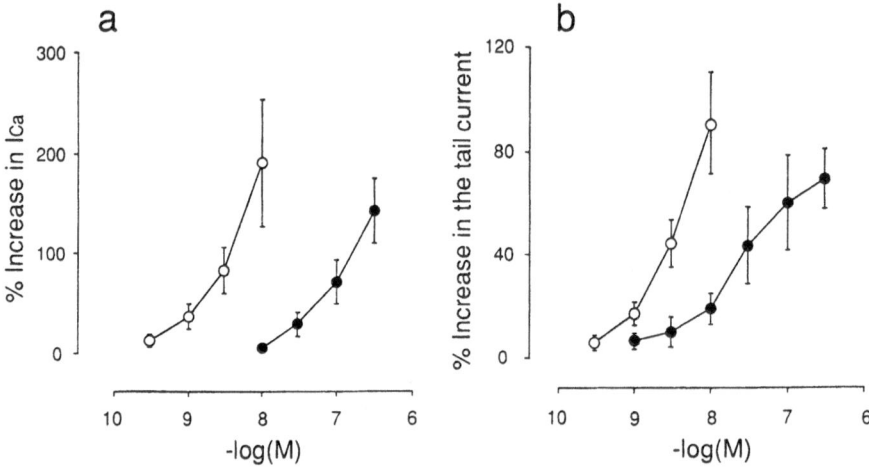

FIG. 5a,b. Concentration–response curves to isoproterenol (*open circles*) and NKH-477 (*solid circles*) for increasing I_{Ca} in the Cs/Cs condition (**a**) and the outward tail current in Co^{2+}-Tyrode solution (**b**). I_{Ca} was elicited by clamp pulses from −30 to 0 mV, and the outward tail current was elicited by clamp pulses from −30 to +70 mV. Values are percent increases from values before application of the drug. Data represent means ± SE of 4–6 cells. (Modified from Harada and [17] with permission)

apparent [18]. As shown in Fig. 2(d–f), 10 nM isoproterenol increased the outward tail current but 100 nM T-1583 failed to do so. Summarized results (Fig. 3) show that the threshold concentration of isoproterenol to increase the outward tail current was 1 nM, and this was identical to that for increasing I_{Ca} (see Fig. 3). The slopes of the concentration–response curves for isoproterenol and T-1583 were 24.5% and 36.7%/log unit dose, respectively.

The concentration that produced a 30% increase in the amplitude of the outward tail current ($EC_{30\%}I_K$) was 11.3 nM (confidence limit, 7.25–19.4 nM) for isoproterenol. On the other hand, high concentrations of T-1583 were required to produce an apparent increase in I_K; the threshold concentration of T-1583 was 100 nM. The $EC_{30\%}I_K$ for T-1583 was 443 nM (confidence limit, 162–5160 nM). Although $EC_{30\%}I_K$ and $EC_{75\%}I_{Ca}$ for isoproterenol were very close (11.3 vs. 8.11 nM), $EC_{30\%}I_K$ for T-1583 was markedly higher than $EC_{75\%}I_{Ca}$ for T-1583 (433 vs. 68.7 nM).

Effects of Isoproterenol and NKH-477 on the Outward Tail Current

Effects of isoproterenol and NKH-477 on the outward tail current were examined in the absence of I_{Ca}. I_{Ca} was abolished by Co^{2+} (0.9 mM) substituted for 0.9 mM Ca^{2+} in normal Tyrode solution. To obtain concentration–response relationships, the outward tail current was obtained by clamp pulses from −30 to +70 mV. In the Co^{2+}-Tyrode solution, isoproterenol and NKH-477 increased the outward tail current in a concentration-dependent manner just as in the normal condition (see Fig. 5). The threshold concentration of isoproterenol to incease the outward tail current was 0.3 nM, and this was identical to that for increasing I_{Ca} (see Figs. 4 and 5).

However, the threshold concentration of NKH-477 for increasing the outward tail current was ~1 nM, and this concentration was tenfold or more lower than that for increasing I_{Ca} (Fig. 5). Slopes of the concentration–response curves for isoproterenol and NKH-477 were 73.5% and 40.2%/log unit concentration, respectively. To evaluate the potency of the drugs on the outward tail current, we calculated the concentration that produced a 40% increase in the amplitude of the outward tail current ($EC_{40\%}I_K$). $EC_{40\%}I_K$ was 2.25 nM (confidence limit, 1.09–4.65 nM) for isoproterenol and 30.6 nM (confidence limit, 19.3–48.6 nM) for NKH-477. Although $EC_{40\%}I_K$ and $EC_{100\%}I_{Ca}$ for isoproterenol were very close (2.25 vs 2.97 nM), $EC_{40\%}I_K$ for NKH-477 was clearly less than $EC_{100\%}I_{Ca}$ for NKH-477 (30.6 vs 143 nM).

Discussion

We examined differences in the threshold concentration of the β-adrenoceptor agonists isoproterenol and T-1583 for increasing I_{Ca} and I_K in single ventricular cells of the guinea pig heart. I_{Ca} was increased by isoproterenol in a concentration-dependent manner. The threshold concentration for increasing the current was 1 nM. I_K was also increased in a concentration-dependent manner by isoproterenol, and the threshold concentration was the same as that for I_{Ca} (see Fig. 3). The potencies of isoproterenol for increasing I_{Ca} and I_K, given as $EC_{75\%}I_{Ca}$ and $EC_{30\%}I_K$, respectively, were calculated from the concentration–response curves. The ratio of calculated $EC_{30\%}I_K$ to $EC_{75\%}I_{Ca}$ for isoproterenol was 1.39; that is, β-adrenoceptor stimulation by isoproterenol results in increases in I_{Ca} and I_K in the same concentration range. T-1583 also increased I_{Ca} and

I_K in a concentration-dependent manner, and the threshold concentration for increasing I_{Ca} was 1 nM (Fig. 3).

The threshold concentration of T-1583 for increasing I_K, however, was 100 nM (Fig. 3); that is, the threshold concentration of T-1583 for increasing I_K was approximately 100 times higher than that for increasing I_{Ca}. The potencies of T-1583 for increasing I_{Ca} and I_K, namely, $EC_{75\%}I_{Ca}$ and $EC_{30\%}I_K$, were calculated from the concentration-response curves, and the ratio of $EC_{30\%}I_K$ to $EC_{75\%}I_{Ca}$ was 6.3. The ratio indicates that T-1583 was a less potent activator of I_K than I_{Ca}.

The differential activation by T-1583 of I_{Ca} and I_K might result from differences in the receptor subtype specificity of the drug because isoproterenol stimulates both β_1- and β_2-adrenoceptors but T-1583 can only stimulate β_1-adrenoceptors at the concentration range used in these experiments [10]. However, this is an unlikely explanation because β_2-adrenoceptors are not present or are not coupled with adenylate cyclase in ventricular cells of the guinea pig heart [19,23,24]. One possible explanation for the difference in threshold concentrations is that a selective β_1-adrenoceptor agonist, T-1583, at low concentrations may stimulate β_1-adrenoceptors and activate adenylate cyclase located in a compartment closely linked to calcium ion channels.

On the other hand, isoproterenol may diffusely stimulate β_1-adrenoceptors, activate adenylate cyclase, and increase cAMP in compartments over and above those related to calcium ion channels. A diffusely increased cAMP may be able to augment I_K because I_K was increased with relatively high concentrations of T-1583 (Figs. 2 and 3). This view is supported by the evidence that in canine ventricular muscles, isoproterenol produced positive inotropic effects with large increments in cAMP levels while T-1583 induced comparable positive inotropic effects accompanied by smaller increases in cAMP levels [10]. Moreover, T-1583 increased the force of contraction with smaller increases in the myocardial oxygen consumption and in coronary blood flow [25,26].

Although we did not measure cAMP levels, small increases in cAMP elicited by a selective β_1-adrenoceptor agonist just enough to increase I_{Ca} may not be enough to augment I_K, or the selective β_1-adrenoceptor agonist may increase cAMP levels in specific compartments closely linked to I_{Ca} but not to I_K. The latter possibility is more probable because the compartmentalization of cAMP-mediated hormone actions has already been proposed [27]. Occupancy of some cell membrane hormone receptors leads to cAMP accumulation and subsequently activates protein kinase in specific subcellular compartments in cardiac muscles [28] and in arterial smooth muscles [29].

The idea of the specific subcellular compartment is further supported by the following experiments. The threshold concentration of NKH-477 for increasing I_K (1 nM) was clearly lower than that for increasing I_{Ca} (10 nM) (see Figs. 4 and 5). The potencies of NKH-477 for increasing I_{Ca} and I_K, given as $EC_{100\%}I_{Ca}$ and $EC_{40\%}I_K$, were 143, and 30.6 nM, respectively. The ratio of calculated $EC_{100\%}I_{Ca}$ to $EC_{40\%}I_K$ for NKH-477 was 4.68. The ratio indicates that NKH-477 was a less potent activator of I_{Ca} than I_K. In cell-free systems, the EC_{50} value of NKH-477 for adenylate cyclase activation (2.3 μM) was similar to that of forskolin (1.7 μM) but the efficacy was approximately two-fold greater than that of forskolin [15]. Therefore, the differences just described are not characteristics of NKH-477 for activation of adenylate cyclase because NKH-477 increases cAMP much more than does forskolin.

As shown in Fig. 5, the concentration–response curve of NKH-477 for I_K reached almot maximla at 0.3 μM. High concentration of forskolin derivatives may reduce I_K

independently of changes in adenylate cyclase activity. For example, forskolin at high concentration reduced the open probability and mean open time of K$^+$ channels of PC12 cells [30], whose I_K displays electrical characteristics like that in ventricular cells of the guinea pig heart. Forskolin at low concentrations ($<1\,\mu M$) stimulates I_K channels and at high concentrations ($10-120\,\mu M$) inhibits the channels [31]. This explanation is also consistent with the recent report of forskolin derivatives, one of which caused significant negative chronotropic and inotropic effects at 30 mM in isolated guinea pig right atria [32]. However, it is still not possible to explain why I_K is more sensitive to modification by direct stimulation of adenylate cyclase than is I_{Ca}.

Temperature-dependent modulation of I_{Ca} and I_K channels by β-adrenoceptor were examined in patch-clamped guinea pig ventricular myocytes [33]. The results indicated that regulation of cardiac potassium but not calcium channels involves a temperature-dependent step that occurs after activation of the catalytic subunit of cAMP-dependent protein kinase. Although modulation produced by isoproterenol, forskolin, and cAMP was more effective in enhancing I_{Ca}, I_K was more sensitive to modulation by interally applied catalytic subunit of cAMP-dependent protein kinase than I_{Ca}. It might be suggested that I_K channels, but not I_{Ca} channels, can be regulated by a diverse group of phosphorylating enzymes. However, a possible explanation for the difference obtained in our results is that direct and diffuse stimulation of adenylate cyclase by NKH-477 may increase cAMP in compartments over and above those related to Ca^{2+} channels Weishaar et al. [34] reported that cAMP and cAMP-dependent protein kinase might be compartmentalized within the cardica cell.

In conclusion, small increases in cAMP elicited by a selective $β_1$-adrenoceptor agonist that are just enough to increase I_{Ca} may not be enough to augment I_K, or the selective $β_1$-adrenoceptor agonist may increase cAMP levels in specific compartments closely linked to I_{Ca} but not to I_K, and direct diffuse stimulation of adenylate cyclase may increase cAMP in compartments over and above those related to Ca^{2+} channels. These results suggest that a simple signal transduction pathway from β-adrenoceptors to I_{Ca} and I_K channels mediated through adenylate cyclase and cAMP-dependent protein kinase is not sufficient to explain these differences, and indicate that increases in I_{Ca} and I_K elicited by $β_1$-adrenoceptor stimulation appear to be generated by different biophysical mechanisms. Further studies are needed to clarify the underlying mechanisms to explain such discrepancies.

References

1. Reuter H (1974) Localization of beta adrenergic receptors, and effects of noradrenaline and cyclic nucleotides on action potentials, ionic currents and tension in mammalian cardiac muscle. J Physiol (Lond) 242:429–451
2. Tsien RW, Giles W, Greengard P (1972) Cyclic AMP mediates the effects of adrenaline on cardiac Purkinje fibres. Nature New Biol 240:181–183
3. Brown HF, Noble SJ (1974) Effects of adrenaline on membrane currents underlying pacemaker activity in frog atrial muscle. J Physiol (Lond) 238:51P–53P
4. Trautwein W, Hescheler J (1990) Regulation of cardiac L-type calcium current by phosphorylation and G proteins. Annu Rev Physiol 52:257–274
5. Walsh KB, Kass RS (1988) Regulation of a heart potassium channel by protein kinase A and C. Science 242:67–69
6. Freeman LC, Kwok W-M, Kass RS (1992) Phosphorylation-independent regulation of cardiac I_K by guanine nucleotides and isoproterenol. Am J Physiol 262(31):H1298–H1302

7. Yatani A, Brown AM (1991) Channel control (scientific correspondence). Nature 354:363–364

8. Hartzell HC, Fishmeister R (1992) Direct regulation of cardiac Ca^{2+} channels by G protein: neither proven nor necessary? Trends Pharmacol Sci 131:380–385

9. Nakajima H, Nagao T, Sato M, Kiyomoto A (1975) Pharmacological properties of a new selective adrenergic β_1-stimulant, α-(3,4,5-trimethoxyphenethylaminomethyl)-3,4-dihydroxybenzylalcohol hydrochloride (T-1583). Jpn J Pharmacol 25:22P

10. Yanagisawa T, Ishii K, Hashimoto H, Taira N (1989) Differential coupling to positive inotropic responses to cyclic AMP produced by stimulation of β_1- and β_2-adrenergic receptors. J Cardiovasc Pharmacol 13:64–75

11. Manalan AS, Besch HR Jr, Watanabe AM (1981) Characterization of [^{3}H] ($\pm$)carazolol binding to β-adrenergic receptors. Application to study of β-adrenergic receptor subtypes in canine ventricular myocardium and lung. Circ Res 49:326–336

12. Metzger H, Linder E (1981) The positive inotropic-acting forskolin, a potent adenylate cyclase activator. Arzneim-Forsch 31:1248–1250

13. Seamon KB, Daly JW (1981) Forskolin: a unique diterpene activator of cyclic AMP-generating system. J Cyclic Nucleotide Res 1:201–224

14. Fujita A, Takahira T, Hosono M, Nakamura K (1992) Improvement of drug-induced cardiac failure by NKH477, a novel forskolin derivative, in the dog heart-lung preparation. Jpn J Pharmacol 58:375–381

15. Hoshono M, Takahira T, Fujita A, Fujihara R, Ishizuka O, Tatee T, Nakamura K (1992) Cardiovascular and adenylate cyclase stimulant properties of NKH477, a novel water-soluble forskolin derivative. J Cardiovasc Pharmacol 19:625–634

16. Iijima T, Imagawa J, Taira N (1990) Differential modulation by beta adrenoceptors of inward calcium and delayed rectifier potassium current in single ventricular cells of guinea pig heart. J Pharmacol Exp Ther 254:142–146

17. Harada K, Iijima T (1994) Differential modulation by adenylate cyclase of Ca^{2+} and delayed K^+ current in ventricular myocytes. Am J Physiol 266(35):H1551-H1557

18. Iijima T, Taira N (1987) Membrane current changes responsible for the positive inotropic effect of OPC-8212, a new positive inotropic agent, in single ventricular cells of the guinea pig heart. J Pharmacol Exp Ther 240:657–662

19. Iijima T, Taira N (1989) β_2-Adrenoceptor mediated increase in the slow inward calcium current in atrial cells. Eur J Pharmacol 163:357–360

20. Hamill PO, Marty A, Neher E, Sakmann B, Sigworth FJ (1981) Improved patch-clamp techniques for high-resolution current recording from ells and cell-free membrane patches. Pflügers Arch 391:85–100

21. McDonald TF, Trautwein W (1978) The potassium current underlying delayed rectification in cat ventricular muscle. J Physiol (Lond) 274:217–246

22. Iijima T, Irisawa H, Kameyama M (1985) Membrane currents and their modification by acetylcholine in isolated single atrial cells of the guinea-pig. J Physiol (Lond) 359:485–501

23. Hedberg A, Minneman KP, Molinoff PB (1980) Differential distribution of beta-1 and beta-2 adrenergic receptors in cat and guinea-pig heart. J Pharmacol Exp Ther 212:503–508

24. Engel G, Hoyer D, Berthold R, Wagner H (1981) ($\pm$)[^{125}Iodo]cyanopindolol, a new ligand for β-adrenoceptors: identification and quantitation of subclasses of β-adrenoceptors in guinea pig. Naunyn-Schmiedebergs Arch PHarmacol 317:277–285

25. Hosono M, Satoh K, Taira N (1988) T-1583 forskolin are similar in their cardiac effects and dissimilar in their vascular effects. Cardiovasc Drugs Ther 2:245–253

26. Yokoyama H, Imagawa J, Satoh K, Taira N (1989) Selective β_1-receptor full agonist, T-1583, increases cardiac contractility with less increase in myocardial oxygen consumption than isoproterenol in heart rate-controlled isolated canine heart preparations. Jpn J Pharmacol 49:59P

27. Earp HS, Steiner AL (1978) Compartmentalization of cyclic nucleotide-mediated hormone action. Annu Rev Pharmacol Toxicol 18:431–459

28. Hayes JS, Brunton LL (1982) Functional compartments in cyclic nucleotide action. J Cyclic Nucleotide Res 8:1–16
29. Rubanyi G, Galvas P, DiSalvo J, Paul RJ (1986) Eicosonoid metabolism and β-adrenergic mechanisms in coronary arterial smooth muscle: potential compartmentation of cAMP. Am J Physiol 250:C406–C412
30. Hoshi T, Garber SS, Aldrich RW (1988) Effects of forskolin on voltage-gated K^+ channels is independent of adenylate cyclase activation. Science 240:1652–1655
31. Harvey RD, Hume JR (1989) Autonomic regulation of a chloride current in heart. Science 244:983–985
32. Hubbard JW, Conway PG, Nordstrom LC, Hartman HB, Lebedinsky Y, O'Malley GJ, Kosley RW Jr (1991) Cardiac adenylate cyclase activity, positive chronotropic and inotropic effects of forskolin analogs with either low, medium or high binding site affinity. J Pharmacol Exp Ther 256:621–627
33. Walsh KB, Begenisich TB, Kass RS (1988) B-Adrenergic modulation of cardiac ion channels: differential temperature sensitivity of potassium and calcium current. J Gen Physiol 93:841–854
34. Weishaar RE, Kobaylarz-Singer DC, Quade MM, Kaplan HR (1988) Role of cyclic-AMP in regulating cardiac muscle contractility: novel pharmacological approaches to modulating cyclic-AMP degradation by phosphodiesterase. Drug Dev Res 12:119–129

Molecular and Functional Heterogeneity of Inward Rectifier Potassium Channels in the Brain and Heart

Naohiko Takahashi[1], Ken-ichirou Morishige[2], Mitsuhiko Yamada[1], Chikako Kondo[1], and Yoshihisa Kurachi[1]

Summary. Three background inward rectifier potassium channels were isolated from a mouse brain cDNA library. Based on their amino acid sequences and the electrophysiological properties of currents expressed in *Xenopus* oocytes, we designated them IRK1, IRK2, and IRK3. The amino acid sequences of IRK2 and IRK3 share 70% and 61% identity with IRK1, respectively. *Xenopus* oocytes injected with cRNAs derived from these clones expressed K^+ currents, which showed classical inward rectifier potassium channel characteristics at the whole-cell current level and were blocked by Ba^{2+} and Cs^+ in a concentration- and voltage-dependent manner. In patch-clamp experiments with $150\,mM$ K^+ in the pipette, the single-channel conductance of IRK1 was ~22 pS; of IRK2, ~34 pS; and of IRK3, ~13 pS. Northern blot analysis revealed that the mRNAs for IRK1 and IRK3 were predominantly expressed in the forebrain rather than in the cerebellum, and vice versa in the case of IRK2. IRK1 and IRK2, but not IRK3, were expressed in the heart. These results demonstrate that the IRK family (IRKs) is composed of multiple genes, which may play diverse functional roles in various organs, including the brain and heart.

Key words. Molecular cloning—Potassium channel—*Xenopus* oocytes—Inward rectification—Patch clamp

Introduction

Inward rectifier potassium channels play a significant role in the maintenance of the resting membrane potential, in regulating the duration of the action potential, and in controlling the excitability of a variety of cell types [1,2]. A complementary DNA encoding inward rectifier potassium channel (IRK1) has been cloned from a mouse macrophage cell line [3], which shows considerable homology with an ATP-regulated potassium channel (ROMK1) cloned from the outer medulla of rat kidney [4]. The G-protein-regulated muscarinic potassium channel (GIRK1 or KGA) cloned from rat heart [5,6] possesses essentially the same molecular structure; all these channels have two putative membrane-spanning segments with one pore-forming region.

[1] Department of Pharmacology II and [2] Department of Obstetrics and Gynecology, Faculty of Medicine, Osaka University, Suita, Osaka 565, Japan

Northern blot analysis demonstrated that the mRNA for IRK1 is expressed in the brain [3,7]. Because the brain has multiple and complex functions, it could be postulated that brain cells express multiple homologous sequences of IRK1 proteins. In this study, to test this premise we hybridized, using IRK1 as a probe, a mouse brain cDNA library under a condition of mild stringency. We have isolated the second and third members of the IRK family (IRKs), IRK2 and IRK3 [8,9].

Materials and Methods

Screening of Mouse Brain cDNA Library

A mouse brain cDNA library (Stratagene, La Jolla, CA, USA) was screened under a mild stringency condition using a fragment of IRK1 [3] as a probe [7–9]. Phage clones were screened with [α-^{32}P] cytidine triphosphate- (CTP-) labeled probes. Hybridization and DNA sequencing were performed as described [7–9].

Functional Expression of IRKs in Xenopus oocytes

The obtained positive clones were transcribed in vitro by T_3 RNA polymerase after digestion with appropriate restriction enzymes. These transcripts were dissolved in sterile water and injected into manually defoliculated oocytes (50 nl of 500 ng/µl). After injection, oocytes were incubated in a modified Barth solution at 18°C, and electrophysiological studies were undertaken 48–96 h later. Experiments were performed at room temperature (20°–22°C). Two-electrode voltage-clamp experiments were carried out with a commercially available amplifier (Turbo Clamp TEC 01C, Tamm, Germany) using microelectrodes which, when filled with 3 M KCl, had resistances of 0.5–1.5 MΩ. Oocytes were bathed in a solution that contained 90 mM KCl, 3 mM MgCl$_2$, 5 mM hydroxy ethylpiperazine ethane sulfonic acid (HEPES) (pH 7.4), and 300 µM niflumic acid to block endogenous chloride current. Oocytes were voltage clamped at various holding potentials, and voltage steps of 1.2-s duration were applied to the cells in 10-mV increments every 5 s. Single-channel recordings were performed in the cell-attached patch configuration using a patch clamp amplifier (Axopatch 200A, Axon Instruments, Foster City, CA, USA; or EPC-7, List Electronic, Darmstadt, Germany). Both pipette and bathing solutions contained 140 mM KCl, 1.4 mM MgCl$_2$ and 10 mM HEPES (pH 7.4). Electrophysiological data were stored on videotapes using a PCM data recording system (VR-10B, Instrutech, New York, NY, USA) and subsequently replayed for computer analysis (EP Analisis, Human Intelligence, Rochester, MN, USA).

Northern Blot Analysis of IRKs

Pieces of various tissues (forebrain, cerebellum, heart, kidney, and leg skeletal muscle) were isolated from 15-day fetal, 3-day neonatal, and 6-week-old adult female BALB/c mice. Total RNAs were extracted by the guanidium thiocyanate method [10], and poly (A)+ RNAs were isolated using Oligotex-dT mRNA kit (QIAGEN, Chatsworth, CA, USA). Aliquots of 3 µg poly (A)+ RNA were separated by electrophoresis in 1.0% agarose gel and blotted onto a Hybond-N nylon membrane (Amersham, Arlington Heights, IL, USA). Hybridization was conducted as described [7–9].

Results

Molecular Cloning of IRKs

After screening of 6×10^5 mouse brain cDNA clones, we obtained three positive full-length clones. Sequence analysis revealed that one is a cDNA identical to IRK1 and another two are homologous cDNAs that share 69% and 59% nucleotide identity with IRK1 [3]. We designated these homologous cDNAs IRK2 and IRK3, respectively, on the basis of their amino acid sequences and the electrophysiological properties of the expressed currents [7–9,11]. Each nucleotide sequencing of IRK1, IRK2, and IRK3 revealed open reading frames encoding proteins of 428, 427, and 445 amino acids, respectively. The Kyte–Doolittle hydropathy plot [12] indicates that these three clones have two membrane-spanning hydrophobic segments (M1 and M2) with one pore-forming region (H5). In Fig. 1, the amino acid sequences of IRK2 and IRK3 are compared with that of IRK1. At the pore-forming region (H5), IRK1, IRK2, and IRK3 show differences from each other at only one amino acid residue.

Electrophysiological Characteristics of IRKs

Figure 2 illustrates the results obtained from *Xenopus* oocytes that had been injected with cRNAs derived from IRK1, IRK2, and IRK3 at 48 h before the recording. With 90 mM of extracellular K^+ ($[K^+]_0$), hyperpolarizing voltage steps from a holding potential of 0 mV revealed rapid activation of an inward large current that showed slowly developed voltage-dependent inactivation at hyperpolarizing voltages. The inactivation of IRK2 current was usually most prominent, which is not evident in this particular example. On depolarization, the currents showed a pronounced inwardly rectifying property. As $[K^+]_0$ was lowered from 90 mM to 20 and 10 mM, the slope conductance of expressed currents was decreased [7–9,11]. The reversal potentials of the expressed currents were in good agreement with the equilibrium potential for K^+ (E_K) values predicted from the Nernst equation at various $[K^+]_0$. External Ba^{2+} and Cs^+ induced a concentration- and voltage-dependent block of the expressed currents [7–9,11].

Single-channel currents of IRK1, IRK2, and IRK3 were recorded in the cell-attached configuration. Each current was observed only in the inward direction and thus showed a strong inwardly rectifying property. As shown in Fig. 3, however, the mean slope conductances of IRK2 (34 pS) [8] and IRK3 (13 pS) [9] were found to be significantly different from that of IRK1 channel (22 pS) [3,7]. Steady-state open probability (P_o) of the IRK2 channel decreased with hyperpolarization, while that of the IRK1 or IRK3 remained constant [8]. The detailed gating kinetic analysis strongly indicates that the increase of long closed gaps (>200 ms) between clusters of the channel burst openings, as shown in Fig. 2, is mainly responsible for the prominent reduction of steady-state P_o at hyperpolarized potential in the case of IRK2 [8].

Tissue Distribution and Developmental Time-Course of mRNAs for IRKs

We conducted Northern blot analysis of IRK1, IRK2, and IRK3 in various mouse tissues. The expression of each clone in the forebrain and cerebellum is shown in Fig. 4. The abundance of mRNAs for IRK1 and IRK3 was much higher in the forebrain

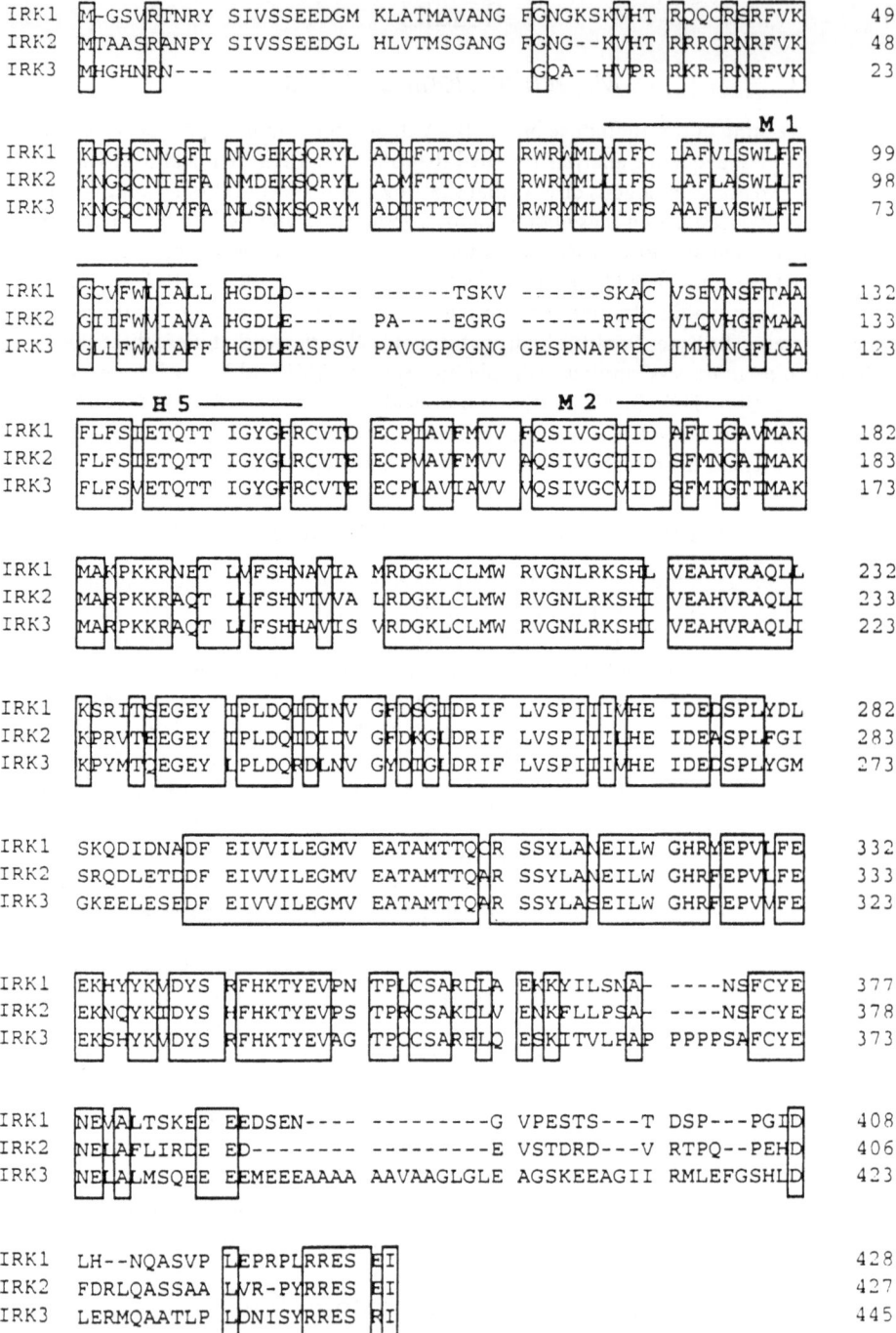

```
IRK1  M-GSVRTNRY  SIVSSEEDGM  KLATMAVANG  FGNGKSKVHT  RQQCRSRFVK      49
IRK2  MTAASRANPY  SIVSSEEDGL  HLVTMSGANG  FGNG--KVHT  RRRCRNRFVK      48
IRK3  MHGHNRN---  ----------  ----------  -GQA--HVPR  RKR-RNRFVK      23

                                                  ——————————— M 1
IRK1  KDGHCNVQFI  NVGEKGQRYL  ADIFTTCVDI  RWRAMLVIFC  LAFVLSWLFF      99
IRK2  KNGQCNIEFA  NMDEKSQRYL  ADMFTTCVDI  RWRYMLLIFS  LAFLASWLLF      98
IRK3  KNGQCNVYFA  NLSNKSQRYM  ADIFTTCVDT  RWRYMLMIFS  AAFLVSWLFF      73

      ———————————                                              —
IRK1  GCVFWLIALL  HGDLD-----  ------TSKV  ------SKAC  VSEVNSFTAA     132
IRK2  GIIFWMIAVA  HGDLE-----  PA----EGRG  ------RTFC  VLQVHGFMAA     133
IRK3  GLLFWWIAFF  HGDLEASPSV  PAVGGPGGNG  GESPNAPKFC  IMHVNGFLGA     123

      ——— H 5 ———                  ——————————— M 2 ———————————
IRK1  FLFSIETQTT  IGYGFRCVTD  ECPLAVFMVV  FQSIVGCHID  AFIIGAVMAK     182
IRK2  FLFSIETQTT  IGYGLRCVTE  ECPMAVFMVV  AQSIVGCHID  SFMNGAIMAK     183
IRK3  FLFSMETQTT  IGYGFRCVTE  ECPLAVIAVV  VQSIVGCMID  SFMIGTIMAK     173

IRK1  MAKPKKRNET  LMFSHNAVIA  MRDGKLCLMW  RVGNLRKSHL  VEAHVRAQLL     232
IRK2  MARPKKRAQT  LLFSHNTVVA  LRDGKLCLMW  RVGNLRKSHI  VEAHVRAQLI     233
IRK3  MARPKKRAQT  LLFSHHAVIS  VRDGKLCLMW  RVGNLRKSHI  VEAHVRAQLI     223

IRK1  KSRITSEGEY  IPLDQIDINV  GFDSGIDRIF  LVSPIIIMHE  IDEDSPLYDL     282
IRK2  KPRVTEEGEY  IPLDQIDIDV  GFDKGLDRIF  LVSPIIILHE  IDEASPLFGI     283
IRK3  KPYMTQEGEY  LPLDQRDLNV  GMDIGLDRIF  LVSPIIIMHE  IDEDSPLYGM     273

IRK1  SKQDIDNADF  EIVVILEGMV  EATAMTTQCR  SSYLANEILW  GHRMEPVLFE     332
IRK2  SRQDLETDDF  EIVVILEGMV  EATAMTTQAR  SSYLANEILW  GHRFEPVLFE     333
IRK3  GKEELESEDF  EIVVILEGMV  EATAMTTQAR  SSYLASEILW  GHRFEPVMFE     323

IRK1  EKHYYKVDYS  RFHKTYEVPN  TPLCSARDLA  EKKYILSNA-  ----NSFCYE     377
IRK2  EKNQYKIDYS  HFHKTYEVPS  TPRCSAKDLV  ENKFLLPSA-  ----NSFCYE     378
IRK3  EKSHYKVDYS  RFHKTYEVAG  TPCCSARELQ  ESKITVLPAP  PPPPSAFCYE     373

IRK1  NEVALTSKEE  EEDSEN----  ---------G  VPESTS---T  DSP---PGID     408
IRK2  NELAFLIRDE  ED--------  ---------E  VSTDRD---V  RTPQ--PEHD     406
IRK3  NELALMSQEE  EEMEEEAAAA  AAVAAGLGLE  AGSKEEAGII  RMLEFGSHLD     423

IRK1  LH--NQASVP  LEPRPLRRES  EI                                     428
IRK2  FDRLQASSAA  LVR-PYRRES  EI                                     427
IRK3  LERMQAATLP  LDNISYRRES  RI                                     445
```

FIG. 1. Alignment of the deduced *IRK1* [3], *IRK2* [8], and *IRK3* [9] protein sequences. Identical amino acid residues are *boxed*. Proposed transmembrane segments *M1*, *M2*, and potential pore-forming region *H5* are indicated by *lines*. *IRK*, inward rectifier potassium channels

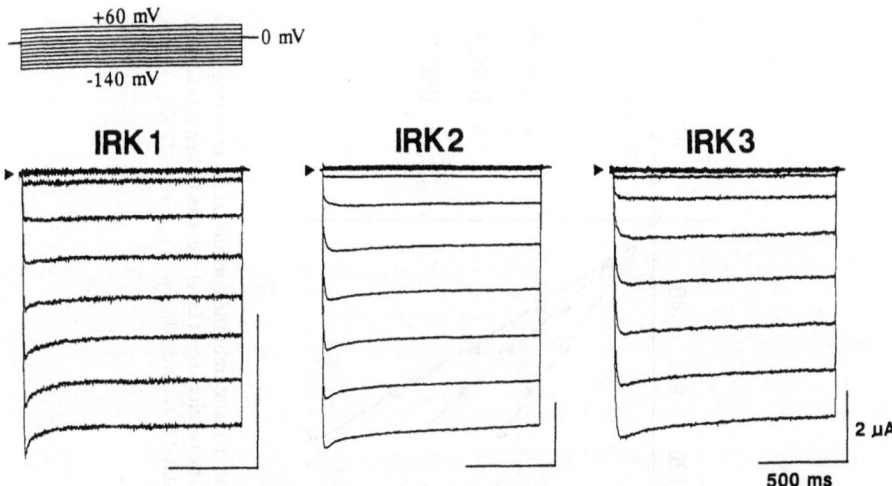

FIG. 2. Cell currents recorded from *Xenopus* oocytes expressing the IRKs, which were obtained by subtracting the currents during the 100 μM Ba²⁺ from the control currents. Potential ranged from −140 to +60 mV in 20-mV increments

than in the cerebellum, and vice versa in the case of IRK2. On the other hand, IRK1 and IRK2, but not IRK3, were expressed in the heart [8,9].

The developmental expression levels of IRK1 and IRK2 mRNAs in the heart were also analyzed by Northern blot. Figure 5 shows the results obtained at the indicated developmental stages. The expression levels of mRNAs for IRK1 and IRK2 are already substantial in the 15-day fetus, and the levels were unchanged throughout all developmental stages studied.

Discussion

In this study, we described amino acid sequences, electrophysiological characteristics, and the tissue distributions of IRK1, IRK2, and IRK3 cloned from a mouse brain cDNA library. When expressed in *Xenopus* oocytes, these three cloned channels exhibited classical inward rectifier potassium channels characteristics indistinguishable from each other. However, the single-channel conductance of IRK2 (34 pS) and IRK3 (13 pS) channels were distinct from that of IRK1 (22 pS) [8,9]. The tissue distributions of mRNAs for these three channels examined by Northern blot analysis were also distinctive. In the brain, the abundance of mRNA for IRK2 was much higher in the cerebellum than in the forebrain, and vice versa in the cases of IRK1 and IRK3 [8,9]. These results suggest that each IRK channel is expressed differentially in various parts of the mouse brain and may play similar but distinct functional roles. IRK2 and IRK3 as well as IRK1 probably possess two membrane-spanning domains with a putative pore-forming region (H5). The H5 region of IRK2 and IRK3 contains amino acids virtually identical with those of IRK1 with the exception of one residue. This one exception may cause the difference of single-channel conductance, because MacKinnon and Yellen [13] suggested that one amino acid variability in the H5 region is sufficient to account for the difference in single-channel conductance of *Shaker*-related potassium channels. The decrease of the steady-state P_o at hyperpolarized

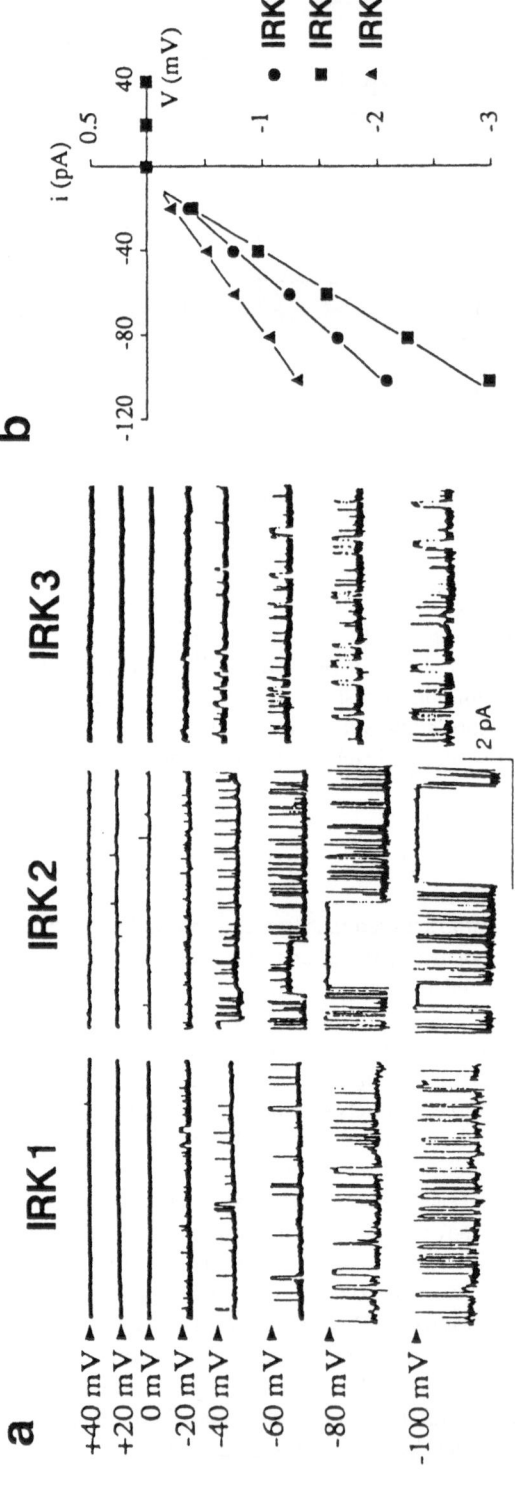

FIG. 3a,b. Single-channel recordings from cell-attached membrane patches of *Xenopus* oocytes expressing the IRKs. Membrane current traces recorded at the membrane potential values are indicated to the left of each trace. *Arrows* to the right of certain traces indicate the patch current level recorded when all channels were closed. Each of these patches appeared to contain one channel. Current–voltage relationships of the channel **b**. records shown in a. *Circles*, IRK1; *squares*, IRK2; *triangles*, IRK3

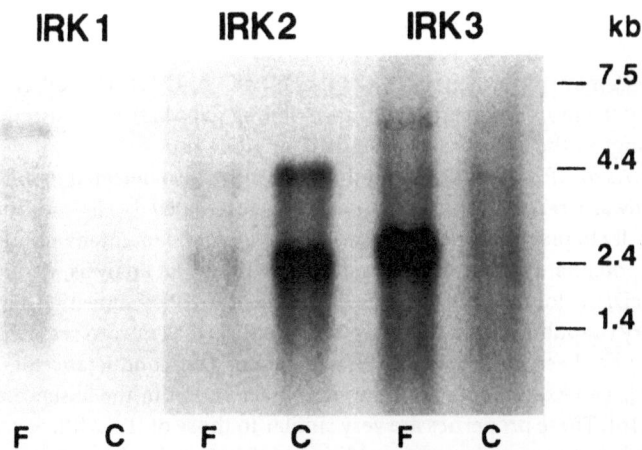

FIG. 4. Northern blot analysis of IRKs in the brain. RNA sample concentrations were determined by absorbance at 260 nm, and 3 µg poly(A)+ RNA was separated on a 1.0% agarose-formamide gel and transferred to a nylon membrane. A major band of 5.5-kb IRK1 mRNA, two bands of 4.3- and 2.4-kb IRK2 mRNAs, and one major band of 2.7-kb and the other weak band of 5.5-kb IRK3 mRNAs were detected. The positions of RNA markers are shown to the *right* of blots. *F*, Forebrain; *C*, cerebellum

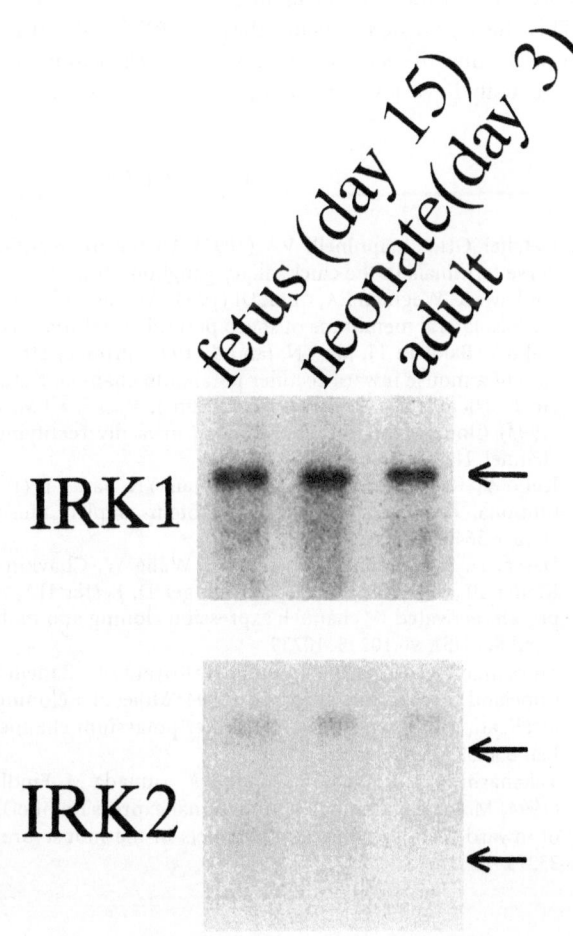

FIG. 5. Developmental time-course of IRK1 and IRK2 mRNAs in the heart. The mRNAs from the three stages of the heart indicated were hybridized with the same probes used in Fig. 4. A major band of 5.5-kb IRK1 mRNA and two bands of 4.3- and 2.4-kb IRK2 mRNAs are indicated with *arrows*

potentials was more prominent in IRK2 than in IRK1 or IRK3. This difference may be explained by the more frequent appearance of long gaps between clusters of channel burst openings in the IRK2 than in the IRK1 or IRK3 [8].

The mRNAs for IRK1 and IRK2, but not IRK3, were also detected in the heart [8,9], where an inward rectifier potassium channel (designated i_{K1}) is indicated electro-physiologically to play an important role, especially in the maintenance of the resting membrane potential [14–16]. In addition to Northern blot analysis, we have isolated two partial cDNA clones corresponding to IRK1 and IRK2 by screening a mouse heart cDNA library (unpublished results). The dominant cardiac inward rectifier potassium channel (i_{K1}) has been reported to have a single-channel conductance of ~40 pS with 150 mM [K^+]$_0$ and exhibit voltage-dependent inactivation in the absence of blocking cations [15,16]. These properties are very similar to those of IRK2 [8]. Several electro-physiological studies suggest that, in addition to the 40-pS i_{K1} channel, inward rectifier potassium channels with conductances less than 40 pS also exist in cardiac myocytes, especially in fetal or neonatal cells [17–19]. IRK1 might correspond to some of these small-conductance inward rectifier potassium channels. In this study, however, the expression levels of mRNAs for IRK1 and IRK2 in the heart were unchanged from 15-day fetal to 6-week-old adult stages. Further studies are necessary to clarify the possible molecular diversity, functional roles and developmental regulation of cardiac inward rectifier potassium channels.

This study provided evidence that the IRK family (IRKs) is composed of multiple genes. The inward rectifier potassium channels belonging to the IRKs may distribute differentially in various cells and play diverse functional roles.

References

1. Fletcher GH, Chiappinelli VA (1992) An inward rectifier is present in presynaptic nerve terminals in the chick ciliary ganglion. Brain Res 575:103–112
2. Ishikawa T, Wegman EA, Cook DI (1993) An inwardly rectifying potassium channel in the basolateral membrane of sheep parotid secretory cells. J Membr Biol 131:193–202.
3. Kubo Y, Baldwin TJ, Jan YN, Jan LY (1993) Primary structure and functional expression of a mouse inward rectifier potassium channel. Nature 362:127–133
4. Ho K, Nichols CG, Lederer WJ, Lytton J, Vassilev PM, Kanazirska MV, Hebert SC (1993) Cloning and expression of an inwardly rectifying ATP-regulated potassium channel. Nature 362:31–38
5. Kubo Y, Reuveny E, Slesinger PA, Jan YN, Jan LY (1993) Primary structure and funtional expression of a rat G-protein-coupled muscarinic potassium channel. Nature 364:802–806
6. Dascal N, Schreibmayer W, Lin NF, Wang W, Chavkin C, DiMagno L, Labarca C, Kieffer BL, Gaveriaux-Ruff C, Trollinger D, Lester HA, Davidson N (1993) Atrial G protein-activated K$^+$ channel: expression cloning and molecular properties. Proc Natl Acad Sci USA 90:10235–10239
7. Morishige K, Takahashi N, Findlay I, Koyama H, Zanelli JS, Peterson C, Jenkins NA, Copeland NG, Mori N, Kurachi Y (1994) Molecular cloning, functional expression and localization of a novel inward rectifier potassium channel in the mouse brain. FEBS Lett 336:375–380
8. Takahashi N, Morishige K, Jahangir A, Yamada M, Findlay I, Koyama H, Kurachi Y (1994) Molecular cloning and functional expression of cDNA encoding a second class of inward rectifier potassium channels in the mouse brain. J Biol Chem 269:23274–23279

9. Morishige K, Takahashi N, Jahangir A, Yamada M, Koyama H, Zanelli JS, Kurachi Y (1994) Molecular cloning and functional expression of a novel brain-specific inward rectifier potassium channel. FEBS Lett 346:251–256

10. Chirgwin JM, Przybyla AE, MacDonald RJ, Rutter WJ (1979) Isolation of biologically active ribonucleic acid from sources enriched in ribonuclease. Biochemistry 18:5294–5299

11. Koyama H, Morishige K, Takahashi N, Zanelli JS, Fass DN, Kurachi Y (1994) Molecular cloning, functional expression and localization of a novel inward rectifier potassium channel in the rat brain. FEBS Lett 341:303–307

12. Kyte J, Doolittle RF (1982) A simple method for displaying the hydropathic character of a protein. J Mol Biol 157:105–132

13. MacKinnon R, Yellen G (1990) Mutations affecting TEA blockade and ion permeations in voltage-activated K$^+$ channels. Science 250:276–279

14. Hille B (1992) Ionic channels of excitable membranes. Sinauer, Sunderland, pp 127–130

15. Sakmann B, Trube G (1984) Conductance properties of single inwardly rectifying potassium channels in ventricular cells from guinea-pig heart. J Physiol 347:641–657

16. Kurachi Y : Voltage-dependent activation of the inward-rectifier potassium channel in the ventricular cell membrane of guinea-pig heart. J Physiol 366:365–385

17. Wahler G (1990) Appearance of large conductance inward rectifying K channels during postnatal development of the rat ventricle. Biophys J 57:512a

18. Josephson IR, Sperelakis N (1989) Developmental changes in the inwardly-rectifying K$^+$ current. Circulation 80:II-144

19. Chen F, Wetzel GT, Friedman WF, Klitzner TS (1991) Single-channel recording of inwardly rectifying potassium currents in developing myocardium. J Mol Cell Cardiol 23:259–267

Activation of Cardiac Adenosine Triphosphate-Sensitive K⁺ Channels: An Obligatory Pathway for the Cardioprotection Afforded by Ischemic and Pharmacological Preconditioning

Icilio Cavero[1], Claudie Hecquet[2], Yasmine Djellas[2],
Véronique Gollot-Robert[1], and Michel Mestre[1]

Summary. The role of ATP-sensitive K⁺ channels (K_{ATP}) in protecting the myocardium from ischemic damage was explored. In the in vitro paced (2 Hz) guinea pig right-ventricular wall, which was perfused through the cannulated right coronary artery, ischemia/reperfusion injury was produced by suspending perfusion of oxygenated Tyrode solution for 30 min and then reinstalling it for 60 min. Aprikalim (AP), a K⁺ channel opener ($0.1 \mu M$), and 90-s ischemia (PC, preconditioning stimulus) were applied singly or together (AP + PC) before starting the 30-min ischemic period. The effects of glibenclamide ($1 \mu M$) alone or preceding AP + PC were also assessed. The parameters measured were resting (RT) and developed (DT) tension, and the duration of the action potential at 50% repolarization (APD_{50}). In control, AP-, or PC-pretreated preparations, ischemia produced a similarly rapid decline of DT, no substantial elevation of RT, and a progressive shortening of APD_{50}. After 60-min reflow, DT remained depressed by 55%, RT increased by 45% (in the AP group, only 18%) and APD_{50} fully recovered its preischemia values. Glibenclamide reduced APD_{50} shortening without affecting the kinetics of contractility loss during ischemia. At the end of reperfusion, glibenclamide-pretreated preparations recovered their contractility slightly less than control preparations. The application of both AP and 90-s PC did not influence the effects of ischemia but reduced significantly (by ~30%) the postischemic depression of DT, as well as the increase in RT, at the end of reperfusion. Thus, combining a concentration of AP and a duration of ischemic stress, which delivered singly do not curtail ischemia/reperfusion injury, improved substantially the recovery of contractile function. This salutary effect was negated by glibenclamide. Thus, activation of ATP-sensitive K⁺ channels mediates this protection independently of an acceleration of contractile failure at the onset of ischemia. In conclusion, the opening of ATP-sensitive K⁺ channels may constitute a natural mechanism by which the myocardium, if it is preconditioned by ischemia or by pharmacological agents, can be protected against the deleterious consequence of a prolonged ischemic insult.

[1] Rhône-Poulenc Rorer, Pharmaceutical Research Vitry-Alfortville Research Center, 94403 Vitry-sur-Seine, France
[2] Department of Pharmacology, University of Illinois, Medical Center, 835 South Wolcott Avenue, Chicago, IL 60612-7343, USA

Key words. Cardioprotection—Action potential duration—Aprikalim—ATP-Sensitive K+ channels—Ischemic preconditioning—Glibenclamide

Introduction

Cardiac myocytes have a high rate of energy turnover, which allows them to fulfill their main function, the development of mechanical work necessary to deliver blood flow to each body tissue. This metabolic feature renders the heart extremely dependent on oxygen, an essential substrate for the efficient biosynthesis of high-energy phosphates. Ischemic insults, even of brief duration, thus trigger a chain of events encompassing the contractile, electrical, and metabolic function of the heart [1-3]. First, developed contractile tension rapidly declines to become virtually nil within 15 min after oxygen deprivation. This effect is accompanied by electrical dysfunction, which at the single myocyte level consists mainly of a progressive shortening of the action potential. This action potential shortening, which is attributed to the activation of outward K+ currents, leads ultimately to the disappearance of the Ca^{2+}-dependent plateau phase of the action potential. If ischemia persists for more than 20 min, diastolic tension starts to rise slowly and ischemic contracture occurs. The failure of the ischemic myocardium to maintain its normal relaxed state is a warning that the energy stores necessary for preserving myocyte viability are dropping to critical levels and, in the absence of rapid reoxygenation, the biological integrity of the cell is being jeopardized.

The prominence of ischemic heart disease in developed countries has triggered research efforts addressed at understanding the effects of ischemia on the cardiac myocyte. Concurrently, means to reduce or prevent the outcome of ischemia have been searched and proposed because this condition is not always the outcome of a pathological event, often, it is unavoidably associated with current surgical procedures such as percutaneous transluminal coronary angioplasty or cardiopulmonary bypass for cardiac valve replacement, large vessel repair, or heart transplantation. Therefore, a real need exists for identifying therapeutic means for enhancing or prolonging the tolerance of discrete myocardial regions or the entire heart against transient periods of oxygen deprivation so that recovery of function can ensue smoothly and rapidly at reoxygenation.

A characteristic response of cardiac myocytes to ischemia is the activation of plasmalemma K+ channels. These adenosine triphosphate- (ATP-) sensitive potassium (K_{ATP}) channels are gated by the metabolic state of the cell (ATP/ADP [adenosine diphosphate] ratio) and are probably not operational at all in the healthy myocardium [4,5]. Since the discovery of the K_{ATP} channel more than 10 years ago, this channel has been the subject of great interest, concerning first its possible physiological function, then its pharmacological manipulation with openers such as aprikalim or blockers such as glibenclamide [6], and more recently, its involvement in cardioprotection.

The term ischemic preconditioning refers to the endogenous capacity of the cardiac myocyte to rapidly adapt to, and enhance its resistance to, oxygen deficit. The physiological signals that activate this mechanism are one or more brief ischemic episodes followed by reperfusion. These signals appear to drive the cardiac myocyte into an emergency metabolic state such that the onset and the extent of electromechanical disturbances and necrotic lesions produced by a subsequent prolonged period of ischemia are attenuated and delayed [7,8]. The opening of K_{ATP} channels on cardiac myocytes appears to mediate the remarkable cardioprotective effects of ischemic preconditioning in dogs, rabbits, pigs, guinea pigs, and humans [9–12].

This investigation was designed to verify whether effective cardiac preconditioning could be obtained by combining a subthreshold concentration of the K^+-channel opener aprikalim [6,12] with a subthreshold duration of ischemia, so that when delivered singly, these stimuli do not afford cardioprotection. Furthermore, the possible involvement of ATP-sensitive K^+ channels in the results obtained was also determined by using glibenclamide, a specific blocker of these channels. The preparation selected for these studies was the guinea pig right-ventricular wall, which was perfused under in vitro conditions through the cannulated right coronary artery. A consistent ischemia/reperfusion injury is easily produced on contractile and electrophysiological parameters by suspending temporarily the delivery of the perfusion fluid to the tissue [13].

Methods and Materials

Guinea pigs (Hartley strain) weighing 600–900 g were placed under ether anesthesia. The thorax was opened and the heart quickly excised and placed in freshly prepared Tyrode solution (composition in mM: NaCl 136; KCl 4, CaCl$_2$ 1.8; MgCl$_2$ 0.5; NaHCO$_3$ 24, NaH$_2$PO$_4$ 0.35; glucose 11.1; pH = 7.35), which was bubbled continuously with 95% O$_2$ and 5% CO$_2$ (Po$_2$ > 500 mmHg) and kept at room temperature (22°C). The right coronary artery was cannulated under a binocular microscope in less than 2 min and perfusion immediately begun (1.5 ml/min). If the cannulation took longer than 2 min, the preparation was discarded because it may have been ischemically preconditioned. Thereafter, the atria were removed. The right ventricle, dissected from the heart, was then, immersed in a 20-ml bath chamber and perfused with the foregoing solution thermoregulated at 35.5° ± 0.5°C.

The coronary flow (generally ~1.5 ml/min) was set to yield a perfusion pressure of 45 ± 5 mmHg, which was measured from a side-arm cannula located close to the tip of the catheter perfusing the coronary artery. The solution within the bath was the same as that used for perfusing the preparation and was renewed at a rate of 15 ml/min. To measure the contractile force, the apex of the ventricle was connected to a force-displacement transducer (Gould, model UC-2, Gould Electronique, Ballainvilliers, France) via a nylon thread; the base of the ventricle was pinned to the floor of the perfusion chamber (endocardium face down) with microsurgical needles. The ventricle was electrically paced (train of rectangular pulses at frequency 2 Hz, duration 2 ms, and intensity twice threshold amperage ~3–6 mA) through an insulated bipolar electrode. Developed tension (in milligrams) measured under isometric conditions was displayed on a polygraph (Gould 8000-s) after appropriate preamplification and amplification. Resting tension was adjusted throughout a 30- to 45-min stabilization period to values (generally 400–700 mg) that optimized developed tension.

The transmembrane action potential was determined by impaling epicardial myocytes with standard glass microelectrodes that were filled with 3M KCl (15–20 MΩ) and coupled to an amplifier (Biologic VF-180, Biologic, Claix, France) via Ag/AgCl wire. The analogic tracing of the action potential was displayed on a digital oscilloscope (Tektronic 5228, Tektronix, Les Ulis, France) and digitized with an A/D converter to calculate the values of the action potential duration measured at 50% of the repolarization phase (APD_{50}, ms). Resting tension (RT) and developed tension (DT) values were determined from the polygraph tracing.

After an appropriate initial stabilization period (30–45 min), four groups of preparations were perfused with a Tyrode solution containing the vehicle (VE_1) of glibenclamide for 10 min. Then, each of these groups was immediately perfused with Tyrode solution containing aprikalim (0.1 μM) or its vehicle (VE_2) for 10 min, followed by a 10-min washout, or subjected to a 90-s no-flow ischemia followed by 8.5 min of reflow (PC). Two additional groups of preparations were perfused with Tyrode solution containing glibenclamide (1 μM) for 10 min followed immediately by a 10-min perfusion with Tyrode solution containing the vehicle of aprikalim (VE_2) or aprikalim (0.1 μM) plus PC (Fig. 1). All these groups of preparations (n = 4–10) (except an additional series used to study the stability of the preparation in normoxic conditions) were exposed to 30-min no-flow ischemia after the foregoing treatments by arresting the delivery of the oxygenated Tyrode solution. During this ischemic period, the solution delivered to the bath chamber was bubbled with 95% N_2 and 5% CO_2.

At the end of the ischemic period, a 60-min reflow was initiated by gradually restoring perfusion flow so that perfusion pressure attained preischemia values at a rate of ~15 mmHg/min over 3 min. During the first 2 min of the reflow period, ventricular pacing was suspended to minimize the occurrence of reperfusion arrhythmias. Evidently, at the reflow, the solution superfusing the preparation was reoxygenated.

Analysis of Results

All results are reported as means ± standard error of the means (means ± SEM). The effects produced by each treatment at the end of the 30-min ischemia or 60-min reperfusion are given as absolute values or as percentages of absolute values measured immediately before initiating ischemia. The significance ($P < .05$) of responses between groups was assessed with a non-paired t-test.

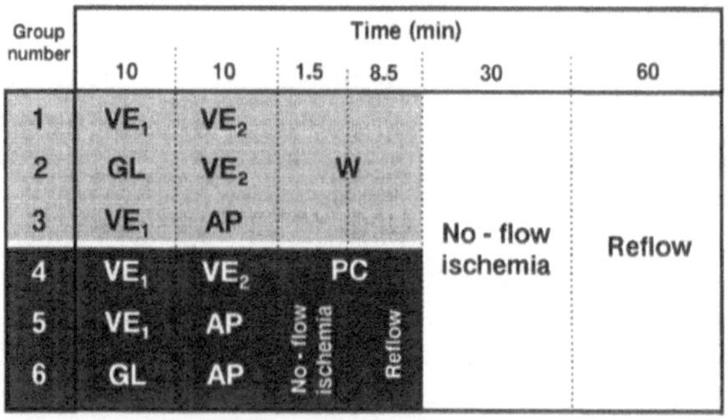

Group number	Time (min)					
	10	10	1.5	8.5	30	60
1	VE_1	VE_2				
2	GL	VE_2	W			
3	VE_1	AP			No - flow ischemia	Reflow
4	VE_1	VE_2	PC			
5	VE_1	AP	No - flow ischemia	Reflow		
6	GL	AP				

FIG. 1. Flowchart of the experimental procedure. Glibenclamide (*GL*) or its vehicle (*VE₁*) and aprikalim (*AP*) or its vehicle (*VE₂*) were added to the perfusion fluid. These treatments were perfused sequentially for 10 min and followed by 10-min reflow. Ischemic preconditioning (*PC*) consisted of a 1.5-min period of no-flow ischemia followed by reflow (8.5 min). *W*, washout period

Drugs

Aprikalim was initially dissolved in distilled water (8 mg/6 ml) under continuous sonication. Glibenclamide (4.9 mg) was initially dissolved in 0.2 ml NaOH (0.1 N) and then diluted under continuous sonication by the slow addition of distilled water (4.8 ml). Appropriate aliquots of these stock solutions were diluted with Tyrode solution.

Results

Effects of 90-min Perfusion with Oxygenated Tyrode Solution

The values of DT, RT, and APD_{50} in control guinea pig perfused right-ventricle preparations underwent minor fluctuations during a 90-min period of perfusion with oxygenated Tyrode solution (Fig. 2).

Effects of 30-Min No-Flow Ischemia and 60-Min Reflow in Vehicle-Pretreated Preparations

Application of 30-min no-flow ischemia was accompanied by a decline in developed contractile force that was of rapid onset. Indeed, after only 60 s of ischemia this parameter had already decreased by 37% ± 3% ($n = 10$) and became virtually nil 15–20 min after ischemia started. As soon as reflow was reinstalled, tension started to develop again. Most of the partial recovery in contractile function occurred during the initial 30 min of reflow, but this parameter remained substantially depressed 55% ± 1%, $n = 10$) below preischemia values at the end of the reflow period (Figs. 3 and 4).

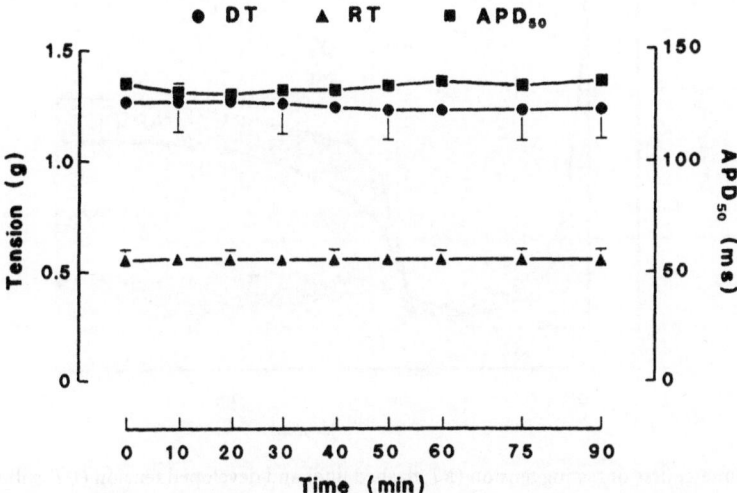

FIG. 2. Time-course of the developed tension (*DT*; circles), resting tension (*RT*; triangles), and duration of action potential at 50% of the repolarization phase (*APD*$_{50}$; squares) in guinea pig right-ventricular walls ($n=4$) during 90-min perfusion with oxygenated Tyrode solution. Results are reported as percentage changes from values measured immediately before starting ischemia

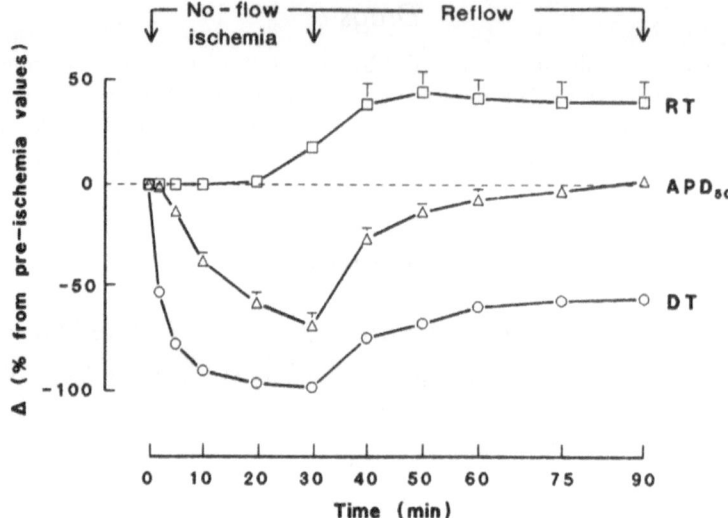

FIG. 3. Time-course of the resting tension (*RT, squares*), developed tension (*DT, circles*), and duration of action potential at 50% of the repolarization phase (*APD$_{50}$*, triangles) during 30-min no-flow ischemia and 60-min reflow in guinea pig right-ventricular walls (*n* = 10). Results are reported as percentage changes from values measured immediately before starting ischemia, which were 533 ± 29 mg, 1250 ± 120 mg, and 140 ± 3 ms for RT, DP, and APD$_{50}$, respectively. The effects on each parameter at the end of 30-min ischemia was a significant (*P* > .05, *t*-test) response. Similarly, at the end of reperfusion RT and DT were significantly changed

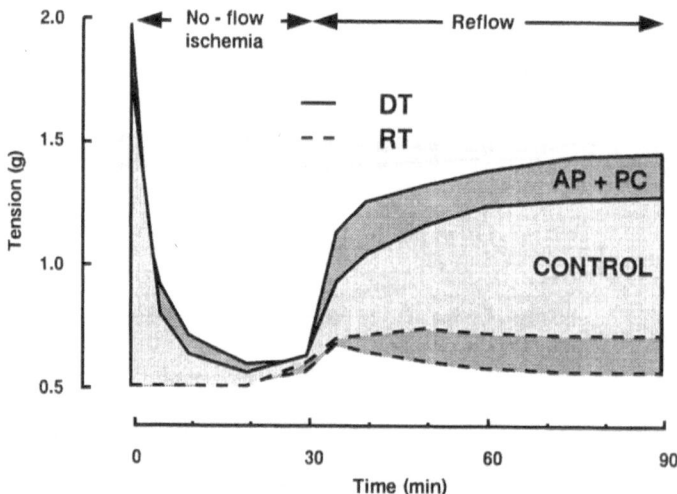

FIG. 4. Time-course of resting tension (*RT*, dashed line) and developed tension (*DT*, solid line) during 30-min no-flow ischemia and 60-min reflow in guinea pig right-ventricular walls either treated with the aprikalim solvent (control) (*n* = 10) or successively treated with aprikalim (0.1 μM) + 90-s ischemic preconditioning (*n* = 8). Standard errors on the points measured (each 5 min) were less than 5%

This means that contractile function recovered only 45% ± 1% of its preischemia values.

Resting tension did not undergo marked changes during the first 20 min of ischemia; during the subsequent 10 min, it increased slightly. This contracture increased maximally (54% ± 3% over preischemia values) during the initial 10 min of the reflow period and then subsided slightly (Figs. 3 and 4). APD_{50} started to decrease 3 min after the start of no-flow ischemia, when developed force was already depressed by more than 60%. This shortening attained a maximum at the end of 30-min ischemia. APD_{50} recovered entirely its preischemia values at the end of 60 min of reflow (Fig. 3).

Effects of 30-min No-Flow Ischemia and 60-min Reflow in Preparations Receiving Aprikalim and 90-s Ischemic Stress Singly or in Combination

A 10-min perfusion (followed by 10-min washout) of the guinea pig right-ventricular wall with oxygenated Tyrode solution containing a small concentration (0.1 μM) of aprikalim or the application of a 90-s no-flow period of ischemia followed by a short (8.5-min) reperfusion period (preconditioning stimulus) before ischemia did not

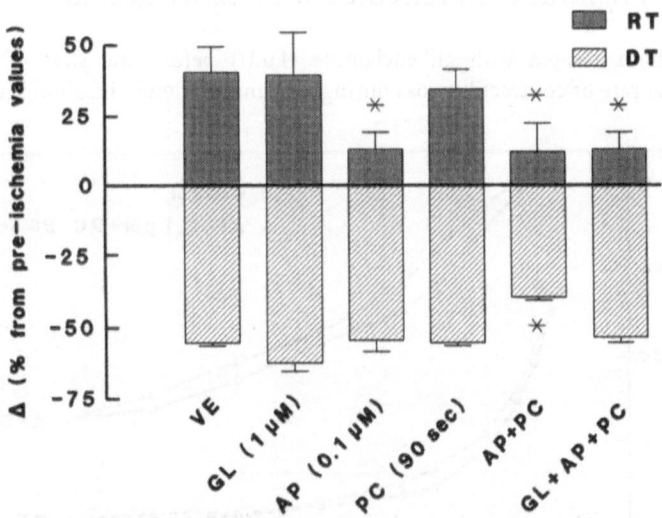

FIG. 5. Resting tension (RT, dark shading) and developed tension (DT, light hatching) values measured in the guinea pig right-ventricular wall ($n = 6$–10/group) at the end of a 60-min reflow period following a 30-min no-flow ischemia. The preparations were treated with the vehicles of glibenclamide and aprikalim (control group, VE), glibenclamide (GL), or aprikalim (AP, 0.1 μM), or were subjected to a 90-s ischemic insult followed by 8.5-min reflow (PC, preconditioning), or were successively treated with AP + PC before starting a 30-min ischemia followed by 60-min reflow. AP + PC were also studied in a group of preparations that were given glibenclamide. (For more details on the experimental procedure, see Fig. 1.) Asterisk indicates that the response is significantly different from that measured in the control group (VE). Preischemia values were similar for all group (DT, 1360 ± 90 mg; RP, 526 ± 10 mg; means of 6 individual group means)

modify the time-course of developed tension and APD_{50} during a 30-min ischemia and a 60-min reperfusion, as compared to control preparations. However, aprikalim $(0.1\,\mu M)$, but not 90-s ischemic preconditioning, curtailed significantly the increase in RT observed in control preparations (Figs. 4 and 5). When the two stimuli (aprikalim, $0.1\,\mu M$, and 90-s ischemic stress) were both applied sequentially to the same preparation before starting ischemia, the loss of contractile tension and the shortening of APD_{50} were not different from those produced by aprikalim, its vehicle (control), or the 90-s preconditioning stress applied singly before starting ischemic stress. Thus, the curves describing the time-course of the decrease in contractile force and of the shortening of APD_{50} during the 30-min ischemic period in vehicle (control) or aprikalim plus 90-s ischemic preconditioning-treated preparations were virtually identical (Fig. 6). However, in preparations that were treated with aprikalim plus 90-s preconditioning, DT was significantly less depressed than it was in control preparations or in preparations pretreated with aprikalim or PC along at the end of the 60-min reperfusion period (see Figs. 4 and 5). Furthermore, the combination of the two treatments curtailed the elevation in RT during reflow that was observed in control and 90-s preconditioned preparations (Figs. 4 and 5).

Effects of 30-min No-Flow Ischemia and 60-min Reflow in Preparations Pretreated with Glibenclamide

In preparations treated with glibenclamide $(1\,\mu M)$ before the start of no-flow ischemia, the rate of contractility loss during a 30-min ischemic insult did not differ

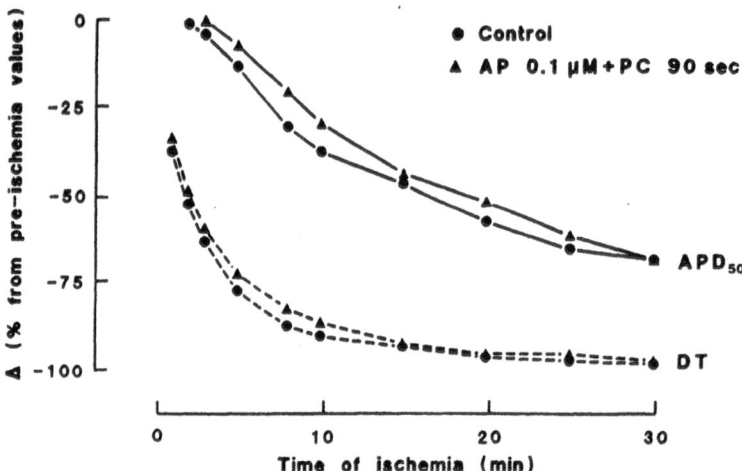

FIG. 6. Decreases in contractile force *(DT)* and in action potential duration *(APD_{50})* during 30-min no-flow ischemia in control *(n = 9)* guinea pig right-ventricular wall and in preparations pretreated with aprikalim $(0.1\,\mu M)$ for 10 min plus 90-s preconditioning stimulus *(PC)* before ischemia *(n = 8)*. Preischemia values were $1250 \pm 130\,g$ for the control group *(circles)* and $110 \pm 3\,ms$ for DT *(triangles, dashed line)* and ADP_{50} *(triangles, solid line)*, respectively; for the AP + PC-treated group, values were $1520 \pm 140\,g$ and $141 \pm 4\,ms$. No significant difference was detected for any time reading between control and AP $0.1\,\mu M$ + PC 90s for both DT and ADP_{50}

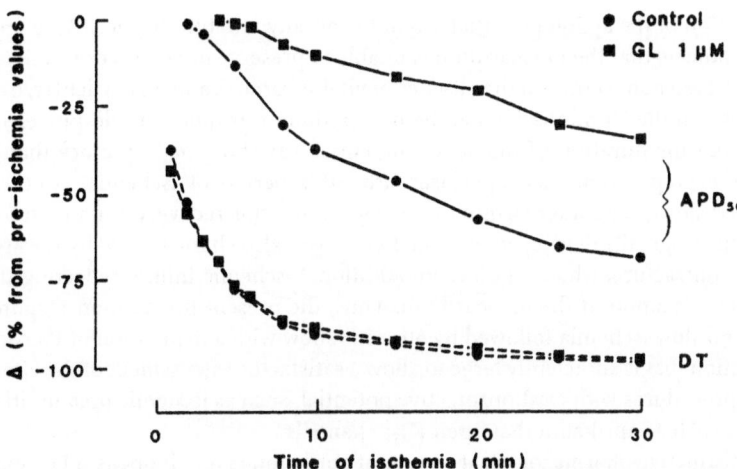

FIG. 7. Decreases in contractile force (*DT*) and in action potential duration (*APD$_{50}$*) during 30-min no-flow ischemia in control (*n* = 10) guinea pig right-ventricular wall and in preparations pretreated with glibenclamide (*GL*, 1 μM, (*squares*)) 10 min before ischemia (*n* = 8). Preischemia values were 1250 ± 130 g for the control group (*circles*) and 140 ± 3 ms for DT (*dashed lines*) and APD$_{50}$ (*solid lines*), respectively; for the GL-treated group they were 1480 ± 120 g and 140 ± 4 ms. No significant difference was detected for any time reading between the DT measured in control and GL-pretreated preparation; however, all the represented values for APD$_{50}$ after GL were significantly (*P* < .05, *t*-test) higher than in the control group

from that measured in control (vehicle-pretreated) preparations. However, in these preparations, shortening of APD$_{50}$ during ischemia was markedly reduced (Fig. 7). At the end of the 60-min reflow period, the developed contractile tension was slightly less than in matched control preparations. However, the increase in RT was of similar magnitude as measured in vehicle-treated preparations (Fig. 5).

Effects of Glibenclamide on the Cardioprotection Afforded by Applying Both Aprikalim and a 90-s Ischemic Stress

The improvement in the recovery of contractility during reperfusion found in preparations that received only the combined treatment of aprikalim and a 90-s ischemic period was not observed with preparations that had been pretreated with glibenclamide before combined treatment. However, glibenclamide did not modify the beneficial effects on resting tension produced by aprikalim and a brief ischemic period (see Fig. 5).

Discussion

Our in vitro guinea pig right ventricle, perfused with physiological salt solution through the cannulated right coronary artery, responded to a prolonged no-flow ischemic period with electromechanical alterations that consisted of a fall in contractility and a shortening in the duration of action potential measured with a microelectrode impaled in epiventricular myocytes. A significant degree of contractile failure (50%) occurred within the first 2 min after the start of no-flow ischemia. At this time, the duration of the action potential did not show any notable change. These findings clearly indicate that the myocardium is unable to preserve intact its contractile properties for even a short time in the absence of vital substrates and, in particular, oxygen. At the end of the 30-min ischemia, the myocardium was quiescent despite electrical pacing and the duration of the action potential was shortened by more than 60%. When the preparation was reperfused after this period of ischemia, contractility recovered slowly, and after 60 min of reoxygenation, this recovery amounted to only 45% of the originally developed tension. Reflow was also characterized by the appearance of contracture, which signifies an additional ischemic injury, reflecting the incomplete relaxation of the myocardium. Thus, the present preparation responds to 30-min no-flow ischemia followed by 60-min reflow with a depression of its contractile function that is sufficiently large to allow a satisfactory assessment of the effectiveness of procedures with cardioprotective potential, such as ischemic preconditioning or drugs such as aprikalim that open K_{ATP} channels.

The distinctive pharmacological feature of aprikalim is that it opens ATP-sensitive K^+ channels in vascular and cardiac muscle. By virtue of this property, aprikalim, at appropriate concentrations or doses, can produce vasorelaxation and enhance the resistance of the myocardium to oxygen deprivation in both in vitro and in vivo models of ischemia/reperfusion injury [6,12,14]. Indeed, in the in vitro perfused rat heart model, aprikalim improves the recovery of contractility at reperfusion and lessens the loss of intracellular lactate dehydrogenase caused by an ischemic stress [15]. Similarly, in vivo aprikalim accelerates the recovery of myocardial contractility after an appropriate ischemic insult producing sustained stunning [16] and reduces the extent of the necrotic region that is normally found in the canine heart subjected to a 60- to 90-min occlusion of a main coronary artery followed by a prolonged period of reperfusion [17]. In addition to these observations, we have already reported that a short 10-min perfusion of the in vitro perfused right ventricle of guinea pigs with 1 μM aprikalim 10 min before starting 30-min ischemia improves recovery of contractility (61% ± 2%, $n = 10$, of the preischemia value against 45% ± 1%, $n = 10$, in control) and attenuates substantially the elevation of resting tension at reperfusion [18].

The beneficial effects of aprikalim in these various animal models of ischemia/reperfusion injury were always prevented by the ATP-sensitive K^+-channel blocker glibenclamide [12,18]. This provides clear and strong pharmacological evidence that ATP-sensitive K^+ channels are either directly or indirectly involved in mediating the cardioprotective effects of aprikalim. This mechanism of cardioprotection is similar to that afforded by ischemic preconditioning in dogs, guinea pigs, and rabbits as well as humans [12]. Thus, our perfused guinea pig right ventricle, when preconditioned with 5-min no-flow ischemia, recovered its contractile activity (67% ± 2%, $n = 8$ of the preischemia value compared to 45% ± 1%, $n = 10$, in control) at the end of the 60-min reperfusion period significantly better than nonpreconditioned preparations [19]. Thus, this ischemic preconditioning stimulus afforded virtually the same degree of cardioprotection as did aprikalim perfused at 1 μM for 10 min before prolonged ischemia was initiated [19]. Pretreating the preparations with glibenclamide negated the cardioprotective effects of ischemic preconditioning [19].

Overall, these results strongly support the proposal that aprikalim and ischemic preconditioning share at least one obligatory cellular pathway for protecting the heart against ischemia, the opening of ATP-sensitive K^+ channels [6,9,10,12]. To confirm this, we tested whether the coapplication of two stimuli, namely aprikalim (0.1 μM) and ischemic preconditioning (90-s ischemia), chosen such that when delivered singly before a prolonged ischemia their intensity would not be sufficient to improve the recovery of contractile function, would together afford such a cardioprotection. Indeed, the application of both procedures sequentially provided a cardioprotective effect as great as that found with a sufficiently long preconditioning stimulus (5-min no-flow ischemia) or a sufficiently high concentration of aprikalim ($1\,\mu M$) [18,19]. Thus, in the guinea pig heart the cardioprotection afforded by these two distinct stimuli results from some endogenous mechanism that can drive the heart into an emergency metabolic state of enhanced resistance to ischemia/reperfusion injury.

Our results were directly confirmed by a recent study by Yao and Gross [20], who demonstrated that a brief activation of the cardiac K$_{ATP}$ channels with an intracoronary infusion of a low, noncardioprotective dose of the K$_{ATP}$-channel opener bimakalim sensitizes the mechanism of ischemic preconditioning. This small dose of bimakalim lowered the threshold of the heart for an effective preconditioning ischemia so that a 3-min coronary artery occlusion, which was insufficient to precondition intact hearts, markedly reduced infarct size to nearly the same extent as did preconditioning with 10 min of coronary artery occlusion followed by reperfusion in anesthetized dogs. Thus, under in vivo [20] and in vitro (our data) conditions, it is possible to effectively precondition the heart to better tolerate prolonged ischemia if a subthreshold duration of preconditioning ischemia is applied after a subthreshold dose of a K$^+$-channel opener.

We further provide experimental evidence, which was not presented by Yao and Gross [20], that it is the opening of ATP-sensitive channels that mediates the synergistic cardioprotection of a subthreshold concentration of a K$^+$-channel opener combined with a subthreshold duration of preconditioning ischemia. Indeed, glibenclamide pretreatment prevented this synergistic beneficial effect. Interestingly, the concentration of glibenclamide we used reduced the shortening of action potential duration, which normally takes place during a prolonged ischemia as a consequence of the opening of ATP-sensitive K$^+$ channels. This indicates that glibenclamide at the concentration studied exerted the desired pharmacological activity.

Noma [4] had postulated that the activation of K$_{ATP}$ channels and the associated decline in action potential duration would restrain Ca^{2+} influx through voltage-activated L-type Ca^{2+} channels. This, in turn, would reduce the free intracellular calcium concentration, which is necessary for the development of myocardial contractile activity. Thus, by inhibiting the mechanical activity of the heart, the opening of K$_{ATP}$ channels would, according to Noma [4], indirectly preserve part of the high-energy phosphate pools, thereby maintaining ionic homeostasis during ischemic stress, and prolong the biological integrity of the ischemic myocyte.

This appealing theory has been repeatedly advanced in recent years to explain the cardioprotective effects associated with the opening of K$_{ATP}$ channels by K$^+$-channel openers, as well as ischemic preconditioning, because it was indirectly supported by the observation that the cardioprotective effect of these procedures was often accompanied by an accelerated shortening of the action potential [9,13,21,22]. Nonetheless, an attentive examination of our time-courses of the loss of contractility and of the shortening of the action potential (which, to our knowledge, never has been done before) casts serious doubts on the argument of Noma [4] and its wide acceptance. Indeed, our heart preparations lost most of their contractility during the onset of ischemia at a time when the duration of the action potential was not yet substantially shortened.

It may be correctly argued that our measurement of the action potential on epiventricular cells does not reflect the electrical state of the inner myocardium, which contributes most to the development of contractile force and which probably suffers ischemic injury more rapidly than the epiventricular cells. Nonetheless, if the opening of K_{ATP} channels and the consequent shortening of the action potential were responsible for the initial marked loss of contractility during the first minutes of ischemia, then glibenclamide treatment, which delayed the ischemia-induced shortening of the action potential, should also have delayed mechanical failure at the onset of ischemia. However, this did not happen in our experiments (Fig. 5). In this context the recent results reported by Yao and Gross [22] are of particular interest. These authors demonstrated that bimakalim can reduce infarct size at a dose that does not accelerate the shortening of the action potential at the onset of prolonged ischemia.

On the basis of all these experimental observations, we conclude that the cardioprotection afforded by ischemic preconditioning and aprikalim against ischemia/reperfusion injury is not obligatorily linked to the saving of high-energy phosphates resulting from an accelerated mechanical failure at the onset of the ischemic stress. This conclusion, however, does not necessarily contradict the pharmacological evidence that the opening of K_{ATP} channels is a mechanism of cardioprotection. Indeed, our results support such a possibility, although we refute that the opening of K_{ATP} mediates the saving of high-energy phosphates via an accelerated loss of myocardial contractility at the onset of the ischemic insult.

Convincing experimental evidence is available showing that the ischemically [8,23] and pharmacologically [24] preconditioned heart uses less energy during a prolonged ischemic stress than the nonpreconditioned heart. Thus, ischemic preconditioning and K^+ channel openers, by virtue of the opening of cardiac K_{ATP} channels, drive the heart into a metabolic state that allows the running of basic cell survival processes more efficiently than normal. This enhances the tolerance of the heart against ischemia and, therefore, a pharmacologically or ischemically preconditioned heart can be expected to suffer quantitatively less ischemia/reperfusion injury than that of a nonpreconditioned heart. An evident corollary to this conclusion is that a preconditioned heart will withstand oxygen deprivation for a longer period than a nonpreconditioned heart.

Acknowledgments. The authors warmly thank Ms. Evelyne Chazot for her patient secretarial work, Ms. Nicole Massa and Mr. Jean-Michel Guillon for their expert preparation of the drawings and finally Dr. Karen Pepper for her professionalism in remarkably improving our style and Prof. Garrett Gross for his careful critical reading of the manuscript.

References

1. Allen DG, Orchard CH (1987) Myocardial contractile function during ischemia and hypoxia. Circ Res 60:153–168
2. Karmazyn M (1990) Ischemic and reperfusion injury in the heart. Cellular mechanisms and pharmacological interventions. Can J Physiol Pharmacol 69:719–730
3. Carmeliet E (1978) Cardiac transmembrane potentials and metabolism. Circ Res 42:577–587
4. Noma A (1983) ATP-regulated K^+ channels in cardiac muscle. Nature 305:147–148
5. Coetzee WA (1992) ATP-sensitive potassium channels and myocardial ischemia: why do they open? Cardiovasc Drug Ther 6:201–208
6. Escande D, Cavero I (1993) Potassium channel openers in the heart. In: Escande D, Standen N (eds) K^+ Channels in cardiovascular medicine. Springer-Verlag, Paris, pp 225–244

7. Murry CE, Jennings RB, Reimer KA (1986) Preconditioning with ischemia: a delay of lethal cell injury in ischemic myocardium. Circulation 74:1124–1136
8. Walker DM, Yellon DM (1992) Ischaemic preconditioning: from mechanisms to exploitation. Cardiovasc Res 26:734–739
9. Gross GJ, Yao Z, Auchampach JA (1994) Role of ATP-sensitive potassium channels in ischemic preconditioning. In: Przyklenk K, Kloner RA, Yellon DM (eds) Ischemic preconditioning and the concept of endogenous cardioprotection. Klewer Academic, Norwell, MS, pp 125–135
10. Paratt JR, Kane KA (1994) K$_{ATP}$ channels in ischaemic preconditioning. Cardiovasc Res 28:783–787
11. Tomai F, Crea F, Gaspardone A, Versaci F, De Paulis R, Penta de Peppo A, Chiariello L, Gioffrè PA (1994) Ischemic preconditioning during coronary angioplasty is prevented by glibenclamide, a selective ATP-sensitive K$^+$ channel blocker. Circulation 90:700–705
12. Cavero I, Djellas Y, Guillon JM (1995) Ischemic myocardial cell protection conferred by the opening of ATP-sensitive potassium channels. Cardiovasc Drug Ther 9 (suppl 2):245–255
13. Cole WC, McPherson CD, Sontag D (1991) ATP-regulated K$^+$ channels protect the myocardium against ischemia/reperfusion damage. Circ Res 69:571–581
14. Gross GJ, Auchampach JA (1992) Role of ATP-dependent potassium channels in myocardial ischaemia. Cardiovasc Res 26:1011–1016
15. Grover GJ, Dzwonczyk S, Sleph PG (1990) Reduction of ischemic damage in isolated rat hearts by the potassium channel opener RP 52891. Eur J Pharmacol 191:11–18
16. Auchampach JA, Maruyama M, Cavero I, Gross GJ (1992) Pharmacological evidence for a role of ATP-dependent potassium channels in myocardial stunning. Circulation 86:311–319
17. Auchampach JA, Cavero I, Gross GJ (1992) Nicorandil attenuates myocardial dysfunction associated with transient ischemia by opening ATP-dependent potassium channels. J Cardiovasc Pharmacol 20:765–771
18. Djellas Y, Mestre M, Cavero I (1993) Aprikalim protection against ischemic injury occurs with an accelerated decrease in action potential duration but not in myocardial contractility. Circulation 88:I-632 (Abstract)
19. Hecquet C, Mestre M, Cavero I (1994) Synergistic cardioprotective effect of a subthreshold concentration of aprikalim and a subthreshold ischemic preconditioning stress. Circulation 90:I-48 (Abstract)
20. Yao Z, Gross GJ (1994) Activation of ATP-sensitive potassium channels lowers threshold for ischemic preconditioning in dogs. Am J Physiol 267:H1888–H1894
21. Escande D, Cavero I (1992) K$^+$ channel openers and "natural" cardioprotection. Trends Pharmacol Sci 13:269–272
22. Yao Z, Gross GJ (1994) Effects of the K$_{ATP}$ channel opener bimakalim on coronary blood flow, monophasic action potential duration, and infarct size in dogs. Circulation 89:1769–1775
23. Murry CE, Richard VJ, Reimer KA, Jennings RB (1990) Ischemic preconditioning slows energy metabolism and delays ultrastructure damage during a sustained ischemic episode. Circ Res 66:913–931
24. Grover GJ, Newburger J, Sleph PG, Dzwonczyk, Taylor SC, Ahmed SZ, Atwal KS (1991) Cardioprotective effects of the potassium channel opener cromakalim: stereoselectivity and effects on myocardial adenine nucleotides. J Pharmacol Exp Ther 257:156–162

Regulation of Rundown and Reactivation of Cardiac ATP-Sensitive K⁺ Channels

MASAYASU HIRAOKA[1], TETSUSHI FURUKAWA[2], TOHRU SAWANOBORI[1], and TEIICHI YAMANE[1]

Summary. In inside-out patch recordings of guinea pig ventricular myocytes under ATP-free conditions, activity of the ATP-sensitive K⁺ channels (K_{ATP}) decreased with time (spontaneous rundown) or by application of Ca^{2+} (Ca^{2+}-induced rundown). Application of a phosphatase inhibitor, okadaic acid, did not influence rundown and its time-course. After rundown, K_{ATP} channels were reactivated by a short exposure to Mg-ATP and subsequent washout. Treatments of the patches with inhibitors of various serine or threonine protein kinases did not prevent the reactivation by Mg-ATP. ATP analogues that were not hydrolyzed or were only poorly hydrolyzable could not reactivate rundown channels. The degree of channel recovery was dependent on the duration and concentration of Mg-ATP exposure. Any products of hydrolysis by ATP or other nucleotide triphosphate were unable to reactivate rundown channels. Fluorescein 5-isothiocyanate (FITC), which has a high specificity for ATP and interacts with lysine residues of the nucleotide-binding site on various ATPases, inhibited K_{ATP}-channel activity. These results suggest that hydrolysis of ATP and its energy may be utilized for reactivation of rundown K_{ATP} channels, but protein phosphorylation by serine/threonine protein kinases appears not to be involved in channel reactivation.

Key words. ATP-Sensitive K⁺ channels (K_{ATP})—Rundown and reactivation of K_{ATP}—ATP hydrolysis—Ventricular myocytes—Mg-ATP

Introduction

The ATP-sensitive K⁺ channel (K_{ATP}) has the unique property that strong inhibition is provided by increased internal ATP; under ATP-free conditions, however, the channel activity decreases with time, a process known as rundown [1–7]. This rundown of channel activity is restored by a short exposure to Mg-ATP and its subsequent removal [5,7–9]. Therefore, for maintenance of channel activity of K_{ATP} to be in an operable state, the presence of ATP is required. The process of channel inhibition seems not to be mediated by ATP hydrolysis or phosphorylation, because both free ATP and Mg-ATP were equally effective for inhibition and nonhydrolyzable ATP

[1]Department of Cardiovascular Diseases and [2]Autonomic Physiology, Medical Research Institute, Tokyo Medical and Dental University, 1-5-45 Yushima, Bunkyo-ku, Tokyo 113, Japan

analogues could also be effective [1,5,7]. Reactivation of the rundown channel, however, could only be achieved by Mg-ATP, and nonhydrolyzable ATP analogues seemed not to replace the action of Mg-ATP [5,7-9]. This has led to the suggestion that Mg-dependent phosphorylation may be necessary to maintain K_{ATP} in an operative state, but neither direct evidence for supporting this explanation nor identification of a protein kinase involved in this process has been presented. Because K_{ATP} plays an important role for pathophysiological functions of the heart, clarification of the mechanism of the channel rundown and reactivation is essential for understanding its function and pathophysiological role.

Rundown and Reactivation of K_{ATP} in Ventricular Myocytes

When the internal face of an inside-out patch membrane of guinea pig ventricular myocytes was exposed to ATP-free conditions, the activity of K_{ATP} was fully activated initially but later gradually decreased with time ("rundown" of the channel activity). Time-course and degree of rundown varied among different patches. Most of our preparations completely lost their activity after 20-30 min in ATP-free conditions, but a short application of Mg-ATP to the internal side of the membrane patch induced a reactivation of the channel activity on removal of Mg-ATP. Application of divalent cations such as Ca^{2+}, or Mg^{2+} in relatively high concentrations, could also induce channel rundown [10-12]. We also demonstrated that internal Ca^{2+} greater than $10\,\mu M$ induced quick rundown, and Ca^{2+}-induced rundown channels were also reactivated by Mg-ATP [13,14].

Proteolytic treatment of the internal face of membranes could prevent or reverse spontaneous or Ca^{2+}-induced rundown [13,15], perhaps by cleaving the inactivation gate of K_{ATP} that is modulated by Ca^{2+}. Trypsin has also been shown to abolish the inhibitory action of sulfonylurea, glibenclamide [16]. Glibenclamide and Ca^{2+} may, therefore, modulate a common gating mechanism. Proteolytic modification of a channel protein or an associated unit does not abolish the inhibition of K_{ATP} by ATP [13,15]. These observations indicate that the channel gate for ATP inhibition is different from the second inactivating gate, which is also modulated by ATP.

Because replenishment of the channel activity by ATP could not be achieved by the free form of ATP or nonhydrolyzable ATP analogues, phosphorylation and dephosphorylation of channel proteins were suggested to be involved in the process of rundown and reactivation [5,8,9], although some questions have been posed as to this interpretation [11,12,17,18]. Therefore, we first tested the effects of inhibition of a protein phosphatase that might be present in the excised patches on rundown of channel activity. Application of the phosphatase inhibitor okadaic acid [19] to patches in ATP-free conditions, however, did not affect the time-course of rundown, nor did its pretreatment have any influence on rapid development of Ca^{2+}-induced rundown and subsequent reactivation (Fig. 1). Our observation was also confirmed in mouse skeletal muscle [20]. These results appear to contradict the idea that phosphatase and Ca^{2+} are involved in channel rundown. Several reports have shown that most divalent cations can induce channel rundown, with Ca^{2+} being most potent, followed by Mg^{2+} and Co^{2+} [10-12]. There are no known protein phosphatases to be activated by divalent cations, which is in accord with the interpretation that the dephosphorylation process may not be involved in rundown of K_{ATP} channels.

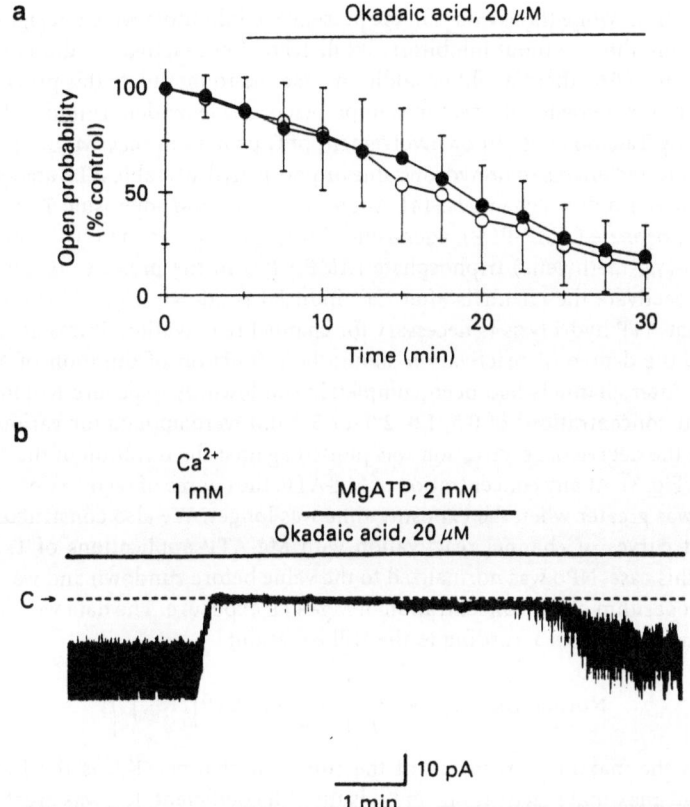

FIG. 1a,b. Effects of a protein phosphatase inhibitor, okadaic acid, on spontaneous- and Ca^{2+}-induced rundown of channel activity. a The probability of channel opening measured at −50 mV every 2.5 min after excision of membrane patch. Measurement was made from a 30-s recording; open probability was expressed as a percentage of the value immediately after excision. *Solid circles*, control ($n = 7$); *open circles*, in the presence of okadaic acid ($n = 4$). Application of okadaic acid did not affect the time-course of decline in channel open probability compared to that in the control. b In the presence of okadaic acid, superfusion of 1 mM Ca^{2+} induced quick and complete rundown of channel activity in 15 s; application of 2 mM Mg-ATP could restore channel activity. The concentration of free Ca^{2+} in the intracellular solution was 10^{-7} M in both a and b except during perfusion with 1 mM Ca^{2+} (b). (Reproduced from [13] with permission)

Reactivation of K$_{ATP}$ by Mg-ATP May Be Not Related to Channel Phosphorylation

To test the phosphorylation hypothesis for reactivation, we examined effects of inhibitors of various serine or threonine protein kinases on Ca^{2+}-induced rundown channel [14]. All the inhibitors tested (1 μM protein kinase inhibitor, 50 μM H8, 5 μM KT5720, 20 μM H7, 5 μM KN62, 20 μM W7, and 5 μM staurosporine), however, did not prevent reactivation of K$_{ATP}$ by Mg-ATP, compared to those in the control. Namely, compared to the channel open probability (NPo) before application of Ca^{2+} as 100%, its value after reactivation by Mg-ATP was 76% ± 14% in the absence of a protein kinase inhibitor, while these values in the presence of inhibitors were not significantly different from those without inhibitors. While NPo after reactivation did not reach a value close to 100%, there might be additional factors to modulate this process other than an Mg-ATP-dependent one; for example, excision-dependent rundown has been suggested by Takano et al. [9] or involvement of G protein in reactivation [21].

We next tested effects of nohydrolyzable or poorly hydrolyzable ATP analogues on reactivation of rundown channels [14]. Applications of 2 mM adenosine 5'-(β,γ-methylene) triphosphate (AMP-PCP), adenosine 5'-0-(3-thiotriphosphate)(ATPγS), or adenosine 5'-(γ,β-methylene) triphosphate (AMP-CPP) in the presence of 2 mM Mg^{2+} failed to reactivate the channels after Ca^{2+}-induced rundown (Fig. 2). These results suggest that ATP hydrolysis is necessary for channel reactivation. if this assumption is correct, the degree of reactivation should be a function of duration of Mg-ATP exposure. After channels had been completely rundown by exposure to 1 mM Ca^{2+}, Mg-ATP at concentrations of 0.5, 1.0, 2.0, or 5.0 mM were applied for various durations, and the degree of reactivation was plotted against the duration of the Mg-ATP exposure (Fig. 3). At any concentration of Mg-ATP, the degree of recovery of rundown channels was greater when the exposure time was longer. We also constructed dose-dependent curves of channel reactivation with Mg-ATP applications of 1, 2, 3, or 5 min. In this case, NPo was normalized to the value before rundown and was plotted against a logarithm of the concentration of Mg-ATP exposure. The data were fitted by a least-squares analysis according to the Hill equation:

$$\text{Normalized } NP_0 = a - a \Big/ \left\{ 1 + \left(\left[\text{Mg-ATP} \right] \Big/ K_{1/2} \right)^n \right\}$$

where a is the maximum recovery of the rundown channel, $K_{1/2}$ is the [Mg-ATP] causing half-maximal reactivation, and n is the Hill coefficient. $K_{1/2}$ was greater when the duration of Mg-ATP exposure was shorter, and the value of the Hill coefficient was smaller when the exposure time was shorter. Thus, the degree of channel reactivation by Mg-ATP seems to be a function of the duration of Mg-ATP exposure. Effects of various products of ATP hydrolysis [inorganic monophosphates (Pi), diphosphates (PPi), adenosine diphosphate (ADP), and adenosine monophosphate (AMP)] were examined as to whether they might reactivate rundown channels. All the products of ATP hydrolysis except a low concentration of ADP (100 μM), however, were shown to be ineffective for reactivation. In contrast to Mg-ATP, 100 μM ADP could reactivate the channel to a certain degree during its exposure but not after its washout. Therefore, reactivation of K$_{ATP}$ by Mg-ATP appears to be different from activation of the channel by a low concentration of ADP [22–24].

Specificity of ATP over Other Nucleotide Triphosphates on Reactivation of K$_{ATP}$

Specificity of ATP for reactivation of channels was tested by examining the effects of other nucleotide triphosphates on Ca^{2+}-induced rundown channels [14]. Application of 2 mM guanosine triphosphate (GTP), cytidine triphosphate (CTP), uridine triphosphate (UTP), inosine triphosphate (ITP), or deoxythymidine triphosphate dTTP in the presence of 2 mM Mg^{2+} could not reactivate rundown channels, indicating a high specificity of ATP for reactivation. Fluorescein 5-isothiocyanate (FITC) is known to react with the nucleotide-binding sites on various ATPases with a high specificity for

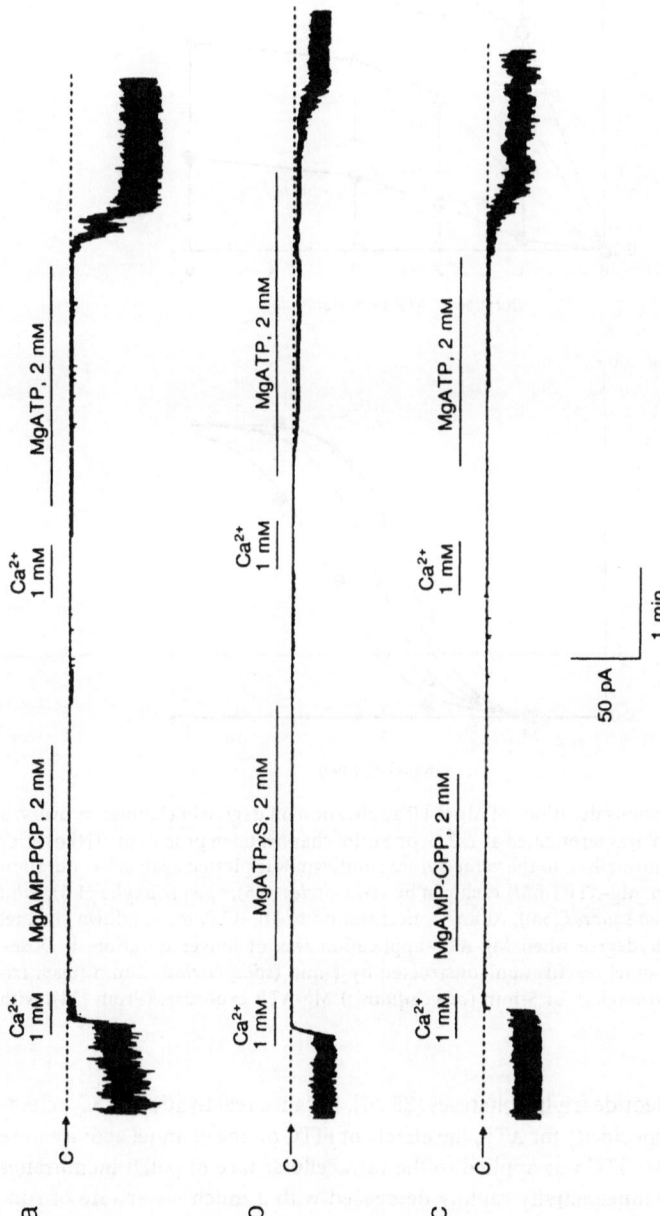

Fig. 2a–c. Effects of nonhydrolyzable or poorly hydrolyzable ATP analogues on reactivation of the rundown ATP-sensitive K^+ K_{ATP} channels. After complete rundown was induced by exposure to 1 mM Ca^{2+}, 2 mM Mg^{2+} plus 2 mM adenosine monophosphate-AMP-PCP (a), ATPγs (b), or AMP-CPP (c) was applied to the intracellular side of membrane patches for 3 min in the presence of Mg^{2+} and then washed out. None of these ATP analogues could reactivate rundown channels, but Mg-ATP could reactivate rundown channels almost completely (right side of each trace). (From [14], with permission)

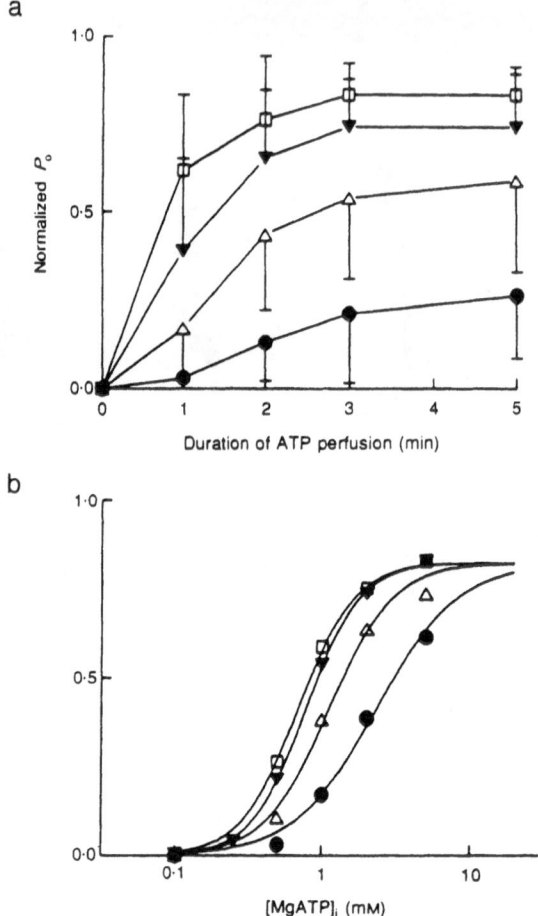

FIG. 3a,b. Effects of various durations of Mg-ATP application on degree of channel recovery. a Application of Mg-ATP was terminated at 1, 2, 3, or 5 min; channel open probability (NPo) after washout of Mg-ATP, normalized to the value before rundown, was plotted against the duration of Mg-ATP application. Mg-ATP (mM) is shown by *solid circles* (0.5); *open triangles* (1.0); *solid triangles* (2.0); and *open squares* (5.0). At any concentration of Mg-ATP, the rundown channel recovered to a greater degree when Mg-ATP application was of longer duration. b Dose–response curves of channel reactivation constructed by 1-min (*solid circles*), 2-min (*open triangles*), 3-min (*solid triangles*), or 5-mm (*open squares*) Mg-ATP exposure. (From [14], with permission)

ATP over other nucleotide triphosphatases [25,26]. Because reactivation of K_{ATP} channels showed a high specificity for ATP, the effects of FITC on the channel activity were studies. When 50 μM FITC was applied to the intracellular face of patch membranes before rundown, channel activity rapidly decreased with a much faster rate of rundown than that without FITC. Channel activity did not recover after washout of FITC, and reactivation by Mg-ATP was markedly reduced compared to the control. It has been shown that FITC reacts with the lysine residue of the nucleotide-binding sites on various ATPases with high specificity for ATP [25–28]. Our results may be interpreted that the binding of Mg-ATP to a site containing a lysine residue of the channel protein or associated unit plays a key role for reactivation, possibly through allosteric interaction. This binding site may not be related to the ATP-binding site for channel inhibition. Further studies are necessary for the clarification of this assumption with structural confirmation of K_{ATP} channels.

Possible Mechanism for Reactivation of K_{ATP} by Mg-ATP

The possible involvement of ATP hydrolysis in channel recovery suggests at least three possible models: (a) one or more ATP hydrolysis products are directly responsible for reactivation; (b) hydrolysis energy may cause conformational changes of the channel protein, resulting in the removal of the Ca^{2+}-induced channel inhibition; and (c) the phosphorylation of a target protein is responsible for the removal of the Ca^{2+}-induced inhibition. The results described here rule out the first possibility. Although our findings are based on indirect proofs and might provide circumstantial evidence, they can reasonably be interpreted that phosphorylation, at least through serine/threonine protein kinases, is not involved in reactivation of K_{ATP} channels. Thus, the third possibility may be excluded. Although our studies do not explain the detailed mechanism of action of the involvement of ATP hydrolysis in channel reactivation, hydrolysis energy may be utilized for this process. In line with this explanation, one attractive hypothesis is attributed to the process of cytoskeletal assembly, which has also been shown to require ATP hydrolysis [29,30]. Evidence has been presented that various ion channels are regulated by the cytoskeleton [31–34], and certain treatments such as removal of ATP and the presence of micromolar or higher Ca^{2+}, which cause rundown of K_{ATP}, are known to sever cytoskeletal filaments [35,36]. Our preliminary and ongoing experiments gave favorable results for the involvement of the actin filament assembly in reactivation. Further studies are necessary for clarification of this important question.

Acknowledgment. This work was supported by a Grant-in-Aid from the Ministry of Education, Science and Culture of Japan to M.H.

References

1. Noma A (1983) ATP-Regulated K+ channels in cardiac muscle. Nature 305:147–148
2. Trube G, Heschler J (1984) Inward rectifying channels in isolated patches of the heart cell membrane: ATP-dependence and comparison with cell-attached patches. Pflügers Arch 401:178–184
3. Kakei M, Noma A, Shibasaki T (1985) Properties of adenosine-triphosphate-regulated potassium channels in guinea-pig ventricular cells. J Physiol (Lond) 363:441–462
4. Findlay I, Dunne MJ, Petersen OH (1985) ATP-sensitive inward rectifier and voltage- and calcium-activated K+ channels in cultured pancreatic islet cells. J Membr Biol 88:165–172
5. Ohno-Shosaku T, Zünkler BJ, Trube G (1987) Dual effects of ATP on K+ currents of mouse pancreatic β-cells. Pflügers Arch 408:133–138
6. Spruce AE, Standen NB, Stanfield PR (1987) Studies of the unitary properties of adenosine-5'-triphosphate-regulated potassium channels of frog skeletal muscle. J Physiol (Lond) 382:213–236
7. Ashcroft FM (1988) Adenosine 5'-triphosphate-sensitive potassium channels. Annu Rev Neurosci 11:97–118

8. Findlay I, Dunne MJ (1986) ATP maintains ATP-inhibited channels in an operational state. Pflügers Arch 407:238–240

9. Takano M, Qin D, Noma A (1990) ATP-dependent decay and recovery of K⁺ channels in guinea pig cardiac myocytes. Am J Physiol 258:H45–H50

10. Findlay I (1987) ATP-sensitive K⁺ channels in rat ventricular myocytes are blocked and inactivated by internal divalent cations. Pflügers Arch 410:313–320

11. Findlay I (1988) Calcium-dependent inactivation of the ATP-sensitive K⁺ channel of rat ventricular myocytes. Biochim Biophys Acta 943:297–304

12. Kozlowski RZ, Ashford MLJ (1990) ATP-sensitive K⁺-channel run-down is Mg²⁺ dependent. Proc R Soc Lond B Biol Sci 240:397–410

13. Furukawa T, Fan Z, Sawanobori T, Hiraoka M (1993) Modification of the adenosine 5'-triphosphate-sensitive K⁺ channel by trypsin in guinea-pig ventricular myocytes. J Physiol (Lond) 466:707–726

14. Furukawa T, Virág L, Furukawa N, Sawanobori T, Hiraoka M (1994) Mechanism for reactivation of the ATP-sensitive K⁺ channel by MgATP complexes in guinea-pig ventricular myocytes. J Physiol (Lond) 479:95–107

15. Porks P, Ashcroft FM (1993) Modification of K–ATP channels in pancreatic β-cells by trypsin. Pflügers Arch 424:63–72

16. Nichols CG, Lopatin AN (1993) Trypsin and α-chymotrypsin abolish glibenclamide sensitivity of K_{ATP} channels in rat ventricular myocytes. Pflügers Arch 422:617–619

17. Albitz R, Kammermeier H, Nilius B (1990) Free energy of ATP-hydrolysis fails to affect ATP-dependent potassium channels in isolated mouse ventricular cells. J Mol Cell Cardiol 22:183–190

18. de Weille JR, Müller M, Lazdunski M (1992) Activation and inhibition of ATP-sensitive K⁺ channels by fluorescein derivatives. J Biol Chem 267:4557–4563

19. Bialojan C, Takai A (1988) Inhibitory effect of a marine-sponge toxin, okadaic acid, on protein phosphatases. Specificity and kinetics. Biochem J 256:283–290

20. Hussain M, Wareham AC (1994) Rundown and reactivation of ATP-sensitive potassium channels (K_{ATP}) in mouse skeletal muscle. J Membr Biol 141:257–265

21. Kirsch GE, Codina J, Birnbaumer L, Brown AM (1990) Coupling of ATP-sensitive K⁺-channels to A1 receptors by G-proteins in rat ventricular myocytes. Am J Physiol 259:H820–H826

22. Findlay I (1988) Effects of ADP upon the ATP-sensitive K⁺ channel in rat ventricular myocytes. J Membr Biol 101:83–92

23. Lederer WJ, Nichols CG (1989) Nucleotide modulation of the activity of rat heart ATP-sensitive K⁺ channels in isolated membrane patches. J Physiol (Lond) 419:193–211

24. Tung RT, Kurachi Y (1991) On the mechanism of nucleotide diphosphate activation of the ATP-sensitive K-channel in ventricular cell of guinea-pig. J Physiol (Lond) 437:239–256

25. Muallem S, Karlish SJD (1983) Catalytic and regulatory ATP-binding sites of the red cell Ca²⁺ pump studied by irreversible modification with fluorescein isothiocyanate. J Biol Chem 258:169–175

26. Abbott AJ, Amler E, Ball WJ Jr (1990) Immunochemical and spectroscopic characterization of two fluorescein 5'-isothiocyanate labelling sites on Na⁺, K⁺-ATPase. Biochemistry 30:1692–1701

27. Scott TL (1985) Distances between the functional sites of the $(Ca^{2+} + Mg^{2+})$-ATPase of sarcoplasmic reticulum. J Biol Chem 260:14421–14423

28. Farley RA, Faller LD (1985) The amino acid sequence of an active site peptide from the H,K-ATPase of gastric mucosa. J Biol Chem 260:3899–3901

29. Korn ED, Carlier MF, Pantaloni D (1987) Actin polymerization and ATP hydrolysis. Science 238:638–644

30. Stossel TP (1993) On the crawling of animal cells. Science 260:1086–1094

31. Cantiello HF, Stow JL, Prat AG, Ausiello DA (1991) Actin filaments regulate epithelial Na⁺ channel activity. Am J Physiol 261:C883–C888

32. Johnson BD, Byerly L (1993) A cytoskeletal mechanism for Ca²⁺ channel metabolic dependence and inactivation by intracellular Ca²⁺. Neuron 10:797–804

33. Galli A, DeFelice LJ (1994) Inactivation of L-type Ca channel in embryonic chick ventricle cell: dependence on the cytoskeletal agents colchicine and taxol. Biophys J 67:2296–2304

34. Wang WH, Cassola I, Giebisch G (1994) Involvement of actin cytoskeleton in modulation of apical K channel activity in rat collecting duct. Am J Physiol 267:F592–F598

35. Korn ED (1982) Actin polymerization and its regulation by proteins from nonmuscle cells. Physiol Rev 62:672–737

36. Janmey PA (1994) Phosphoinositides and calcium as regulators of cellular actin assembly and disassembly. Annu Rev Physiol 56:169–191

The Pharmacology of Potassium Channel Superfamilies: Modulation of K_{ATP} and BK_{Ca}

GILLIAN EDWARDS and ARTHUR H. WESTON

Summary. Two K-channel superfamilies, distinguished by the presence of either two or six transmembrane-spanning segments, respectively, in their pore-forming α-subunits, are now recognized. The pharmacology of the ATP-sensitive K channel (K_{ATP}), which is widely distributed in the cardiovascular system, is extensive and well studied. K_{ATP} is opened by a variety of agents, typified by levcromakalim, and inhibited by glibenclamide, although the mechanisms by which these and related drugs modulate K_{ATP} is not understood. Both in vitro and in vivo, most openers of K_{ATP} so far described are somewhat vascular selective, but selective agents that target other specific tissues or organs are under development. Pharmacological studies on the large-conductance, Ca-sensitive K channel (BK_{Ca}) are at a relatively early stage. This channel can be opened by agents such as dehydrosoyasaponin-1 and NS1619, and inhibited by alkaloids like penitrem A and the toxins charybdotoxin and iberiotoxin. Although in vivo studies with agents such as NS1619 are at an early stage, relatively few effects on the cardiovascular system have so far been reported.

Key words. Potassium channels—K_{ATP}—BK_{Ca}—Pharmacology—Tissue selectivity

Introduction

Potassium (K) channels form the most diverse group of known ion channels [1], and they are of critical importance in regulating the excitability of those cells which form the cardiovascular system. The generally high intracellular K concentration ($[K^+]_i$, approximately 150 mM) in smooth and cardiac muscle and in neurones contrasts with the typical extracellular concentration of this ion ($[K^+]_o$, 5 mM). Because the basal membrane potential of the cells of the cardiovascular system lies in the range −50 to −60 mV, the opening of K channels produces hyperpolarization toward −90 mV, the K equilibrium potential. For the past 10–15 years, attempts have been made to exploit these basic biophysical properties by developing synthetic molecules that can open K channels and induce a state of quiescence [2]. Such agents were originally relatively selective for the ATP-sensitive K channel (K_{ATP}) [2], but it is now possible to open the large-conductance Ca-sensitive K channel (BK_{Ca}) with a variety of molecules [3]. The purpose of this chapter is to overview these developments and to comment on their significance from the standpoint of possible therapeutic applications.

School of Biological Sciences, University of Manchester, Manchester M13 9PT, UK

K-Channel Structure

Much is now known about the structure of the pore-forming α-subunits of K channels. Injection of the nucleic acid sequences that encode these subunits into *Xenopus* oocytes or into mammalian cell lines results in the expression of functional K channels. Furthermore, the manner in which the protein is folded into the membrane has been predicted from hydrophobicity plots. On this basis, the major K-channel subtypes seem to fall into two main groups or superfamilies (Fig. 1), the pore-forming α-subunits of which constitute either six (superfamily 1) or two (superfamily 2) membrane-spanning regions, respectively [4,5]. In addition, a protein that induces a very slowly activating K current (I_{Kmin}) when expressed in *Xenopus* oocytes has also been identified. Presumably any resulting channel (K_{min}) is multimeric, but this bears no resemblance to other K-channel types. This protein may thus not form a channel itself but may rather act as an activator of endogenous (silent) channels [6].

Superfamily 1

This family comprises the voltage-sensitive K channels and includes the delayed rectifier K channels (K_V), A-type K channels (K_A), and BK_{Ca} [7–9]. The α-subunits for these channels probably consist of six membrane-spanning α-helical regions (S1–S6) joined by intracellular and extracellular linkers and with both *N*- and *C*-termini located intracellularly (see Fig. 1). Mutagenesis experiments have permitted the identification of those regions of the protein that are probably involved in the formation of the pore, composed of the membrane-dipping S5–S6 linker region (P) together with part of S6 and the S4–S5 linker. Similar experiments have identified the amino acid sequences that are important for ion selectivity, for calcium sensitivity, and particularly for the voltage-sensor region (S4).

Functional K channels are formed by the association of multiple (probably four) α-subunits, which may be the product of a single gene (forming a homomultimer) or of different genes from within the same family (heteromultimer). Thus a voltage-sensitive K channel could be formed by the association of a *Shaker*-related Kv1.1 protein with, for example, a *Shaker*-related Kv1.4 protein, but not with products of the *Shab* (Kv2.n), *Shaw* (Kv3.n), or *Shal* (Kv4.n) genes. The ability of the channel-forming α-subunits to associate as heteromultimeric complexes may be an indication that

---

→

FIG. 1. Typical features of the Ca-sensitive (BK_{Ca}) and ATP-sensitive (K_{ATP}) potassium (K) channels. *Upper panel*: current–voltage (I–V) relationships exhibited by whole-cell currents showing the typical outwardly rectifying characteristics of the current $I_{BK(Ca)}$ and the mild inwardly rectifying properties of the current $I_{K(ATP)}$. Note that the threshold potential for $I_{BK(Ca)}$ is usually positive of the potassium equilibrium potential, E_K. *Lower panels*: probable topology of the α- and β-subunits of BK_{Ca} and of K_{ATP} and its associated sulfonylurea receptor. Each α-subunit of BK_{Ca} comprises six α-helical, membrane-spanning segments (*rectangles*, S1–S6) with the voltage sensor at S4 (*black rectangle*). P, pore region. Four α-subunits probably combine in a tetramer to form a functional channel. Each α-subunit of BK_{Ca} is associated with a β-subunit that modifies channel gating properties. Each α-subunit of K_{ATP} is composed of only two membrane-spanning regions. As with BK_{Ca}, the functional arrangement is believed to be tetrameric. The sulfonylurea receptor shown is the 140-kDa glibenclamide-binding site with two nucleotide-binding folds (*NBF*), each containing one Walker A and one Walker B region. (From [4,5,7–10,14,16,17])

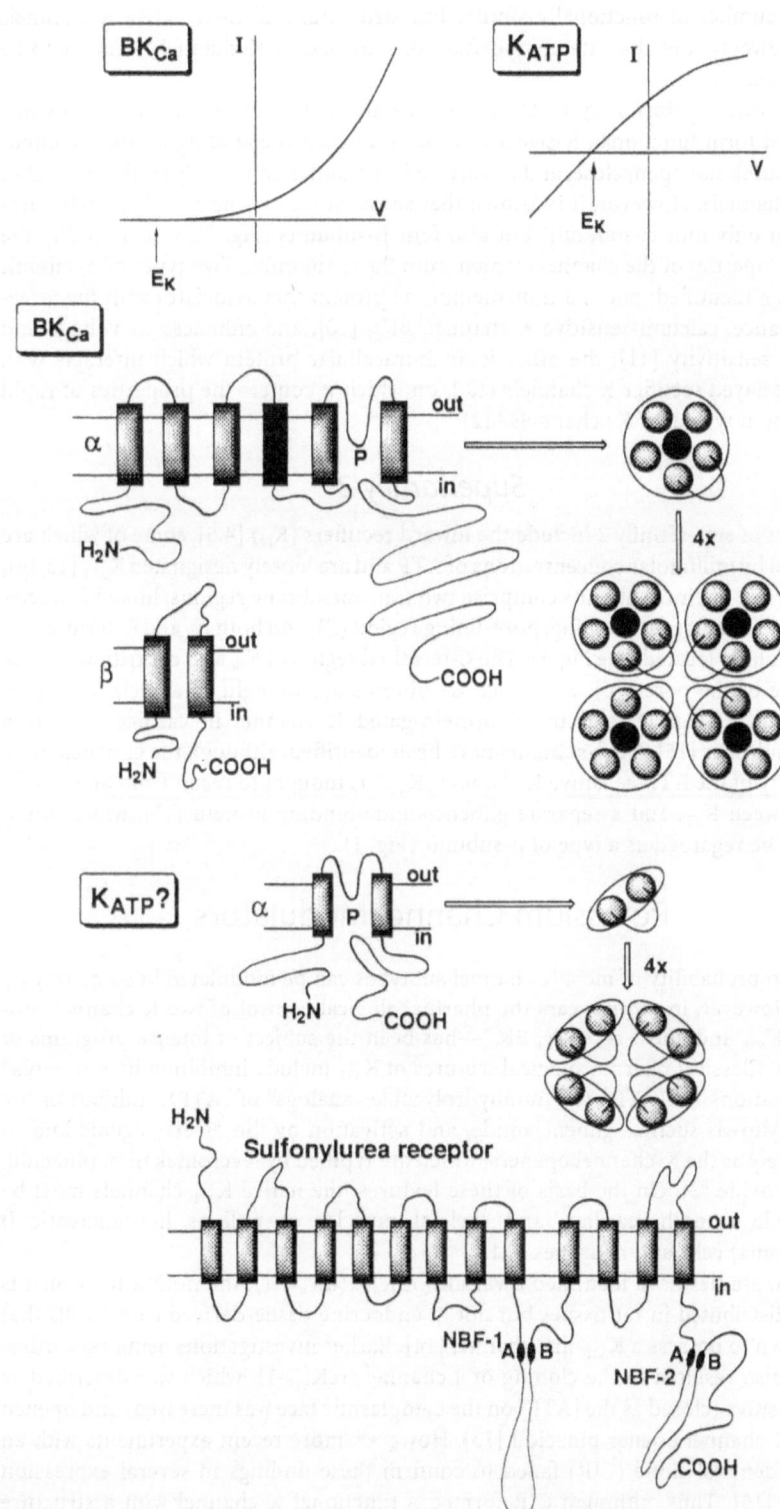

a large number of functionally similar but structurally distinct native K channels exist. However, the absolute composition of most native K channels remains to be established.

In various expression systems, the homo- and heterotetrameric complexes just described form functional, K-selective channels which (depending on their component α-subunits) open, close, and inactivate in a manner apparently similar to that of native channels. However, it is known that some native or wild-type channels comprise not only four α-subunits, but also four β-subunits (Fig. 1), which modify the gating properties of the channel formed from the α-subunits. Two types of β-subunit have been identified; one is a transmembrane protein that associates with the large-conductance, calcium-sensitive K channel, BK_{Ca} [10], and enhances its voltage and calcium sensitivity [11]; the other is an intracellular protein which interacts with cloned delayed rectifier K channels (K_V), on which it confers the properties of rapid inactivation typical of K_A channels [12].

Superfamily 2

Members of superfamily 2 include the inward rectifiers (K_{IR}) [4,5], some of which are inhibited by millimolar concentrations of ATP and are loosely designated K_{ATP} [13,14], but see [15]. Their α-subunits comprise two transmembrane regions, linked extracellularly by a membrane-dipping, pore-lining region (P), and both N- and C-termini are intracellularly located (see Fig. 1). The C-terminal region of K_{IR} also contributes to the structure of the pore [16]. Four such α-subunits are thought to associate to form the channels (Fig. 1), and the G-protein-gated K channel in cardiac atria is a heteromultimer [15]. No β-subunits have been identified, although the glibenclamide sensitivity of the ATP-sensitive K channel (K_{ATP}) is thought to result from an interaction between K_{ATP} and a separate glibenclamide-binding protein [17], which could perhaps be regarded as a type of β-subunit (Fig. 1).

Potassium Channel Modulators

The open probability of most K-channel subtypes can be modulated in some way by drugs. However, in recent years the pharmacological control of two K-channel subtypes—K_{ATP} and, most recently, BK_{Ca}—has been the subject of intense programs of research. Classical pharmacological features of K_{ATP} include inhibition by millimolar concentrations of ATP_i (or nonhydrolyzable analogs of ATP), inhibition by sulphonylureas such as glibenclamide, and activation by the diverse agents known collectively as the K-channel openers, which are typified by levcromakalim, pinacidil, and diazoxide [2]. On the basis of these features, the native K_{ATP} channels must be present in smooth, cardiac, and skeletal muscles as well as in pancreatic β (insulinoma) cells and neurones [2,18].

Recent studies have identified a variant of K_{ATP} (uK_{ATP}-1), the mRNA for which is widely distributed in rat tissues but not in endocrine tissue-derived clonal cells that are known to possess a K_{ATP}-like channel [14]. Earlier investigations using rat cardiac muscle also resulted in the cloning of a channel (rcK_{ATP}-1), which was described as ATP sensitive (closed as the [ATP] on the cytoplasmic face was increased) and opened by the K-channel opener pinacidil [13]. However, more recent experiments with an almost identical clone (CIR) failed to confirm these findings in several expression systems [15]. Thus, although CIR formed a functional K channel with a structure characteristic of superfamily 2, no evidence of "K_{ATP}-like" properties was obtained [15]. Such findings led Krapivinsky and co-workers [15] to conclude that the structure of K_{ATP} was still unknown.

Irrespective of this controversy, K_{ATP} is voltage- and calcium insensitive, and its unitary conductance is relatively low [2,18]. In contrast, BK_{Ca} is very sensitive to both voltage and calcium, its unitary conductance is high, and it belongs to superfamily 1 [8,9]. Thus K_{ATP} is "available" over the whole range of physiological potentials, but the open probability of BK_{Ca} is very low at potentials negative to $0\,mV$ unless $[Ca^{2+}]_i$ increases (see Fig. 1).

Openers of K_{ATP}

The identification, almost a decade ago, that the mechanoinhibitory effect of BRL 34915 (cromakalim, Fig. 2) could be attributed to the opening of a K channel [19] highlighted the potential usefulness of such a mechanism as a means of reducing cellular excitability. Although nicorandil (Fig. 2) was the first compound to be described with K-channel-opening properties, its pharmacology was complicated by the presence of a nitrate group that additionally endowed it with the properties of a nitrovasodilator [20,21]. Subsequently, diazoxide, minoxidil sulfate, and pinacidil, originally classed as hypotensive agents of unknown mechanism of action, were also identified as K-channel openers [2,22]. The general pharmacology of these agents has been comprehensively reviewed [2,22–24].

The majority of the K-channel openers available today are analogs of these early compounds. Their actions are usually inhibited by glibenclamide, from which it has been concluded that their target K channel is K_{ATP} [2,22], the regulation of which is discussed in the chapter by Hiraoka et al., this volume. Binding studies suggest that the K_{ATP}-channel openers may interact at a common site [25] (see also chapter by Quast et al., this volume), and the basic features of a pharmacophore characteristic of many synthetic openers of K_{ATP} have been proposed [26] (Fig. 2).

Role of Nucleoside Diphosphates

It has been known for some time that the nucleoside diphosphate, adenosine diphosphate (ADP), opposes the inhibitory effects of $[ATP]_i$ on K_{ATP}. Such an observation has led to the view that the open probability of K_{ATP} under physiological conditions is regulated by the $[ATP]_i : [ADP]_i$ ratio, rather than by a simple change in $[ATP]_i$ alone [2,18].

Recent studies using isolated cells from rabbit portal vein have led to the proposal [27] that K_{ATP} is, in fact, regulated physiologically by nucleoside diphosphates rather than by ATP. The basis of such a view was that inside-out membrane patches from the rabbit portal vein only showed openings of K_{ATP} when nucleoside diphosphates were present. Similarly, the K-channel opener pinacidil was relatively ineffective unless a nucleoside diphosphate was present [27]. Broadly similar observations have been previously reported using inside-out patches from cardiac muscle after K channels in the patches had been allowed to run down [28,29]. On the basis of these studies in cardiac muscle and of those using rat portal vein in which ATP- and K-channel opener-sensitive K currents could be obtained in the absence of nucleoside diphosphates [31,32], it seems possible that the cells isolated from the rabbit portal vein [27] were in a run-down condition, leading to the erroneous conclusion that K_{ATP} is primarily regulated by nucleoside diphosphates.

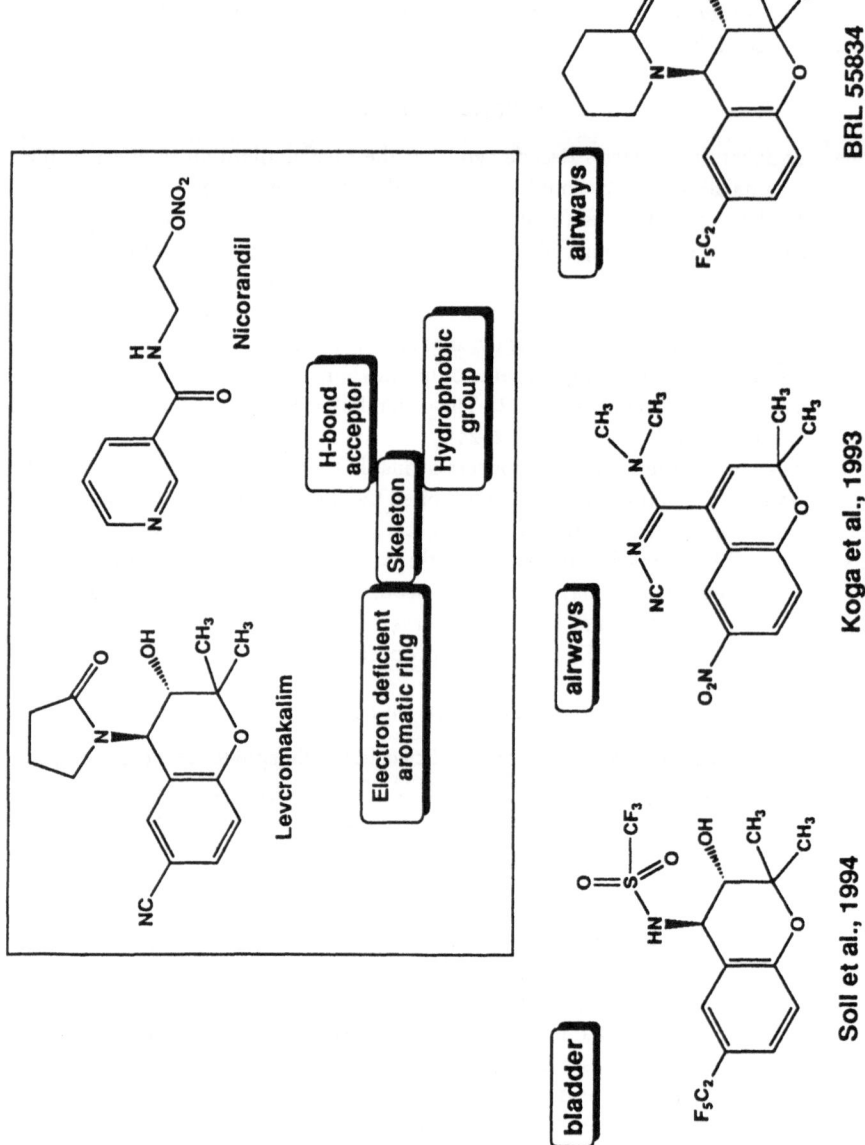

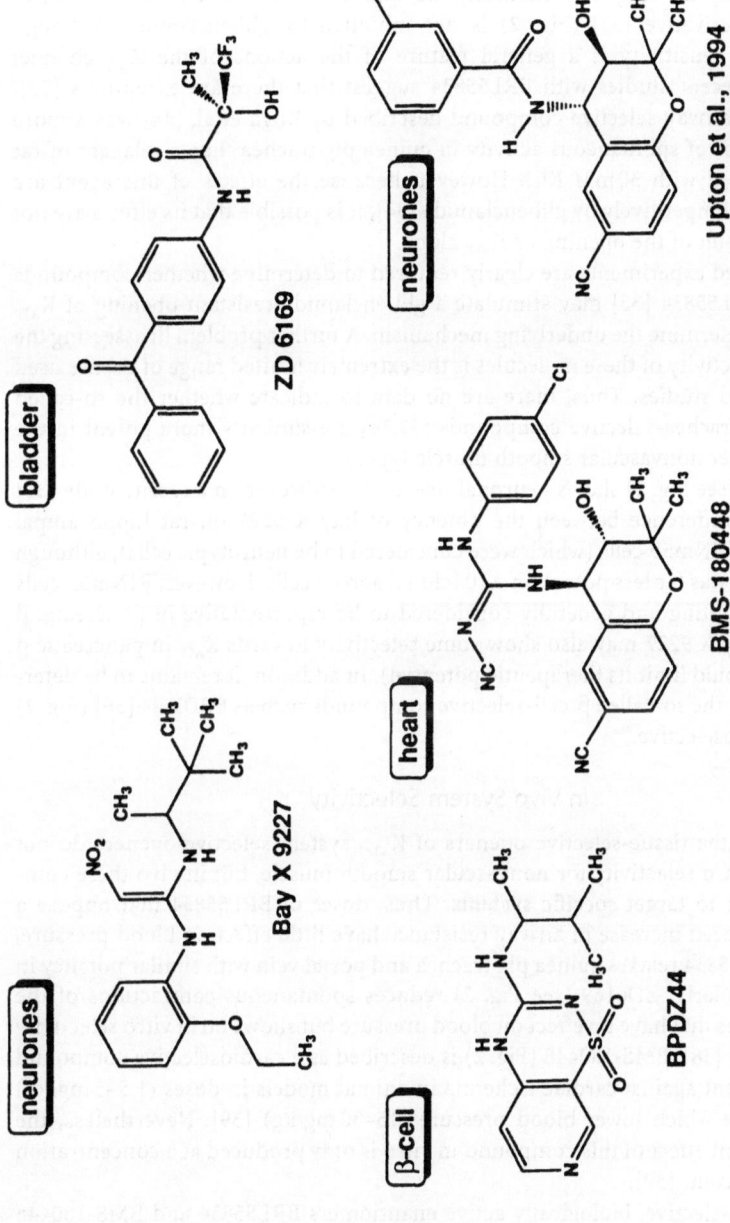

FIG. 2. Postulated basic pharmacophore for openers of K_{ATP} [42], together with structures of molecules with varying degrees of tissue and system selectivity

In Vitro Tissue-Selective K_{ATP}-Channel Openers

Most K-channel openers, typified by levcromakalim, the biologically active enantiomer of the racemate cromakalim (see Fig. 2), show some vascular selectivity in vitro
[22]. Although there are reports of tissue-selective compounds, data concerning these
are scarce and it is not certain whether their biological effects are achieved by
an action solely on K_{ATP}. For example, the relaxant effect of a bladder-selective
benzopyran derivative [33] (Fig. 2) is not inhibited by glibenclamide. Although
glibenclamide sensitivity is a general feature of the actions of the K_{ATP}-channel
openers [2], recent studies with BRL55834 suggest that there are exceptions [33].
Similarly, the airway-selective compound described by Koga et al. [34] was a more
potent inhibitor of spontaneous activity in guinea pig trachea than a relaxant of rat
aorta contracted with 30 mM KCl. However, because the effects of this agent are
inhibited noncompetitively by glibenclamide [34], it is possible that its effects are not
entirely the result of the opening of K_{ATP} alone.

More detailed experiments are clearly required to determine whether compounds
other than BRL55834 [33] may stimulate a glibenclamide-resistant opening of K_{ATP}
and, if so, to determine the underlying mechanism. A further problem in assessing the
true tissue selectivity of these molecules is the extremely limited range of tissues used
in the reported studies. Thus, there are no data to indicate whether the so-called
bladder- and trachea-selective compounds [32,34] are similarly more potent in the
heart or in other nonvascular smooth muscle types.

Bay X 9227 (see Fig. 2) shows neuronal selectivity. However, in a recent study [35]
there was no difference between the potency of Bay X 9227 on rat hippocampal
neurones and RINm5F cells (which were considered to be neurotypic cells), although
the compound was far less potent on A10 (clonal aortic) cells. However, RINm5F cells
are insulin secreting and generally considered to be representative of pancreatic β
cells. Thus, Bay X 9227 may also show some selectivity towards K_{ATP} in pancreatic β
cells (which would limit its therapeutic potential). In addition, it remains to be determined whether the so-called β-cell-selective compounds such as BPDZ 44 [36] (Fig. 2)
are also "neuroselective."

In Vivo System Selectivity

In contrast to the tissue-selective openers of K_{ATP}, system-selective openers do not
show any in vitro selectivity for nonvascular smooth muscle, but in vivo these compounds appear to target specific systems. Thus, doses of BRL55834 that oppose a
histamine-induced increase in airway resistance have little effect on blood pressure,
although BRL55834 relaxes guinea pig trachea and portal vein with similar potency in
vitro [37]. Similarly, ZD6169 (see Fig. 2) reduces spontaneous contractions of the
bladder in doses that have no effect on blood pressure but shows no in vitro selectivity
for the bladder [38]. BMS-180448 (Fig. 2) is described as a cardioselective compound
that is protectant against cardiac ischemia in animal models in doses (1.5–3 mg/kg)
less than those which lower blood pressure (15–30 mg/kg) [39]. Nevertheless, the
cardioprotectant effect of this compound in vitro is only produced at a concentration
that is vasorelaxant [39].

The system-selective, biologically active enantiomers BRL55834 and BMS-180448
possess the 3S,4R configuration of levcromakalim, and relatively little biological activity is associated with the corresponding 3R,4S enantiomers for each of these three

agents. Surprisingly, although the 3S,4R configuration of fluorobenzoylamino benzopyran recently described by Upton and co-workers [40] is a hypotensive agent, oral administration of the 3R,4S enantiomer increases the maximal electroshock seizure threshold in mice at a dose (10 mg/kg) that has no effect on rat blood pressure [40].

The basis for the in vivo system selectivity in the absence of in vitro tissue selectivity remains to be established. Although it is assumed that such a property may have a pharmacokinetic basis, other factors may be important, and in some instances the glibenclamide sensitivity of reported system-selective effects is unknown.

Inhibitors of K_{ATP}

The sulfonylureas, typified by glibenclamide (Fig. 3), are hypoglycemic agents that stimulate insulin secretion by a complex mechanism which may include stimulation of the glycolytic pathway as well as the inhibition of K_{ATP} in pancreatic β cells [2]. Lack of inhibition by glibenclamide is usually taken to indicate that K_{ATP} is not involved. However, the recent finding that the effects of the benzopyran BRL55834 are partially glibenclamide resistant, yet phentolamine sensitive, questions this belief [33] (Fig. 4).

Recent studies using photo-affinity labeling have identified a membrane-bound sulfonylurea (SU) binding site with an M_r of 140 kDa [17]. The topology of this site (see Fig. 1) shows it to be a member of the ATP-binding cassette superfamily [41], members of which are transporters. This raises the distinct possibility that agents like glibenclamide which bind to the SU receptor inhibit K_{ATP} indirectly by modifying the transport of some endogenous substance that normally functions to modulate K_{ATP}. The possibility that this substance effectively increases the intracellular ATP concentration, $[ATP_i]$, in the vicinity of the channel and that this might contribute to its inhibitory effect on K_{ATP} should not be overlooked. The finding that glibenclamide loses its ability to inhibit K_{ATP} under certain conditions of metabolic inhibition [42] would support such an indirect inhibitory effect.

Several SU binding sites exist [43], and the location of the 140-kDa unit [17] seems to be on an intracellular organelle [44]. As modification of the 140-kDa receptor in humans leads to a defined medical condition (familial persistent hyperinsulinemic hypoglycemia of infancy) [45], this receptor clearly plays a role in modulating glycemia. However, whether it is the only such site with this function remains to be established.

Benzoic acid derivatives of glibenclamide, such as meglitinide and AZ-DF 265 (Fig. 3), both of which lack the sulfonylurea moiety, are also capable of inhibiting K_{ATP} and stimulating insulin secretion [2]. Because there are no reports of such agents modifying glycolysis, it is possible that these act by a mechanism that does not involve increased ATP synthesis. Further experiments are required to determine their effects on K_{ATP} in the presence of metabolic inhibitors.

Two inhibitors of K_{ATP} that exhibit tissue selectivity are 5-hydroxydecanoate and ZM181,037 (see Fig. 3). The former appears to inhibit only K_{ATP}, and in cardiac muscle it has a preference for ischemic tissue [46]. In contrast, ZM181,037 antagonizes the stimulatory effects of cromakalim on ^{86}Rb efflux in rat detrusor and portal vein without increasing plasma glucose in vivo [47].

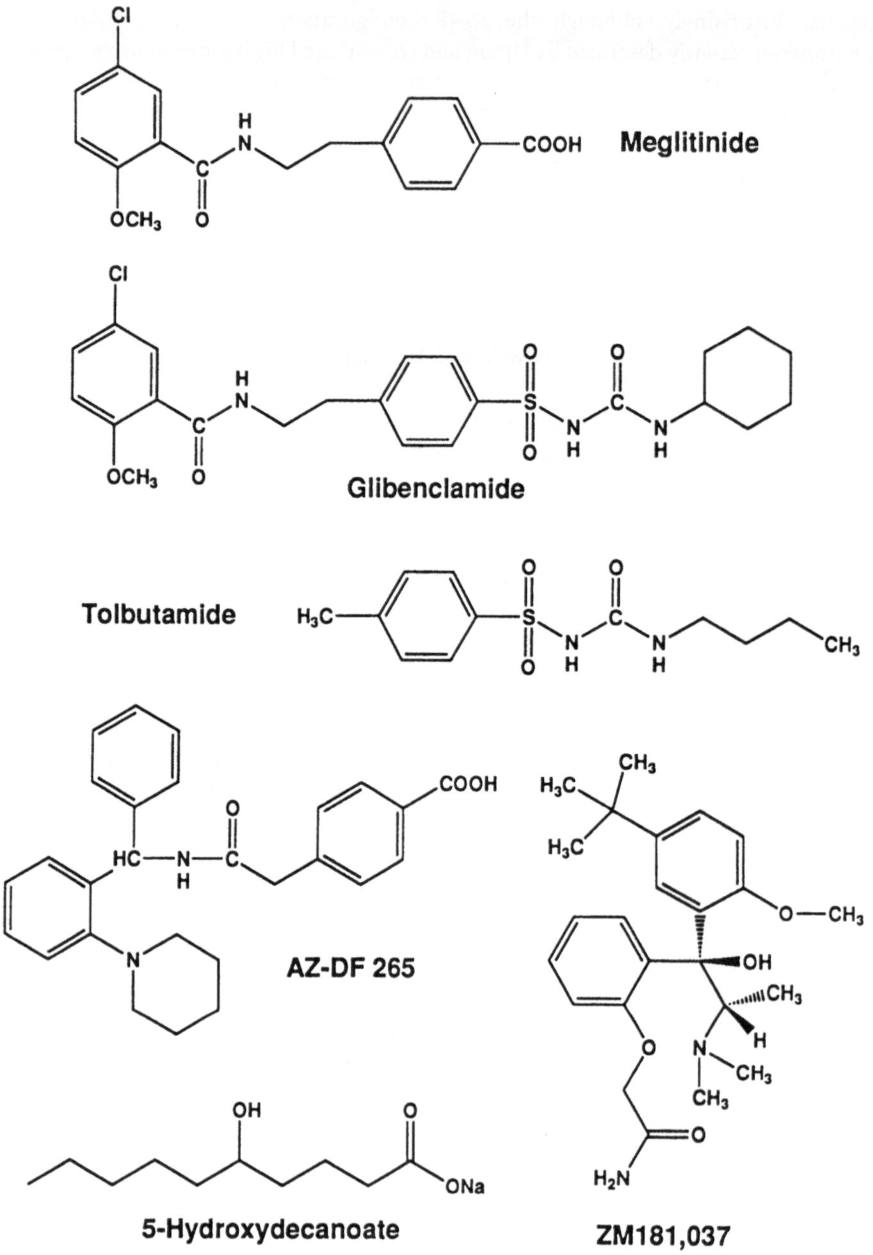

FIG. 3. Chemical structures of inhibitors of K_{ATP}

Openers of BK_{Ca}

Several compounds capable of opening BK_{Ca} have now been described (Fig. 5), but there are few data concerning the in vivo effects of such agents. BK_{Ca} is found in virtually all tissues, and because of its large conductance, the opening of just a few of these channels in cells could produce very marked hyperpolarization. However, the

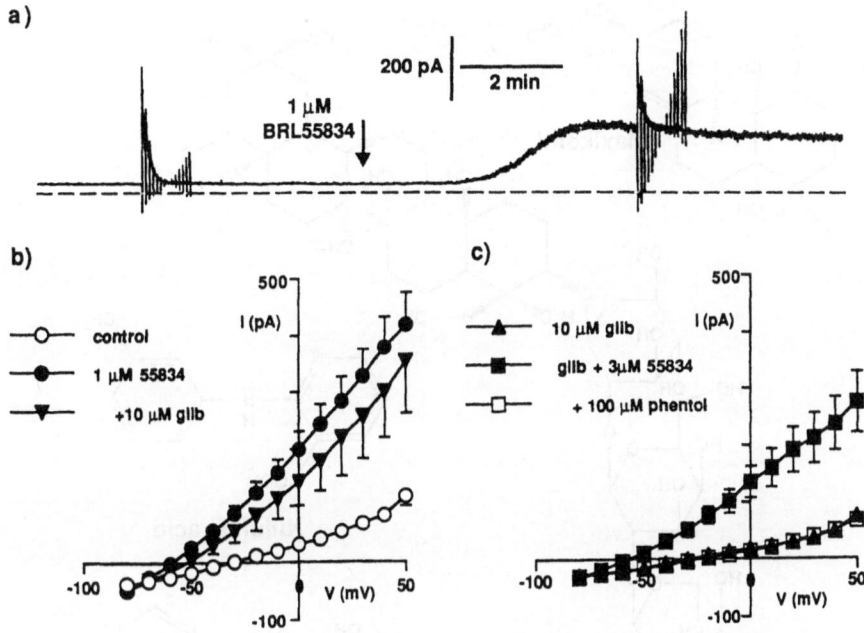

FIG. 4a–c. Glibenclamide-resistant effects of the K_{ATP} opener BRL55834. **a,** In a freshly isolated portal vein cell held at $-10\,mV$ under voltage-clamp conditions, exposure to BRL55834 ($1\,\mu M$) generated a typical noisy increase in current at the holding potential. Stepping protocols (from $-80\,mV$ to $+50\,mV$) elicited before and during exposure to BRL55834 show the characteristics of the induced current; **b** and **c,** mean current–voltage (I–V) relationships obtained from five cells under different conditions. In **b,** the BRL55834-induced current (*solid circles*) is largely resistant to subsequent exposure to glibenclamide (*triangles*) (*open circles,* control). In **c,** BRL55834 is still able to evoke substantial current even with prior exposure to glibenclamide (*solid squares*). However, subsequent exposure to the K_{ATP} inhibitor phentolamine (*open squares*) totally abolishes the effects of BRL55834, indicating that the channel opened by BRL55834 is K_{ATP}. *Dashed line,* zero current. (Adapted from [35] with permission)

threshold potential at which BK_{Ca} opens may vary in different tissues. Thus BK_{Ca} is thought to play a more important role in determining the resting membrane potential of nonvascular smooth muscle (e.g., trachealis and bladder) than of vascular smooth muscle [48,49]. Therefore, it seems feasible that BK_{Ca} openers could affect these tissues in concentrations that would have little effect on the normal vasculature. However, in pathological conditions associated with excessive smooth muscle contractility, such as irritable bowel, unstable bladder, and vasospastic angina, the $[Ca^{2+}]_i$ is likely to be greater than in normally active tissue. Such tissues could be rather sensitive to openers of BK_{Ca}, and thus the selective opening of BK_{Ca} might be relatively easy to achieve in spite of the ubiquity of the channel itself. Furthermore, BK_{Ca} may be important in regulating neurotransmitter release and thus openers of this channel may prove to be useful in the treatment of conditions associated with excessive neuronal discharge, such as epilepsy.

The NeuroSearch Series

NS004 (NeuroSearch, Glostrup, Denmark) opens the large-conductance Ca-sensitive K channel in GH_3 cells and channels expressed by the *Slo* gene in *Xenopus* oocytes

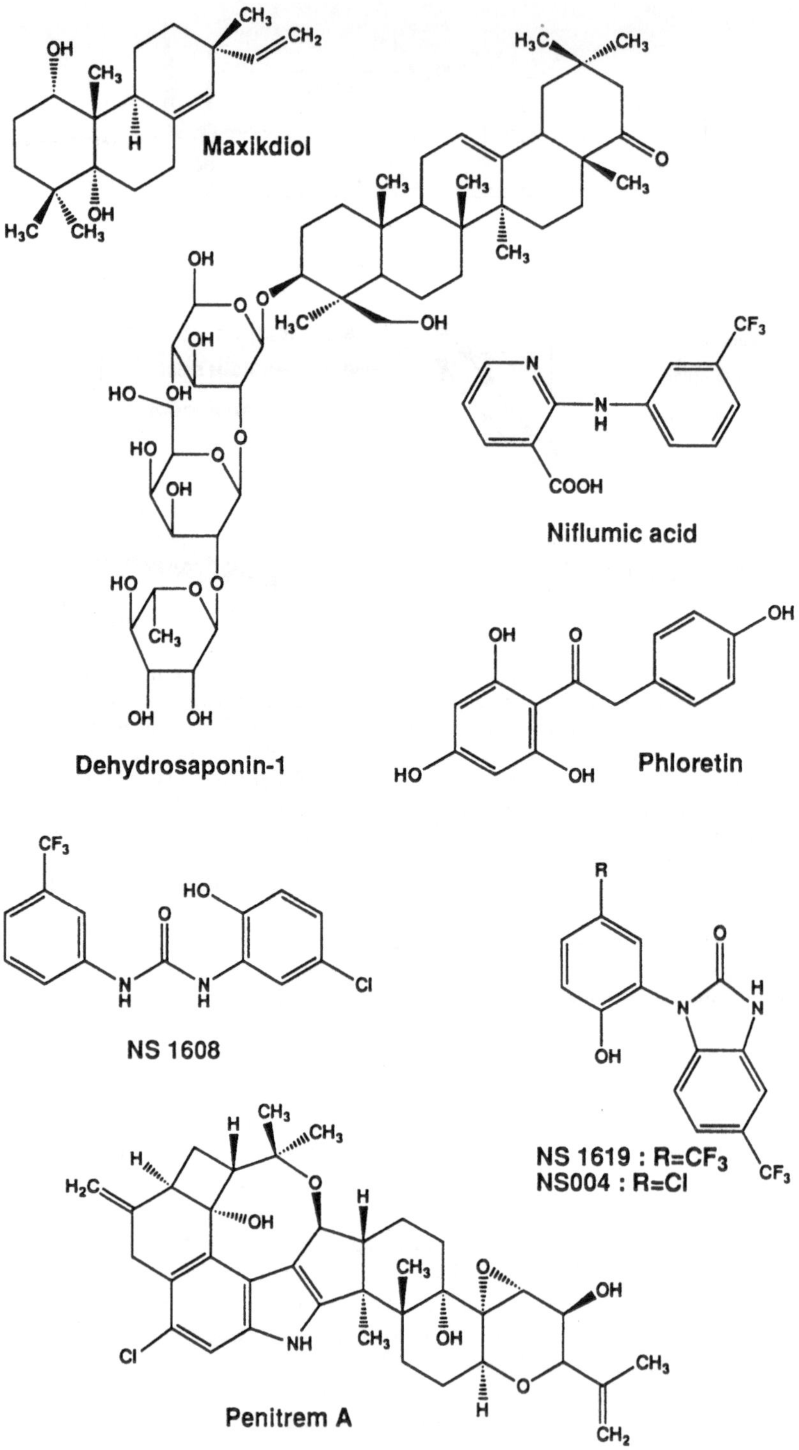

FIG. 5. Chemical structures of modulators of BK$_{Ca}$

[50]. In addition, the open probability of BK_{Ca} channels derived from rat cortex and incorporated into lipid bilayers is increased over a range of potentials in the presence of NS004, suggesting that this compound shifts the voltage sensitivity of the channel [50].

NS1619 (Fig. 5), a derivative of NS004, is also an efficacious opener of BK_{Ca} in a variety of tissues [3]. Its stimulatory effects on BK_{Ca} (Fig. 6) in the rat portal vein are calcium independent and appear to result from a shift of the voltage activation threshold in a hyperpolarizing direction [51]. The effects of NS004 and NS1619 on BK_{Ca} are antagonized by various inhibitors of this channel including charybdotoxin, iberiotoxin, and penitrem A [3,51]. NS1608 is a recently described molecule related to NS1619 in both structure and actions [52].

The sites of action of these NeuroSearch compounds remain to be determined, although both NS004 and NS1619 are membrane permeable and are capable of activating BK_{Ca} when applied either intra- or extracellularly. The ability of NS004 to stimulate the opening of BK_{Ca} in lipid bilayers [50] would be consistent with a direct effect of this K-channel opener on BK_{Ca}. However, NS1619 and the chemically related molecules phloretin and niflumic acid (see Fig. 4) have inhibitory effects on numerous other channels [51,53,54]. Indeed, the inability of penitrem A (Fig. 5) to antagonize

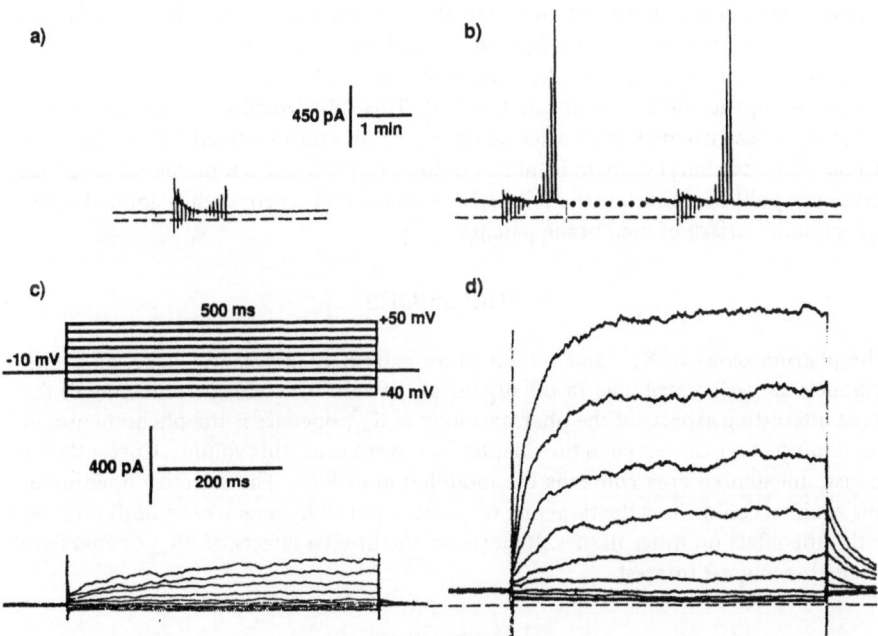

FIG. 6a–d. Typical effects of NS1619 in freshly isolated cells from rat portal vein held at −10 mV under whole-cell clamp conditions. a Control currents obtained on stepping from −10 mV to potentials in the range −80 mV to +50 mV in 10-mV steps. b Currents evoked in the same cell after 10-min exposure to NS1619 (20 μM). Note the marked increased in evoked current magnitude and the outwardly rectifying character of the responses. c and d Currents identical to those described in a and b, but recorded on a faster timebase; those evoked on stepping to −80, −70, −60, and −50 mV have been removed for clarity. The NS1619-induced current was charybdotoxin sensitive. *Dashed line*, zero current. (Adapted from [53] with permission)

the mechanoinhibitory effect of NS1619 in the rat portal vein [51] and the ability of NS1619 to relax 80 mM KCl-contracted rat aorta suggest that its effects may be related to the inhibition of calcium currents rather than to the opening of K channels [51].

NS004 also modifies the activity of channels other than BK_{Ca}. For example, this agent is the first *opener* of cystic fibrosis transmembrane regulator (CFTR) channels to be described [55]. In addition, NS004 reduces outward current flow through a variety of cloned voltage-sensitive K channels expressed in *Xenopus* oocytes [50]. Despite their effects on numerous channel types, neither NS004 nor NS1619 (at doses to 30 mg/kg) reduces blood pressure in either normal or spontaneously hypertensive rats (S-P Olesen, 1995, personal communication). Nevertheless, the firing frequency of dopaminergic neurones is reduced by 30 mg/kg NS1619 (ip) (S-P Olesen, 1995, personal communication). It remains to be determined whether this is an effect on BK_{Ca}, and if so, whether NS1619 shows some selectivity for this channel in neurones.

The Soyasaponins and Maxikdiol

Dehydrosoyasaponin-1 (DHS-1, Fig. 5) is an opener of BK_{Ca} that was isolated from the medicinal herb *Desmodium adscendens* [56]. Unfortunately, the poor membrane permeability of this compound renders it effective only after intracellular application and thus precludes any therapeutic potential. Nevertheless, it may be a useful tool with which to provide an insight into the regulation of channel gating. DHS-1 is of additional interest because it is the first compound that has been found to open a K channel via an interaction with the β-subunit of BK_{Ca} [11,56].

Another opener of BK_{Ca} is maxikdiol [59]. This dihydroxyisoprimane derivative (see Fig. 5) was isolated from a fermentation broth and identified by its ability to displace labeled charybdotoxin from its binding site [57]. The few biological data that have been published indicate that, like DHS-1, maxikdiol is active when applied to the cytoplasmic surface of membrane patches.

Conclusions

The pharmacology of K_{ATP} and BK_{Ca} is at an extremely interesting stage, and both channels are well distributed in the organs of the cardiovascular system. One of the most interesting aspects of the pharmacology of K_{ATP} openers is the phenomenon of cardioprotection, discussed in the Chapter by Cavero et al., this volume. Currently the largest unexplored area concerns the modulation of BK_{Ca}. The selective opening of this channel could allow the targeting of neurones or of hyperactive smooth muscles with little effect on other tissues. Reports on the in vivo effects of BK_{Ca} openers are awaited with great interest.

References

1. Rudy B (1988) Diversity and ubiquity of K⁺ channels. Neuroscience 25:729–749
2. Edwards G, Weston AH (1993) The pharmacology of ATP-sensitive potassium channels. Annu Rev Pharmacol Toxicol 33:597–637
3. Olesen S-P (1994) Activators of large-conductance Ca²⁺-dependent K⁺ channels. Exp Opin Invest Drugs 3:1181–1188
4. Jan LY, Jan YN (1990) How might the diversity of potassium channels be generated? Trends Neurosci 13:415–419

5. Kubo Y, Baldwin TJ, Jan YN, Jan LY (1993) Primary structure and functional expression of a mouse inward rectifier potassium channel. Nature 362:127–133

6. Attali B, Guillemare E, Lesage F, Honoré E, Romey G, Lazdunski M, Bahanin J (1993) The protein IsK is a dual activator of K^+ and Cl^- channels. Nature 365:850–852

7. Pongs O (1992) Molecular biology of voltage-dependent potassium channels. Physiol Rev 72:S69–S88

8. Butler A, Tsunoda S, McCobb DP, Wei A, Salkoff L (1993) mSlo, a complex mouse gene encoding "maxi" calcium-activated potassium channels. Science 261:221–224

9. Latorre R (1994) Molecular workings of large conductance (maxi) Ca^{2+}-activated K^- channels. In: Peracchia C (ed) Handbook of membrane channels: molecular and cellular physiology. Academic, New York, pp 79–102

10. Knaus HG, Garcia-Calvo M, Kaczorowski GJ, Garcia ML (1994) Subunit composition of the high conductance calcium-activated potassium channel from smooth muscle, a representative of the mSlo and slowpoke family of potassium channels. J Biol Chem 269:3921–3924

11. McManus OB, Helnis LM, Pallanck L, Ganetzky B, Swanson R, Reid JL (1995) Functional role of the β-subunit of high conductance calcium-activated potassium channels. Neuron 14:1–20

12. Dolly JO, Rettig J, Scott VES, Parcej DN, Wittkat R, Sewing S, Pongs O (1994) Oligomeric and subunit structures of neuronal voltage-sensitive K^+ channels. Biochem Soc Trans 22:473–478

13. Ashford MLJ, Bond CT, Blair TA, Adelman JP (1994) Cloning and functional expression of a rat heart K_{ATP} channel. Nature 370:456–459

14. Inagaki N, Tsuura Y, Namba N, Masuda K, Gonoi T, Horie M, Seino Y, Mizuta M, Seino S (1995) Cloning and functional characterization of a novel ATP-sensitive potassium channel ubiquitously expressed in rat tissues, including pancreatic islets, pituitary, skeletal muscle and heart. J Biol Chem 270:11

15. Krapivinsky G, Gordon EA, Wickman K, Velimirovic B, Krapivinsky L, Clapham DE (1995) The G-protein-gated atrial K^+ channel I_{KACh} is a heteromultimer of two inwardly rectifying K^+-channel proteins. Nature 374:135–141

16. Taglialatela M, Wible BA, Caporaso R, Brown AM (1994) Specification of pore properties by the carboxy terminus of inwardly rectifying K^+ channels. Science 264:844–847

17. Aguilar-Bryan L, Nichols CG, Wechsler SW, Clement JP, Boyd AE, Gozález G, Herrera-Sosa H, Nguy K, Bryan J, Nelson DA (1995) Cloning of the β-cell high affinity sulfoylurea receptor: a regulator of insulin secretion. Science 268:423–426

18. Ashcroft SJH, Ashcroft FM (1990) Properties and functions of ATP-sensitive K-channels. Cell Signalling 2:197–214

19. Hamilton TC, Weir SW, Weston AH (1986) Comparison of the effects of BRL34915 and verapamil on electrical and mechanical activity in rat portal vein. Br J Pharmacol 88:103–111

20. Taira N (1989) Nicorandil as a hybrid between nitrates and potassium channel activators. Am J Cardiol 63:18J–24J

21. Frampton J, Buckley MM, Fitton A (1992) Nicorandil: a review of its pharmacology and therapeutic efficacy in angina pectoris. Drugs 44:625–655

22. Edwards G, Weston AH (1994) Effect of potassium channel modulating drugs on isolated smooth muscle. In: Szekeres L, Papp J Gy (eds) Handbook of experimental pharmacology, vol 111. Springer, Heidelberg, pp 469–531

23. Hamilton TC, Berrahee A, Moen JS, Price RK, Ramji JV, Clapham JC (1993) Levcromakalim. Cardiovasc Drug Rev 11:199–222

24. Gopalakrishnan M, Janis RA, Triggle DJ (1993) ATP-sensitive K^+ channels—pharmacologic properties, regulation and therapeutic potential. Drug Dev Res 28:95–127

25. Manley PW, Quast U, Andres H, Bray K (1993) Synthesis of and radioligand binding studies with a tritiated pinacidil analogue–receptor interactions of structurally different classes of potassium channel openers and blockers. J Med Chem 36:2004–2010

26. Atwal KS (1994) Pharmacology and structure-activity relationships for K-ATP modulators: tissue-selective K-ATP openers. J Cardiovasc Pharmacol 24(suppl 4):S12–S17
27. Zhang H, Bolton TB (1995) Activation by intracellular GDP, metabolic inhibition and pinacidil of a glibenclamide-sensitive K-channel in smooth muscle cells of rat mesenteric artery. Br J Pharmacol 114:662–672
28. Tung RT, Kurachi Y (1991) On the mechanism of nucleotide diphosphate activation of the ATP-sensitive K$^+$ channel in ventricular cell of guinea-pig. J Physiol 437:239–256
29. Terzic A, Findlay I, Hosoya Y, Kurachi Y (1994) Dualistic behaviour of ATP-sensitive K$^+$ channels toward intracellular nucleoside diphosphates. Neuron 12:1049–1058
30. Noack Th, Edwards G, Deitmer P, Weston AH (1992) Potassium channel modulation in rat portal vein by ATP depletion: a comparison with the effects of levcromakalim (BRL 38227). Br J Pharmacol 107:945–955
31. Edwards G, Ibbotson T, Weston AH (1993) Levcromakalim may induce a voltage-independent K-current in rat portal veins by modifying the gating properties of the delayed rectifier. Br J Pharmacol 110:1037–1048
32. Soll RM, Dollings PJ, McCaully RJ, Argentieri TM, Lodge N, Oshiro G, Colatsky T, Norton NW, Zebrick D, Havens C, Halaka N (1994) N-Sulfonamides of benzopyran-related potassium channel openers—conversion of glyburide insensitive smooth muscle relaxants to potent smooth muscle contractors. Bioorg & Med Chem Lett 4:769–773
33. Edwards G, Schneider J, Niederste-Hollenberg A, Noack Th, Weston AH (1995) Effects of BRL55834 in rat portal vein and bovine trachea: evidence for the induction of a glibenclamide-resistant, ATP-sensitive potassium current. Br J Pharmacol 115:1027–1037
34. Koga H, Sato H, Ishizawa T, Kuromaru K, Nabata H, Imagawa J, Yoshida S, Sugo I (1993) N,N-Disubstituted benzopyran-4-(N'-cyano)carboxamidines, cromakalim analogs with selective activity for guinea pig trachealis. Bioorganic & Med Chem Lett 3:1111–1114
35. Hunnicutt EJ, Davis JN, Chisholm JC (1994) A new glibenclamide-insensitive neuroselective hyperpolarizing agent. Eur J Pharmacol 261:R1–R3
36. Pirotte B, Antoine MH, Detullio P, Hermann M, Herchuelz A, Delarge J, Lebrun P (1994) A pyridothiadiazine (BPDZ 44) as a new and potent activator of ATP-sensitive K$^+$ channels. Biochem Pharmacol 47:1381–1386
37. Bowring NE, Arch JRS, Buckle DR, Taylor JF (1993) Comparison of the airways relaxant and hypotensive potencies of the potassium channel activators BRL-55834 and levcromakalim (BRL-38227) in vivo in guinea-pigs and rats. Br J Pharmacol 109:1133–1139
38. Grant TL, Ohnmacht CJ, Howe BB (1994) Anilide tertiary carbinols: a novel series of K$^+$ channel openers. Trends Pharmacol Sci 15:402–404
39. Atwal KS, Grover GJ, Ahmed SZ, Ferrara FN, Harper TW, Kim KS, Sleph PG, Dzwonczyk S, Russell AD, Moreland S, McCullough JR, Normandin DE (1993) Cardioselective anti-ischemic ATP-sensitive potassium channel openers. J Med Chem 36:3971–3974
40. Upton N, Evans JM, Thompson M, Blackburn TP (1994) New fluorobenzoylamino benzopyrans as potential anticonvulsant agents. Epilepsia 35(suppl 7):76
41. Greenberger LM, Ishikawa Y (1994) ATP-binding cassette protein. Common denominators between ion channels, transporters and enzymes. Trends Cardiovasc Med 4:193–198
42. Findlay I (1993) Sulphonylurea drugs no longer inhibit ATP-sensitive K$^+$ channels during metabolic stress in cardiac muscle. J Pharmacol Exp Ther 266:456–467
43. Müller G, Hartz D, Pünter J, Ökonomopulos R, Kramer W (1994) Differential interaction of glimepiride and glibenclamide with the β-cell sulfonylurea receptor. I. Binding characteristics. Biochim Biophys Acta 1191:267–273
44. Ozanne SE, Guest PC, Hutton JC, Hales CN (1995) Intracellular localization and molecular heterogeneity of the sulphonylurea receptor in insulin-secreting cells. Diabetologia 38:277–282

45. Thomas PM, Cote GJ, Wohlik N, Haddad B, Matthew PM, Rabl W, Aguilar-Bryan L, Gagel RF, Bryan J (1995) Mutations in the sulfonylurea receptor gene in familial persistent hyperinsulinemic hypogylcemia of infancy. Science 268:426–429

46. McCullough JR, Normandin DE, Conder ML, Sleph PG, Dzwonczyk S, Grover GJ (1991) Specific block of the anti-ischemic actions of cromakalim by sodium 5-hydroxydecanoate. Circ Res 69:949–958

47. Kau ST, Zografos P, Do ML, Halterman TJ, McConville MW, Yochim CL, Trivedi S, Howe BB, Li JHY (1994) Characterization of ATP-sensitive potassium channel-blocking activity of Zeneca ZM181,037, a eukalemic diuretic. Pharmacology 49:238–248

48. Grant TL, Zuzack JS (1991) Effects of K^+ channel blockers and cromakalim (BRL 34915) on the mechanical activity of guinea pig detrusor smooth muscle. J Pharmacol Exp Ther 259:1158–1164

49. Small RC, Berry JL, Cook SJ, Foster RW, Green KA, Murray MA (1993) Potassium channels in airways. In: Chung KF, Barnes PJ (eds) Pharmacology of the respiratory tract: experimental and clinical research. Dekker, New York, pp 137–176

50. McKay MC, Dworetzky SI, Meanwell NA, Olesen S-P, Reinhart PH, Levitan IB, Adelman JP, Gribkoff VK (1994) Opening of large-conductance calcium-activated potassium channels by the substituted benzimidazolone NS004. J Neurophysiol (Bethesda) 71:1873–1882

51. Edwards G, Niederste-Hollenberg A, Schneider J, Noack Th, Weston AH (1994) Ion channel modulation by NS 1619, the putative BK-Ca channel opener, in vascular smooth muscle. Br J Pharmacol 113:1538–1547

52. Olesen S-P, Moldt P, Pedersen O (1994) Urea and amide derivatives and their use in the control of cell membrane potassium channels. Patent application WO94/22807, October 13, 1994

53. Koh D-S, Reid G, Vogel W (1994) Effect of the flavoid phloretin on Ca^{2+}-activated K^+ channels in myelinated nerve fibres of Xenopus laevis. Neurosci Lett 165:167–170

54. Ottolia M, Toro L (1994) Potentiation of large conductance K_{Ca} channels by niflumic, flufenamic, and mefamic acids. Biophys J 67:2272–2279

55. Gribkoff VK, Champigny G, Barbry P, Dworetzky SI, Meanwell NA, Lazdunski M (1994) The substituted benzimidazolone NS004 is an opener of the cystic fibrosis chloride channel. J Biol Chem 269:10983–10986

56. McManus OB, Harris GH, Giangiacomo KM, Feigenbaum P, Reuben JP, Addy ME, Burka JF, Kaczorowski GJ, Garcia ML (1993) An activator of calcium-dependent potassium channels isolated from a medicinal herb. Biochemistry 32:6128–6133

57. Singh SB, Goetz MA, Zink DL, Dombrowski AW, Polishook JD, Garcia ML, Schmalhofer W, McManus OB, Kaczorowski GJ (1994) Maxikdiol: a novel dihydroxyiso-primane as an agonist of maxi-K channels. J Chem Soc Perkin Trans 1:3349–3352

Modulation of ATP-Sensitive K+ Channels in Rat Aorta and Kidney

Ulrich Quast, Claudia Linde, Cornelia Löffler,
and Friedrich Metzger

Summary. ATP-sensitive K+ channels (K_{ATP} channels) are gated by the ratio of ATP to nucleoside diphosphates, blocked by sulfonylureas such as glibenclamide (GBC), and opened by K_{ATP}-channel openers like cromakalim and P1075. After a short review of the vascular K_{ATP} channel, we describe their modulation in rat aorta by protein kinases A and C (PKA, PKC) in binding studies with [³H]P1075, in ⁸⁶Rb+ efflux experiments (as a reflection of K+-channel opening), and in vasorelaxation assays. The results show that PKA sensitizes the preparation for channel activation by openers while PKC inhibits channel opening by P1075 without preventing the vasorelaxant effect. The binding of [³H]P1075 to its drug receptor remains unaffected by PKA and PKC, suggesting that the binding step may be several steps upstream from the channel opening. In the kidney, K_{ATP} channels of the vascular type modulate renin secretion from juxtaglomerular cells; a different subtype of K_{ATP} channels has been described in several tubular segments where they contribute to electrolyte homeostasis. Binding studies with [³H]P1075 in intact metabolically competent glomeruli showed the existence of a high-affinity receptor for the K_{ATP} channel openers with pharmacological properties resembling those of the receptor in rat aorta; in addition, two classes of binding sites were found for [³H]GBC. The potential relevance of these binding sites is discussed.

Key words. K_{ATP} Channels—Protein kinase A—Protein kinase C—[³H]P1075 binding—[³H]glibenclamide binding—Rat aorta—Rat glomeruli

Introduction: K_{ATP} Channels

Adenosine triphosphate-(ATP-) sensitive K+ channels (K_{ATP} channels) are found in excitable tissues such as the heart, skeletal and smooth muscle, neurons, pancreatic β cells [1,2], and the rat adenohypophysis, but also in tissues like kidney epithelium or the follicular cells surrounding the *Xenopus* oocyte (for references, see [3]). These constitute a heterogeneous class of K+ channels that are closed by ATP binding to an intracellular binding site; they open when ATP dissociates from this site or when Mg²⁻ salts of nucleoside diphosphates (NDP) such as magnesium-adenosine diphosphate (Mg-ADP) and magnesium-guanosine diphosphate (Mg-GDP) bind to an activatory site different from the inhibitory ATP site.

Department of Pharmacology, University of Tübingen, D-72074 Tübingen, Germany

The opening of K_{ATP} channels is regulated by the quotient of ATP/NDP; thus, these channels link cellular excitability to the metabolic state of the cell [1–4]. The activity of K_{ATP} channels is modulated by phosphorylation [1–5]. A characteristic feature of K_{ATP} channels is their inhibition by sulfonylureas such as glibenclamide with widely varying affinities in different tissues [1–5]. In many tissues, the K_{ATP} channels are opened by a structurally heterogeneous class of compounds, the K_{ATP}-channel openers, which includes nicorandil [an agent that also acts as a nitrate, increasing cyclic guanosine monophosphate (cGMP)], minoxidil sulphate, pinacidil, diazoxide, cromakalim, and aprikalim [1–5]. Under quasi-physiological conditions, the different K_{ATP} channels exhibit single-channel conductances ranging from 15 to 40 pS and slight inward rectification [1,4].

The molecular structure of the K_{ATP} channel is currently under discussion [6]. The four pore-forming α-subunits probably belong to the superfamily of inwardly rectifying K^+ (K_{IR}) channels [6]. Two quite different members have been proposed as the α-subunit of the channel [7,8]; most interestingly, neither one is sensitive to inhibition by glibenclamide [7,8]. It is therefore assumed that the native K_{ATP} channel may be a heteromultimer of four (possibly different) K_{IR} α-subunits, probably including the sulfonylurea receptor as regulator [6]. Two high-affinity sulfonylurea-binding proteins have been purified: one of them is a 38-kDa protein [9]; the other, a 140-kDa protein, has recently been cloned from a β-cell line and shown to belong to the ABC (ATP-binding cassette) protein superfamily; however, this protein has 13 transmembrane segments instead of the usual 12 segments [10].

The physiological role of K_{ATP} channels depends on the tissue. In the pancreatic β cell, K_{ATP} channels regulate insulin release in response to the plasma glucose level. The sulfonylureas are blockers optimized for this channel in the β cell and are of major importance in the treatment of non-insulin-dependent diabetes [1]. In many tissues, K_{ATP} channels are in the closed state under physiological conditions; they open when the tissue is metabolically compromised; that is, the quotient of ATP/NDP falls. Their opening clamps the cell in the resting state, thus saving ATP and helping the cell to survive. The fact that the K_{ATP}-channel openers act on precisely the K^+ channel that opens under ischemic and hypoxic conditions may explain the therapeutic benefit found with these compounds in animal models of cardioprotection and intermittent claudication [5].

K_{ATP} Channels in the Vasculature

At first sight the physiological role of K_{ATP} channels in vascular smooth muscle may appear unclear because the Mg-NDP/Mg-ATP ratio in vascular myocytes under physiological conditions keeps the channel in the closed state. However, in some vascular beds these channels are opened by vasorelaxant neurotransmitters and hormones, probably via activation of a G protein. Opening of K_{ATP} channels mediates the relaxation of the coronary vasculature by adenosine, prostacyclin, or its analogue iloprost, and of mesenteric arterioles by calcitonin gene-related peptide (see references in [2–4]). In contrast, the contribution of K_{ATP}-channel opening to the vasorelaxant effect of the endothelium-derived hyperpolarizing factor(s) (EDHF) seems to remain controversial [4]. There is convincing evidence to show that these channels are opened by depletion of intracellular ATP or an increase in Mg-NDP (references in [2–4]), thus affording relaxation of vascular tone in and increased blood supply to ischemic tissue.

Vascular Effects of the K$_{ATP}$-Channel Openers

Opener Binding and Channel Opening

The direct manifestation of K$^+$-channel opening is a K$^+$ current which, in smooth muscle under physiological conditions, is directed outward, leading to hyperpolarization of the cell. This K$^+$ efflux can also be observed in tracer efflux experiments using ^{42}K$^+$ or ^{86}Rb$^+$ (for reviews, see [4,5]). The mechanism by which the K$_{ATP}$-channel openers activate the channel in vascular smooth muscle is still a matter of debate [4,5]. Binding assays using the tritiated pinacidil analog [^{3}H]P1075 in rings of rat aorta suggest that the major K$_{ATP}$-channel openers bind to the same target (but possibly to different sites at this target) to elicit their effects [11,12]. The sulfonylurea glibenclamide binds to a site different from and negatively allosterically coupled to the [^{3}H]P1075-binding site [11]. The biochemical characterization of the drug receptor for the openers has been hampered by the fact that binding is lost on homogenization of the tissue [12]; however, recently Groppi and co-workers [13] have succeeded in identifying a 48-kDa protein as the drug receptor in photo affinity-labeling studies in a smooth muscle cell line. The question of whether the drug receptor of the channel openers is an α-subunit of the K$_{ATP}$ channel or a different protein must remain open until the drug receptor is cloned. The fact that K$_{ATP}$-channel openers are able to open K$_{ATP}$ channels in isolated patches from vascular smooth muscle cells (see references in [4]) does not necessarily imply a direct action of these compounds on the channel because the isolated patch may contain proteins other than the α-subunits important for channel modulation.

Smooth Muscle Relaxation

The hyperpolarization of smooth muscle leads to relaxation, and the K$_{ATP}$-channel openers have been instrumental in the study of the relationship between membrane potential and the contractility of smooth muscle [14]. First, hyperpolarization clamps the cell at sufficiently negative values to prevent depolarization-induced Ca^{2+} entry by voltage-sensitive Ca^{2+} channels [15]; in this respect the openers may be looked at as indirect Ca^{2+} channel blockers. In addition, the K$_{ATP}$-channel openers, by their hyperpolarizing action, inhibit the agonist-induced accumulation of IP$_3$, thus interfering with agonist-stimulated Ca^{2+} mobilization from intracellular stores; they also reduce the intracellular Ca^{2+} concentration in vascular smooth muscle at rest and decrease the Ca^{2+} sensitivity of the contractile elements in strips of canine coronary artery (see references in [14]). The precise mechanism by which hyperpolarization of the cell membrane regulates these phenomena remains to be established. The ability of the K$_{ATP}$-channel openers to inhibit both the agonist-induced mobilization of Ca^{2+} from intracellular stores, and the increase in Ca^{2+} sensitivity of the contractile apparatus predicts that the smooth muscle relaxant profile of these compounds will differ from that of the Ca^{2+} antagonists and explains earlier findings that the K$_{ATP}$ openers relax contractions that do not depend on depolarization-induced Ca^{2+} entry (see references in [14]).

Other studies using the K$^+$-channel blockers tedisamil, Ba^{2+}, and Rb$^+$ show, however, that most of the K$^+$ channels opened by the K$_{ATP}$-channel openers can be blocked without much effect on smooth muscle relaxation. This suggests that the openers possess mechanisms of vasorelaxation that are independent of plasmalemmal K$_{ATP}$-channel opening. One such mechanism is the (partial) inhibition of intracellular

Ca^{2+} store refilling, produced by (lev)-cromakalim in vascular tissues (see review, [14]).

The vasorelaxant effect of the K_{ATP} channel shows two characteristic traits: first, it is abolished in media containing high concentrations of K^+ [15], and second, it is inhibited by the sulfonylureas, in particular, glibenclamide [16]. Glibenclamide inhibits both the K^+-channel opening and the vasorelaxant effects of the K_{ATP}-channel openers at similar concentrations [16]. This implies that the "additional" mechanisms of vasorelaxation (which are independent of plasmalemmal K_{ATP}-channel opening) are also sensitive to depolarization and to glibenclamide.

The antagonism by glibenclamide of the vasorelaxant and channel-opening effects of the K_{ATP} openers often displays a competitive appearance (see, e.g., [16]); however, as mentioned, kinetic studies have shown that the openers and glibenclamide are not strictly competitive with one another but that they bind to two different sites which are negatively allosterically coupled [11]. In vascular smooth muscle, concentrations $\geq 100\,nM$ are required to produce substantial inhibition of the vasorelaxant and $^{86}Rb^+$ efflux stimulating effects of the K_{ATP}-channel openers [16]. At these concentrations, however, but even more so in the micromolar range, glibenclamide has numerous additional effects unrelated to K_{ATP}-channel blockade (see references in [17]).

The complex relationship between the K^+ channel opening and the vasorelaxant effects of openers as well as the mode of inhibition of various compounds and mechanisms are shown in Fig. 1. Note that an indirect mechanism of action of the openers is assumed.

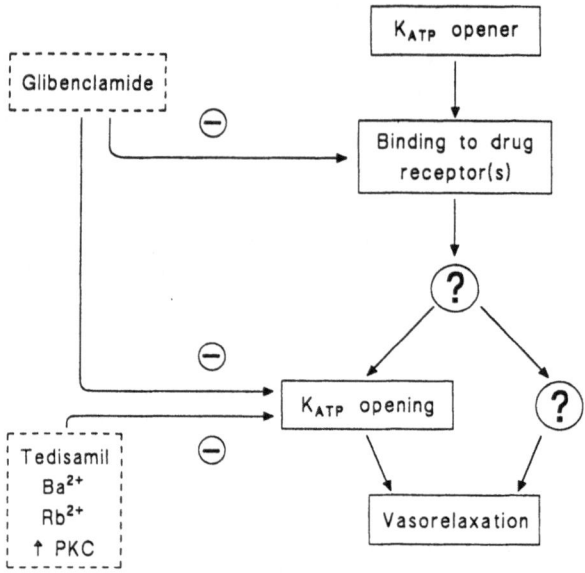

FIG. 1. ATP-sensitive K^+ (K_{ATP}) channel openers and vasorelaxation. The binding of the openers to their drug receptor induces (unknown) changes in the cell, leading to K_{ATP}-channel opening, hyperpolarization, and vasorelaxation. In addition, the openers induce vasorelaxation by yet poorly identified pathways that are independent of K_{ATP}-channel opening. The sulfonylureas like glibenclamide are unique among the inhibitors of the K_{ATP}-channel openers because they inhibit the binding of the openers and block the channel. The other inhibitors such as tedisamil, Ba^{2+}, Rb^+, and phorbol esters block the channel but do not prevent vasorelaxation (see text for details). *PKC*, protein kinase C

Modulation of K$_{ATP}$ Channels in Rat Aorta by
Protein Kinases A and C

In many tissues, cyclic AMP-dependent phosphorylation seems to be necessary to keep K$_{ATP}$ channels in a functional state and to prevent "rundown" of the channel [1,2]. There is some controversy whether phosphorylation by protein kinase A (PKA) alone is sufficient to open K$_{ATP}$-channels (see references in [18]).

In a recent study in rat isolated aorta, we used the potent pinacidil analog P1075 as the K$^+$-channel opener; opening of K$_{ATP}$-channels was assessed by measuring the increase in the rate constant of ^{86}Rb$^+$ efflux from the preparation in response to P1075 [18]. Stimulation of PKA by dibutyryl-cAMP, forskolin, and isobutylmethylxanthine (IBMX) augmented the K$^+$-channel-opening effect of P1075 (see Fig. 2a for IBMX). The lower trace in Fig. 2a shows that glibenclamide (1 μM) abolished the ^{86}Rb$^+$ efflux induced by P1075 in the presence of IBMX (100 μM), indicating that this efflux is passing entirely through K$_{ATP}$-channels. In addition, the effect of IBMX was (partially) reversed by the kinase inhibitor H 89, suggesting that it was mediated by activation of PKA [18]. IBMX induced a leftward shift in the concentration–^{86}Rb$^+$ efflux curve of P1075 without changing the maximum, suggesting that increased cAMP levels sensitized the preparation for the effect of the K$^+$-channel opener [18]. Interestingly, specific binding of [^{3}H]P1075 was unaffected by IBMX (Fig. 2b).

In a subsequent study we investigated the effect of protein kinase C (PKC) stimulation by phorbol esters like phorbol dibutyrate (PDBu) on the effects of P1075 (Linde and Quast, unpublished data). As shown in Fig. 3a, PDBu (30 nM) reduced P1075-induced ^{86}Rb$^+$ efflux to 33% of control; at 100 nM this inhibition was complete (data not shown). The presence of 100 nM PDBu increased the tension induced by noradrenaline (100 nM) and greatly slowed down the time-course of P1075-induced vasorelaxation; however, the concentration–relaxation curve of P1075 at equilibrium was only slightly shifted to the right (Fig. 3b). Binding of [^{3}H]P1075 was unchanged by PDBu to 1 μM, the highest concentration tested (not shown).

It is concluded that in rat isolated aorta PKA and PKC modulate K$_{ATP}$-channel opening in opposite directions. In this respect the channel in rat aorta resembles the K$_{ATP}$ channels described in rabbit mesenteric artery [19] and in the follicular cells of the *Xenopus* oocyte [20]; in contrast to these, however, the channel in rat aorta is not opened by PKA activation. The data with PKC stimulation provide a further example that (essentially complete) inhibition of channel opening has only minor effects on the vasorelaxant potency of the K$_{ATP}$-channel openers (see previous section and Fig. 1). The fact that binding of [^{3}H]P1075 is unchanged by stimulation of PKA and PKC suggests that the binding step may be several steps upstream from channel opening (Fig. 1).

K$_{ATP}$ Channels in the Kidney

Evidence for K$_{ATP}$ channels in the kidney has been found in the vas afferens and in the tubular system. In pithed rats in which cardiovascular reflexes are absent, infusion of glibenclamide lowered plasma renin activity but administration of K$_{ATP}$-channel openers increased renin levels in a glibenclamide-sensitive manner [21]. In cell cultures enriched in juxtaglomerular (renin-secreting) cells, the K$_{ATP}$-channel opener, cromakalim, increased renin secretion in a concentration-dependent fashion [22].

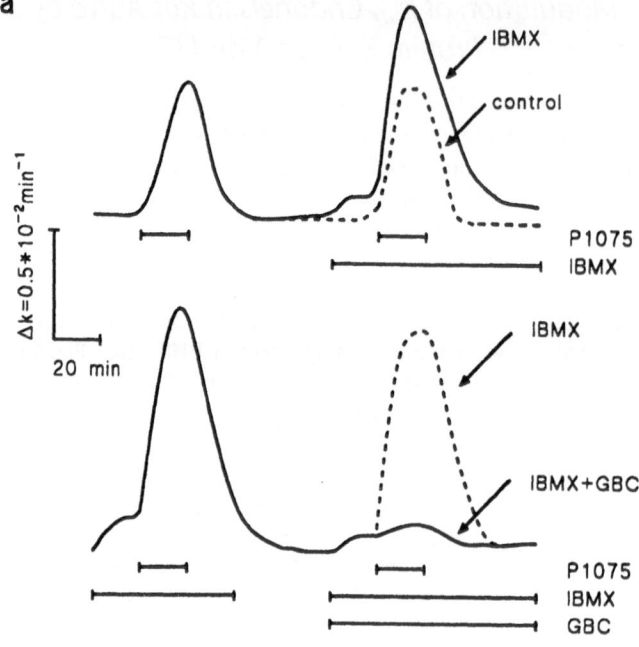

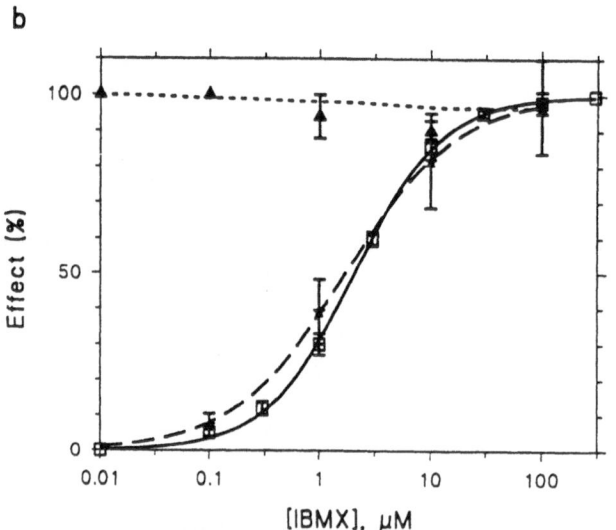

FIG. 2a,b. Interaction of isobutylmethylxanthine (*IBMX*) with P1075 in rat aorta. a Original traces of the rate constant, k, of $^{86}Rb^+$ efflux, which is a good qualitative measure of the membrane permeability to K^+. *Upper trace*: P1075 (50 nM) was superfused twice for 20 min; the second stimulation was performed in the absence (*control, broken line*) or in the presence of IBMX (100 μM); IBMX doubled the response to P1075 as assessed by the area under the k *vs* time curve. *Lower trace*: inhibition by glibenclamide (*GBC*). The preparation was stimulated twice by IBMX (100 μM) and P1075 (50 nM); the second stimulation was performed in the absence (*control, broken line*) or presence of GBC (1 μM). Substances were applied as indicated by the

a

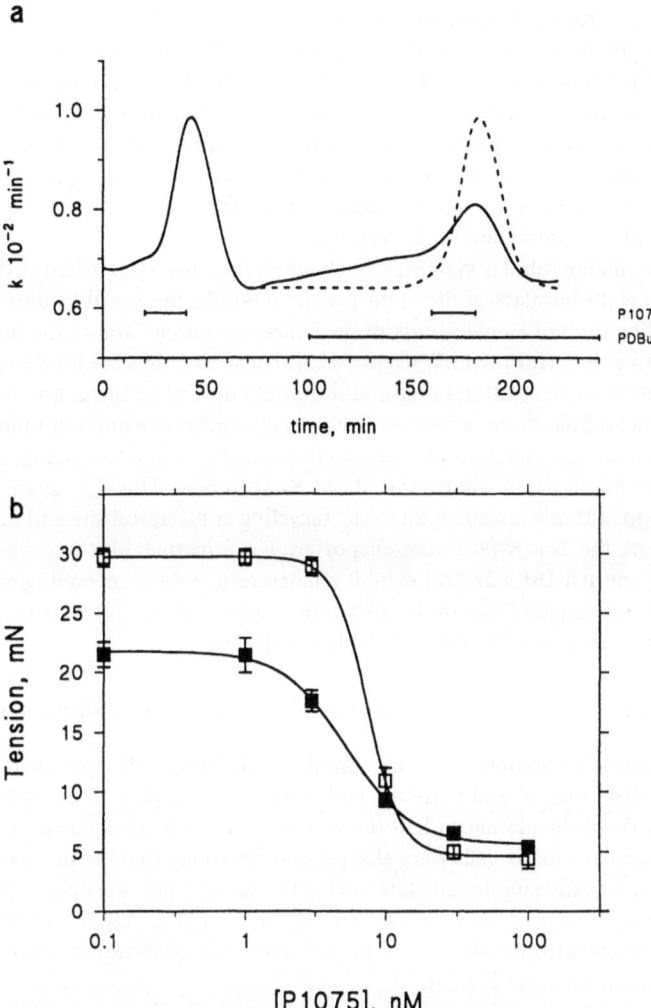

b

FIG. 3a,b. Effect of phorbol dibutyrate (*PDBu*) on P1075-induced $^{86}Rb^+$ efflux and vasorelaxation. a Mean trace showing the effect of P1075 (50 nM) superfused twice for 20 min; the second stimulation was performed in the absence (control, *broken line*) or in the presence of PDBu (30 nM). PDBu led to a slow increase in basal tracer efflux and inhibited the response to P1075 by 66% ± 4% of control. b Vasorelaxant effect of P1075 on noradrenaline- (100 nM) induced tone in the absence (*full square*) and presence of PDBu (100 nM, *open square*). PDBu increased noradrenaline-induced tension by 40%, greatly slowed down the relaxation kinetics (not shown), and shifted the vasorelaxation curve from 5.3 nM to 7.4 nM; the Hill coefficient increased from 1.9 to 3.7

←——————————————————————————————————————

FIG. 2a,b. *Continued*

respective *bars*. Note the small increases in $^{86}Rb^+$ efflux produced by IBMX alone, which are discussed elsewhere. b Effects of IBMX on noradrenaline- (100 nM) induced tone of rat aorta (*open square*), P1075-induced $^{86}Rb^-$ efflux (*star*), and specific binding of [^{3}H]P1075 (*triangle*). Note that vasorelaxation and potentiation of P1075-induced channel opening occur at similar concentrations of IBMX; specific binding of [^{3}H]P1075 is not affected

These findings strongly suggest that juxtaglomerular cells (which are derived from vascular smooth muscle cells) are endowed with K_{ATP} channels that participate in the regulation of renin release. It is well known that the rate of renin secretion is inversely coupled to the intracellular Ca^{2+} concentration (the "calcium paradox" [23]). To explain the effects of K_{ATP}-channel modulation on renin secretion, one may assume that, as in smooth muscle cells, opening of K_{ATP} channels in juxtaglomerular cells reduces the intracellular Ca^{2+} concentration but blockade increases $[Ca^{2+}]_i$; these changes would then modulate renin secretion.

In the mammalian tubular system, K_{ATP} channels have been described at the single-channel level at the basolateral site of the proximal tubule, the apical membrane of the thick ascending limb of Henle's loop, of the collecting tubule, and of the inner medullary collecting duct (for reviews, see [3,24,25]. These channels are inhibited by ATP in the millimolar concentration range and show mild inward rectification; the channel in the proximal tubule shows a low sensitivity to glibenclamide and tolbutamide. The K_{ATP} channel in the proximal tubule plays an important role in K^+ recycling, the one in the collecting tubule is an important site of K^+ secretion. The K_{ATP} channel in the ascending loop of Henle is important for K^+ recycling at the apical site and the normal functioning of the $Na^+/K^+/2Cl^-$ cotransporter. K_{ATP}-channel blockers like gliben-clamide [26] and ICI 181, 037 [27] exhibit a natriuretic potassium-saving effect, and indirect evidence suggests that these eukalemic diuretic actions result from blockade of K_{ATP} at the thick ascending limb of Henle's loop [26].

Binding Studies with K_{ATP}-Channel Modulators in Rat Glomeruli

The glomerulus is a complex structure containing different cell types such as endo-thelial, epithelial (visceral and parietal), and mesangial cells [28]. In our preparation, about 10%–15% of the glomeruli had the vascular pole still attached so that a small amount of vascular muscle cells were also present. Provided that the preparation was kept in a metabolically competent state during the experiment, the opener [³H]P1075 bound to a single class of sites with an affinity of $3 nM$ (Fig. 4a). This binding was inhibited by openers from different chemical classes with inhibition constants similar to those found in rat aorta [12,29].

Although all openers inhibited specific [³H]P1075 binding completely, gliben-clamide inhibited binding to only 72%, with an inhibition constant ($K_i = 720 nM$) [29] similar to the value determined in aortic strips [12]. This shows that the receptor for the K_{ATP}-channel openers in the glomerulus has a pharmacological profile similar to that in the vasculature. Although it is presently unknown on which cell population of the glomerulus the drug receptor is located, the following two observations suggest that it is associated with the mesangial cells: (i) the [³H]P1075 binding capacity of the glomeruli for [³H]P1075 was reasonably high (10 fmol/mg protein, i.e., about 1/6 of that in aorta), and (ii) binding was not reduced in prepara-tions in which no vessels were attached to the glomeruli. It is well known that mesangial cells are derived from smooth muscle cells and contribute about 30% to the total cell number of the glomerulus [28]. On the other hand, we have not found specific [³H]P1075 binding in primary cultures of mesangial cells after 3–4 weeks; this failure, however, may be the result of culture conditions. Thus, more work is neces-sary to determine the localization of the receptor for the K_{ATP}-channel openers in the glomerulus.

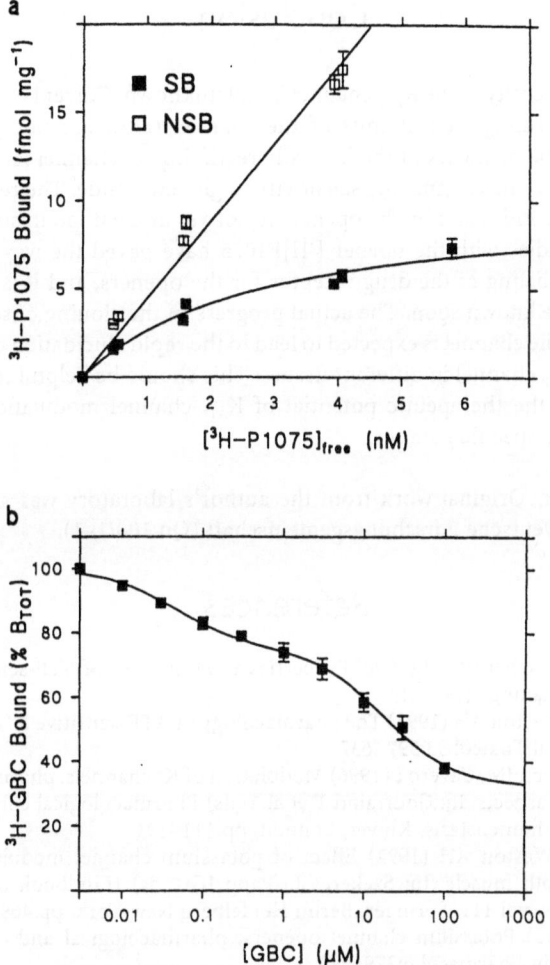

FIG. 4. Binding of K$_{ATP}$-channel modulators in metabolically competent rat glomeruli. a Specific binding (*SB*) and nonspecific binding (*NSB*) of [³H]P1075 [SB (*solid squares*), NSB (*open squares*) in fmol/mg protein] as a function of the free label concentration. Analysis of SB reveals a single class of sites with $K_D = 3\,nM$ and a binding capacity (B_{max}) of 10 fmol/mg protein. b Inhibition of [³H]glibenclamide ([³H]GBC, 0.6 nM) binding by (unlabeled) GBC. The curve fit shows two classes of sites with affinities of $43 \pm 11\,nM$ and $20 \pm 6\,\mu M$, which displace 25% and 42% of total binding (70 fmol/mg protein), respectively

In metabolically competent glomeruli, [³H]glibenclamide ([³H]GBC) bound to two classes of sites: the first, with $K_D = 45\,nM$ and $B_{max} \approx 1.3$ pmol/mg protein, and the second, with $K_D = 25\,\mu M$ and $B_{max} \approx 1000$ pmol/mg protein (Fig. 4b). The binding capacity of the high-affinity glibenclamide sites is more than 100 times that of the P1075 sites, and the low-affinity sites are again much more numerous; thus, it is no surprise that the K$_{ATP}$-channel openers do not interfere with glibenclamide binding in this preparation. If the glomeruli are not gassed with carbogen or if cell metabolism is inhibited, glibenclamide binding to both sites is greatly reduced (data not shown). The further characterization of the glibenclamide-binding sites is in progress.

Conclusion

The molecular identity of the K_{ATP} channel is still unknown. Current evidence suggests that the pore-forming (α-)subunits of the channel (although not yet definitively identified) may be members of the inwardly rectifying K^+-channel family; additional subunits confer to the channel the sensitivity to glibenclamide. The regulation of the channel by nucleotides and by the openers is not yet understood in structural terms. The binding studies with the opener [^{3}H]P1075 have paved the way for the recent photo-affinity labeling of the drug receptor for the openers, and it is hoped that its structure may be known soon. The actual progress in the cloning of several putative components of the channel is expected to lead to the rapid elucidation of the structure of the native K_{ATP} channel in different tissues. This should be helpful in finding novel ways to exploit the therapeutic potential of K_{ATP}-channel modulation in different tissues in a more specific manner.

Acknowledgment. Original work from the author's laboratory was supported by a grant from the Deutsche Forschungsgemeinschaft (Qu 100/1–1).

References

1. Ashcroft SJH, Ashcroft FM (1990) Properties and functions of ATP-sensitive K^+-channels. Cell Signalling 2:197–214
2. Edwards G, Weston AH (1993) The pharmacology of ATP-sensitive K^+ channels. Annu Rev Pharmacol Toxicol 33:597–637
3. Quast U, Guillon JM, Cavero I (1996) Modulation of K^+ channels: pharmacological and therapeutical aspects. In: Godfraind T et al. (eds) Pharmacological control of calcium an potassium homeostasis. Kluver, London, pp 111–121
4. Edwards G, Weston AH (1994) Effect of potassium channel modulating drugs on isolated smooth muscle. In: Szekeres L, Papp JG (eds) Handbook of experimental pharmacology, vol 111. Springer, Berlin Heidelberg New York, pp 469–531
5. Quast U (1992) Potassium channel openers: pharmacological and clinical aspects. Fundam & Clin Pharmacol 6:279–293
6. Krapivinsky G, Gordon EA, Wickman K, Velimirovic B, Krapivisnky L, Clapham DE (1995) The G-protein-gated atrial K^+ channel I_{KACh} is a heteromultimer of two inwardly rectifying K^+-channel proteins. Nature 374:135–141
7. Ashford MLJ, Bond CT, Blair TA, Adelman JP (1994) Cloning and functional expression of a rat heart K_{ATP} channel. Nature 370:456–459
8. Inagaki N, Tanura Y, Namba N, Masuda K (1995) Cloning and functional characterization of a novel ATP-sensitive potassium channel ubiquitously expressed in rat tissues, including pancreatic islets, pituitary, skeletal muscle and heart. J Biol Chem 270:5691–5694
9. Schwanstecher M, Löser S, Chudziak F, Panten U (1994) Identification of a 38-kDa high affinity sulfonylurea-binding peptide in insulin-secreting cells and cerebral cortex. J Biol Chem 269:17768–17771
10. Aguilar-Bryan L, Nichols CG, Wechsler SW, Clement JP, Boyd AE, González G, Herrera-Sosa H, Nguy K, Bryan J, Nelson DA (1995) Cloning of the β cell high-affinity sulfonylurea receptor: a regulator of insulin secretion. Science 268:423–429
11. Bray KM, Quast U (1992a) A specific binding site for K^+ channel openers in rat aorta. J Biol Chem 267:11689–11692
12. Quast U, Bray KM, Andres H, Manley PW, Baumlin Y, Dosogne J (1993) Binding of the K^+ channel opener [^{3}H]P1075 in rat isolated aorta: relationship to functional effects of openers and blockers. Mol Pharmacol 43:474–481

13. Thomasco LM, Gadwood RC, Groppi VE, Wolfe ML, Hsi RSP, Easter JA (1994) Synthesis and biological activitity of a tritiated cyanoguanidine photoaffinity probe for ATP-sensitive potassium channels. Presented at the 208th American Chemical Society meeting, Washington, DC, August 21–24, 1994

14. Quast U (1993) Do the K$^+$ channel openers relax smooth muscle by opening K$^+$ channels? Trends Pharmacol Sci 14:332–336

15. Hamilton TC, Weir SW, Weston AH (1986) Comparison of the effects of BRL 34915 and verapamil on electrical and mechanical activity in rat portal vein. Br J Pharmacol 88:103–111

16. Quast U, Cook NS (1989) In vitro and in vivo comparison of two K$^+$ channel openers, diazoxide and cromakalim, and their inhibition by glibenclamide. J Pharmacol Exp Ther 250:261–270

17. Quast U (1995) Effects of potassium channel activators in isolated blood vessels. In: Evans JM, Hamilton TC, Stemp G (eds) Potassium channels and their modulators: from synthesis to clinical experience. Taylor and Francis, London, pp 173–195

18. Linde C, Quast U (1995) Potentiation of P1075-induced K$^+$ channel opening by stimulation of adenylate cyclase in rat isolated aorta. Br J Pharmacol 115:515–521

19. Quayle JM, Bonev AD, Brayden JE, Nelson MT (1994) Calcitonin gene-related peptide activated ATP-sensitive K$^+$ currents in rabbit arterial smooth muscle via protein kinase. J Physiol 475:9–13

20. Honoré E, Lazdunski M (1991) Hormone-regulated K$^+$ channels in follicle-enclosed oocytes are activated by vasorelaxing K$^+$ channel openers and blocked by antidiabetic sulfonylureas. Proc Natl Acad Sci USA 88:5438–5442

21. Richer C, Pratz J, Mulder P, Mondot S, Giudicelli, JF, Cavero I (1990) Cardiovascular and biological effects of K$^+$ channel openers, a class of drugs with vasorelaxant and cardioprotective properties. Life Sci 47:1693–1705

22. Ferrier CP, Kurtz A, Lehner P, Shaw SG, Pusterla C, Saxenhofer H, Weidmann P (1989) Stimulation of renin secretion by potassium-channel activation with cromakalim. Eur J Clin Pharmacol 36:443–447

23. Kurtz A (1990) Cellular control of renin secretion. Rev Physiol Biochem Pharmacol 113:1–40

24. Wang W, Sackin H, Giebisch G (1992) Renal potassium channels and their regulation. Annu Rev Physiol 54:81–96

25. Giebisch G (1993) Diuretic action of potassium channel blockers. Eur J Clin Pharmacol 44(suppl 1):S3–S5

26. Clark MA, Humphrey SJ, Smith MP, Ludens JH (1993) Unique natriuretic properties of the ATP-sensitive K$^+$-channel blocker glyburide in conscious rats. J Pharmacol Exp Ther 265:933–937

27. Kau ST, Zografos P, Do ML (1994) Characterization of ATP-sensitive potassium channel-blocking activity of ZENECA ZM 181,037, a eukalemic diuretic. Pharmacology 49:238–248

28. Taugner R, Hackenthal E (1989) The juxtaglomerular apparatus: structure and function. Springer, Heidelberg

29. Metzger F, Albinus M, Quast U (1995) A specific binding site for openers of the ATP-sensitive potassium channel in rat isolated glomeruli. Naunyn-Schmiedebergs Arch Pharmacol 351(suppl 1):R92

Note added in proof: The K$_{ATP}$ channel in pancreatic β cells has meanwhile been cloned (Inagaki et al. (1995) Science 270:1166–1170). Further studies on [^{3}H]P1075 binding to glomeruli strongly suggest that specific binding is located on the vascular endings and not on mesangial cells (Metzger and Quast, submitted to J Pharmacol Exp Ther).

Part 2
Mechanisms of Vascular Regulation

Regulation of Vascular Tone

THÉOPHILE GODFRAIND, NICOLE MOREL, OLIVIER FERON,
CHANTAL DESSY, and SALVATORE SALOMONE

Summary. In physiological or pathophysiological conditions, vascular tone is regulated by various neural, endocrine, paracrine, and autocrine factors that may exert immediate or delayed effects. In this chapter, we report experiments undertaken to characterize immediate effects by examining the role of endothelium-derived relaxing factors (EDRFs) and of endothelin. We also summarize studies on long-term effects by examining calcium channels and regulation of vascular tone in hypertension, considering comparison of contractile properties of arteries from normotensive and hypertensive rats and their relation with calcium channels. We discuss the following points: differences in postcontraction tone, in response to Ca^{2+}-channel activator, in the effect of amlodipine added in vitro on the Bay K 8644 concentration–effect curve, and in dihydropyridine-binding sites. We show the influence of salt loading on the cardiac and renal preproendothelin-1mRNA expression and on its consequences in stroke-prone spontaneously hypertensive rats, and report its blood pressure-independent inhibition by lacidipine, a long-lasting calcium antagonist.

Key words. Vascular tone—Hypertension—Remodeling—Calcium antagonists—Endothelin gene expression

Introduction

In physiological or pathophysiological conditions, vascular tone is regulated by various neural, endocrine, paracrine, and autocrine factors that may exert immediate or delayed effects. The immediate effects may be studied in vitro by examining the smooth muscle tone resulting from contractile or relaxing stimuli evoked by the exposure of the preparation to a combination of various agents diluted in the perfusion fluid to reach the same concentration as that present in the biophase. The delayed effects may be studied ex vivo if appropriate controls are available. This means that a physiological condition should be compared to a pathophysiological one, assuming that the pathological state may result from an abnormal expression of regulatory factors. Such a situation is provided by hypertension, in which elevated blood pressure may be normalized by a variety of specific agents acting on different systems, which indicates that several factors may be the cause of elevated blood pressure.

Laboratoire de Pharmacologie, Université Catholique de Louvain, B-1200 Brussels, Belgium

Therefore, we have compared ex vivo vessels isolated from hypertensive or normo-tensive rats submitted to various diets with or without calcium antagonists. The use of calcium antagonists is based not only on historical background, considering our pioneering role in this field [1], but mainly on the widespread acceptance of their efficiency in the management of hypertension. Indeed, calcium translocation from outside to inside the cell through voltage-operated calcium channels is a major mechanism involved in signal transduction processes maintaining a prolonged in-crease in vascular tone, and its blockade may achieve blood pressure reduction. Several reports have shown that secondary delayed effects of hypertension such as cardiovascular hypertrophy are blunted after prolonged calcium antagonist treatment [2].

It may be assumed that vascular smooth muscle is the primary target for the antihypertensive action of calcium antagonists. In view of the observation that an appropriate drug regimen of the new generation of calcium antagonists produces blood pressure reduction in hypertensive but not in normotensive states [2–4], we have examined whether the modulation of voltage-operated Ca channels could be affected in hypertension. Because calcium antagonists, in addition to their immediate action on vascular smooth muscle, do exert long-term effects on factors responsible for structural changes in the organs of the cardiovascular system, we have examined whether, if in addition to inhibition of vasoconstriction, they could inhibit the gene expression of some growth factors. Because endothelin is both a vasoconstrictor and a growth factor, special attention has been devoted to this agent, to its interaction with endothelium-derived nitric oxide (EDNO) and adrenergic agents, and to the expression of its gene.

Characterization of Immediate Effects

There are several examples in the literature showing that combination between ago-nists may lead to potentiation: for instance, responses to noradrenaline are potenti-ated by serotonin, as initially shown by de la Lande et al. [5] and later confirmed by Van Nueten et al. [6]. Also, the response to noradrenaline may be enhanced by the neuropeptide Y [7], an effect believed to play an important pathological role. In this report, we focus on the action of low doses of endothelin-1 (ET-1) and on endothelium derived relaxing factors (EDRFs) because endothelium dysfunction is present in hypertension [8].

Role of EDRFs

Since Furchgott and Zawadzki [9] first described the endothelium-dependent relax-ation to acetylcholine in the aorta of the rabbit, it has been established that the endothelium can mediate, wholly or partly, the relaxing effect of a large number of agents [10,11]. This effect of the endothelium is mediated by the release of EDRFs, both nonpeptide and peptide substances including endothelium-derived NO (EDNO) [12], endothelium-derived hyperpolarizing factor (EDHF), a factor of still unknown chemical structure [13], prostacyclin, and C-type natriuretic peptide. Interestingly, these EDRFs are released by the action of the same agonists, although it is not yet clear if this action involves the same subtype of receptors.

The ratio between EDNO and EDHF effect does seem to differ among the vascula-ture. Relaxation is more EDHF dependent in resistance arteries than in conduit arteries, but this cannot be established as a rule, because there are also differences according to the anatomical origin of the arteries. The mechanism by which EDNO mediates vascular relaxation is likely to be activation of soluble guanylate cyclase, leading to an elevation of the content of guanosine 3′:5′-cyclic monophosphate (cGMP) in vascular smooth muscle [14–16]. We examine here the complex action of cGMP at the cellular level. EDHF hyperpolarizes smooth muscle cells by increasing the smooth muscle K^+ conductance and moving the membrane potential closer to the equilibrium potential for K^+ [17].

Endothelium activation not only produces vasodilatation but also modulates the contraction induced by a wide variety of vasoconstrictor agonists. The endothelium markedly modifies the response to vasoconstrictor agonists in canine and porcine coronary arteries and in the aorta of rat and rabbit [18,19]. Such a modulation may involve several factors, including the contractile machinery, calcium influx, and intracellular calcium release [20–22].

Endothelium removal in the isolated aorta of the rat enhances the contractile response to different α-adrenergic agonists, especially partial agonists, which only cause weak contractions in intact preparations [22]. When comparing concentration–response curves from different α-adrenergic agonists in the presence and the absence of endothelium, it appears that removal of the endothelium shifts the concentration–response curves to the different agonists to the left, with an enhancement of the maximal developed tension. This effect is most pronounced for oxymetazoline, clonidine, and UK14,304; these compounds have only a negligible effect in the presence of endothelium.

The role of NO in this effect was assessed in experiments designed to mimic an increase in tissue content of cGMP by incubation with the lipophilic analogue 8-bromo-cGMP. In the absence of endothelium, 8-bromo-cGMP ($0.1\,mM$) causes a shift to the right of the concentration–response curve to noradrenaline, with a significant depression of the maximal response, similar to that obtained in the presence of endothelium. This suggested that endothelium removal increases the efficacy of agonists by increasing the receptor reserve, a hypothesis forwarded by Alosachie and Godfraind [23], using the method of Furchgott and Bursztyn [24], based on partial receptor inactivation by phenoxybenzamine. The affinity of noradrenaline for its receptors, expressed by K_A values, was almost the same in the presence and absence of endothelium, amounting to 1.37×10^{-7} and $1.36 \times 10^{-7}\,M$, respectively. However, there was a marked shift to the left of the curve, representing the contractile response to noradrenaline as a function of receptor occupation, after removal of the endothelium, indicating the presence of a greater receptor reserve in preparations without endothelium. In intact preparations, 19% of the receptors were needed to produce 50% of the maximal response; however, in preparations without endothelium, only 3% of the receptor population was needed to produce the same effect. The calculated relative intrinsic efficacy for noradrenaline in the absence of endothelium was sevenfold higher that in its presence. These findings indicate that the endothelium controls the efficacy of the α-adrenergic agonists (Fig. 1).

In rat aorta, the contractile response to noradrenaline $10^{-8}\,M$ developed by aortic rings without endothelium is sixfold higher than the force developed by preparations with endothelium. A similar amplification of the response is observed in preparations treated with methylene blue ($3 \times 10^{-6}\,M$ for 10 min). Treatment of the aortas without endothelium with 8-bromo-cGMP ($10^{-4}\,M$) reduces the contractile response to noradrenaline. Removal of the endothelium evoked a small but significant increase of

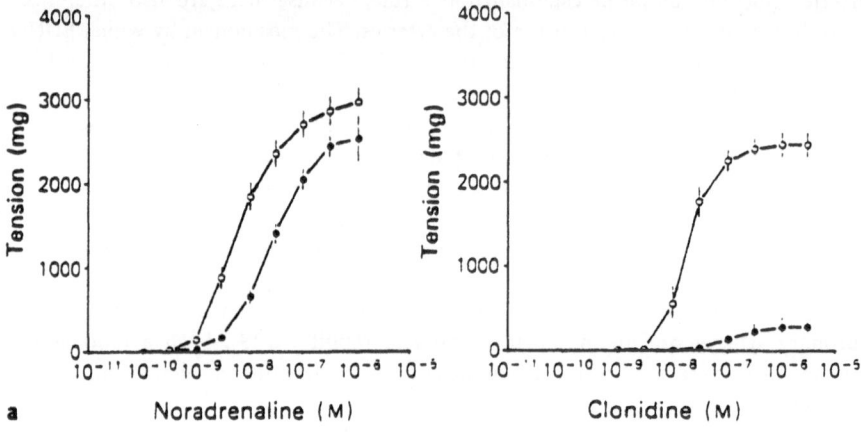

a   Noradrenaline (M)   Clonidine (M)

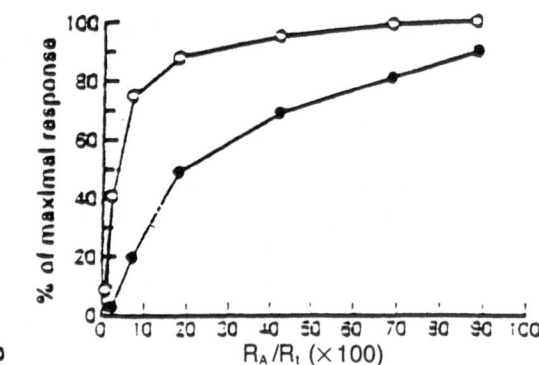

b

FIG. 1a,b. Enhanced responsiveness of rat isolated aorta to adrenoceptor stimulation after removal of endothelial cells. **a** Comparison of cumulative concentration–effect curves with (*solid circles*) and without (*open circles*) endothelium elicited by noradrenaline (*left panel*) and clonidine (*right panel*) in rat isolated aorta. **b** Contractile responses to noradrenaline in rat isolated aorta as a function of receptor occupation in tissues with (*solid circles*) and without (*open circles*) endothelium. *RA/Rt*, proportion of receptors occupied. (Modified from [19] and from [23])

[45]Ca entry in unstimulated preparations. The noradrenaline-dependent [45]Ca entry is twofold higher in preparations without endothelium than in those with endothelium (Fig. 2). Treatment with methylene blue ($3 \times 10^{-6} M$ for 30 min) of the preparations with endothelium also enhances the noradrenaline-dependent [45]Ca entry to levels similar to those found in preparations without endothelium.

These observations show that the endothelium modulates both [45]Ca entry and the contraction evoked by noradrenaline. This modulation is related to efficacy of the adrenergic agonists. Thus, the efficacy of an agonist is, at least in part, related to the gating of calcium channels [20]. However, this effect on calcium influx is not the unique action of cGMP on the agonist-evoked calcium movements in smooth muscle. It indeed has been shown by Lang and Lewis [21,22] that another effect of

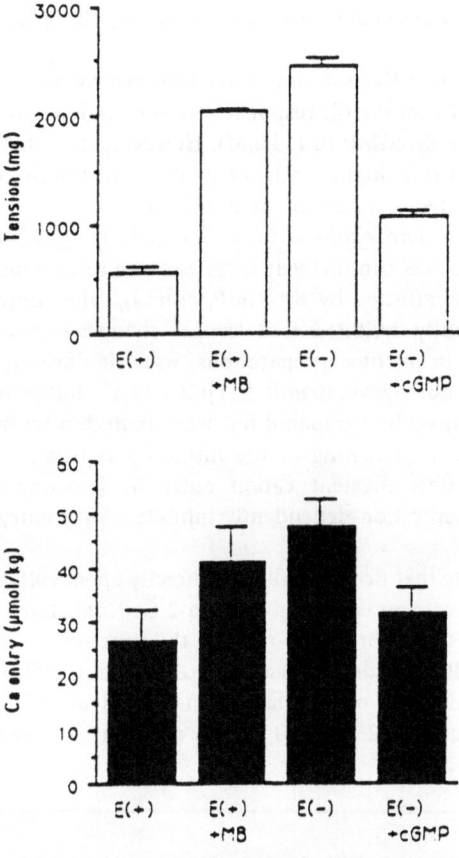

FIG. 2. Endothelium-derived relaxation factor (EDRF) and cyclic guanosine monophosphate (cGMP) control gating of noradrenaline-operated calcium channels in vascular smooth muscle. *Upper panel:* tonic contractile force (expressed in milligrams) developed by rings of rat aorta stimulated with noradrenaline ($10^{-8} M$). *E(+)*, preparations with intact endothelium treated with methylene blue for 10 min before noradrenaline; *E(−)*, preparations in which endothelium was removed; *E(−) + cGMP*, preparations in which endothelium was removed and treated with 8-bromo-cGMP (0.1 mM for 30 min before noradrenaline). *Lower panel:* ^{45}Ca influx (expressed in nmol/kg wet weight) in preparations treated with noradrenaline ($10^{-8} M$ for 2 min). (Modified from [20])

cGMP is to inhibit agonist-induced inositol 1,4,5-trisphosphate production, which leads to inhibition of intracellular calcium release and to the associated increase in vascular tone.

The action of the increase of cellular cGMP on both Ca signal and contraction has been examined recently in our laboratory [25] and compared to the pharmacological action of NO donors, which is usually attributed to a cellular rise in cGMP. Because this hypothesis is, however, based only on indirect evidence, we have studied the effects of cGMP on Ca^{2+} movements and contraction in rat isolated endothelium-denuded aorta stimulated by KCl depolarizing solution using the permeant analog 8-bromo-cGMP (Br-cGMP). Isometric contraction and fura-2 Ca^{2+} signals were measured simultaneously in preparations treated with Br-cGMP and with verapamil. The activation of calcium channels was estimated by measuring the quenching rate of the intracellular fura-2 signal by Mn^{2+} and by the depolarization-dependent influx of $^{45}Ca^{2+}$.

Stimulation with 67 mM KCl solution evoked an increase in cytosolic Ca^{2+} concentration ([Ca^{2+}]cyt) and a contractile response that were inhibited by pretreatment with verapamil (0.1 µM) or Br-cGMP (0.1–1 mM). However, the inhibition of the fura-2 Ca^{2+} signal was significantly higher with verapamil than with Br-cGMP, although the contraction was inhibited to a similar extent (Fig. 3).

When preparations were exposed to a K^+-depolarizing solution in which the calcium concentration was cumulatively increased, the related increase in the fura-2 Ca^{2+} signal was barely affected by Br-cGMP, although the contractile tension was strongly and significantly inhibited. Cellular Ca^{2+} changes were also estimated with $^{45}Ca^{2+}$. $^{45}Ca^{2+}$ influx in resting preparations was significantly reduced by Br-cGMP (0.1 mM) but not by verapamil (0.1 µM); $^{45}Ca^{2+}$ influx in KCl-depolarized preparations was reduced by verapamil but was unaffected by Br-cGMP. Measurements of Mn^{2+}-induced quenching of the intracellular fura-2 signal showed that Br-cGMP did not affect divalent cation entry in K^+-stimulated preparations, while verapamil concentration-dependently inhibited Mn^{2+} entry stimulated by K^+ depolarization (Fig. 4).

Such results indicate that Br-cGMP did not directly affect voltage-dependent Ca^{2+}-channel gating in the rat aorta. For a given fura-2 Ca^{2+} signal, the contraction is less in preparations exposed to Br-cGMP than in the untreated ones, suggesting that the activation of cGMP-dependent kinases reduces the contractile efficacy of calcium. Furthermore, the reduction of depolarization-dependent $^{45}Ca^{2+}$ uptake reported with sodium nitroprusside [26], a NO donor, was not observed with biologically

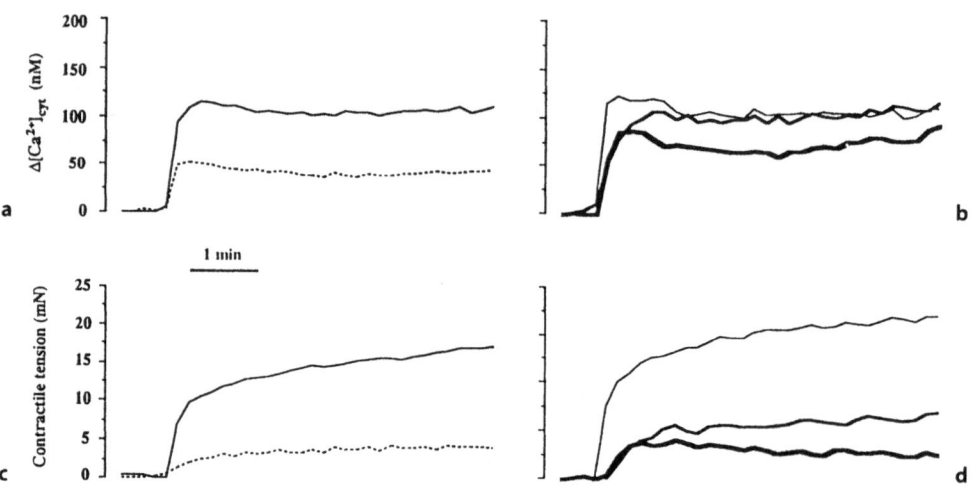

FIG. 3a–d. Effects of 8-bromo-cGMP (Br-cGMP) and verapamil on depolarization-evoked Ca^{2+} signal and contraction in rat aorta. Effects of verapamil (0.1 µM) and Br-cGMP (0.1–1 mM) on 67 mM KCl-stimulated calcium signals (Δ[Ca^{2+}]$_{cyt}$; **a,b**) and contractile tension (**c,d**). **a,c** *Solid line*, untreated preparation; *dashed line*, 0.1 µM verapamil-treated preparation. **b,d** *Thin line*, untreated preparation; *thicker line*, 0.1 mM Br-cGMP-treated preparation; *thickest line*, 1 mM Br-cGMP-treated preparation. (Modified from [25])

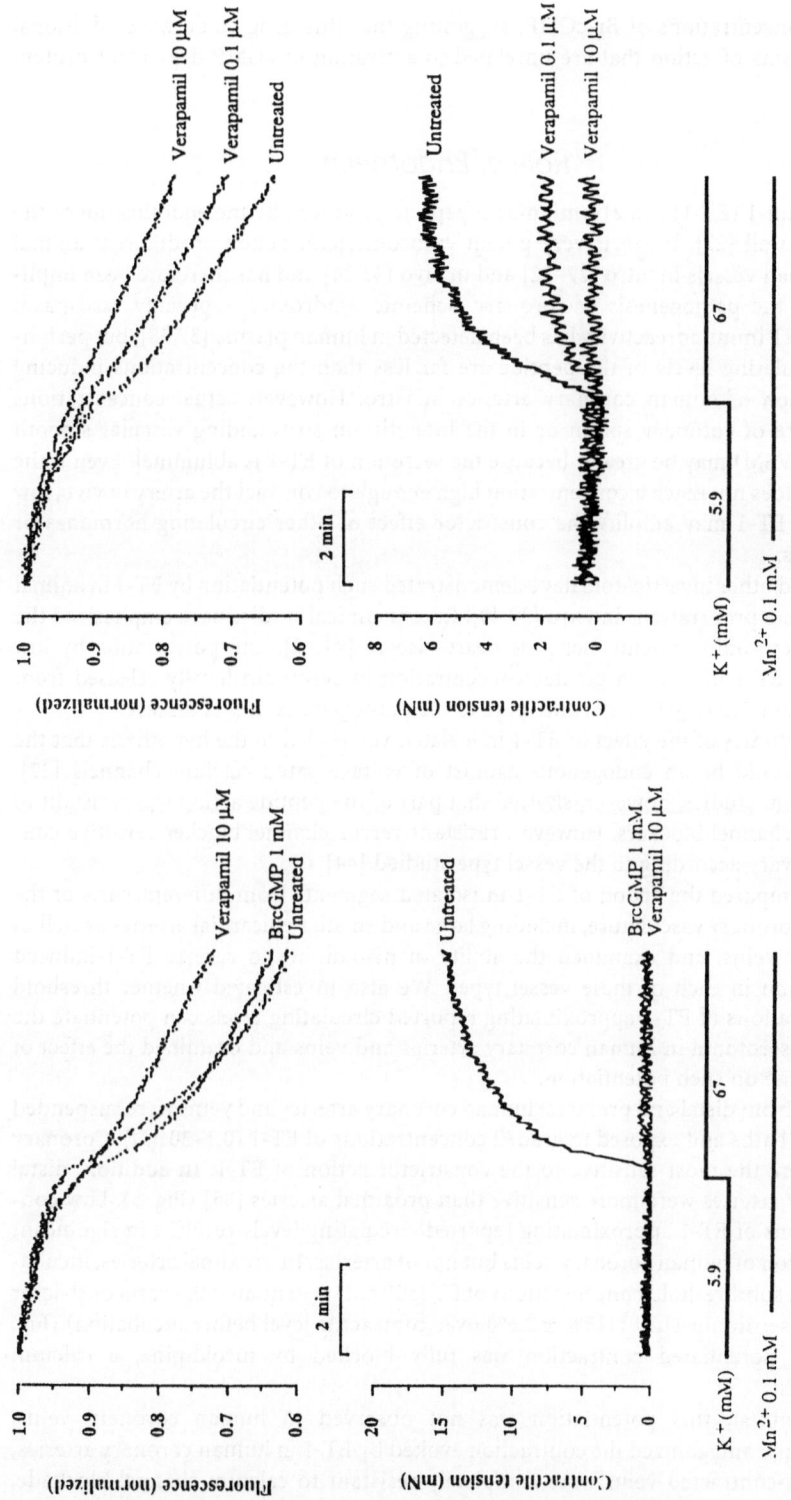

FIG. 4. Effects of 8-bromo-cGMP and verapamil on Mn²⁺-induced quenching of fura-2 fluorescence and contraction in rat aorta. *Left panel:* effects of 1 mM Br-cGMP and 10μM verapamil. *Right panel:* effects of verapamil (0.1 μM and 10μM). (Mondified from [25])

active concentrations of Br-cGMP, suggesting that this drug could have additional mechanisms of action that are unrelated to activation of cGMP-dependent protein kinase.

Role of Endothelin

Endothelin-1 (ET-1) is a 21-amino-acid peptide produced by the endothelium of the vascular wall [27]. It exerts very potent vasoconstrictor action on different animal and human vessels in vitro [27–32] and in vivo [33,34] and has therefore been implicated in the pathogenesis of coronary ischemic syndromes, especially vasospasm [35,36]. ET immunoreactivity has been detected in human plasma [37,38], but peripheral circulating levels of the peptide are far less than the concentrations inducing contraction of human coronary arteries in vitro. However, actual concentrations at the site of coronary spasm or in the interstitium surrounding vascular smooth muscle (VSM) may be greater because the secretion of ET-1 is abluminal. Even if the peptide does not reach a concentration high enough to contract the artery in vivo, low levels of ET-1 may amplify the constrictor effect of other circulating hormones or autacoids.

We and other investigators have demonstrated such potentiation by ET-1 in animal and human preparations in vitro [39,40]. Recent clinical studies have emphasized the role of serotonin in acute ischemic heart disease [41,42], and potentiation by low levels of ET-1 of a much greater concentration of serotonin locally released from activated platelets [43] may contribute to the pathogenesis of this disease.

Early studies of the effect of ET-1 in isolated vessels led to the hypothesis that the peptide could be an endogenous agonist of voltage-gated calcium channels [27]. Subsequent studies, however, showed that part of the peptide action was resistant to calcium channel blockers. However, resistant versus channel blocker-sensitive contraction vary according to the vessel type studied [44].

We compared the action of ET-1 in isolated segments from different parts of the human coronary vasculature, including large and smaller epicardial arteries as well as coronary veins, and examined the ability of nisoldipine to reverse ET-1-induced contraction in each of these vessel types. We also investigated whether threshold concentrations of ET-1 approximating reported circulating levels can potentiate the effect of serotonin in human coronary arteries and veins and examined the effect of nisoldipine on such potentiation.

Rings from distal and proximal human coronary arteries and veins were suspended in organ baths and exposed to graded concentrations of ET-1 (0.1–30 nM). Coronary veins were the most sensitive to the constrictor action of ET-1. In addition, distal coronary arteries were more sensitive than proximal arteries [45] (Fig. 5). Low concentrations of ET-1 approximating reported circulating levels resulted in significant contraction of human coronary veins but not of arteries. In proximal arteries, incubation with subthreshold concentrations of ET (300 pM) potentiated the vasoconstrictor effect of serotonin 1 μM (115% ± 2.6% over contractile level before incubation) (Fig. 6). This potentiated contraction was fully blocked by nisoldipine, a calcium antagonist.

In contrast, this potentiation was not observed in human coronary veins. Nisoldipine antagonized the contraction evoked by ET-1 in human coronary arteries, but ET-1-contracted veins were completely resistant to calcium channel blockade. Difference in sensitivity to nisoldipine in distal and proximal coronary arteries and

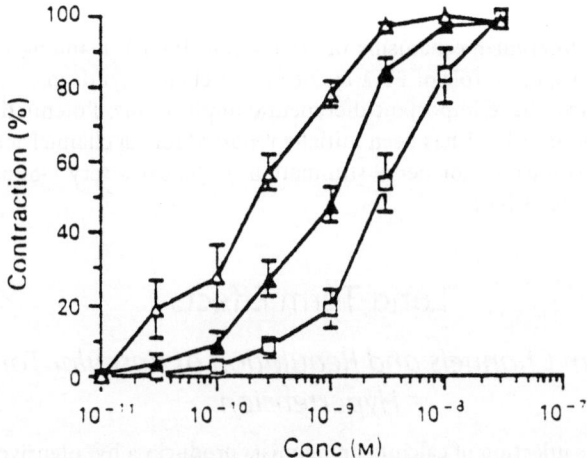

FIG. 5. Evidence for heterogeneity of endothelin-evoked response in human coronary artery. Concentration–response curves for endothelin-1 (ET-1) in human left-anterior descending coronary artery. Rings were prepared from segment 5 (*squares*; n = 7), segment 6 (*solid triangles*; n = 20), and the more distal part of segment 8 (*open triangles*; n = 6). (Modified from [45])

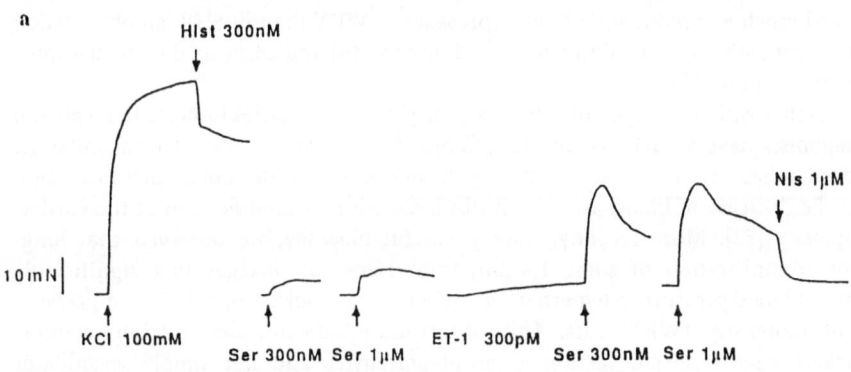

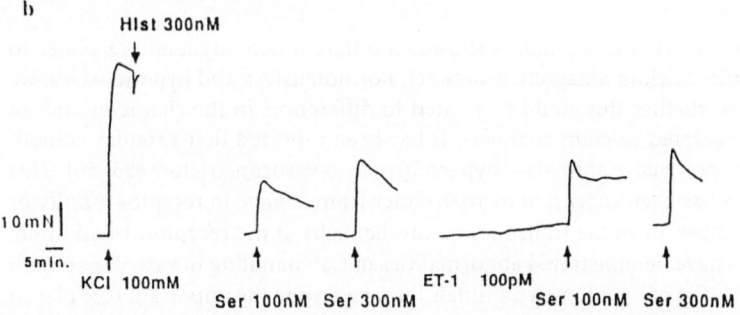

FIG. 6a,b Effect of nisoldipine (*Nis*) on contractions potentiated by endothelin-1 (*ET-1*) in human isolated coronary arteries and veins. Typical recording of contraction of a human proximal artery segment (a) and a human coronary vein segment (b) with two concentrations (0.3–1 μM) of serotonin (*Ser*) before and after 90-min incubation with a subthreshold concentration (100–300 pM) of ET-1. *Hist*, histamine. (Modified from [92])

veins suggests different mechanisms of contraction for ET-1 among these vessels. Because of the suspected role of ET-1 in coronary ischemic syndromes, this differential sensitivity may have important therapeutic implications. Potentiating action of low concentrations of ET-1 has been initially reported for Ca channel activator in rat aorta [39] and confirmed for nerve stimulation in the ear artery [46] as well as for catecholamine effects [40].

Long-Term Effects

Calcium Channels and Regulation of Vascular Tone in Hypertension

The intravenous injection of calcium antagonists produces a hypotensive effect more pronounced in hypertensive than in normotensive animals. In conscious rats, Ishii et al. [47] have observed that a similar decrease of blood pressure was evoked by nifedipine at doses much lower in spontaneously hypertensive (SHR) than in Wistar Kyoto (WKY) rats. Knorr and Garthoff [48] have compared the activity of nitrendipine and hydralazine on the blood pressure of SHR and WKY. They observed that the vasodilator hydralazine was equipotent in both strains, but that nitrendipine evoked much less reduction of blood pressure in WKY than in SHR, an observation consistent with recent clinical studies in humans [49] and confirmed with lacidipine and amlodipine [50].

Together with hemodynamic observations [51], these studies indicate that calcium antagonists have an activity profile different from classical arteriolar vasodilators. Indeed, it has been reported that during chronic administration of a calcium antagonist the decrease of blood pressure is observed without modification of the cardiac frequency [52]. More recently, after a careful bioassay, we observed that long-term administration of some 1,4-dihydropyridines at dosages that significantly reduced blood pressure in hypertensive (SHR) rats did not change the blood pressure of normotensive (WKY) rats. This observation indicates that calcium channel blockers have a specific action as antihypertensive and not simply vasodilator agents, which is consistent with the observation that they are powerful remodelling agents able to suppress cardiac and vascular hypertrophy of hypertensive animals [2,4].

Because these in vivo observations showed a different hemodynamic response to dihydropyridine–calcium antagonists between normotensives and hypertensives, we have examined whether this could be related to differences in the characteristics of their voltage-operated calcium channels. It has been reported that vascular smooth muscle from hypertensive animals is hypersensitive to vasoconstrictors [53–56]. This hyperreactivity has been suggested to arise either from change in receptor affinity or in receptor number, or in the transduction mechanisms of the receptor. In addition, several reports have demonstrated abnormalities of Ca^{2+} handling in vascular smooth muscle cells (SMCs) of hypertensive animals that, regarding the important role played by Ca^{2+} in the regulation of vascular tone, could be responsible for marked change in vessel reactivity [57,58]. Different observations have suggested that voltage-dependent Ca^{2+} channels could be altered in vessels from hypertensive rats. The first argument for the implication of a change in Ca^{2+} channels in hypertension is the blood pressure-lowering effect of Ca^{2+} antagonists [51,59]. Those drugs have also been shown to suppress the myogenic active tone displayed by blood vessels from hypertensive rats [58,60].

We have investigated the changes occurring in the functional responses to Ca^{2+} channel modulation in arteries from SHR. Seeking the cause of those modifications, different hypotheses were tested. The existence of a change in the receptor properties of the Ca^{2+} channels was tested by measuring the binding of a dihydropyridine Ca^{2+} channel blocker.

Comparison of Contractile Properties of Arteries from Normotensive and Hypertensive Rats and Their Relation with Calcium Channels

Post-contraction Tone

When arteries of SHR are pre-contracted by exposure to 100 mM KCl solution and thereafter transferred into a physiological solution, they show long-lasting elevation of their tone. The amplitude of this post-contraction tone, which is absent in arteries from normotensive rats, is related to the age of the rat, being much higher in older than in younger rats. This vessel tone is suppressed after preincubation of the arteries with the dihydropyridine Ca^{2+}-channel blockers nisoldipine and amlodipine, and is absent in aortas from SHR treated with doses of amlodipine and nisoldipine that inhibit the development of hypertension [2,4] (Fig. 7). The post-contraction tone of SHR arteries is greatly attenuated when the arteries are submitted to successive long-lasting stimulations by KCl solution. These observations indicate that a labile factor could be responsible for this anomalous tone, which may be related to a reduced threshold for activation of calcium channels in SHR vessels, a conclusion consistent with their increased responsiveness to calcium channel activators.

Response to Ca^{2+}-Channel Activator in Arteries of Hypertensive Rats

Several reports [53,60] have shown that arteries isolated from hypertensive rats present an increased sensitivity to the Ca^{2+}-channel activator Bay K 8644, which is known to produce a contraction of vascular smooth muscles by increasing the probability of opening of voltage-operated Ca^{2+} channels [61]. Figure 8 shows the concentration–response curves to Bay K 8644 measured in aortic rings of 20-week-old normotensive WKY and SHR in the presence of N^{ω}-nitro-L-arginine (L-NNA, 100 μM)

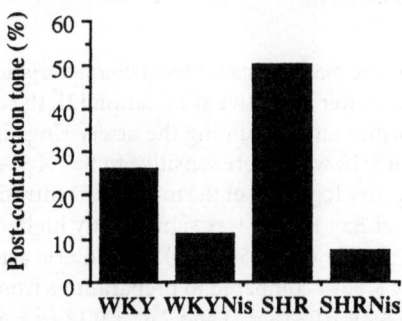

FIG. 7. Post-contraction tone of aortic rings from spontaneously hypertensive (*SHR*) and normotensive Wistar Kyoto (*WKY*) rats measured 5 min after changing the 100 mM KCl solution in the bath to a physiological solution. Post-contraction tone was significantly higher in SHR than in WKY aortic rings. Chronic treatment of the rats by nisoldipine (*SHRNis-WKYNis*) significantly reduced the post-contraction tone. (Modified from [2])

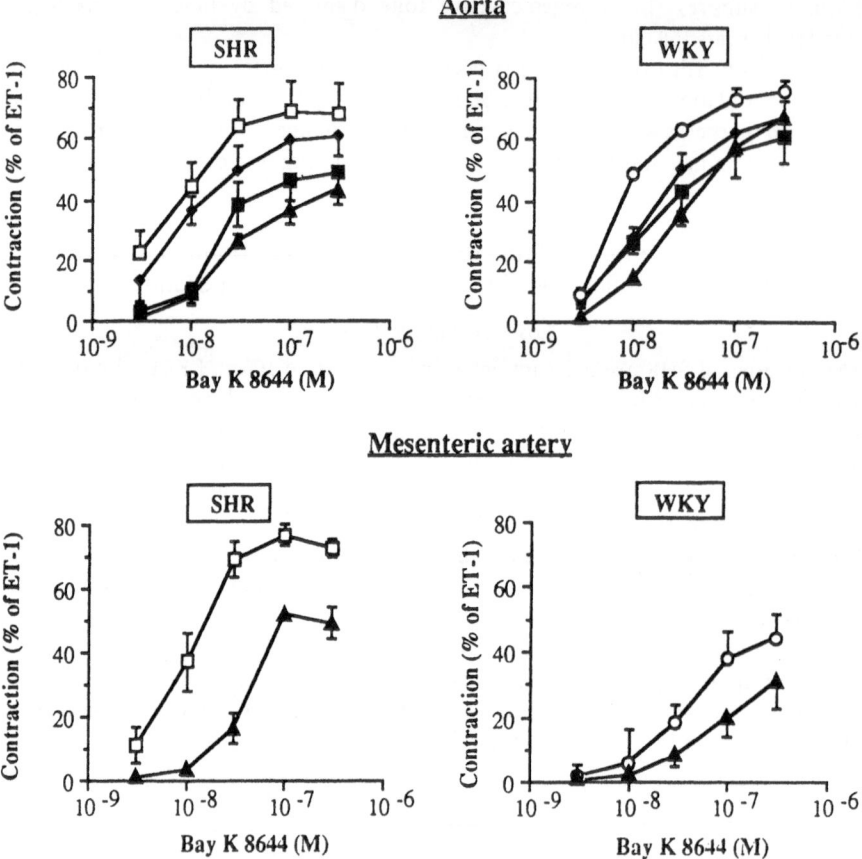

FIG. 8. Cumulative concentration–response curves to Bay K 8644 in aorta and mesenteric artery rings from spontaneously hypertensive (SHR) and normotensive Wistar Kyoto (WKY) rats in the absence and the presence of amlodipine. Bay K 8644 contractions were induced in the presence of N-nitro-L-arginine (100 μM) and 9 (aorta) or 12.5 (mesenteric artery) mM KCl and in the absence (*open symbols*) or presence of amlodipine 1 nM (*diamond*), 3 nM (*square*), and 10 nM (*triangles*). (Modified from [4])

to block the synthesis of nitric oxide. Because most characteristics of the arteries from hypertensive rats disappear after repetitive stimulation [2], the contractions to Bay K 8644 were first elicited 60 min after mounting the artery rings in the organ baths. In these conditions, aortas of SHR were more sensitive to Bay K 8644 than were aortas of WKY. The pD_2 value (negative log value of the molar concentration producing 50% of the maximum response) of Bay K 8644 was significantly higher is SHR (8.06 ± 0.07) compared to WKY (7.67 ± 0.09) ($P > .05$, $n = 6$). Mesenteric arteries from SHR were also more sensitive to Bay K 8644 compared to preparations from WKY. pD_2 values of Bay K 8644 were equal to 8.2 ± 0.07 ($n = 7$) and 7.62 ± 0.13 ($n = 6$; $P > .05$) in SHR and WKY, respectively (Fig. 8).

Effect of Amlodipine Added In Vitro on the BAY K 8644 Concentration–Effect Curve

The effect of an in vitro incubation of the aortic rings in the presence of various concentrations of the Ca-antagonistic dihydropyridine amlodipine was also examined. As illustrated in Fig. 8, the preincubation of aortas isolated from WKY for 120 min in physiological solution with amlodipine (1–10 nM) shifted the concentration–response curve of Bay K 8644 to the right without producing a significant decrease in the maximum response. However, in the same conditions, in aortas from SHR the Bay K 8644 curve shift to the right was more pronounced than in WKY, and the maximum response to Bay K 8644 was significantly depressed.

Results were analyzed as noncompetitive antagonism as described by Kenakin [62]. This analysis of the data yielded the following values for the apparent K_B for amlodipine: 3.9 ± 0.7 nM ($n = 4$) and 1.3 ± 0.3 nM ($n = 4$) ($P > .05$) in WKY and SHR aortas, respectively, which were approximately four times lower than the K_i values obtained in radioligand-binding studies. Figure 8 also illustrates the effect of the in vitro preincubation of mesenteric arteries in the presence of amlodipine 10 nM. In agreement with the results with aortas, amlodipine was a more potent inhibitor of the Bay K 8644-induced contraction in SHR than in WKY mesenteric artery rings.

Dihydropyridine-Binding Sites

There is no agreement in radioligand-binding studies to show that a modification in the receptor for dihydropyridine Ca^{2+}-channel blockers occurs in SHR, causing the higher sensitivity of SHR arteries to Ca^{2+} channel modulators. Chatelain et al. [63] reported that the dihydropyridine-binding site density increased in cardiac membrane preparations from 24-week-old SHR compared to normotensive WKY. However, no significant difference was found by other authors in 1,4-dihydropyridine binding site densities between hearts from normotensive and hypertensive animals [2,64,65].

We measured the $[^3H](+)$isradipine-specific binding in segments of intact aortas and mesenteric arteries to preserve the cellular factors that regulate the activity of Ca^{2+} channels in vivo. Saturation curves of $[^3H](+)$isradipine binding were established in aortic rings from WKY and SHR bathed in 100 mM KCl solution. In both strains, the analysis of the binding data showed the presence of an homogeneous population of specific binding sites. No difference was noted either in the dissociation constant (K_D) or in maximum binding (B_{max}) value between the two strains (K_D, 53 ± 6.9 pM and 62 ± 13 pM; B_{max}, 4.8 ± 0.4 and 4.5 ± 0.5 fmol/mg wet weight, in SHR and WKY aortas, respectively).

The binding of dihydropyridines is voltage dependent: according to the modulated receptor model, the binding affinity of dihydropyridine Ca^{2+} antagonists varies with the state of the Ca^{2+} channel, the inactivated state of the channel in arteries presenting a higher affinity than the resting state of the channel [66]. In aortas from both WKY and SHR, the specific binding of $[^3H](+)$isradipine (at a free concentration of 100 pM, a concentration close to its K_D value) was dependent on the concentration of KCl in the medium (Fig. 9). The maximum specific binding was obtained in the presence of 100 mM KCl and did not differ in aortas from WKY or SHR, in agreement with saturation experiments. At KCl concentrations less than 20 mM, however, the specific binding was significantly greater in aortas from SHR compared to WKY ($P < .05$). Similar results were obtained in the superior mesenteric artery.

Because there was no difference in B_{max} between depolarized artery preparations from SHR and WKY, the difference observed in unstimulated arteries may be related to a higher proportion of inactivated channels in SHR aortas. According to the equation $1/K_{app} = h/K_R + (1-h)/K_I[28]$, where K_R and K_I are the dissociation constants for the resting and inactivated channel, respectively, K_R being greater than K_I, K_{app} the appar-

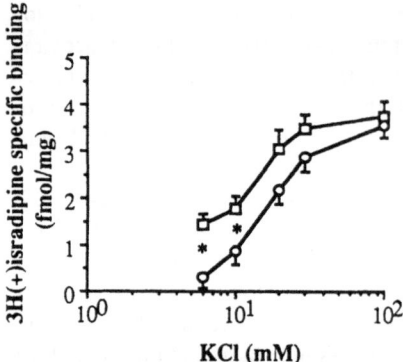

FIG. 9. Influence of KCl concentration in the medium on the specific binding of ^{3}H(+)-isradipine in aortic rings from spontaneously hypertensive (SHR, *squares*) and normotensive Wistar Kyoto (WKY, *circles*) rats. (Modified from [4])

ent dissociation constant, and h the proportion of the inactivated channels, we estimated that in aortas bathed in physiological solution the proportion of inactivated channels is less than 10% in WKY and about 30% in SHR. This difference in binding of dihydropyridine (DHP) between SHR and WKY may be related to the difference in resting membrane potential that has been noted between SHR and WKY aortic SMCs, SHR aortic SMCs being depolarized by about 10 mV compared to WKY aortic SMCs [4].

Influence of Salt Loading on the Cardiac and Renal Preproendothelin-1 mRNA Expression in Stroke-Prone Spontaneously Hypertensive Rats and Its Blood Pressure-Independent Inhibition by Lacidipine

It has been proposed that ET-1 may play a role in the pathophysiology of hypertension, but plasma ET-1 concentrations in experimental and human hypertension are similar or slightly higher than in normotensive controls [67]. Kurihara et al. [68] have recently reported that ET-1$^{+/-}$ heterozygous mice, which produce lower plasma levels of endothelin-1 than wild-type mice, develop elevated blood pressure. It could therefore be that ET-1 plays a more important role in the regulation of vascular resistance as an autocrine/paracrine effector than as a circulating factor.

Among effects that would not be mediated through circulating ET-1, pathophysiological involvement of ET-1 production has recently been suggested in renal and cardiac tissues. Hoffman et al. [69] have claimed that because of the diuretic and natriuretic effect of endothelin [70,71] it is conceivable that a renal deficiency of the peptide causes volume-overload hypertension. As for the role of ET-1 in the heart, ET-1 was shown to stimulate hypertrophy and contractility of cultured rat cardiomyocytes [72], associated with the induction of muscle-specific gene transcripts [73]. Moreover, an association between salt sensitivity and a greater incidence of renal failure and cardiac hypertrophy has been described in some groups of hypertensive patients [74,75].

As reported recently by us [76], the age-related increase of systolic blood pressure (SBP) in salt-loaded stroke-prone spontaneously hypertensive rats (SL-SHRSP) was not different from that of non-salt-loaded-(NS) SHRSP, so that blood pressure values after 6 weeks of NaCl treatment were not significantly different between these two groups (Table 1). At the opposite extreme, salt loading significantly induced cardiac hypertrophy, as shown by the measurements of ventricle to: body weight ratio (Table 1). Northern blot analysis of total RNA extracted from rat ventricles and kidneys using a specific probe for preproendothelin-1 (preproET-1) revealed a single band of 2.3 kb, in agreement with the size of preproET-1 transcripts previously described [27]. Densitometric scanning of the autoradiograms showed that the cardiac expression of preproET-1 mRNA was 3.4-fold more elevated in 14-week-old SPSHR-SL than in age-matched SPSHR-NS ($P < .01$). No significant difference in the expression of the gene of preproET-1 was detected from the kidney of these two types of rats (Fig. 10). This finding together with the observation that the SBP was not significantly different in each group is in agreement with the hypothesis proposed by Hoffman et al. [69] that the level of renal ET-1 is closely related to the blood pressure level.

A most interesting conclusion from our study, however, is that the SBP modulation may not be advanced to explain the production of ET-1 in salt-loaded rat ventricles and the significant increase of cardiac hypertrophy in these same rats. In different publications [75], it has been suggested that a trophic effect of sodium on cardiac mass may be superimposed on that of pressure load imposed on the left ventricle in essential hypertension. From our data, ET-1, which is known to act in a paracrine/

TABLE 1. Biometric parameters of non-salt-loaded (NS) and salt-loaded (SL) stroke-prone spontaneously hypertensive rats (SHRSP).

Lacidipine dosage (mg kg⁻¹ day⁻¹)	Blood pressure (mm Hg)	Ventricle to body weight ratio (mg/g)	Aorta weight/ length (mg/mm)
SHRSP-NS			
0 ($n = 7$)	235.9 ± 9.3	3.28 ± 0.05	0.789 ± 0.021
0.3 ($n = 7$)	241.9 ± 6.1	3.15 ± 0.05	0.770 ± 0.028
SHRSP-SL			
0 ($n = 7$)	241.9 ± 16.2	3.75 ± 0.12*	0.918 ± 0.026*
0.3 ($n = 7$)	264.1 ± 10.2	3.40 ± 0.06**	0.841 ± 0.020***

*, $P < .01$, vs SHR-NS lacidipine, 0; ***, $P < .05$; **, $P < .01$, vs SHR-SL lacidipine, 0.

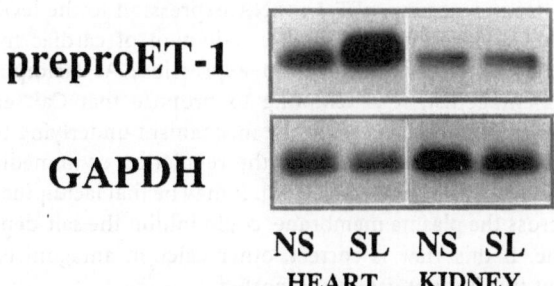

preproET-1

GAPDH

NS SL NS SL
HEART   KIDNEY

FIG. 10. Influence of salt loading on cardiac and renal preproendothelin-1(*preproET-1*) mRNA expression in stroke-prone spontaneously hypertensive rats (SPSHR). Analysis of preproET-1 mRNA expression in heart and kidney of SHRSP under the influence of sodium load is shown by Northern blot analysis of total RNA, extracted from ventricles and kidneys of salt-loaded (*SL*) and non-salt-loaded (*NS*) SHRSP and hybridized with ³²P-labeled cDNA probe for rat preproET-1 and glyceraldehyde 3-phosphate dehydrogenase (*GAPDH*). (Modified from [76])

autocrine manner in growth regulation through induction of immediate-early genes [77], could therefore be considered as one of the missing links between dietary salt intake and blood pressure-independent cardiac hypertrophy. We cannot exclude that the cardiac ET-1 level in the model of genetically hypertensive rats is not in part dependent on the SBP level. Nevertheless, Larivière et al. [78] showed that vascular hypertrophy and increased production of immunoreactive ET-1 were found in the vessels of salt-loaded mineralocorticoid-dependent hypertensive rats and not of spontaneously hypertensive rats, but they did not provide information on renal ET-1 expression.

The mechanism for the salt-induced production of ET-1 in the heart of SPSHR may be related to any of the different stimuli that increase the expression of ET-1 mRNA transcripts. Interestingly, Ang II-induced hypertrophy of cultured rat cardiomyocytes was shown to be partially blocked by an endothelin receptor antagonist [79]. More-over, Sung et al. [80] have recently demonstrated that Ang-II stimulated the release of immunoreactive endothelin from cultured vascular SMCs. Cardiac-specific regulation of the renin-angiotensin system could therefore mediate local responses such as the induction of ET-1 production. However, dietary salt excess is known to reduce plasma renin activity in SHRSP [81], and this could be the same for the tissular renin activity although enhancement of the brain renin-angiotensin system following long-term salt loading has been reported in spontaneously hypertensive rats [82]. Thus, the role of the tissular renin-angiotensin system still needs to be better characterized after salt loading.

The age-related increase of SBP was not altered by salt loading or lacidipine treatment as shown by the SBP values in the different groups of SPSHR at the 13th week of age (see Table 1). However, our data [83] showed, interestingly, that lacidipine at the daily dosage of $0.3\,\mathrm{mg\,kg^{-1}}$ reduced cardiovascular hypertrophy in salt-loaded rats (SPSHR-SL) ($P < .05$), but was without significant action on ventricle and aorta weights in non-salt-loaded rats (SPSHR-NS) (Table 1). This confirms that the protective properties of lacidipine are not necessarily related to a reduction of SBP. Furthermore, no significant effect on cardiac mass was observed in non-salt-loaded rats, indicating that this low dose of lacidipine specifically blunted salt-dependent mechanisms.

Northern blot analysis of total RNA extracted from rat ventricles using a specific probe for preproET-1 revealed that lacidipine treatment (daily dosage of $0.3\,\mathrm{mg\,kg^{-1}}$) reduced the salt-dependent preproET-1 mRNA expression to the level of untreated SPSHR-NS (Fig. 11). This suggests that the reduction of cardiac hypertrophy by lacidipine was related to reduction of ET-1 expression. As lacidipine is a highly selective calcium antagonist, it is tempting to propose that Ca^{2+} entry blockade through the plasma membrane could be the mechanism underlying this inhibition. Calcium influx is known to be involved in the regulation of immediate-early gene transcription induced by ET-1 and Ang II [84]. It may be that lacidipine, by regulating calcium fluxes across the plasma membrane, could inhibit the salt-dependent induction of ET-1 gene. If this view is correct, other calcium antagonists should exert similar effects, but this has not yet been reported.

Alternatively, so-called secondary properties of L-type calcium channel blockers could account for the inhibition of ET-1 expression in ventricles of lacidipine-treated rats. For instance, perturbation resulting from the interaction of a highly lipophilic drug such as lacidipine with the plasma membrane may physically affect the activity of membrane proteins. Roth et al. [85] have reported that the protein kinase C signal transduction pathway, known to cause protooncogene expression, could be

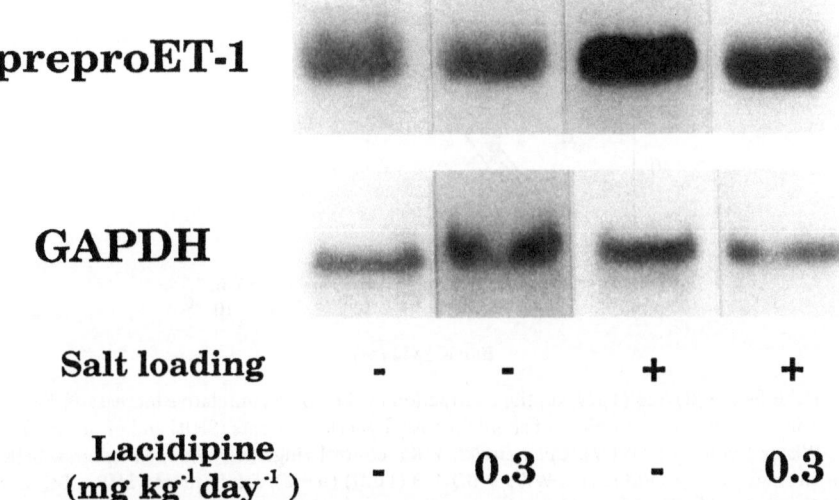

preproET-1

GAPDH

| Salt loading | - | - | + | + |
| Lacidipine (mg kg⁻¹day⁻¹) | - | **0.3** | - | **0.3** |

FIG. 11. Inhibition by lacidipine of salt-dependent endothelin gene expression in stroke-prone spontaneously hypertensive rats (SHRSP). Northern blot analysis of total RNA (20 μg/lane), extracted from ventricles of SHRSP and hybridized with ^{32}P-labeled cDNA probe for rat preproET-1 and GAPDH, shows the effects of salt loading and lacidipine daily treatment. (Modified from [83])

perturbated by a high concentration of a dihydropyridine into lipid bilayers. It will be necessary to examine the effect of lacidipine on ET-1 gene expression in isolated cells to see if the action here reported is a direct one or is mediated through a neuroendocrine pathway sensitive to both salt loading and lacidipine.

The Functional Consequences of the Overexpression of ET-1 in the Cardiovascular System

The role of endothelin in the pathogenesis of hypertension is a matter of controversy [70], and although ET-1 at subthreshold concentration does potentiate the action of drugs acting through L-type calcium channels, there is no clear demonstration that the effects reported earlier under Long-Term Effect may be related to ET-1. However, significant increase in the immunoreactive ET-1 content and in preproET-1 gene expression have been found in vessels from deoxycorticosterone acetate- (DOCA-) salt hypertensive rats [86], suggesting that endothelin could be increased in some cases of hypertension. Involvement of endothelin in the pathogenesis of hypertension is suggested by the observation that BQ-123, an antagonist of the endothelin ET_A receptor [87], produces a significant decrease in blood pressure in stroke-prone spontaneously hypertensive rats [88] and in transgenic renin hypertensive rats (A Knorr, personal communication).

To investigate whether endothelin could be involved in the hyperreactivity of arteries from SHR, we measured the influence of the endothelin antagonist BQ-123 on the contraction induced by Bay K 8644 in the aorta from 20-week-old WKY and SHR in the presence of L-NNA [90]. We observed that BQ-123 (1 μM) shifted the dose-response curve of SHR aortic rings to Bay K 8644 to the right but had no significant effect on the contraction evoked by Bay K 8644 in WKY aortic rings (Fig. 12). The pD_2

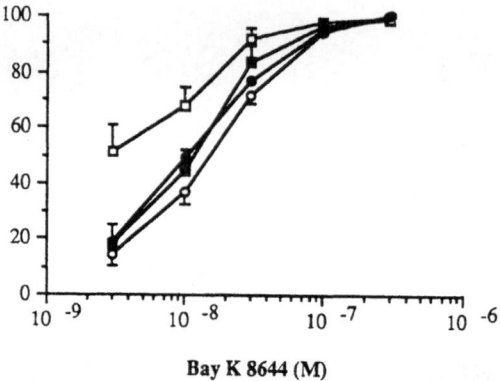

Bay K 8644 (M)

FIG. 12. Effect of BQ-123 (1 μM) on the contraction evoked by a cumulative increase in Bay K 8644 concentration in aortic rings of spontaneously hypertensive rats (SHR) and of normotensive Wistar Kyoto rats (WKY). *Open circles*, WKY control rings (*n* = 6); *open squares*, SHR control rings (*n* = 7); *solid circles*, WKY + BQ-123 (1 μM) (*n* = 6); *solid squares*, SHR + BQ-123 (1 μM) (*n* = 7). (Modified from [4])

values of Bay K 8644 were 7.86 ± 0.04 and 7.98 ± 0.02 (*n* = 6) in WKY aortas in the absence and presence of BQ-123, respectively, and 8.51 ± 0.16 and 7.99 ± 0.07 (*n* = 7; *P* < .05) in SHR aortic rings in the absence and presence of BQ-123, respectively [89].

Such a result suggests that endothelin could play a role in the hyperreactivity of Ca^{2+} channels in SHR aorta; therefore, we have designed other experiments to test this hypothesis by studying properties of arteries isolated from animals with an increased ET-1 gene expression.

We have examined the reactivity of arteries isolated from stroke-prone SP sodium-loaded rats. Those arteries were studied when we observed a marked increase in preproendothelin mRNA levels in the cardiovascular system, 6 weeks after sodium load and just before the appearance of the stroke lesions. The responsiveness of those arteries was influenced by sodium load, as shown by the higher sensitivity of the basilar artery to the contracting action of Bay K 8644. Interestingly, we observed, as reported previously, that there was no further increase in blood pressure in these animals, and the simultaneous measurement of the response of the resistance mesenteric artery showed that there was no difference in responsiveness between salt-loaded and other rats, indicating that the higher sensitivity was located in the cerebral circulation, which is pathologically sensitive to salt. This indicates that endogenous endothelin like exogenous endothelin increases vessel reactivity and that this might be relevant to its pathophysiological action.

Concluding Remarks

Experimental results summarized here demonstrate that at a low threshold level ET-1, which has been implicated in pathological states, may markedly influence the reactivity of blood vessels to vasoconstrictors and increase the tone of the preparation. This may occur when its expression is enhanced by diet manipulation, which aggravate the pathological state of animals. It must be emphasized that in such conditions, when the reactivity of vessels is increased there is also tissue remodeling characterized by cardiac and vascular hypertrophy. It has been discussed by other authors that such changes may have important functional consequences in vivo [90,91]. In this chapter it has also been shown that calcium channel blockers not only are agents able to inhibit vasoconstrictor responses, but are also able to inhibit the induction of genes such as the ET-1 gene. That this novel property may be observed at drug regimens which do not influence blood pressure means that the effect of growth factor may be separated from the effect of vasoconstrictors in a disease such as hypertension, and gives a rationale for a therapy of hypertension beyond the control of vascular tone. Our results also indicate that the control of endothelin gene expression could provide an appropriate therapy for some diseases including cardiac ischemia and stroke. The therapeutic action of calcium antagonists in those conditions could also be related to an effect beyond the control of vascular tone, for instance, the overexpression of the ET-1 gene.

References

1. Spedding M, Paoletti R (1992) Classification of calcium channels and the sites of action of drugs modifying channel function. Pharmacol Rev 44:363–376
2. Godfraind T, Kazda S, Wibo M (1991) Effects of a chronic treatment by nisoldipine, a calcium antagonistic dihydropyridine, on arteries of spontaneously hypertensive rats. Circ Res 68:674–682
3. Micheli D, Ratti E, Toson G, Gaviraghi G (1991) Pharmacology of lacidipine, a vascular-selective calcium antagonist. J Cardiovasc Pharmacol 17:S1–S8
4. Morel N, Godfraind T (1994) Selective interaction of the calcium antagonist amlodipine with calcium channels in arteries of spontaneously hypertensive rats. J Cardiovasc Pharmacol 24:524–533
5. de la Lande IS, Cannell VA, Waterson JG (1966) The interaction of serotonin and noradrenaline on the perfused artery. Br J Pharm Pharmacol 28:255–272
6. Van Nueten JM, Janssen PAJ, Van Beek J, Xhonneux T, Verbeuren TJ, Vanhoutte PM (1981) Vascular effects of ketanserin (R 41 486), a novel antagonist of 5-HT2 serotonergic receptors. J Pharmacol Exp Ther 218:217–230
7. Tschopl M, Miller RC, Pelton TJ, Stoclet JC, Bucher B (1993) Vasoconstrictor effects of various neuropeptide Y analogues on the rat tail artery in the presence of phenylephrine. Br J Pharmacol 110:1098–1104
8. Inagami T, Naruse M, Hoover R (1995) Endothelium as an endocrine organ. Annu Rev Physiol 57:171–89
9. Furchgott RF, Zawadzki JV (1980) The obligatory role of endothelial cells in the relaxation of arterial smooth muscle by acetylcholine. Nature 288:373–376
10. Furchgott RF (1984) The role of endothelium in the responses of vascular smooth muscle to drugs. Annu Rev Pharmacol Toxicol 24:175–197
11. Ignarro LJ, Kadowitz PJ (1985) The pharmacological and physiological role of cyclic GMP in vascular smooth muscle relaxation. Annu Rev Pharmacol Toxicl 25:171–191
12. Palmer RMJ, Ferrige AG, Moncada S (1987) Nitric oxide release accounts for the biological activity of endothelium-derived relaxing factor. Nature 327:524–526
13. Feletou M, Vanhoutte PM (1987) Relaxation of canine coronary artery to electrical stimulation: limited role of free radicals. Am J Physiol 253:H884–H889
14. Diamond J, Chu EB (1983) Possible role for cyclic GMP in endothelium dependent relaxation in rabbit aorta by acetylcholine. Comparison with nitroglycerin. Res Commun Chem Pathol Pharmacol 41:369–381
15. Holzmann S (1982) Endothelium induced relaxation by acetylcholine associated with large rises in cyclic GMP in coronary arterial strips. J Cyclic Nucl Res 8:409–419
16. Rapoport RM, Martin BD, Murad F (1983) Endothelium dependent relaxation in rat aorta may be mediated through cyclic GMP dependent protein phosphorylation. Nature 306:174–176

17. Garland CJ, Plane F, Kemp BK, Cocks TM (1995) Endothelium-dependent hyperpolarization: a role in the control of vascular tone. Trends Pharmacol Sci 16:23–30
18. Cocks TM, Angus JA (1983) Endothelium-dependent relaxation of coronary arteries by noradrenaline and serotonin. Nature 305:627–630
19. Eglème C, Godfraind T, Miller RC (1984) Enhanced responsiveness of rat isolated aorta to clonidine after removal of the endothelial cell. Br J Pharmacol 81:16–18
20. Godfraind T (1986) EDRF and cyclic GMP control gating of receptor-operated calcium channels in vascular smooth muscle. Eur J Pharmacol 126:341–343
21. Lang D, Lewis MJ (1989) Endothelium-derived relaxing factor inhibits the formation of inositol trisphosphate by rabbit aorta. J Physiol (Lond) 411:45–52
22. Lang D, Lewis MJ (1991) Endothelium-derived relaxing factor inhibits the endothelin-1-induced increase in protein kinase C activity in rat aorta. Br J Pharmacol 104:139–144
23. Alosachie I, Godfraind T (1986) Role of cyclic GMP in the modulation by endothelium of the adrenolytic action of prazosin in rat isolated aorta. Br J Pharmacol 89:525–532
24. Furchgott RF, Bursztyn P (1967) Comparison of dissociation constants and of relative efficacies of selected agonists acting on parasympathetic receptors. Ann NY Acad Sci 144:882–899
25. Salomone S, Morel N, Godfraind T (1995) Effects of 8-bromo-cyclic GMP and verapamil on depolarization-evoked Ca^{2+} signal and contraction in rat aorta. Br J Pharmacol 114:1731–1737
26. Karaki H, Sato K, Ozaki H, Murakami K (1988) Effects of sodium nitroprusside on cytosolic calcium level in vascular smooth muscle. Eur J Pharmacol 156:259–266
27. Yanagisawa M, Kurihara H, Kimura S, Tomobe Y, Kobayashi M, Mitsui Y, Yazaki Y, Goto K, Masaki T (1988) A novel potent vasoconstrictor peptide produced by vascular endothelial cells. Nature 332:411–415
28. Chester AH, Dashwood MR, Clarke JG, et al (1989) Influence of endothelin on human coronary arteries and localization of its binding site. Am J Cardiol 63:1395–1398
29. Cocks TM, Faulkner NL, Sudhir K, Angus J (1989) Reactivity of endothelin-1 on human and canine large veins compared with large arteries in vitro. Eur J Pharmacol 171:17–24
30. D'Orléans-Just P, Finet M, de Nucci G, Vane JR (1989) Pharmacology of endothelin-1 in isolated vessels: effect of nicardipine, methylene blue, hemoglobin, and gossypol. J Cardiovasc Pharmacol 13 (suppl 5):S19–S22
31. Franco-Cereceda A (1989) Endothelin- and neuropeptide Y-induced vasoconstriction of human epicardial coronary arteries in vitro. Br J Pharmacol 97:968–972
32. Godfraind T, Mennig D, Bravo G, Chalant C, Jaumin P (1989) Inhibition by amlodipine of activity evoked in isolated human coronary arteries by endothelin, prostaglandin F2-alpha and depolarization. Am J Cardiol 64:I58–I64
33. Kiowski W, Lüscher TF, Linder L, Bühler FR (1991) Endothelin-1-induced vasoconstriction in humans. Reversal by calcium channel blockade but not by nitrovasodilators or endothelium-derived relaxing factor. Circulation 83:469–475
34. Vierhapper H, Wagner O, Nowotny P, Waldhausl W (1990) Effect of endothelin-1 in man. Circulation 81:1415–1418
35. Kurihara H, Yoshizumi M, Sugiyama T, et al (1989) The possible role of endothelin-1 in the pathogenesis of coronary vasospasm. J Cardiovasc Pharmacol 13(suppl 5):S132–S137
36. Lüscher TF (1990) Endothelin: key to coronary vasospasm? Circulation 83:701–703
37. Hartter E, Woloszcuk W (1989) Radioimmunoassay of endothelin. Lancet i:909
38. Davenport AP, Ashby MJ, Easton P, Ella S, Bedford J, Dickerson C, Nunez DJ, Capper SJ, Brown MJ (1990) A sensitive radioimmunoassay measuring endothelin-like immunoreactivity in human plasma: comparison of levels in patients with essential hypertension and normotensive control subjects. Clin Sci 78:261–264

39. Godfraind T, Mennig D, Morel N, Wibo M (1989) Effect of endothelin-1 on calcium channel gating by agonists in vascular smooth muscle. J Cardiovasc Pharmacol 13(suppl 5):S112–S117

40. Yang Z, Richard V, Von Segesser L, Bauer E, Stulz P, Turina M, Luscher TF (1990) Threshold concentrations of endothelin-1 potentiate contractions to norepinephrine and serotonin in human arteries. A new mechanism of vasospasm. Circulation 82:188–195

41. Golino P, Piscione F, Willerson JT, Cappelli-Bigazzi M, Focaccio A, Villari B, Indolfi C, Russolillo E, Condorelli M, Chiariello M (1991) Divergent effect of serotonin on coronary-artery dimensions and blood flow in patients with coronary atherosclerosis and control patients. N Engl J Med 324:641–648

42. McFadden EP, Clarke JG, Davies GJ, Kaski JC, Haider AW, Maseri A (1991) Effect of intracoronary serotonin on coronary vessels in patients with stable angina and patients with variant angina. N Engl J Med 324:648–654

43. Houston DS, Shepherd JT, Vanhoutte PM (1986) Aggregating human platelets cause direct contraction and endothelium-dependent relaxation in isolated canine coronary arteries. J Clin Invest 78:539–544

44. Godfraind T (1994) Calcium antagonists and vasodilatation. Pharmacol Ther 64:37–75

45. Godfraind T (1993) Evidence for heterogeneity of endothelin receptor distribution in human coronary artery. Br J Pharmacol 110:1201–1205

46. La M, Rand MJ (1993) Endothelin-1 enhances vasoconstrictor responses to exogenously administered and neurogenically released ATP in rabbit isolated perfused arteries. Eur J Pharmacol 249:133–139

47. Ishii H, Itoh K, Nose T (1980) Different antihypertensive effects of nifedipine in conscious experimental hypertensive and normotensive rats. Eur J Pharmacol 64:21–29

48. Knorr A, Garthoff B (1984) Differential influence of the calcium antagonist nitrendipine and the vasodilator hydralazine on normal and elevated blood pressure. Arch Int Pharmacodyn Ther 269:296–322

49. Meilhac B, Mallion JM, Carre A, Chanudet X, Poggi L, Gosse P, Dollocchio M (1992) Etude de l'influence de l'horaire de la prise sur l'effet antihypertenseur et la tolérance de la nitrendipine chez les patients hypertendus essentiels légers à modérés. Thérapie (Paris) 47:205–210

50. Micheli D, Ratti E, Toson G, Gaviraghi G (1991) Pharmacology of lacidipine, a vascular-selective calcium antagonist. J Cardiovasc Pharmacol 17:S1–S8

51. Kazda S, Knorr A (1990) Calcium antagonists In: Ganten D, Mulrow PJ (eds) Pharmacology of antihypertensive therapeutics. Springer, Berlin Heidelberg New York, pp 301–375

52. Fröhlich ED (1986) Hemodynamic effects of diltiazem in the spontaneously hypertensive rat and in human hypertension. In: Aoki K (ed) Essential hypertension: calcium mechanisms and treatment. Springer, Berlin Heidelberg New York, pp 191–218

53. Hollowa ET, Bohr DR (1973) Reactivity of vascular smooth muscle in hypertensive rats. Circ Res 33:678–685

54. Thompson LP, Bruner CA, Lamb FS, King CM, Webb RC (1987) Calcium influx and vascular reactivity in systemic hypertension. Am J Cardiol 59:29A–34A

55. Boonen HCM, De Mey JGR (1990) Increased calcium sensitivity in isolated resistance arteries from spontaneously hypertensive rats: effects of dihydropyridines. Eur J Pharmacol 179:403–412

56. Bodin P, Travo C, Stoclet JC, Travo P (1993) High sensitivity of hypertensive aortic myocytes to norepinephrine and angiotensin. Am J Physiol 264:C441–C445

57. Kwan CY (1985) Dysfunction of calcium handling by smooth muscle in hypertension. Can J Physiol Pharmacol 63:366–374

58. Sada T, Koike H, Ikeda M, Sato K, Ozaki H, Karaki H (1990) Cytosolic free calcium of aorta in hypertensive rats. Hypertension (Dallas) 16:245–251

59. MacGregor GA, Rotellar C, Markandu ND, Smith SJ, Saguella GA (1982) Contrasting effects of nifedipine, captopril and propranolol in normotensive and hypertensive subjects. J Cardiovasc Pharmacol 4:S358–S362

60. Aoki A, Asano M (1986) Effects of Bay K 8644 and nifedipine on femoral arteries of spontaneously hypertensive rats. Br J Pharmacol 88:221–230

61. Hess P, Lansman JB, Tsien RW (1984) Different modes of Ca channel gating behaviour favoured by dihydropyridine Ca agonists and antagonists. Nature 311:538–544

62. Kenakin TP (1987) Pharmacologic analysis of drug-receptor interaction. In: Pharmacologic analysis of drug-receptor interaction. Raven, New York

63. Chatelain P, Demol D, Roba J (1984) Comparison of [^{3}H]nitrendipine to heart membranes of normotensive and spontaneously hypertensive rats. J Cardiovasc Pharmacol 6:220–223

64. Ishii K, Kano T, Kurobe Y, Ando J (1983) Binding of [^{3}H]nitrendipine to heart and brain membranes from normotensive and spontaneously hypertensive rats. Eur J Pharmacol 88:277–278

65. Galletti F, Rutledge A, Krogh V, Triggle DJ (1991) Age-related changes in Ca^{2+} channels in spontaneously hypertensive rats. Gen Pharmacol 22:173–176

66. Morel N, Godfraind T (1991) Characterization in rat aorta of the binding sites responsible for blockade of noradrenaline-evoked calcium entry and contraction by nisoldipine. Br J Pharmacol 102:467–477

67. Vanhoutte PM (1993) Is endothelin involved in the pathogenesis of hypertension? Hypertension (Dallas) 21:747–751

68. Kurihara Y, Kurihara H, Suzuki H, Kodama T, Maemura K, Nagai R, Oda H, Kuwaki T, Cao WH, Kamada N, Jishage K, Ouchi Y, Azuma S, Toyoda Y, Ishikawa T, Kumada M, Yazaki Y (1994) Elevated blood pressure and craniofacial abnormalities in mice deficient in endothelin-1. Nature 368:703–710

69. Hoffman A, Grossman E, Abassi ZA, Keiser HR (1994) Renal endothelin and hypertension. Nature 372:50

70. Zeidel MI, Kone B, Brady H, Gullans S, Brenner BM (1989) Endothelin, a peptide inhibitor of Na^+-K^+-ATPase in intact renal tubular epithelial cells. Am J Physiol 257:C1101–1107

71. Hoffman A, Grossman E, Keiser HR (1990) Opposite effects of endothelin-1 and big-endothelin-(1–39) on renal functions in rats. Eur J Pharmacol 182:603–606

72. Suzuki T, Hoshi H, Mitsui Y (1990) Endothelin stimulates hypertrophy and contractility of neonatal rat cardiac myocytes in a serum-free medium. FEBS Lett 268:149–151

73. Ito H, Hirata H, Hiroe M, Tsujino M, Adachi S, Takamoto T, Nitta M, Taniguchi K, Marumo F (1991) Endothelin-1 induces hypertrophy with enhanced expression of muscle-specific genes in cultured neonatal rat cardiomyocytes. Circ Res 69:209–215

74. Campese VM (1994) Salt sensitivity in hypertension: renal and cardiovascular implications. Hypertension (Dallas) 23:531–550

75. Beil AH, Schmieder RE, Messerli FH (1994) Salt intake, blood pressure and cardiovascular structure. Cardiovasc Drugs Ther 8:425–432

76. Feron O, Salomone S, Godfraind T (1995) Inhibition by lacidipine of salt-dependent cardiac hypertrophy and endothelin gene expression in stroke-prone spontaneously hypertensive rats. Biochem Biophys Res Commun 210:219–224

77. Battistini B, Chailler P, D'Orléans-Juste P, Brière N, Sirois P (1993) Growth regulatory properties of endothelins. Peptides (Elms ford) 14:385–399

78. Larivière R, Thibault G, Schiffrin EL (1993) Increased endothelin-1 content in blood vessels of deoxycorticosterone acetate-salt hypertensive but not in spontaneously hypertensive rats. Hypertension (Dallas) 21:294–300

79. Ito H, Hirata Y, Adachi S, Tanaka M, Tsujino M, Koike A, Nogami A, Marumo F, Hiroe M (1993) Endothelin-1 is an autocrine/paracrine factor in the mechanism of angiotensin II-induced hypertrophy in cultured rat cardiomyocytes. J Clin Invest 92:398–403

80. Sung CP, Arleth AJ, Storer BL, Ohlstein EH (1994) Angiotensin type 1 receptors mediate smooth muscle proliferation and endothelin biosynthesis in rat vascular smooth muscle. J Pharmacol Exp Ther 271:429–437

81. Volpe M, Rubattu S, Ganten D, Enea I, Russo R, Lembo G, Mirante A, Condorelli G, Trimarco B (1993) Dietary salt excess unmasks blunted aldosterone suppression and sodium retention in the stroke-prone phenotype of the spontaneously hypertensive rat. J Hypertens 11:793–798

82. Yamashita Y, Takata Y, Takishita S, Kimura Y, Fujishima M (1986) Enhancement of brain renin-angiotensin system induced by long-term salt loading in spontaneously hypertensive rats. J Hypertens 4:S361–S363

83. Feron O, Salomone S, Godfraind T (1995) Influence of salt loading on the cardiac and renal preproendothelin-1 mRNA expression in stroke-prone spontaneously hypertensive rats. Biochem Biophys Res Commun 209:161–166

84. Grohe C, Nouskas J, Vetter H, Neyses L (1994) Effects of nisoldipine on endothelin-1- and angiotensin II-induced immediate/early gene expression and protein synthesis in adult rat ventricular cardiomycocytes. J Cardiovasc Pharmacol 24:13–16

85. Roth TM, Keul R, Emmons LR, Horl WH, Block LH (1992) Manidipine regulates the trascription of cytokine genes. Proc Natl Acad Sci USA 89:4041–4075

86. Lariviere R, Day R, Schiffrin EL (1993) Increased expression of endothelin-1 gene in blood vessels of deoxycorticosterone acetate salt hypertensive rats. Hypertension (Dallas) 21:916–920

87. Ihara M, Noguchi K, Saeki T, Fukuroda T, Tsuchida S, Kimura S, Fukami T, Ishikawa K, Nishikibe M, Yano M (1992) Biological profiles of highly potent novel endothelin antagonists selective for the ETA receptor. Life Sci 50:247–255

88. Nishikibe M, Tsuchida S, Okada M, Fukuroda T, Shimamoto K, Yano M, Ishikawa K, Ikemoto F (1993) Antihypertensive effect of a newly synthesized endothelin antago-nist, BQ-123, in a genetic hypertensive model. Life Sci 52:717–724

89. Morel N, Godfraind T (1994) The endothelin ETA receptor antagonist, BQ-123, normalizes the response of SHR aorta to Ca^{2+} channel activator. Eur J Pharmacol 252:R3–R4

90. Struyker-Boudier HAJ, van Bortel LMAB, De Mey JGR (1990) Remodeling of the vascular tree in hypertension: drug effects. Trends Pharmacol Sci 11:240–245

91. Mulvany MJ, Aalkjaer C, Heagerty AM, Nyborg NCB, Strandgaard S (1991) Resistance arteries, structure and function. Excerpta Med Int Cong Ser:905

92. Balligand JL, Godfraind T (1994) Effect of nisoldipine on the contractions evoked by endothelin-1 in human isolated distal and proximal coronary arteries and veins. J Cardiovasc Pharmacol 24:618–625

Smooth Muscle: Control of $[Ca^{2+}]_c$ by the Membrane Potential

GERRIT ISENBERG

Summary. Mechanisms by which the membrane potential can control Ca^{2+}-dependent contractions were studied by a combination of voltage-clamp and Ca^{2+} microfluometry. Ca^{2+} influx and the concentration of cytosolic Ca^{2+} ($[Ca^{2+}]_c$) were measured simultaneously in smooth muscle cells (smc) from the guinea pig, either visceral smc from the urinary bladder or vascular smc from the coronary artery. The first part of this chapter reviews the influence of membrane potential on Ca^{2+} influx through voltage-gated L-type Ca^{2+} channels; the second part describes the Ca^{2+} influx through nonselective cation channels that are activated by acetylcholine, ATP, or stretch. Depolarization-induced Ca^{2+} influx increases $\Delta[Ca^{2+}]_c$ with two components that can be separated by pharmacological interventions. The tonic component can be attributed to the direct effects of Ca^{2+} influx. The phasic component results from Ca^{2+}-induced Ca^{2+} release from the sarcoplasmic reticulum (SR) that amplifies the Ca^{2+} influx. In smc from urinary bladder and from coronary artery, the relative contributions of Ca^{2+} influx and of Ca^{2+} release to depolarization-induced $\Delta[Ca^{2+}]_c$ largely differ.

Key words. Smooth muscle—Membrane current—Intracellular Ca^{2+}—Ca^{2+} influx—Ca^{2+} release

Introduction

Our understanding of the membrane control of the concentration of cytosolic Ca^{2+} ($[Ca^{2+}]_c$) has been significantly improved by the introduction of isolated smooth muscle cells (smc). Ca^{2+} influx is quantified by voltage clamp and changes in $[Ca^{2+}]_c$ by fluorescent indicators in the same cell, knowledge that provides insight in the cellular and molecular events such as the opening of single Ca^{2+} channels or the Ca^{2+}-induced Ca^{2+} release from sarcoplasmic reticulum (SR). This chapter briefly reviews our results on this topic; the literature is too extensive to be referenced. The results are from two types of smc: (1) smc from the urinary bladder, which are excitable and typical of other visceral smc; and (2) smc from the coronary artery, which are nonexcitable and represent vascular smc. I show that the membrane potential controls $[Ca^{2+}]_c$ through similar mechanisms; however, the relative importance of these mechanisms largely differs in these two types of smc.

Department of Physiology, Martin-Luther University of Halle-Wittenberg, D-06097 Halle (Saale), Germany

Membrane Resting and Action Potential

Acutely isolated urinary bladder myocytes have resting potentials of about −50 mV [1]. On electrical stimulation, they generate action potentials (Fig. 1A). After the stimulus, the membrane depolarizes with a slow "pacemaker" depolarization (phase 0) to a threshold at −25 mV. The action potential rises (phase 1) to an overshoot of +20 mV. A rapid repolarization (phase 2) gives the action potential a duration of approximately 15 ms (measured at −20 mV). In vivo, the neurotransmitter acetylcho-

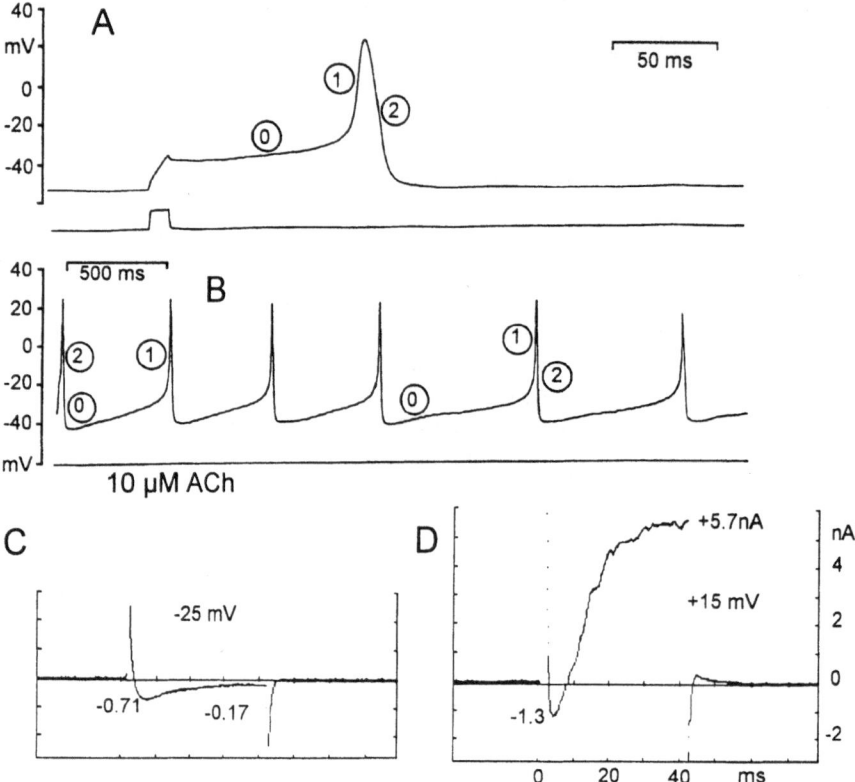

FIG. 1A–D. Action potentials and net membrane currents from a smooth muscle cell (smc) isolated from the urinary bladder of the guinea pig. **A** A small stimulus current (10 ms, 0.2 nA) depolarizes the membrane from the resting potential (−50 mV) to −38 mV. After the stimulus, the membrane does not repolarize but slowly depolarizes (phase 0). When −30 mV is reached, the action potential starts with a fast upstroke (phase 1) to the overshoot (25 mV). From the overshoot, the membrane rapidly repolarizes (phase 2) to the resting potential. **B** Bath application of 10 μM acetylcholine (*horizontal line*) induces a train of action potentials. Note: the most negative potential (−43 mV) turns into a pacemaker-depolarization (phase 0). **C,D** Net membrane currents recorded with the voltage-clamp technique with 44-ms steps depolarizing from −50 to −25 mV (**C**) or +15 mV (**D**). **C** At −25 mV, activation of the Ca^{2+}-channel current I$_{Ca}$ within 5 ms builds up a net negative current surge (−0.71 nA). In the nonclamped cell, the negative current I$_{Ca}$ generates the upstroke of the action potential (phase 1). In the following time, I$_{Ca}$ decays (inactivates) to −0.17 nA. **D** At +15 mV, the negative current surge (−1.3 nA) changes within 8 ms into a large outward potassium current (I$_{K(Ca)}$). In nonclamped cells, the positive I$_{K(Ca)}$ repolarizes the membrane to the resting potential. (From [1] with permission)

line (ACh) induces trains of action potentials. In the presence of ACh, there is not a stable resting potential; the repolarization changes into the pacemaker-depolarization (phase 0), thereby generating the next new action potential [2].

Membrane Currents Generating Action Potentials

Action potentials are generated by the flow of ionic currents through the surface membrane. The voltage-clamp technique measures these membrane currents. In general, inward currents depolarize and outward currents repolarize the membrane, the rate of the voltage change increasing with the current amplitude. A clamp step from -50 mV to -25 mV results in an inward current that peaks to -0.7 nA and then slowly decays with time (Fig. 1C). Later on, this inward current will be identified as a Ca^{2+}-channel current, I_{Ca}. A clamp step to 0 mV initially induces an inward current; after 10 ms, the current changes into an outward current (Fig. 1D) that is a Ca^{2+}-activated K^+ current ($I_{K(Ca)}$). ACh activates an inward current that flows through "nonselective cation channels" (I_{ns}). In the simple example of Fig. 1, the pacemaker depolarization is generated by I_{ns} and I_{Ca}, the rapid upstroke by I_{Ca}, and the repolarization by $I_{K(Ca)}$. In urinary bladder smc, the superimposition of these three time-dependent current components is sufficient for generating rhythmic electrical activity [1].

The density of I_{Ca} (I_{Ca} divided by the cell surface) is about tenfold smaller in coronary than in bladder smc [2], while the density of $I_{K(Ca)}$ is similar or larger. Because a small I_{Ca} is superimposed by a large $I_{K(Ca)}$ (Fig. 2B1), there is not enough net negative membrane current to generate an action potential. The coronary myocyte, however, can generate action potentials when the K^+ channels are blocked, by dialyzing Cs^+ ions from the electrode into the cell (see Fig. 2B3) or by adding Ba^{2+} or tetraethylammonium (TEA$^+$) ions to the bath. Excitability can also be induced by augmentation of I_{Ca}, as by vasopressin [3] or by Ca^{2+}-channel openers such as BayK 8644. Vice versa, excitable bladder smc become nonexcitable when I_{Ca} is reduced with Ca^{2+}-channel blockers (e.g., nifedipine) or when I_K is increased with K^+-channel openers (e.g., lemakalim [4]).

Ca^{2+} Channel Currents (I_{Ca})

Block of K^+ currents changes the net current into I_{Ca}. I_{Ca} disappears if the extracellular Ca^{2+} ions are substituted by Mg^{2+} ions (Fig. 3C). Most smc have an L- and an T-type I_{Ca}. Both currents flow through channels that open and close under the control of the membrane potential. T-type Ca^{2+} channels open between -70 and -20 mV (low-voltage-activated channels) and inactivate completely. The L-type Ca^{2+} channels activate at potentials to -40 mV (high-voltage-activated Ca^{2+} channels) and inactivate only incompletely ([5]; see following). Only the L-type I_{Ca} is blocked by Ca^{2+}-channel antagonists such as nifedipin, gallopamil, or diltiazem.

The gating of single L-type Ca^{2+} channels can be recorded with the patch-clamp technique (Fig. 3A). At -50 mV, the probability for channel openings (P_o) is almost zero, the channel is in the closed state C_1 where it is available for activation. Activation by depolarization to 0 mV induces bursts of short-duration inward currents (-0.4 pA at 0 mV, 2 mM [Ca^{2+}]$_o$, 37°C [6]). The channels do not open instantaneously but after an approximately 4-ms "waiting time." The waiting time suggests that the channel passes a second closed state, C_2, before it enters the open state O. More positive

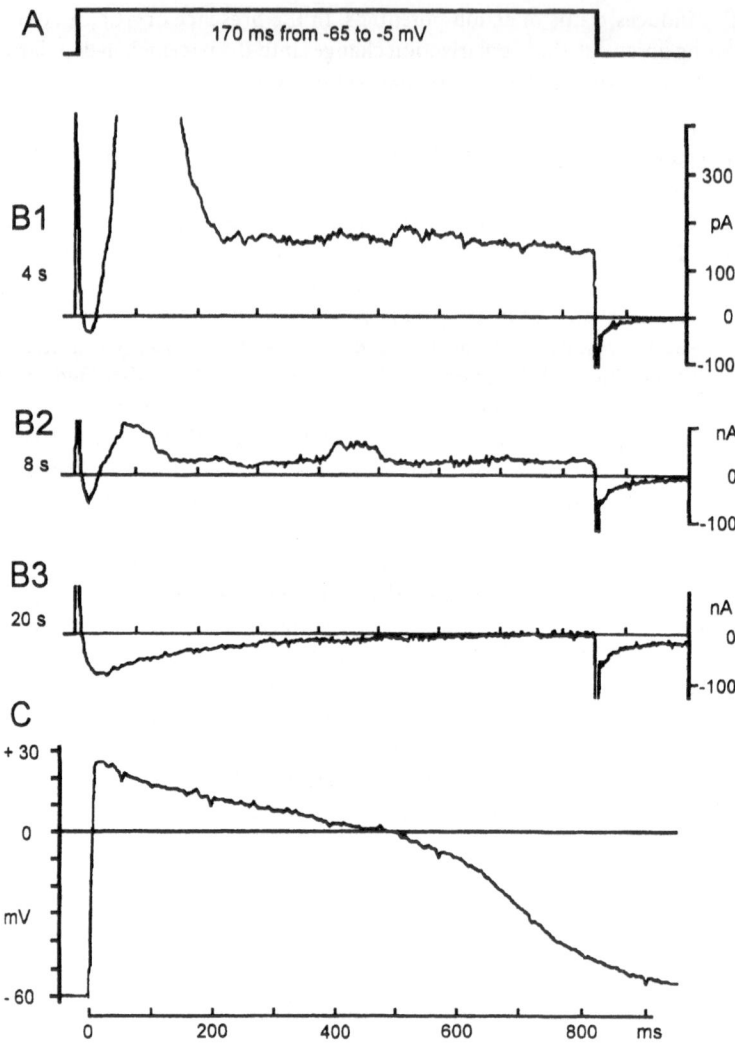

Fɪɢ. 2A–C. Coronary myocytes. **A** Voltage-clamp protocol at the top. **B** Net membrane currents: cell dialysis with Cs⁺ electrode solution reduces or blocks the large $I_{K(Ca)}$, thereby unmasking the I_{Ca} (20 s). The number of seconds at the left (*B1–B3*) indicate the time of Cs⁺ dialysis starting with whole-cell access. **C** When $I_{K(Ca)}$ is blocked, the coronary smc is excitable; it responds to the stimulus with 800-ms long action potentials

potentials shift the distribution between $C_1 \leftrightarrow C_2$ toward C_2 and thereby reduce the waiting time and increase P_o. The burst activity reflects multiple transitions $C_2 \leftrightarrow O \leftrightarrow C_2$.

From O, the channel can pass to the closed inactivated state I. At positive potentials this transition is nearly irreversible, that is, the channel is refractory. As a consequence, P_o decays with time (Fig. 3B; [7]). However, in a potential "window" between -50 and -0 mV, the transitions $O \rightarrow C_2$ and $O \rightarrow I$ compete with each other; that is, reopenings can occur and inactivation remains incomplete. Ca^{2+} influx through incompletely inactivated Ca^{2+} channels is related to the tonic component of $\Delta[Ca^{2+}]_c$ and

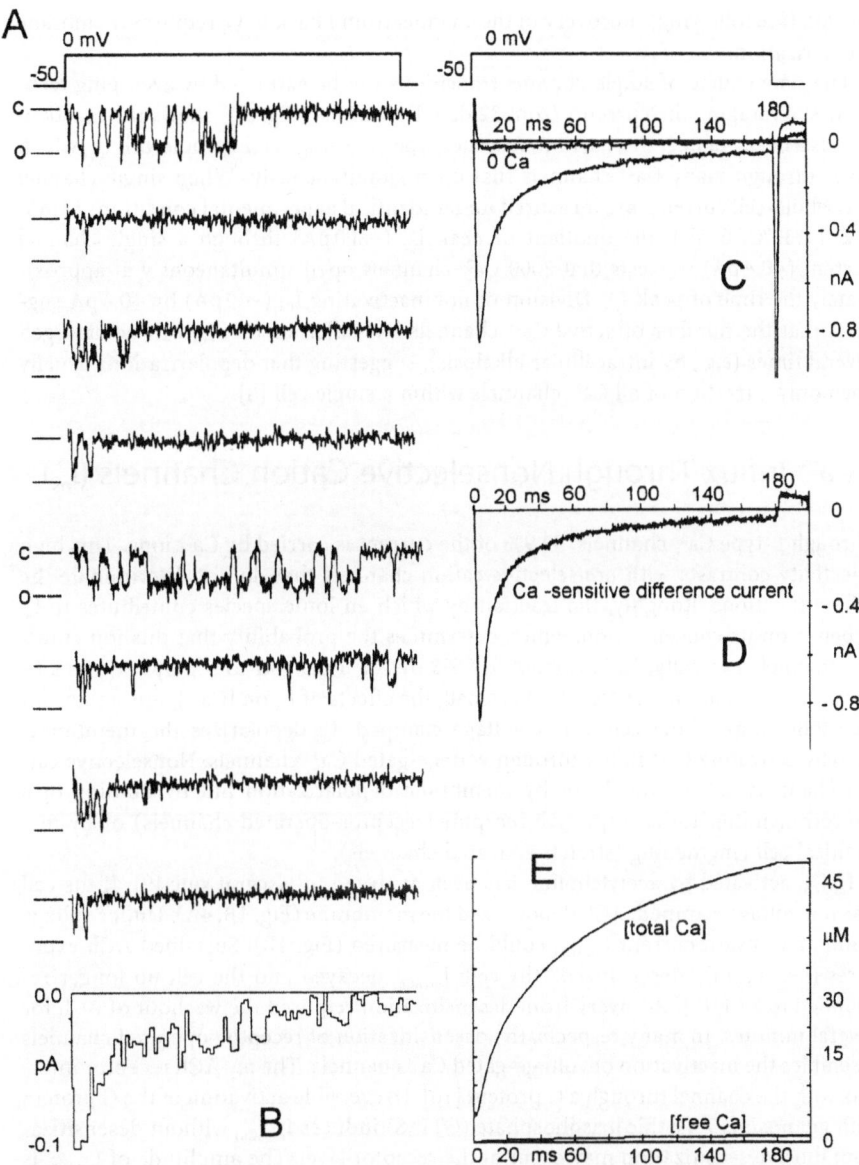

FIG. 3A–E. Gating of L-type Ca²⁺ currents of urinary bladder smc at 36°C and with 2 mM Ca²⁺ as charge carrier. A Single-channel currents during 180-ms depolarizations to 0 mV. Amplitude between closed (*solid line*) and open state (*dotted line*) is −0.4 pA. Blank records without openings have been omitted. B Ensemble average current, 32 consecutive sweeps (blanks included). C Whole-cell current before and after substitution of Ca²⁺ by Mg²⁺. D I$_{Ca}$ is defined as Ca²⁺-sensitive difference current. E Increment in the total cellular calcium concentration [total Ca] estimated from dividing the time integral of I$_{Ca}$ by the Faraday constant 96 500 As·mol⁻¹, the equivalence charge 2, and the cell volume of 8 pl. Only a small fraction of [total Ca] is ionized [free Ca]

tension (see following). Recovery of the channel from I back to C_l requires membrane repolarization.

The time course of single-channel transitions can be extracted by averaging techniques. Averaging the currents from 32 depolarizations (Fig. 3B) shows the inactivation as a decay of negative current. Another type of average is the whole-cell I_{Ca}, which flows through many Ca^{2+} channels that open simultaneously. When single-channel and whole-cell currents are measured under identical experimental conditions (2 mM $[Ca^{2+}]_o$, 37°C, 0 mV), the quotient of peak I_{Ca} (−800 pA) through a single-channel current (−0.4 pA) suggests that 2000 Ca^{2+} channels open simultaneously at approximately the time of peak I_{Ca}. Division of noninactivating I_{Ca} (−40 pA) by −0.4 pA suggests that the number of active Ca^{2+} channels has fallen to 100. I_{Ca} can be enlarged several times (e.g., by intracellular alkalosis), suggesting that depolarizations usually open only a fraction of all Ca^{2+} channels within a single cell [8].

Ca^{2+} Influx Through Nonselective Cation Channels (I_{ns})

Through L-type Ca^{2+} channels, 99.9% of the current is carried by Ca^{2+} ions. This high selectivity contrasts with nonselective cation channels that do not discriminate the different cations. Roughly, the fraction by which an ionic species contributes to I_{ns} depends on its concentration, which determines the probability that this ion enters the channel. Typically, I_{ns} is carried to 95% by Na^+ ions and to 5% by Ca^{2+} ions (− 50 mV). Although this Ca^{2+} fraction is small, the effects of I_{ns} on $[Ca^{2+}]_c$ are significant (see following). If the cell is not voltage clamped, I_{ns} depolarizes the membrane, thereby activating Ca^{2+} influx through voltage-gated Ca^{2+} channels. Nonselective cation channels are activated not by membrane depolarization but by binding of a neurotransmitter to its respective receptor (receptor-operated channels) or by mechanical cell lengthening (stretch-activated channels).

$I_{ns(ACh)}$ activated by acetylcholine has been analyzed in visceral smc [9]. If the cell was not voltage clamped, ACh depolarized the membrane (Fig. 1B, 4A). Under voltage clamp, an inward current $I_{ns(ACh)}$ could be measured (Fig. 4B). Sustained ACh exposures (i.e., 1 min) "desensitized" the cell; $I_{ns(ACh)}$ decayed and the cell no longer responded to ACh [9]. Recovery from desensitization required the washout of ACh for several minutes. In many respects, the desensitization of receptor-operated channels resembles the inactivation of voltage-gated Ca^{2+} channels. The m_2-ACh receptor interacts with the channel through a G protein [10]. Irreversible activation of the G protein with guanosine-5′-[γ-thio]trisphosphate (GTPγS) induces $I_{ns(ACh)}$ without desensitization; thus, desensitization may occur at the receptor level. The amplitude of $I_{ns(ACh)}$ is facilitated severalfold by a rise in $[Ca^{2+}]_c$ from preceding action potentials or I_{Ca} (Fig. 4B). In the absence of ACh, the increase in $[Ca^{2+}]_c$ did not activate $I_{ns(ACh)}$; that is, the channel is Ca^{2+} modulated but not Ca^{2+} activated [9]. Drugs like verapamil or nifedipine that reduce Ca^{2+} influx decrease the augmentation of $I_{ns(ACh)}$ and reduce ACh-induced contraction.

$I_{ns(ATP)}$ is Activated When ATP Binds to Purinergic P_{2x} Receptors

In the urinary bladder and other visceral tissue, ATP is released by stimulation of noncholinergic, nonadrenergic nerves. In vascular tissue, ATP is coreleased with adrenaline. P_{2x} receptors are part of the channel protein [11]. Under voltage-clamp

A

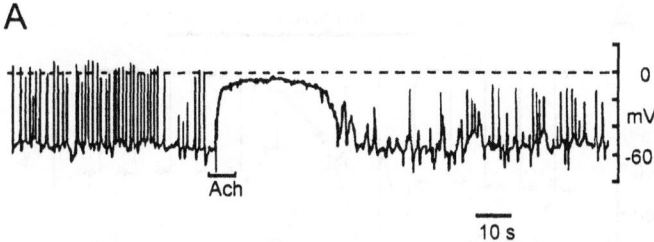

B

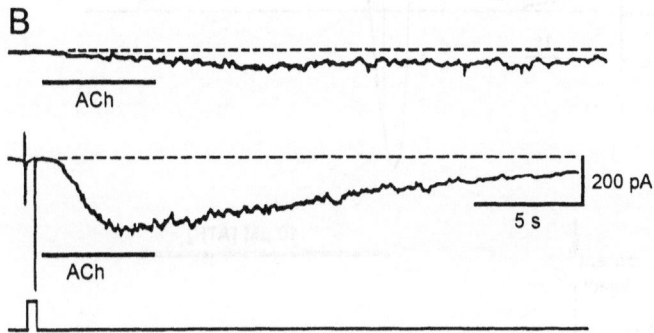

FIG. 4A,B. Ca²⁺ influx resulting from 10 μM acetylcholine (*ACh*); smc from longitudinal layer of guinea pig jejunum. A Current clamp with spontaneous action potentials. A 10-s exposure to ACh induces a sustained depolarization to −5 mV, thereby activating voltage-gated I_{Ca}. B At clamped membrane potential (−50 mV), ACh induces an inward current $I_{ns(ACh)}$ of which 4% is carried by Ca²⁺. Preceding clamp steps to 0 mV and I_{Ca} facilitate the $I_{ns(ACh)}$ severalfold. (From [10] with permission)

conditions (−50 mV), I_{ns} from bath-applied ATP (10 μM) peaked within 1 s and then desensitized. I_{ns} increased [Ca²⁺]$_c$ by about 1 μM. Simultaneous measurements of I_{ns} and Δ[Ca²⁺]$_c$ suggest that about 6% of ATP-gated I_{ns} is carried by Ca²⁺ [12]. There are two mechanisms by which P_{2x} stimulation can cause Ca²⁺ influx. The direct one is the Ca²⁺ permeation through the nonselective channel. The more indirect mechanism is membrane depolarization and activation of voltage-gated L-type Ca²⁺ channels. Figure 5 suggests that the direct mechanism is of greater importance than the indirect one. The ATP-induced Δ[Ca²⁺]$_c$ nearly blocked I_{Ca} (arrows in Fig. 5A). Further, ATP induced an initial small depolarization that rapidly reversed [12]; presumably, the depolarizing effects of I_{ns} were antagonized by [Ca²⁺]$_c$ activation of K⁺ channels.

Stretch-Activated $I_{ns(SAC)}$

Filling the bladder with urine or stretching multicellular trabeculae induces action potentials [13]. In isolated bladder cells, similar effects are seen during mechanical lengthening ("stretch") [14]. The effect was attributed to the stretch activation of nonselective cation channels (SACs). The whole-cell currents (Fig. 6) show $I_{ns(SAC)}$ as an inward current at −50 mV. In addition, they show a reduction of peak I_{Ca} and an increase in $I_{K(Ca)}$ at 0 mV (Fig. 6B; [14]). Presumably, these latter effects are caused by an increase in [Ca²⁺]$_c$ (compare with Fig. 5). Cell lengthening is thought to activate

G. Isenberg

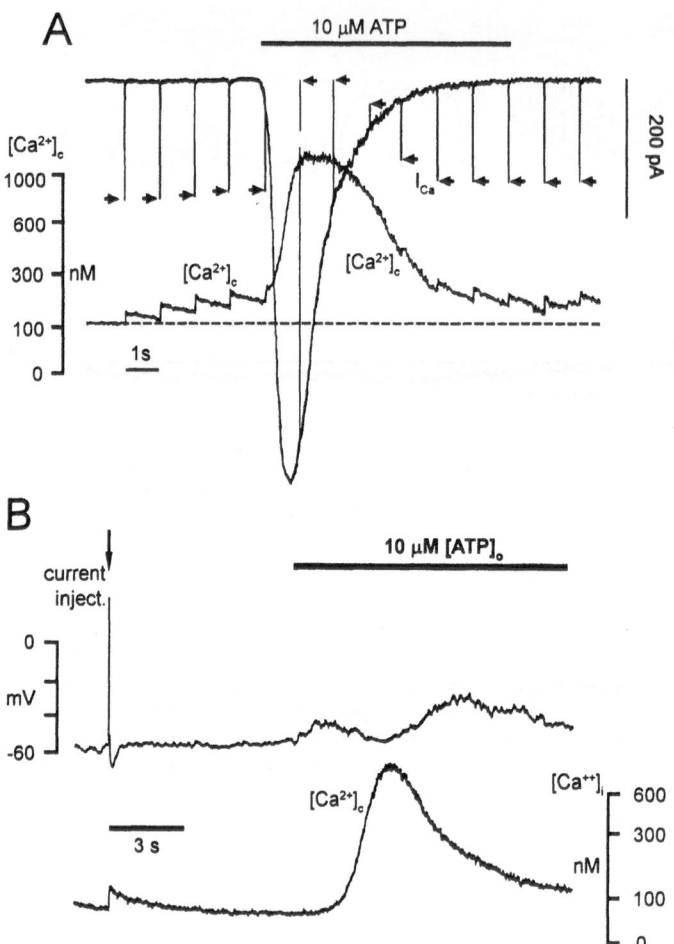

FIG. 5A,B. Ca^{2+} influx and increase in cytosolic Ca^{2+} concentration ($\Delta[Ca^{2+}]_c$) from extracellular ATP in smc from guinea pig urinary bladder. A Voltage clamp to $-50\,mV$. ATP induces a -600-pA inward current $I_{ns(ATP)}$ and suppresses I_{Ca} (peak I_{Ca} marked by *arrows*). $[Ca^{2+}]_c$ increased from resting $100\,nM$ (*dashed line*) to approximately $1000\,nM$. B Current clamp. The single action potential (*arrow labeled current injection*) induced a $50\,nM$ $\Delta[Ca^{2+}]_c$; ATP induced a $800\,nM$ $\Delta[Ca^{2+}]_c$. Note: $\Delta[Ca^{2+}]_c$ turns the initial depolarization into a repolarization, presumably because of Ca^{2+} activation of maxi K^+ channels. (From [12] with permission)

SACs via a deformation of the cytoskeleton that can be mimicked by a slight suction applied to the open end of the patch electrode. On suction, the single-channel currents appeared without measurable delay, and after removal of suction the channel activity promptly disappeared (Fig. 7A; [15]). The open probability of SACs increased with the amplitude of suction along a sigmoidal curve, it saturated at approximately $-5\,kPa$. SACs conducted Na^+ and K^+ ions nearly equally well and only slightly better than Ca^{2+} ions (Fig. 7B; [15]). Thus, Ca^{2+} influx through SACs can increase $[Ca^{2+}]_c$ via the same two mechanisms that have already been discussed for $I_{ns(ACh)}$ and $I_{ns(ATP)}$.

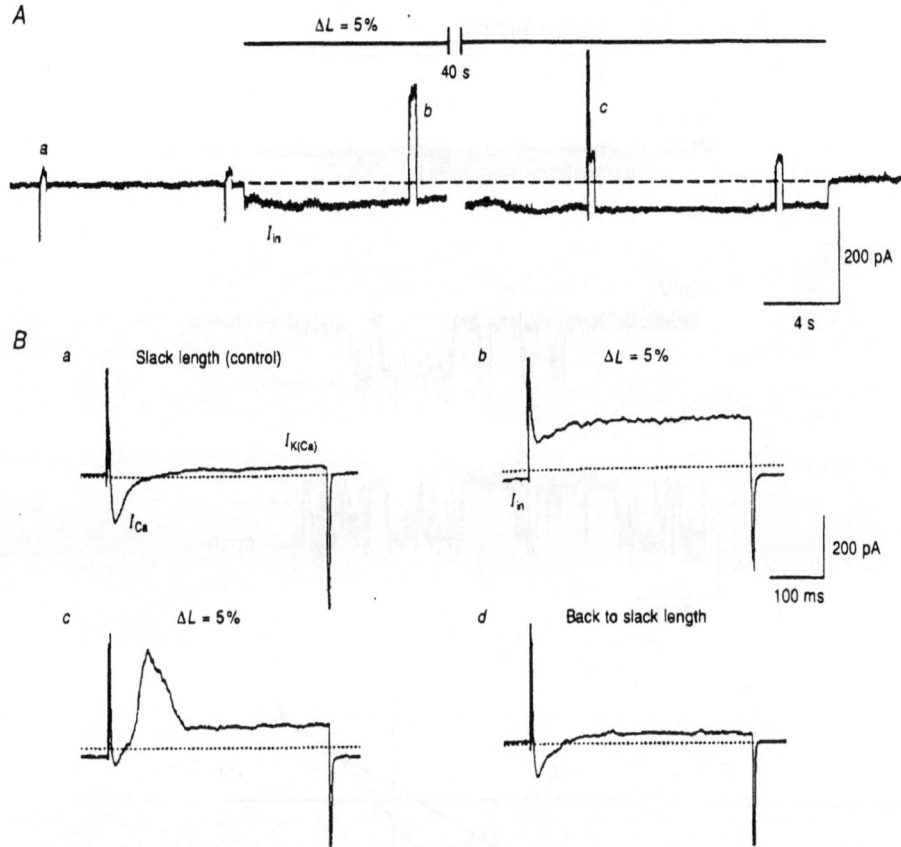

FIG. 6A,B. Ca²⁺ influx induced by a 5% lengthening (stretch) of guinea pig urinary bladder smc. A Induction of a –70-pA net inward current at –50 mV. B During the clamp step to 0 mV, stretch reduces the negative current surge that results from I_{Ca} and increases the outward current at the end of the pulse (*a–d*). Presumably, both effects result from an increase in [Ca²⁺]$_c$. (From [14] with permission)

Ca²⁺ Influx Increments [Ca²⁺]$_c$

The effect of Ca²⁺ influx on the cellular calcium content has been quantified as "increment in the total intracellular calcium concentration" (ΔΣCa). The adjective "total" is used because only a small part of Ca²⁺ influx stays ionized; most of it is bound, sequestered into the SR, or extruded into the extracellular space. ΔΣCa is calculated from Ca²⁺ influx by dividing the time integral of the whole-cell current (e.g., I_{Ca} or the Ca²⁺ fraction of I_{ns}) by the Faraday constant (96 550 As·mol⁻¹), the equivalence charge (2), and the cell volume (e.g., 8 pl). Figure 3E shows ΔΣCa calculated from I_{Ca} during an 180-ms step to 0 mV. ΔΣCa increases at a high rate (500 nM/ms) when I_{Ca} peaks but at a constant low rate (10 nM/ms) after I_{Ca} has been partially inactivated. In comparison, Δ[Ca²⁺]$_c$ has an amplitude about 100-fold lower. Δ[Ca²⁺]$_c$ starts about 5 ms after peak I_{Ca} [16]. Another 5 ms later, Δ[Ca²⁺]$_c$ increases at maximal rate (6 µM/s; Fig. 8).

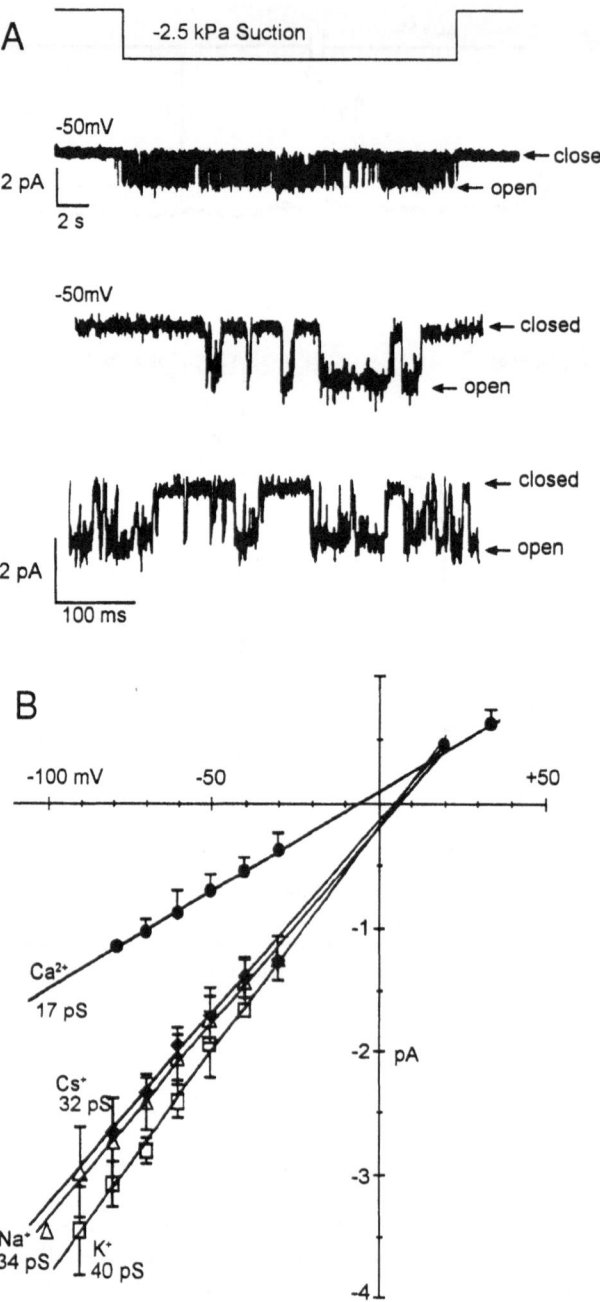

FIG. 7A,B. Currents through stretch-activated channels (SACs) urinary bladder smc. **A** At a patch potential of −50 mV, currents through single SACs were activated by suction to the open end of the patch pipette (negative pressure of −2.5 kPa). **B** The amplitude of single channel currents as function of patch potential. The charge carrier in the pipette, as well as the single-channel conductance, are indicated [concentration: 140 mM for K⁺ (*open squares*), Na⁺ (*open triangles*), Cs⁻ (*solid diamonds*); 10 mM for Ca²⁺ (*solid circles*)]. (From [15] with permission)

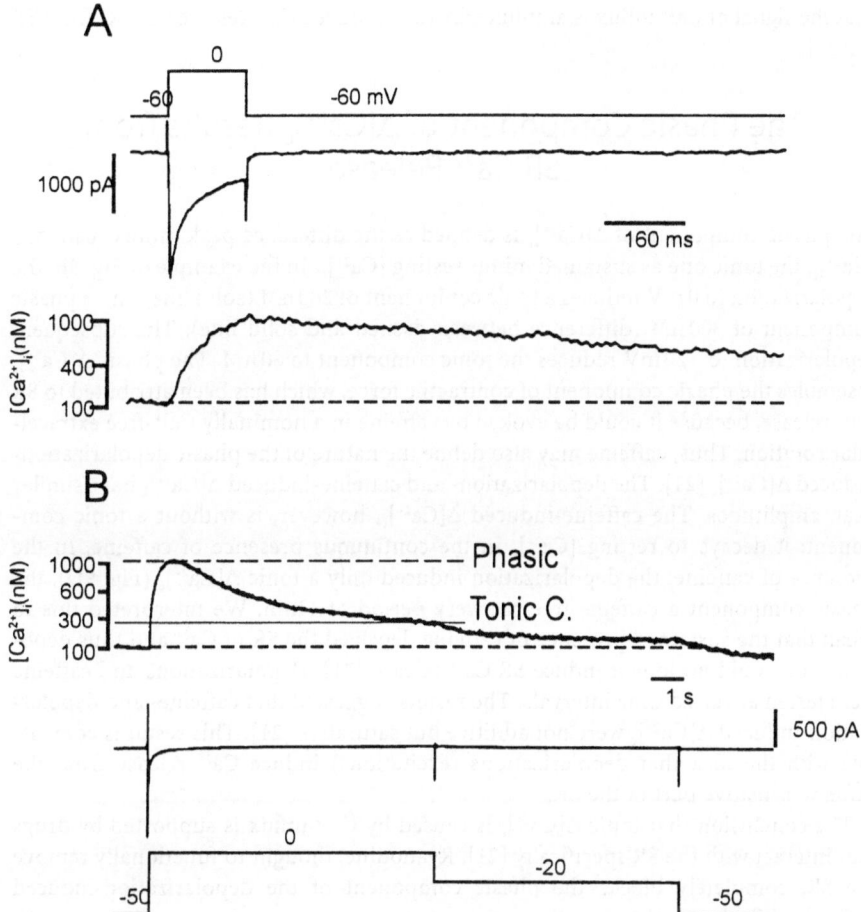

FIG. 8A,B. [Ca²⁺]$_c$ transients in response to voltage-clamp depolarizations. **A** A 160-ms step from −60 to 0 mV induces I_{Ca} and a raise in [Ca²⁺]$_c$ from 120 to 1000 nM. On repolarization to −60 mV, [Ca²⁺]$_c$ slowly returns toward the resting level. **B** The membrane potential was stepped from −50 to 0 mV for 10 s and then to −20 mV for another 10 s before it was repolarized to −50 mV. Note: in addition to the phasic response, there is a significant tonic elevation at the end of the long depolarizations. (From [16] with permission)

After 50 ms, the rate of rise falls, and it becomes zero after 300–500 ms; that is, when ΔΣCa is still rising, [Ca²⁺]$_c$ falls. The differences in amplitude and the time-course of ΔΣCa and Δ[Ca²⁺]$_c$ suggest that Δ[Ca²⁺]$_c$ is not directly caused by Ca²⁺ influx. While the calculated ΔΣCa is a fictitious value, the true cytosolic ΔΣCa$_c$ is reduced by sequestration into the SR and extrusion into the extracellular space.

The ratio of true ΔΣCa$_c$ to Δ[Ca²⁺]$_c$ defines the Ca²⁺ buffer value of the cytosol. ΣCa$_c$ has been measured by X-ray microprobe analysis in the cytosol of urinary bladder cells [17] or of vascular smc [18]. The ratio ΣCa$_c$/Δ[Ca²⁺]$_c$ yields a cytosolic buffer value of 2000 : 1 at rest and of 800 : 1 for a 500-ms depolarization; that is, only 1 or 2 of 2000 total cytosolic calcium atoms are ionized [17]. The result suggests that Ca²⁺ influx and calculated ΔΣCa are too small to account for the rapid rise in Δ[Ca²⁺]$_c$. These differences as well as the dissociation in the time-course of ΔΣCa and Δ[Ca²⁺]$_c$ suggest that the signal of Ca^{2+} influx is amplified by Ca^{2+}-induced Ca^{2+} release (CICR) from SR [19,20].

The Phasic Component of $\Delta[Ca^{2+}]_c$ Results from SR Ca^{2+} Release

The phasic component of $\Delta[Ca^{2+}]_c$ is defined as the difference peak minus sustained $[Ca^{2+}]_c$, the tonic one as sustained minus resting $[Ca^{2+}]_c$. In the example of Fig. 8B, the depolarization to 0 mV induces a tonic component of 200 nM (solid line) and a phasic component of 800 nM (difference between dashed and solid line). The subsequent repolarization to −20 mV reduces the tonic component to 80 nM. The phasic $\Delta[Ca^{2+}]_c$ resembles the phasic component of contractile force, which has been attributed to SR Ca^{2+} release, because it could be evoked by caffeine in a nominally Ca^{2+}-free extracellular solution. Thus, caffeine may also define the nature of the phasic depolarization-induced $\Delta[Ca^{2+}]_c$ [21]. The depolarization- and caffeine-induced $\Delta[Ca^{2+}]_c$ have similar peak amplitudes. The caffeine-induced $\Delta[Ca^{2+}]_c$, however, is without a tonic component; it decays to resting $[Ca^{2+}]_c$ in the continuous presence of caffeine. In the presence of caffeine, the depolarization induced only a tonic $\Delta[Ca^{2+}]_c$ (Fig. 9D), the phasic component a caffeine-free recovery period of 1 min. We interpreted this to mean that the sustained presence of caffeine deprived the SR of Ca^{2+} and thus depolarization could no longer induce SR Ca^{2+} release [21]. Depolarizations and caffeine were tested at varied time intervals. The results suggested that caffeine- and depolarization-induced $\Delta[Ca^{2+}]_c$ were not additive but saturative [21]. This result is compatible with the idea that depolarizations (excitations) induce Ca^{2+} release from the caffeine-sensitive part of the SR.

The conclusion that tonic $\Delta[Ca^{2+}]_c$ is caused by Ca^{2+} influx is supported by drugs that interact with the SR specifically [21]. Ryanodine, thought to functionally remove the SR, completely blocks the phasic component of the depolarization-induced $\Delta[Ca^{2+}]_c$ while the amplitude of the tonic component is almost constant. Thus, $\Delta[Ca^{2+}]_c$ in Fig. 9C at 12 min may be interpreted as a direct effect of Ca^{2+} influx. Vice versa, the difference of $\Delta[Ca^{2+}]_c$ recorded at 2 and 12 min may indicate the contribution of SR Ca^{2+} release. (For problems of such a subtraction method, see [21].) A similar separation comes from experiments with thapsigargin (1 μM), a drug that inhibits the SR-Ca^{2+}-ATPase and thereby the SR Ca^{2+} filling. Thapsigargin abolished the phasic part of the depolarizing-induced $\Delta[Ca^{2+}]_c$. It also slowed down the rate of decay of $\Delta[Ca^{2+}]_c$, as ryanodine did. The effects of ryanodine or thapsigargin link the phasic component of $\Delta[Ca^{2+}]_c$ to the Ca^{2+} release function of the SR. Vice versa, the persistence of the tonic component of depolarization-induced $\Delta[Ca^{2+}]_c$ suggests that this is a direct consequence of Ca^{2+} influx [7,16,21].

The tonic component of depolarization-induced $\Delta[Ca^{2+}]_c$ changes in proportion to the amplitude of noninactivating I_{Ca}. Tonic $\Delta[Ca^{2+}]_c$ increases by increasing the noninactivating I_{Ca} with a change from 2 to 10 mM $[Ca^{2+}]_o$ (Fig. 9A). When noninactivating I_{Ca} is reduced by repolarization from 0 to −20 mV, tonic $\Delta[Ca^{2+}]_c$ is reduced (Fig. 8B). Further, tonic $[Ca^{2+}]_c$ is reduced by Ca^{2+}-channel blockers like nifedipine (1 μM) or verapamil (3 μM; not shown). More generally, modulation of Ca^{2+} influx through noninactivating L-type Ca^{2+} channels is considered to be one important mechanism by which the membrane potential controls tonic $[Ca^{2+}]_c$ and tonic contractions of smooth muscle. Relaxation occurs when Ca^{2+} influx is reduced phar-

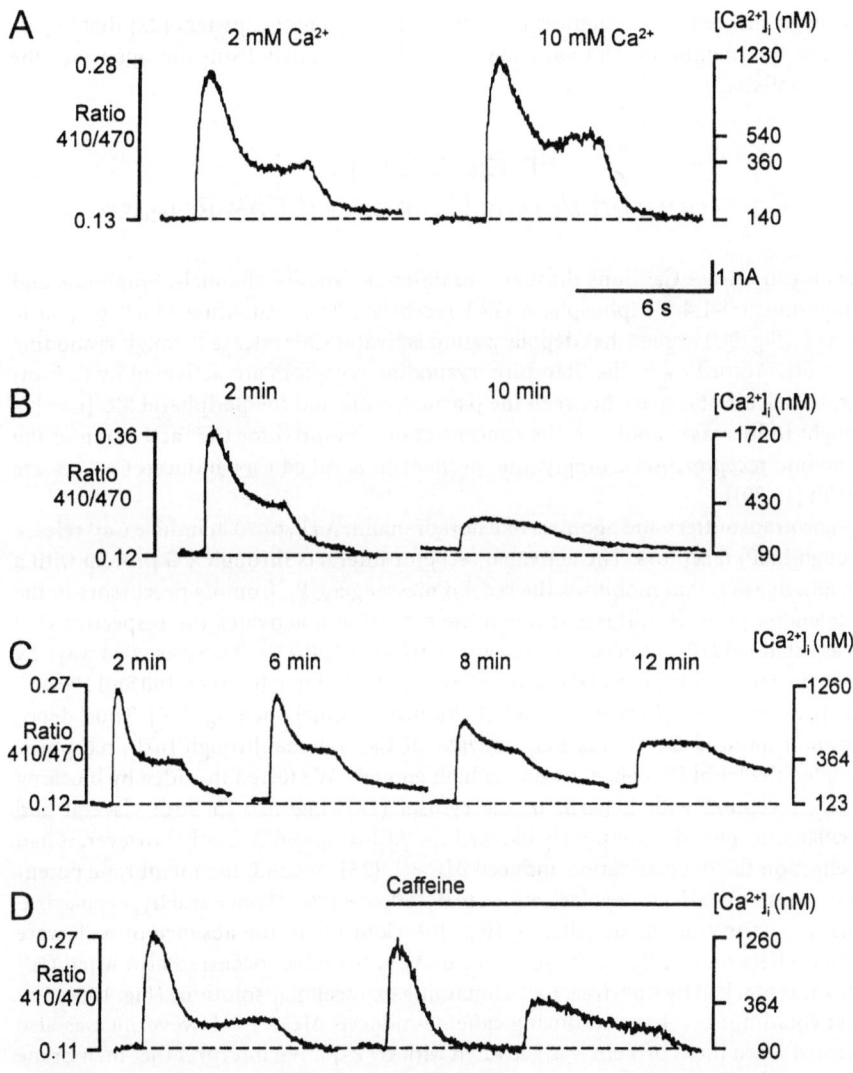

FIG. 9A–D. Depolarization-induced $[Ca^{2+}]_c$ transients: separation of tonic and phasic components. Note: all $[Ca^{2+}]_c$ transients were induced by steps from −60 to 0 mV; tonic component is $[Ca^{2+}]_c$ at end of pulse minus $[Ca^{2+}]_c$ at rest; phasic component is peak $[Ca^{2+}]_c$ minus tonic $[Ca^{2+}]_c$. A Elevation of extracellular $[Ca^{2+}]$ from 2 (*left*) to 10 mM (*right*) increases the tonic component from 360 to 540 nM. B 10 µM thapsigargin was applied through the patch pipette. Phasic $[Ca^{2+}]_c$ was abolished, tonic $[Ca^{2+}]_c$ was reduced, and on repolarization decay was retarded. C Application of 10 µM ryanodine through the patch pipette blocks the phasic component but does not modify the tonic one. D Rapid application of 10 mM caffeine mimics the phasic component. In the continuous presence of caffeine, depolarization can induce only the tonic component. (From [21] with permission)

macologically, as by Ca^{2+}-channel blockers or by K^+-channel openers [22] that hyper-polarize the membrane and shift the L-type Ca^{2+} channels from the open into the closed state.

Phasic $\Delta[Ca^{2+}]_c$: Ca^{2+}-Induced Versus IP_3-Induced Ca^{2+} Release

The SR can release Ca^{2+} ions through two different types of channels, ryanodine and D-myo-inositol-1,4,5-triphosphate (IP_3) receptors. The ryanodine block of phasic $\Delta[Ca^{2+}]_c$ (Fig. 9C) argues that depolarization activates Ca^{2+} release through ryanodine receptors. According to the literature, ryanodine receptors are activated by Ca^{2+} in-flux. Locally, in the space between the plasmalemma and the peripheral SR, $[Ca^{2+}]$ is thought to increase rapidly to the concentrations required for Ca^{2+} activation of the ryanodine receptor. Accordingly, the mechanism is called Ca^{2+}-induced Ca^{2+} release (CICR; [19,20]).

Neurotransmitters and agonists like noradrenalin, ATP, or ACh induce Ca^{2+} release through $InsP_3$ receptors. The activated receptor interacts through a G protein with a phospholipase C that mobilizes the second messenger, IP_3, from its precursors in the sarcolemma [23]. IP_3 diffuses through the cytosol and activates the respective Ca^{2+} release channel (IP_3-induced Ca^{2+} release or IICR; [19,20,23]). There are two ways by which the membrane potential can interfere with IICR. First, between 100 and 500 nM, $[Ca^{2+}]_c$ increases the efficacy by which IP_3 induces channel openings [24]. Thus, depo-larization-induced Ca^{2+} influx may activate SR Ca^{2+} release through $InsP_3$ receptors, provided the basal IP_3 concentration is high enough. We tested this idea by blocking the IP_3 receptors with heparin in the cytosol (1–10 mg/ml). In both visceral and vascular smc, heparin completely blocked the ACh-induced $\Delta[Ca^{2+}]_c$; however, it had no effect on the depolarization-induced $\Delta[Ca^{2+}]_c$ [25]. Second, the membrane poten-tial modulates the IICR; depolarizations to 0, +60, or +100 enhance and hyperpolariza-tions to −100 mV attenuate $\Delta[Ca^{2+}]_c$ (Fig. 10). Controls in the absence of ACh were without effect on $[Ca^{2+}]_c$. In the presence of ACh, the effect occurred also when Ca^{2+} influx was blocked by Ca^{2+}-free, La^{3+}-containing extracellular solutions (Fig. 10B). The effect could not be observed during caffeine-induced $\Delta[Ca^{2+}]_c$. However, it was also recorded when the G protein was activated with GTP-γS. We interpret that membrane depolarization facilitates and hyperpolarization inhibits the liberation of IP_3 from the membrane lipids [25].

Phasic and Tonic $\Delta[Ca^{2+}]_c$ in Coronary Myocytes

In coronary myocytes and other vascular smc, the density of peak I_{Ca} is about tenfold smaller than in the visceral smc from the urinary bladder [2]. Presumably, this small I_{Ca} is unable to trigger a full-sized CICR: depolarization to 0 mV induce a $\Delta[Ca^{2+}]_c$ that peaks to 200 nM at the end of the 6-s pulse. The subsequent caffeine-induced $\Delta[Ca^{2+}]_c$ peaked within 1.5 s to 1200 nM. Thus, on average, depolarizations induced only 10% ± 6% (n = 16) of the caffeine-induced $\Delta[Ca^{2+}]_c$ [21]. Because the small depolarization-induced $\Delta[Ca^{2+}]_c$ was followed by a large caffeine-induced $\Delta[Ca^{2+}]_c$, one can exclude the possibility that the SR was insufficiently Ca^{2+} loaded. Rather, the result was inter-preted to indicate that depolarization-induced Ca^{2+} influx can trigger Ca^{2+} release only

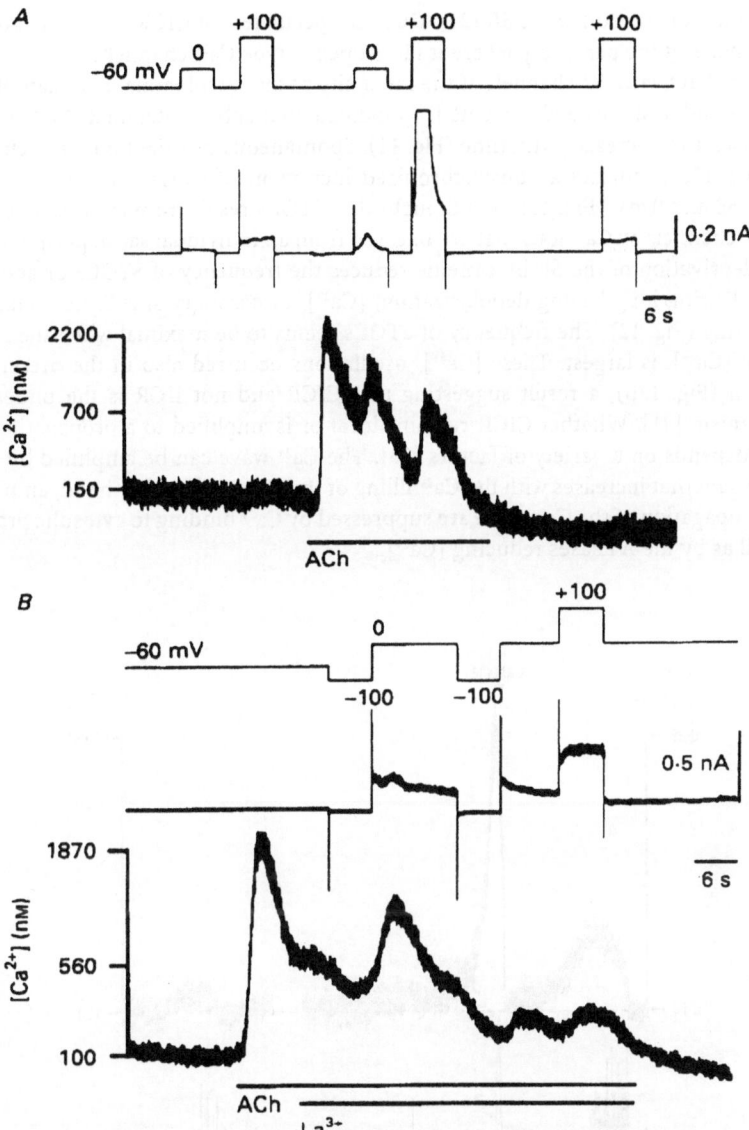

FIG. 10A,B. Coronary smc: ACh-induced $\Delta[Ca^{2+}]_c$ are sensitive to changes in membrane potential independent of Ca^{2+} influx. Nominally Ca^{2+}-free extracellular solution. *Top traces*, voltage-clamp protocol; *middle traces*, net membrane current, mostly $I_{K(Ca)}$; *lower traces*, $[Ca^{2+}]_c$. Exposure to ACh ($10\,\mu M$) or to lanthanum ($3\,mM$) is marked by *horizontal lines*. A In the absence of ACh, the depolarizations to 0 or $+100\,mV$ do not change $[Ca^{2+}]_c$ while they increase $[Ca^{2+}]_c$ during the ACh-induced $\Delta[Ca^{2+}]_c$. Note: in the presence of ACh, the step to $+100\,mV$ induces a $I_{K(Ca)}$ whose peak is largely off the scale. B Block of membrane Ca^{2+} fluxes with Ca^{2+}-free solution containing $3\,mM\ La^{3+}$. In the presence of La^{3+}, hyperpolarization ($6\,s$, $-100\,mV$) reduced $[Ca^{2+}]_c$; however, depolarizations ($12\,s$, $0\,mV$) increased $[Ca^{2+}]_c$. The following changes in membrane potential influenced $[Ca^{2+}]_c$ in a similar but attenuated pattern. Note that La^{3+} suppresses $I_{K(Ca)}$. La^{3+} retarded the decay of the ACh-induced $\Delta[Ca^{2+}]_c$ as if the decay were caused by both La^{3+}-sensitive Ca^{2+} efflux and La^{3+}-insensitive Ca^{2+} reuptake into the sarcoplasmic reticulum (SR). (From [25] with permission)

from a minor fraction of the SR [21]. One can speculate that CICR is activated only at those parts of the periphery where it faces open L-type Ca^{2+} channels.

$\Delta[Ca^{2+}]$ activates K^+ channels at the inner site of the sarcolemma. For example, the caffeine-induced outward currents $I_{K(Ca)}$ indicate that subsarcolemmal $[Ca^{2+}]$ rapidly increases and decreases with time (Fig. 11). Spontaneous transient outward currents (STOCs; [26]) indicate a nonsynchronized increment of subsarcolemmal $[Ca^{2+}]$ at both -50 and $0\,mV$ (Fig. 11). It is thought that STOCs result from the activation of a few K^+ channels by Ca^{2+} ions that are released from an individual sac of peripheral SR. Ca^{2+} deprivation of the SR by caffeine reduces the frequency of STOCs or abolishes them. During long-lasting depolarization, $[Ca^{2+}]_c$ of coronary smc is not stable but oscillating (Fig. 12). The frequency of STOCs seems to be maximal when the rate of rise in $[Ca^{2+}]_c$ is largest. These $[Ca^{2+}]_c$ oscillations occurred also in the presence of heparin (Fig. 12B), a result suggesting that CICR and not IICR is the underlying mechanism [21]. Whether CICR remains local or is amplified to a propagating Ca^{2+} wave depends on a variety of factors [23]. The Ca^{2+} wave can be amplified by CICR with a gain that increases with the Ca^{2+} filling of the SR. On the other hand, amplitude and propagation of the Ca^{2+} wave are suppressed by Ca^{2+} binding to cytosolic proteins as well as by the ATPases reducing $[Ca^{2+}]_c$.

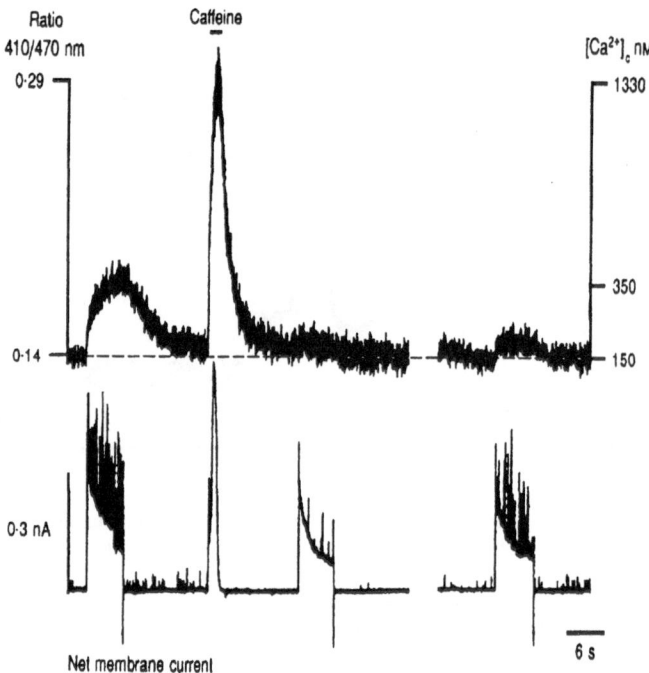

Fig. 11. Coronary smc: comparison of depolarization-with-caffeine-induced $\Delta[Ca^{2+}]_c$. Steps from -50 to $0\,mV$ last 6 s; 10 mM caffeine was puffed onto the cell for 2 s. The third depolarization followed 1 min after washout of caffeine. Note correlation between depolarization-induced $\Delta[Ca^{2+}]_c$ and frequency of spontaneous transient outward currents (STOCs). (From [2] with permission)

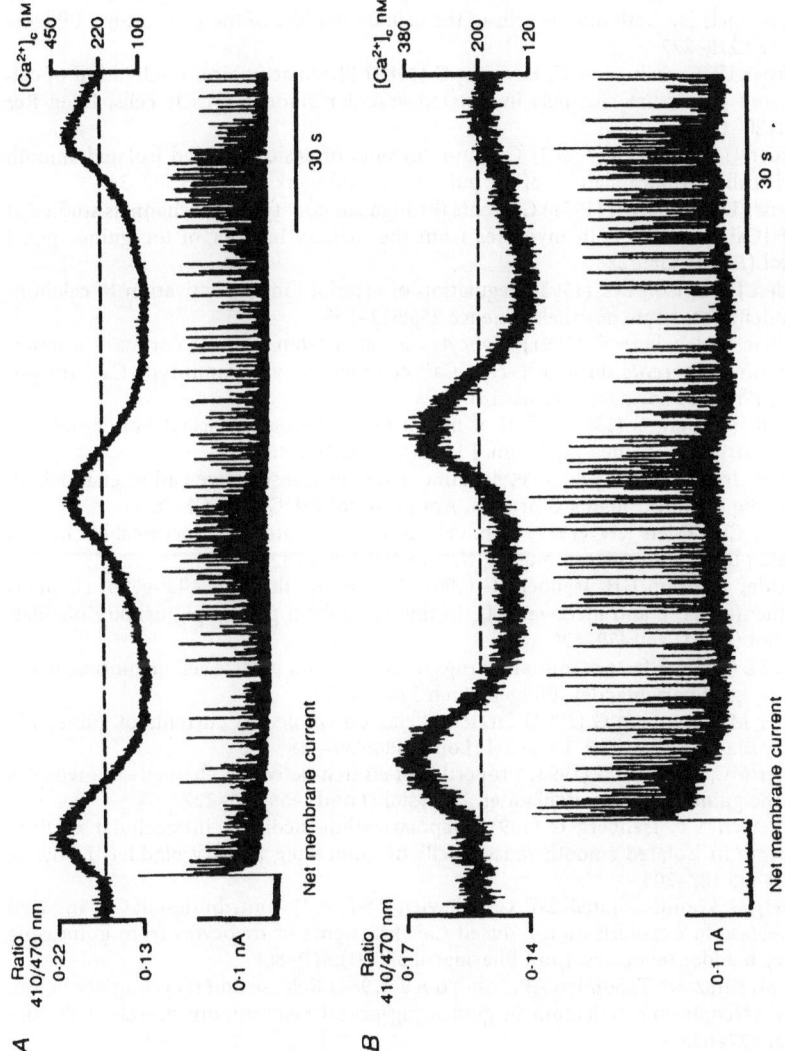

FIG. 12A,B. Coronary smc: Δ[Ca²⁺]ₑ and STOCs in response to 160-s depolarizations from −50 to 0 mV in the absence (A) and in the presence (B) of 5 mg ml⁻¹ heparin in the electrode solution. (From [2] with permission)

References

1. Klöckner U, Isenberg G (1985) Action potentials and net membrane currents of isolated smooth muscle cells (urinary bladder of the guinea-pig). Pflügers Arch 405:329–339
2. Ganitkevich VA, Isenberg G (1995) Efficacy of peak Ca^{2+} currents (I_{Ca}) as trigger of sarcoplasmic reticulum Ca^{2+} release in myocytes from the guinea-pig coronary artery. J Physiol (Lond) 484:307–312
3. Bonev A, Isenberg G (1992) Arginine-vasopressin induces mode-2 gating in L-type Ca^{2+} channels (smooth muscle cells of the urinary bladder of the guinea-pig). Pflügers Arch 420:219–222
4. Klöckner U, Trieschmann U, Isenberg G (1989) Pharmacological modulation of calcium and potassium channels in isolated vascular smooth muscle cells. Drug Res 39(1):120–125
5 Klöckner U, Isenberg G (1985) Calcium currents of cesium loaded isolated smooth muscle cells (urinary bladder of the guinea-pig). Pflügers Arch 405:340–348
6. Klöckner U, Isenberg G (1991) Currents through single L-type Ca^{2+} channels studied at 2 mM $[Ca^{2+}]_o$ and 36°C in myocytes from the urinary bladder of the guinea-pig. J Physiol (Lond) 438:P228
7. Brayden JE, Nelson MT (1992) Regulation of arterial tone by activation of calcium-dependent potassium channels. Science 256:532–535
8. Klöckner U, Isenberg G (1991) Myocytes isolated from porcine coronary arteries: reduction of currents through L-type Ca^{2+} channels by verapamil-type Ca^{2+} antagonists. J Physiol Pharmacol 42:165–181
9. Inoue R, Isenberg G (1990) Effect of membrane potential on acetylcholine-induced inward current in guinea-pig ileum. J Physiol (Lond) 424:57–71
10. Inoue R, Isenberg G (1990) Acetylcholine activates nonselective cation channels in guinea pig ileum through a G protein. Am J Physiol 258:C1173–C1178
11. Benham CD, Tsien RW (1987) A novel receptor-operated Ca^{2+}-permeable channel activated by ATP in smooth muscle. Nature 328:275–278
12. Schneider P, Hopp HH, Isenberg G (1991) Ca^{2+} influx through ATP-gated channels increments $[Ca^{2+}]_i$ and inactivates I_{Ca} in myocytes from guinea-pig urinary bladder. J Physiol (Lond) 440:479–496
13. Creed KE (1971) Effects of ions and drugs on the smooth muscle cell membrane of the guinea-pig urinary bladder. Pflügers Arch 326:127–141
14. Wellner MC, Isenberg G (1994) Stretch effects on whole-cell currents of guinea-pig urinary bladder myocytes. J Physiol (Lond) 480:439–448
15. Wellner MC, Isenberg G (1993) Properties of stretch-activated channels in myocytes from the guinea-pig urinary bladder. J Physiol (Lond) 466:213–227
16. Ganitkevich VY, Isenberg G (1991) Depolarization-mediated intracellular calcium transients in isolated smooth muscle cells of guinea-pig urinary bladder. J Physiol (Lond) 435:187–205
17. Isenberg G, Wendt-Gallitelli MF, Ganitkevich VY (1992) Contribution of Ca^{2+} induced Ca^{2+} release to depolarization-induced Ca^{2+} transients of myocytes from guinea-pig urinary bladder myocytes. Jpn J Pharmacol 58(SII):81P–86P
18. Bond M, Kitazawa T, Somlyo AP, Somlyo AV (1984) Release and recycling of calcium by the sarcoplasmic reticulum in guinea-pig portal vein smooth muscle. J Physiol (Lond) 677–695
19. Endo M, Iino M, Kobayashi T, Yamamoto (1990) Control of calcium release in smooth muscle cells. Prog Clin Biol Res 327:193–204
20. Somlyo AP, Somlyo AV (1994) Signal transduction and regulation in smooth muscle. Nature 372:231–236
21. Ganitkevich VY, Isenberg G (1992) Contribution of Ca^{2+}-induced Ca^{2+} release to the $[Ca^{2+}]_i$ transients in myocytes from guinea-pig urinary bladder. J Physiol (Lond) 458:119–137

22. Standen NB, Quayle JM, Davies NW, Brayden JE, Huang Y, Nelson MT (1989) Hyper-polarizing vasodilators activate ATP-sensitive K$^+$ channels in arterial smooth muscle. Science 245:177-180
23. Berridge MJ (1993) Inositol trisphosphate and calcium signalling. Nature 361:315-325
24. Iino M, Endo M (1992) Calcium-dependent immediate feedback control of inositol 1,4,5-trisphosphate-induced Ca^{2+} release. Nature 360:76-78
25. Ganitkevich VY, Isenberg G (1993) Membrane potential modulates inositol 1,4,5-tris-phosphate-mediated Ca^{2+} transients in guinea-pig coronary myocytes. J Physiol (Lond) 470:35-44
26. Benham CD, Bolton TB (1986) Spontaneous transient outward currents in single visceral and vascular smooth muscle cells of the rabbit. J Physiol (Lond) 381:385-406

Role of Phosphodiesterase III in the Control of Blood Flow

Hiroyoshi Hidaka[1] and Yukio Kimura[2]

Summary. Smooth muscle cells, endothelial cells, and platelets are the main components controlling the blood flow. Disturbance of the functions of these cells causes blood flow abnormalities, and recent studies reveal that elevation of the intracellular level of cyclic adenosine monophosphate (cAMP) may improve this disorder. An increase in cAMP level results from either activation of adenylate cyclase or inhibition of phosphodiesterases (PDEs). PDEs, key enzymes which hydrolyze cAMP to AMP, exist in multiple forms in a wide variety of tissues. The major isozymes in platelets and endothelial cells are PDEIII and PDEIV, respectively. IBMX, a widely used nonselective inhibitor of PDE, increases cAMP in endothelial cells. Nevertheless, this substance has an adverse effect on platelet aggregation with endothelial cells via inhibition of production of PGI_2, the eicosanoide that prevents platelet aggregation via activation of adenylate cyclase. In contrast, cilostazol and cilostamide inhibit PDEIII in a specific manner and do not affect PGI_2 production in endothelial cells. Therefore, cilostamide has a more potent effect on prevention of platelet aggregation. Long-term exposure of platelets to exogenous PGI_2 caused down-regulation of adenylate cyclase and activation of PDE, resulting in a decrease in intracellular cAMP. These findings suggest that chronic treatment with PGI_2 may lessen its antiplatelet action. Cilostamide, which steadily raised the cAMP level via PDEIII inhibition, caused vasodilation and prevented smooth muscle cell proliferation. Intimal thickening after endothelial denudation was effectively blocked by cilostamide. We conclude that the increase in cAMP level through inhibition of PDEIII rather than through adenylate cyclase activation is effective for treatment of blood flow abnormalities.

Key words. Cilostamide—Cilostazol—Platelet—Endothelial cell—Cyclic nucleotide phosphodiesterase

Introduction

Smooth muscle cells (SMCs), endothelial cells (ECs), and platelets (PLTs) are the main cell components controlling blood flow. Several important aspects of control of blood flow including cardiac and vascular muscle contractile function, platelet aggregation,

[1] Department of Pharmacology, Nagoya University School of Medicine, Showa-ku, Nagoya 466, Japan
[2] Tokushima Research Institute, Otsuka Pharmaceutical Co., Ltd., Kawauchi-chou, Tokushima 771-01, Japan

169

and fluid balance are affected by changes in cyclic nucleotide metabolism, and the role of phosphodiesterase (PDE) in regulating these functions has been the subject of considerable investigation. Early efforts in this research area have focused on the biochemical characterization of the different PDEs present in various organs and cells. Subsequent studies have focused on the functional roles of the different enzymes and employed selective inhibitors of the various PDEs.

We reported in 1979 [1] that cilostamide is a selective inhibitor of PDEIII. This compound was 1100 times more potent as an inhibitor of PDE fraction III (PDEIII) than of PDE fraction I (PDEV). These PDEs were purified from platelets. The K_i of cilostamide is one of the lowest of those reported for PDE inhibitors. Cilostamide has therefore been widely used as a pharmacological tool for a selective inhibition of PDEIII. Figure 1 shows the chemical structure of cilostamide and its derivative cilostazol. The compound cilostazol has been newly developed for clinical use as an antithrombotic agent.

Cardiac Contractile Function

The role played by cyclic nucleotides in modulating myocardial contractility has been the subject of intense investigation for nearly 30 years [2,3]. Although a direct role of cyclic guanosine monophosphate (cGMP) in regulating ventricular contractile function has not been demonstrated, the relationship between changes in tissue levels of cyclic adenosine monophosphate (cAMP) and changes in contractility has been clearly documented. Several studies have shown that the positive inotropic response to cAMP results from coordinated phosphorylation of several proteins involved in regulation of intracellular calcium homeostasis. Cyclic AMP also increases the slow inward calcium current in cardiac cells. Although cGMP has little effect on basal calcium current, cGMP can attenuate the effect of cAMP on calcium current. This effect is thought to be mediated by the increase in hydrolysis of cAMP via a PDEII.

Many of the initial findings concerning the involvement of cAMP in regulation of ventricular contractility were obtained using agents that increase cAMP synthesis. cAMP levels can also be increased by inhibiting cyclic nucleotide degradation with PDE inhibitors. Although the nonselective inhibitors theophylline and isobutylmethylxanthine (IBMX) have positive inotropic effects comparable with isoproterenol, differences in positive inotropic effects have been noted among selective PDE inhibitors such as imazodan and rolipram. Thus, although the selective PDEIII inhibitors imazodan, CI-930, and amrinone directly increase contractility when administered to anesthetized dogs, no such increase is observed with the selective PDEIV inhibitors rolipram and Ro 20-1724. Weishaar et al. [4] have suggested

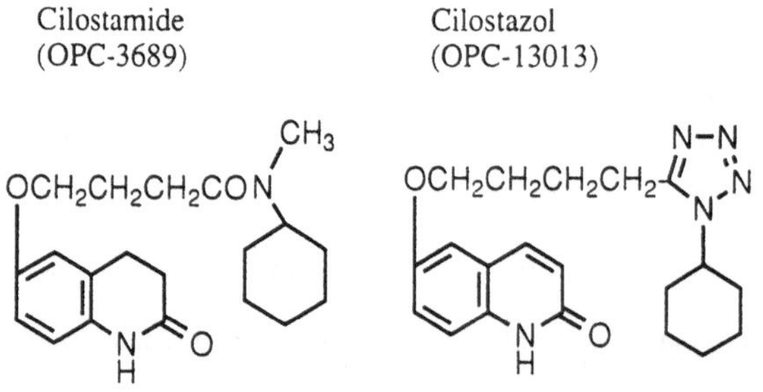

Cilostamide
(OPC-3689)

Cilostazol
(OPC-13013)

FIG. 1. Chemical structures of cilostamide and cilostazol

that this difference in effect results from differences between the intracellular localization of PDEIII and PDEIV in the canine left ventricle, as PDEIII is membrane bound while PDEIV is a soluble agent. This hypothesis is supported by the observation that in those species in which the ventricular PDEIII is soluble (e.g., hamster, guinea pig, rat), the selective PDEIII inhibitor imazodan has a diminished effect on cardiac contractility compared to that in species in which this subclass is membrane bound (e.g., dog, rhesus monkey) (Fig. 2). Similar differences among species in response to selective PDEIII inhibitors have also been reported by Schwartz et al. [5] and Alousi and Farah [6].

These findings suggest that PDEIII plays an important role in regulating ventricular contractility. In addition, the positive inotropic effects of selective PDEIII inhibitors depend on the proportion of enzyme molecules that are membrane bound. This finding suggests that local increases in cAMP in specific intracellular compartments play an important role in modulating the relationship between cAMP and cardiac contractility. Kauffman et al. [7] have shown that PDEIII in canine ventricular muscle is bound to the sarcoplasmic reticulum. Artman et al. [8] have reported specific binding sites for the selective PDEIII inhibitor LY-186126 on isolated sarcoplasmic reticulum vehicles. These findings support the hypothesis that PDEIII regulates the level of cAMP in a local compartment and that regulation of calcium fluxes plays an important role in regulation of venticular contractile function.

Vascular Muscle Contractile Function

Cyclic AMP and calcium ions are ubiquitous intracellular messengers, and there are close interrelationships between these two intracellular regulatory systems. In the case of smooth muscle, cAMP formation may involve stimulation of Ca^{2+} and Na^+

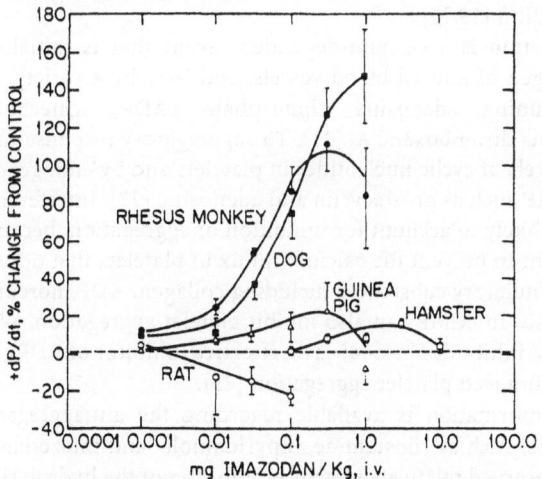

FIG. 2. Relationship between doses of intravenously administered imazodan (CI-914) and myocardial contractility in dog (*solid squares*), rhesus monkey (*solid circles*), guinea pig (*triangles*), golden Syrian hamster (*open squares*), and rat (*open circles*). The procedures used to administer imazodan and measure changes in myocardial contractility were previously described by Weishaar et al. [4]

pumps, inhibition of potential-operated calcium channels, and a decrease in the affinity of myosin light-chain kinase for the Ca^{2+}–calmodulin complex. Increased tissue levels of both cAMP and cGMP are associated with relaxation of vascular smooth muscle. This relaxant effect has been demonstrated in vitro using several approaches, with PDE inhibitors, lipophilic cyclic nucleotide analogues, receptor agonists, and direct-acting adenylate and guanylate cyclase stimulators [9–15]. The relaxant response to cAMP or cGMP is presumably mediated through activation of cyclic nucleotide-specific protein kinase, leading to phosphorylation of proteins associated with regulation of calcium homeostasis in vascular muscle. Increases in cGMP within vascular muscle lead to activation of cell membrane-bound calcium ATPase, resulting in removal of calcium from the cell.

In addition to receptor agonists and cyclase stimulators, inhibitors of cyclic nucleotide PDE have also been employed to characterize the involvement of cAMP and cGMP in regulation of vascular relaxation. The relaxant effects of theophylline and other nonselective PDE inhibitors on isolated arterial and venous smooth muscle have been described. In vitro vascular relaxant effects have also been reported for the selective PDEI inhibitor vinpocetine [16], the selective PDEV inhibitor zaprinast [10], and a number of selective PDEIII inhibitors [17].

Platelet Aggregation

Circulating platelets respond to hemorrhage by changing shape and adhering to the injured area; the thrombus plug thus formed reestablishes the continuity of the vascular endothelium and prevents further bleeding. Although platelet aggregation is an essential part of normal hemostasis, alterations in platelet activity play a significant role in the pathogenesis of coronary artery disease [18]. Enhanced platelet activity may also contribute to poor recovery from arteriovenous graft surgery, stroke, and myocardial infraction [19,20].

Platelet aggregation is a calcium-dependent event that is initially triggered by exposure to collagen of injured blood vessels, and later by a variety of chemotactic substances, including adenosine diphosphate (ADP), catecholamines, and eicosanoids such as thromboxane A_2 [21]. The aggregatory response can be inhibited by increases in levels of cyclic nucleotides in platelets and by endogenous substances that increase cAMP such as prostacyclin and adenosine [22]. Interference with cAMP hydrolysis seems likely to account for inhibition of aggregation, because an increase in cAMP is thought to prevent the calcium influx in platelets that occurs in response to a variety of stimulatory substances including collagen, ADP, norepinephrine, and thrombin. Increases in cGMP can also inhibit platelet aggregation. We showed that the selective PDEV inhibitor MY-5445 is an effective inhibitor of ADP-, collagen-, and arachidonic acid-induced platelet aggregation [23].

Considerable information is available regarding the antiaggregatory effects of the PDE inhibitors, such as cilostamide, dipyridamole, and imazodan. McElroy and Philip [23] also observed relatively selective inhibition of the hydrolysis of cGMP and cAMP in crude human platelet preparations by dipyridamole and related agents, and reported a close correspondence between their tendency to promote relative accumulation of cAMP and their inhibitory effects on platelet adhesion and aggregation. Several inhibitors of platelet aggregation including papaverine, EG-626, theophylline, 2-chloroadenosine, and adenosine also exhibit relatively selective inhibition of human platelet cAMP phosphodiesterase (PDEIII). The PDEV/PDEIII ratios for these inhibitors range from 4.4 to 31.4, while that for cilostamide is 1100. Cilostamide is the most selective PDEIII inhibitor of all reported phosphodiesterase inhibitors.

Pharmacological Characteristics of PDEIII Inhibitors

Cilostamide and cilostazol are potent inhibitors of PDEIII from platelets and aorta, but moderate or weak inhibitors of PDEV from platelets and PDEI from aorta. Cilostamide and cilostazol only minimally inhibit both PDEIV and PDEI from brain.

IBMX is a nonselective PDE inhibitor. If a PDE inhibitor does not inhibit prostaglandin (PGI_2) generation in endothelial cells, it has the great advantage of a synergistic inhibitory effect on platelet aggregation with endogenous adenylate cyclase activator PGI_2 in vitro. However, it has been reported by many investigators that IBMX inhibits not only thromboxane A_2 generation but also PGI_2 generation. Figure 3 shows the effect of cilostazol on platelet aggregation in the presence and absence of endothelial cells. The synergistic effect in the presence of endothelial cells was almost entirely lost in the absence of these cells. When endothelial cell had previously been treated with aspirin, enhancement of the effects of cilostazol by endothelial cells was almost completely eliminated. This effect is thought to result from inhibition of endothelial cell PGI_2 biosynthesis by aspirin. Figure 4 shows the results of a study to determine the effects of cilostazol and aspirin on PG metabolism in terms of percentage changes in 6-keto PGF_1-α; it was found that aspirin markedly decreased thromboxane B_2.

The effects of PDE inhibitors on PGI_2 synthesis and intracellular cAMP levels in human umbilical vein endothelial cells (HUVECs) in the presence or absence of

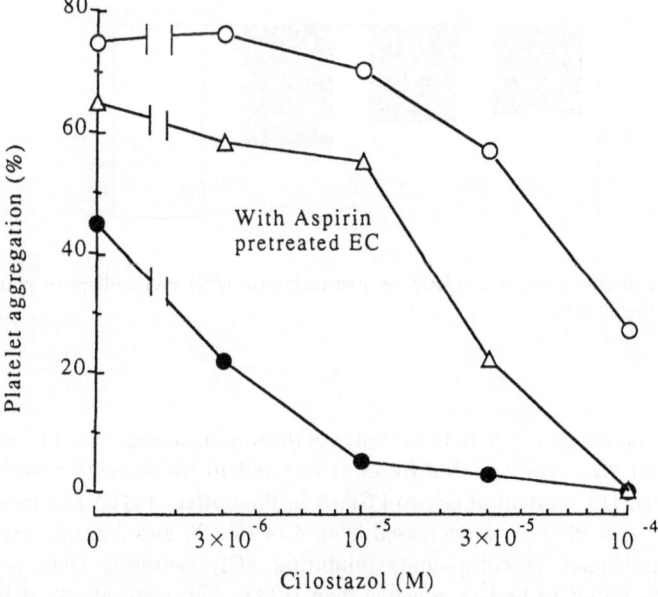

FIG. 3. Inhibitory effect of cilostazol on platelet aggregation in the presence (*solid circles*) or absence (*open circles*) of vascular endothelial cells

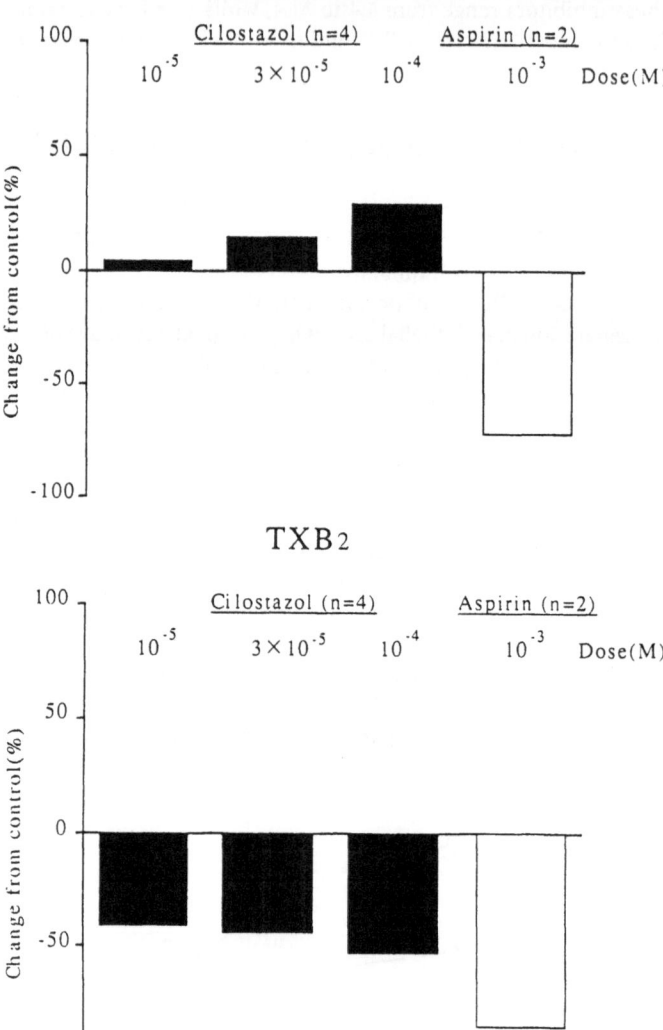

FIG. 4. Effects of cilostazol and aspirin on prostaglandin (*PG*) metabolism in platelets and vascular endothelial cells

thrombin are shown in Fig. 5. In the absence of thrombin, cilostazol at 10^{-5} and $10^{-4} M$ did not inhibit PGI_2 synthesis, but IBMX at 10^{-4} and $10^{-3} M$ did significantly inhibit PGI_2 synthesis. The content of 6-keto PGF_1-α in the buffer of HUVECs treated with IBMX at 10^{-4} and $10^{-3} M$ was decreased from 4.14 to 2.90 and 2.22 ng, respectively. When the potencies of compounds inhibiting PGI_2 synthesis were compared, cilostazol was found to be less effective than IBMX. Cilostazol at $10^{-4} M$ increased cAMP levels from 0.40 to 0.97 pmol per 2.5×10^5 cells, while IBMX at 10^{-4} and $10^{-3} M$

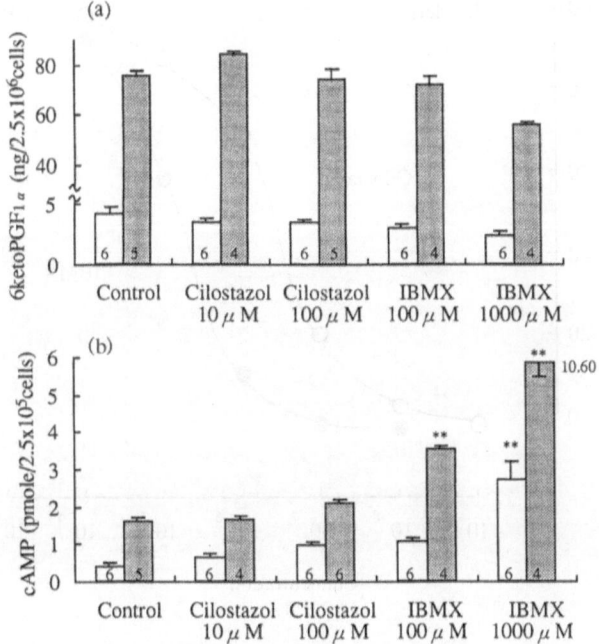

FIG. 5a,b. Effects of cilostazol and IBMX on PGI$_2$ generation (a) and cAMP levels (b) in human umbilical vein endothelial cells HUVECs. Incubation was carried out with (*shaded column*) or without (*unshaded column*) 0.5 U/ml of thrombin. Numbers in columns represent number of experiments. **, Significantly different from control ($P < .01$ by Dunnett's test)

did significantly increase cAMP levels to 1.07 and 2.66 pmol per 2.5 × 10⁵ cells, respectively. The cAMP level of HUVECs treated with cilostazol at 10⁻⁴ M was lower than that of HUVECs treated with IBMX at 10⁻⁴ M. Cilostazol had no effect on PGI$_2$ synthesis in the presence of thrombin, but IBMX significantly inhibited PGI$_2$ synthesis in the presence and in the absence of thrombin. The content of 6-keto PGF$_1$-α in the medium of HUVECs treated with IBMX at 10⁻³ M decreased from 75.0 to 55.2 ng. Cilostazol at 10⁻⁴ M slightly increased the cAMP level from 1.58 to 2.18 pmol per 2.5 × 10⁵ cells. IBMX at 10⁻⁴ and 10⁻³ M significantly increased cAMP levels to 3.54 and 10.60 pmol per 2.5 × 10⁵ cells, respectively.

Cilostazol was found to be less effective than IBMX in increasing cAMP levels and inhibiting PGI$_2$ synthesis in HUVECs stimulated with thrombin. Although most PDE inhibitors inhibit not only platelet aggregation but also PGI$_2$ generation in endothelial cells, cilostazol is quite specific for platelet aggregation. Figure 6 shows the inhibitory effects of cilostazol and IBMX on crude preparations of PDE from platelets and endothelial cells. The dose–response curve for inhibition of PDE from endothelial cells by cilostazol is not simple and has two separate phases. The inhibitory effect of cilostazol on this PDE is weaker than on PDE from platelets. The inhibitory effects of IBMX on those PDE preparations were almost the same as those of cilostazol.

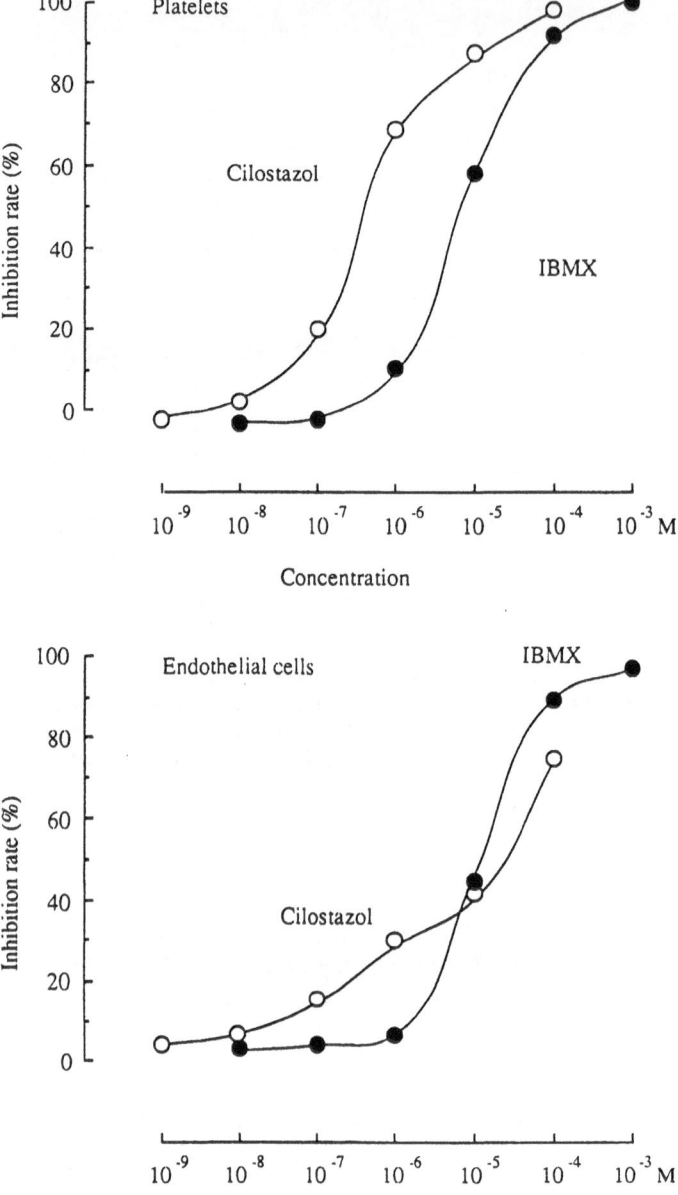

FIG. 6. Inhibitory effects of cilostazol and IBMX on cyclic AMP hydrolyzing activities in crude preparations from platelets and HUVECs

Isolation of Multiple Forms of PDE from Platelets and HUVECs

Three different forms of PDE were isolated from human platelets and designated FI (PDEV), FII (PDEI), and FIII (PDEIII), based on the order of elution from a DEAE-Sephacel column (Fig. 7). In platelets, FI- and FIII-PDEs preferentially hydrolyzed cGMP and cAMP, respectively. FII-PDEs hydrolyzed both cGMP and cAMP with apparently equal affinity, but its hydrolytic activity was less than that of both FI- and FIII-PDE activities. Figure 7b shows that HUVECs also possess three different forms of PDE (FI, FII, and FIII), which elute in a fashion similar to those of human platelets. FI-PDE and FIII-PDE from HUVECs preferentially hydrolyze cGMP and cAMP, respectively, as do those from human platelets. Unlike that from human platelets, HUVEC FII-PDE and FIII-PDE each selectively hydrolyzed cAMP more than cGMP. In addition, the cAMP-hydrolyzing activity of FII-PDE was higher than that of FIII-PDE.

The apparent K_m values of FIII-PDE from platelets and of FII and FIII-PDE from HUVECs were 0.20, 2.0 and 0.39 μM, respectively (Table 1). Inhibition of hydrolysis of cAMP by cGMP was evident for the FIII-PDEs from both human platelets and HUVECs. The FII-PDE from HUVECs was not inhibited by cGMP. Table 2 shows

TABLE 1. Biochemical properties of cAMP-PDEs from human platelets and HUVECs.

Cell origin	PDE	K_m (μM) for cAMP[a]	Effect of cGMP
Human platelets	FI	0.20	Inhibited
HUVECs	FII	2.0	No effect
	FIII	0.39	Inhibited

cAMP, Cyclic adenosine monophosphate; PDE, phosphodiesterase; HUVEC, human umbilical vein endothelial cell.
[a] K_ms were determined using Lineweaver-Burk plots. Enzyme activity was measured using the method of Hidaka and Asano [24].

TABLE 2. IC$_{50}$ Values of cilostazol and IBMX for PDE isozymes from human cells and tissue.

	F-I cGMP	F-II cAMP	F-III cAMP
Platelets			
Cilostazol	14	96	0.19
IBMX	15	36	6.2
Endothelial cells			
Cilostazol	9.2	55	0.71
IBMX	11	14	3.1
Aorta			
Cilostazol	>1000	0.4	

Enzyme activity was measured using the method of Hidaka and Asano [24]. The IC$_{50}$ values (concentration that produced 50% inhibition of substrate hydrolysis) for the PDE inhibitors examined were determined from concentration–response curves.

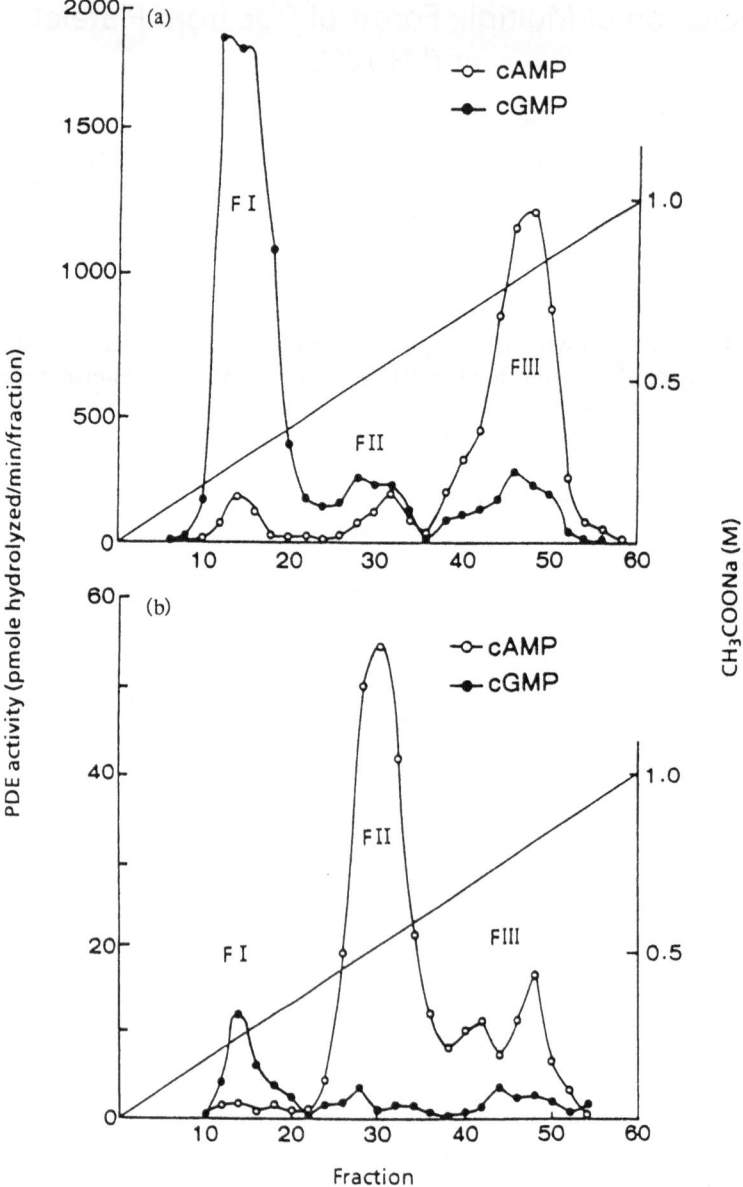

FIG. 7a,b. cAMP and cGMP PDE activities from human platelets (a) and HUVECs (b) in 5.0-ml fractions obtained from a DEAE-Sephacel column with a $0-1.0\,M$ sodium acetate gradient. Substrate concentration was $0.4\,\mu M$ for both cAMP and cGMP [22]

the inhibitory effects of cilostazol and IBMX on PDE isozymes from platelets, endothelium, and aorta.

It is well known that many PDE inhibitors inhibit platelet aggregation by increasing platelet cAMP levels. Both cilostazol and IBMX increase cAMP levels and inhibit platelet aggregation in a concentration-dependent manner. The potencies of cilostazol in increasing platelet cAMP levels and inhibiting platelet aggregation are about 30-fold greater than those of IBMX. Nevertheless, when the potencies in increasing cAMP levels and inhibiting PGI_2 synthesis in HUVECs of the two compounds were compared, cilostazol was found to be less effective than IBMX. These findings are consistent with the decrease in plasma TXB_2 and the 6-keto PGF_1-α/TXB_2 ratio noted after cilostazol treatment in patients with cerebral atherosclerosis. It was hypothesized that IBMX, a nonselective PDE inhibitor, inhibits the functions of both human platelets and HUVECs, and that cilostazol, a selective cAMP-PDE inhibitor, selectively inhibits the function of human platelets.

Effect of Cilostamide on Intimal Thickening

Because cilostamide has been found to increase the cAMP level in SMC, a direct effect of cilostamide in suppressing SMC proliferation is suggested (Fig. 8). Rats underwent balloon angioplasty in a modification of the original aortic balloon injury model described by Baumgartner and Muggli [25]. The left carotid artery was obstructed by passage of a balloon catheter to induce intimal hyperplasia. Two weeks later, a 10-mm portion was excised from the left carotid artery and assayed for DNA content as an index of intimal hyperplasia. The right carotid artery was left intact as a control. As shown in Fig. 9, cilostamide significantly reduced the DNA content of balloon-injured left carotid arteries by 23.0%, 28.0%, and 31.8% in a dose-dependent manner compared to that in the control group.

It is clear that cilostamide strongly inhibits intimal proliferation in vivo. Cilostamide inhibits PDEIII and also inhibits platelet aggregation. Because platelets release large amounts of growth factors such as platelet-derived growth factor (PDGF) and epithelial growth factor (EGF), we had presumed that cilostamide prevented intimal proliferation by inhibiting platelet aggregation. In another experiment using antiplatelet serum (APS) with this rat model, APS had no effect on intimal proliferation although the rats had been thrombocytopenic during the 2-week period. These findings suggested that the platelet activity affects arteries only immediately after they are injured. During the 2 weeks of intimal SMC proliferation, these proliferating SMCs have antithrombotic activity and prevent the adhesion of platelets to the surface of

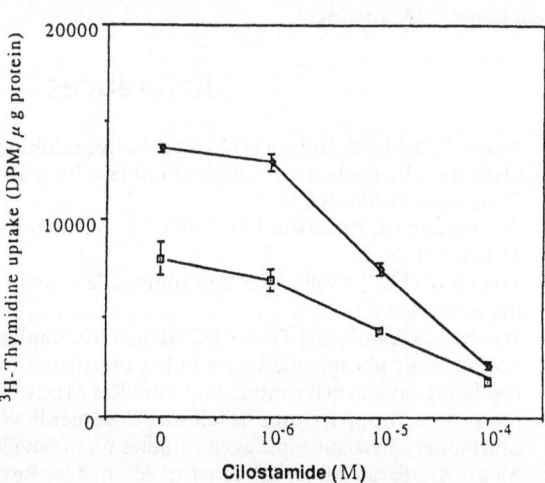

FIG. 8. Effect of cilostamide on rat carotid artery smooth muscle cell proliferation ([³H]thymidine uptake). *Squares with center dot*, without fetal bovine serum (FBS); *triangles*, with FBS

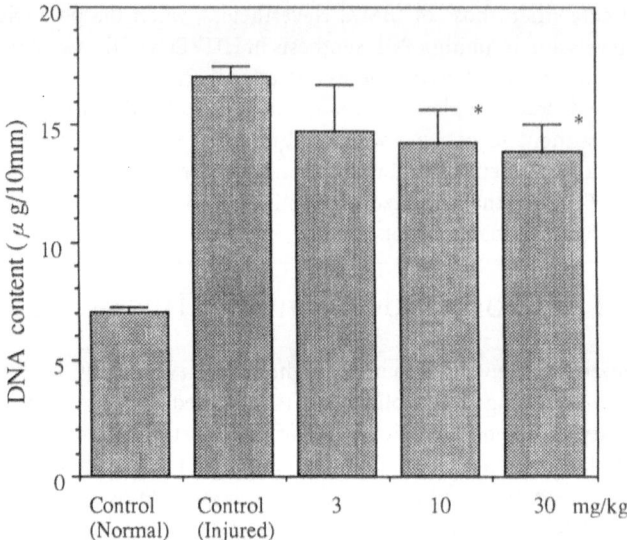

FIG. 9. Effects of cilostamide on intimal thickening in four groups of rats (each, $n = 8$). Cilostamide was administered at 3, 10, or 30 mg/kg body weight at 1 h before balloon catheterization and then twice a day for 2 weeks. DNA content in carotid arteries was determined using a fluorescence method for detection of a marker of intimal thickening

newly proliferating SMC. These findings suggested that platelets do not affect intimal SMC proliferation. Because cilostamide prevented SMC DNA synthesis, cilostamide did not inhibit intimal proliferation by inhibiting platelet aggregation. Cilostamide inhibits intimal proliferation directly by preventing the growth of SMC.

In conclusion, although PDEIII plays an important role in regulating ventricular contraction, platelet aggregation, vascular relaxation, and proliferation of vascular smooth muscle, excessive PDEIII activation results in a blood flow disorder. Given these findings, we believe that inhibition of cAMP hydrolysis by chronic administration of selective PDEIII inhibitors may provide a successful strategy for treatment of such blood flow disorders.

References

1. Asano T, Ochiai Y, Hidaka H (1977) Selective inhibition of separated forms of human platelet cyclic nucleotide phosphodiesterase by platelet aggregation inhibitors. Mol Pharmacol 13:400–406
2. Drummond GI, Anderson RJ (1979) Cyclc nucleotides and cardiac function. Circ Res 44:145–153
3. Tsein RW (1977) Cyclic AMP and contractile activity in heart. Adv Cyclic Nucleotide Res 8:363–420
4. Weishaar RE, Kobylarz-Singer DC, Steffen RP, Kaplan HR (1987) Subclasses of cyclic AMP-specific phosphodiesterase in left ventricular muscle and their involvement in regulating myocardial contractility. Circ Res 61:539–547
5. Schwartz A, Grupp I, Grupp G, Johnson C, Berner P, Wallick E, Imai K, Alousi A (1979) Amrinone: a new inotropic agent, studies on organelle systems. Circulation 60:16
6. Alousi AA, Farah AE (1980) Letter to editor. Circ Res 46:887–888

7. Kauffman RF, Schenck KM, Utterback BG, Crowe VG, Cohen MC (1987) In vitro vascular relaxation by new inotropic agents. Relationship to phosphodiesterase inhibition and cyclic nucleotides. J Pharmacol Exp Ther 242:864–872

8. Artman M, Robertson DW, Mahony L, Thompson WJ (1989) Analysis of the binding sites for the cardiotonic phosphodiesterase inhibitor [^{3}H]LY-186126 in ventricular myocardium. Mol Pharmacol 36:302–311

9. Bohr DF (1973) Vascular smooth muscle updated. Circ Res 32:71–73

10. Kukovetz WR, Holzmann S, Wurm A, Pöch G (1979) Evidence for cyclic GMP-mediated relaxant effects of nitrocompounds in coronary smooth muscle. Naunyn-Schmiedeberg's Arch Pharmacol 310:129–138

11. Mueller E, van Breemen C (1979) Role of intracellular Ca^{2+} sequestration in β-adrenergic relaxation of smooth muscle. Nature 281:682–683

12. Murad F (1986) Cyclic guanosine monophosphate as a mediator of vasodilation. J Clin Invest 78:1–5

13. Silver PJ, Schmidt-Silver C, Disalvo J (1982) β-Adrenergic relaxation and cAMP kinase activation in coronary artery smooth muscle. Am J Physiol 242:H177–H184

14. Sybertz EJ, Desiderio DM, Tetzloff G, Chiu PJS (1986) Phorbol dibutyrate contractions in rabbit aorta: calcium dependence and sensitivity to nitrovasodilators and 8-Br-cyclic GMP. J Pharmacol Exp Ther 239:78–83

15. Vegesna RVK, Diamond J (1983) Comparison of the effects of forskolin and isoproterenol on cyclic AMP levels and tension in bovine coronary artery. Can J Physiol Pharmacol 61:1202–1205

16. Hidaka H, Tanaka T, Itoh H (1984) Selective inhibitors of three forms of cyclic nucleotide phosphodiesterase. Trends Pharmacol Sci 5:237–239

17. Kauffman RF, Schenck KM, Utterback BG, Crowe VG, Cohen MC (1987) In vitro vascular relaxation by new inotropic agents. Relationship to phosphodiesterase inhibition and cyclic nucleotides. J Pharmacol Exp Ther 242:864–872

18. Harker LA (1987) Role of platelets and thrombosis in mechanisms of acute occlusion and restenosis after angioplasty. Am J Cardiol 60:20B–28B

19. Halt JI (1979) Role of blood platelets in coronary artery disease. Am J Cardiol 43:1197–1206

20. Rievey MP, Alexander MR, Taylor JW (1984) Dipyridamole: a critical evaluation. Drug Select Perspect 18:869–880

21. Salzman EW (1972) Cyclic AMP and platelet function. N Engl J Med 286:350–363

22. Hidaka H, Endo T (1984) Selective inhibitors of three forms of cyclic nucleotide phosphodiesterase: basic and potential clinical applications. Adv Cyclic Nucleotide Res 16:245–259

23. McElroy F, Philip RB (1975) Relative potencies of dipyridamole and related agents as inhibitors of cyclic nucleotide phosphodiesterases: possible explanation of mechanism of inhibition of platelet function. Life Sci 17:1479–1494

24. Hidaka H, Asano T (1976) Human blood platelet 3′:5′-cyclic nucleotide phosphodiesterase. Biochim Biophys Acta 429:485–497

25. Baumgartner HR, Muggli R (1976) Adhesion and aggregation: morphological demonstration and quantitation in vivo and in vitro. In: Platelets in biology and physiology, vol 1. North-Holland, Amsterdam, pp 23–60

Hyperpolarization–Relaxation Coupling in Vascular Smooth Muscle: Findings with K+ Channel Openers

Teruyuki Yanagisawa

Summary. Elucidation of the inhibitory mechanisms of hyperpolarization induced by the K+ channel openers levcromakalim, cromakalim, pinacidil, nicorandil, KRN2391, and Ki4032 on Ca^{2+} movement and the force of contraction produced by either the stimulation of thromboxane A_2 receptors or depolarization with high KCl has shown the following. When the plasma membrane is hyperpolarized by K+ channel openers, voltage-dependent L-type Ca^{2+} channels are deactivated and the influx of Ca^{2+} is decreased, as is the case with the KCl-induced Ca^{2+} influx. Hyperpolarization of the plasma membrane also has another inhibitory effect on the membrane-associated enzyme activity of phospholipase C. The production of inositol 1,4,5-trisphosphate (IP_3) and IP_3-induced Ca^{2+} release from intracellular stores, which is related to the stimulation of the agonist receptors, are inhibited by hyperpolarization of the plasma membrane by K+ channel openers. Nicorandil and KRN2391 behave as "N-K hybrids." We have also shown the voltage dependence of the Ca^{2+} sensitivity of contractile elements. Furthermore, membrane hyperpolarization induced by various K+ channel openers relaxed canine coronary arteries more profoundly than decreased $[Ca^{2+}]_i$. Thus, the membrane voltage may regulate intracellular enzyme activities, including contractile elements. This new facet of signal transduction therefore should be considered in the control of vascular tone.

Key words. K+ Channel opener—Cytoplasmic Ca^{2+} concentration—Membrane potential—Enzyme activity—Coronary artery

Introduction

Increasing attention has recently been paid to a group of vasodilators that activate or open K+ channels in vascular smooth muscle and which eventually increase coronary blood flow or lower blood pressure [1]. In vascular smooth muscle cells, the resting membrane potential is less negative than the K+ equilibrium potential (E_K) [2,3].

Elevation of intramural pressure in small arteries was found to cause depolarization and contraction of smooth muscle cell, which is called "myogenic tone" or "autoregulation." In Fig. 1a, the regulatory mechanism in vascular smooth muscle is

Department of Pharmacology, Tohoku University School of Medicine, Aoba-ku, Sendai 980, Japan

shown with the integral relation of three major types of K⁺ channels. The efficiency of
K⁺ channel opening as a modifier of membrane potential is extraordinary (Fig. 1b).
When the membrane is hyperpolarized toward E_K by opening of K⁺ channels, excita-
tion-induced Ca²⁺ influx via voltage-dependent Ca²⁺ channels is thought to decrease
[1–3]. Although intracellular Ca²⁺ concentration ($[Ca^{2+}]_i$) is one of the main determinants of mechanical activity of vascular smooth muscle, various reports have shown
that it is not the only determinant of this activity [4,5], and mechanisms involved in
contractions following receptor stimulation by agonists are far more complex than
those following simple membrane depolarization in vascular smooth muscle [6].
Nevertheless, contractions induced by agonists are effectively inhibited by the K⁺
channel openers cromakalim or aprikalim [7,8]. At present the relaxant action of K⁺
channel openers is generally understood to be a consequence of its ability to hold the
membrane potential of vascular smooth muscle cells close to their E_K [3]. There have
been several reports, however, that cromakalim could exert effects in addition to the
indirect closure (deactivation) of L-type Ca²⁺ channels [8,9].

In this review, we explore the effects of the K⁺ channel openers levcromakalim (BRL
38227, the active enantiomer of cromakalim) [10], cromakalim, pinacidil, nicorandil
[11], KRN2391, and Ki4032 [12–14] on $[Ca^{2+}]_i$ and the force of contraction of isolated
canine coronary arterial smooth muscle contracted with high KCl or the agonist
U46619, a thromboxane A₂ analog, using the fura-2 microfluorimetric method [15].
We further show the possibility of the existence of signaling mechanisms by which the
changes in level of membrane potential by either K⁺ channel openers or altering KCl

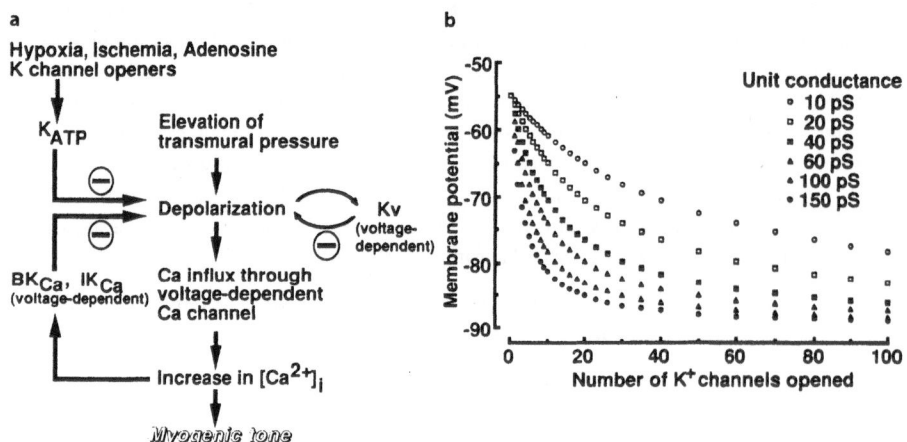

FIG. 1. a Integration of vasodilatory signals (hyperpolarization or repolarization) produced by
the activation of three major types of K⁺ channels to regulate arterial tone (myogenic response).
K_{ATP}, ATP-sensitive K⁺ channel (unit conductance of 5–10 pS); Kv, voltage-dependent K⁺
channel (unit conductance of 50–100 pS or 10–20 pS); B_{KCa} (unit conductance of 100–250 pS) or
I_{KCa} (unit conductance of 18–60 pS), high or intermediate conductance Ca²⁺-activated K⁺ channel. b Relationship between the number of K⁺ channels opened and the increase in membrane
potential. Unit conductance of K⁺ channel is changed from 10 to 150 pS. To calculate the changes
in membrane potential the following assumptions are made in a single vascular smooth muscle:
a total cell ionic conductance of 500 pS, an E_K (equilibrium potential for K⁺) of −90 mV (K⁺$_{out}$/
K⁺$_{in}$, 5 mM/150 mM), an Em (membrane potential) of −55 mV [$g_K \times E_K/(g_K + g_L)$], a K⁺ conductance ($g_K$) of 305 pS, and a leakage conductance (g_L) for all other ions together (Na⁺, Ca²⁺, and
Cl⁻) of 195 pS. (Data adapted and modified from [3,8])

concentration ($[K^+]_o$) in physiological salt solution (PSS) influence the Ca^{2+} sensitivity of contractile elements during the relaxation and contraction phases of high KCl-depolarized canine coronary arterial smooth muscle, even in the absence of agonists or drugs that may change membrane potential in vascular smooth muscle [10,14,16].

Effect of K⁺ Channel Openers on the Membrane Potential

KRN2391 (10^{-7}–$10^{-4} M$) hyperpolarized the membrane of canine coronary arterial smooth muscle cells in a concentration-dependent manner in 5 mM KCl-PSS (5K-PSS) [14]. The resting membrane was hyperpolarized from -52.8 ± 1.1 mV ($n = 13$) to -77.4 ± 1.3 mV ($n = 7$) by $10^{-4} M$. In 30 mM KCl-PSS (30K-PSS), the membrane depolarized to -33.9 ± 0.8 mV ($n = 15$). KRN2391 also hyperpolarized the membrane in 30K-PSS. The membrane potentials in the presence of $10^{-4} M$ KRN2391 were -40.0 ± 1.4 mV ($n = 6$). The membrane potentials in 5K-PSS in the absence and presence of glibenclamide ($10^{-5} M$) were -56.4 ± 5.4 mV and -52.8 ± 5.9 mV ($n = 5$; $P > .05$), respectively. Neither value was significantly different from those in the presence of both glibenclamide and KRN2391 ($10^{-5} M$) (-51.0 ± 6.4 mV) ($n = 5$). Thus, hyperpolarization induced by KRN2391 was blocked by glibenclamide [14].

In 30K-PSS, the application of levcromakalim produced membrane hyperpolarization [10]. The mean membrane hyperpolarization produced by levcromakalim ($10^{-5} M$) was -5.0 ± 0.5 mV ($n = 5$). The reduction of $[K^+]_o$ produced concentration-dependent membrane repolarization. The reduction of $[K^+]_o$ from 30 to 25 mM resulted in repolarization of -4.0 ± 0.4 mV ($n = 4$).

Effects of K⁺ Channel Openers on $[Ca^{2+}]_i$ and the Force of Contraction Induced by High KCl

In canine coronary artery loaded with fura-2, depolarization by 30–90 mM KCl-PSS produced a concentration-dependent increase in $[Ca^{2+}]_i$ and force [15,16]. The observed increase in $[Ca^{2+}]_i$ and force was abolished in Ca^{2+}-free PSS and was verapamil sensitive, thus certainly associated with an increased Ca^{2+} influx through voltage-dependent L-type Ca^{2+} channels [15,16]. In 5K-PSS, levcromakalim, cromakalim, pinacidil, nicorandil, KRN2391, and Ki4032 reduced $[Ca^{2+}]_i$ from the basal level, but the resting tone was not affected. In 30K-PSS, all six K⁺ channel openers reduced both $[Ca^{2+}]_i$ and contraction in a concentration-dependent manner; however, contraction was nearly abolished by pinacidil, nicorandil [11], and KRN2391 [12] at their maximum concentrations where significantly increased $[Ca^{2+}]_i$ levels remained.

The decreases in $[Ca^{2+}]_i$ by six drugs were abolished by glibenclamide or tetrabutylammonium (TBA). When the arterial rings were perfused with 45 mM or higher concentrations of KCl-PSS (>45K-PSS), levcromakalim, cromakalim, or Ki4032 had no effect on either the force of contraction or the increased $[Ca^{2+}]_i$, but pinacidil, nicorandil, or KRN2391 inhibited the force of contraction in a concentration-dependent manner. However, the increased $[Ca^{2+}]_i$ was not changed at all by pinacidil, nicorandil, or KRN2391 [11,12]. Thus, levcromakalim, cromakalim, and Ki4032 are specific K⁺ channel openers compared with pinacidil, nicorandil, and

KRN2391. The effects of K^+ channel openers in reducing the increased $[Ca^{2+}]_i$ may only be achieved when the resultant membrane potential associated with the presence of a raised KCl concentration is less negative than E_K and when the K^+ channel openers can hyperpolarize the membrane to reduce the opening probability of voltage-dependent Ca^{2+} channels.

The procedure to increase $[K^+]_o$ in PSS more than $45\,mM$ is very useful to differentiate K^+ channel openers from Ca^{2+} channel blockers [11,12]. In normal 5K-PSS, K^+ channel openers reduced $[Ca^{2+}]_i$ below the basal level, and such effects induced by levcromakalim, pinacidil, and nicorandil were blocked by TBA or glibenclamide. The reduction of $[Ca^{2+}]_i$ by K^+ channel openers was larger than that by the Ca^{2+} channel blockers verapamil and nicardipine. These results suggest that several kinds of Ca^{2+} channels or Ca^{2+}-permeable channels are open in resting conditions and that hyperpolarization of the plasma membrane by K^+ channel openers is capable of closing these Ca^{2+}-entry pathways.

Nicorandil and KRN2391 Behave as Hybrids Between Nitrates and K^+ Channel Openers

TBA or glibenclamide blocked the ability of nicorandil (10^{-4} and $10^{-3}M$) and KRN2391 (10^{-7}–$10^{-4}M$) to reduce $[Ca^{2+}]_i$ following exposure to $30\,mM$ KCl-PSS, but had a relatively small effect on nicorandil- or KRN2391-induced relaxation [11,12]. KRN2391 was a more potent K^+ channel opener compared with nicorandil; they have the nitroxy group in their molecules. The relaxant effect of nicorandil or KRN2391 was reduced by the guanylyl cyclase inhibitor methylene blue [12,17] and increased cyclic GMP in vascular smooth muscles [18,19]. These reduced the Ca^{2+} sensitivity of contractile proteins [11,12].

The relaxant effect of nicorandil or KRN2391, unrelated with a decrease in $[Ca^{2+}]_i$, was akin to that of nitroglycerin [16]. Thus, it is likely that nicorandil and KRN2391 partly relax smooth muscle cells without reducing the increased $[Ca^{2+}]_i$ following Ca^{2+} influx by depolarization via mechanisms resembling those of nitroglycerin. We would like to call such a vasodilating mechanism an "N–K hybrid," indicating dual, i.e., nitrate (N) and K^+ channel-activating, mechanisms in one molecule [20]. The structure–activity relationships of pyridine derivatives as K^+ channel openers indicate that the nitroxy substituent is very important for not only nitrate activity but also for the potency of K^+ channel openers [21]. Such a structure–activity relationship has been also shown for nicorandil [22].

Effects of K^+ Channel Openers on Ca^{2+} Influx by the Agonist U46619

Thromboxane A_2 is a potent constrictor of vascular smooth muscle as well as a strong inducer of platelet aggregation [23]. U46619 is a stable and full agonist analogue of thromboxane A_2 [24]. The human thromboxane A_2 receptor has been cloned, and its amino acid sequence shows that it is one of the G-protein-coupled receptors [25]. The vasoconstrictor mechanisms of thromboxane A_2 analogues have been proposed as releasing Ca^{2+} from intracellular stores and increasing transmembrane Ca^{2+} influx [26]. The relationship between $[Ca^{2+}]_i$ and force shows that U46619 increases Ca^{2+}

sensitivity of the contractile proteins [6]. The increase in Ca^{2+} sensitivity of contractile proteins by various agonists has been reported in coronary arteries [27,28].

Because the tonic increase in $[Ca^{2+}]_i$ induced by U46619 is abolished by verapamil or removal of $[Ca^{2+}]_o$ [6], it seems to be caused by Ca^{2+} influx through L-type Ca^{2+} channels stimulated by U46619, the same as by histamine [27]. The optimal concentration of $[K^+]_o$ that counteracts both the hyperpolarizing action and the inhibitory effects of cromakalim ($3 \times 10^{-6} M$) on changes in $[Ca^{2+}]_i$ and force induced by U46619 is between 20 and 25 mM [6]. An increase in $[K^+]_o$ is known to increase K^+ conductance of the plasma membrane [29,30]. Thus, the counteracting influence of the increase in $[K^+]_o$ seems to be mainly the result of its membrane depolarization effect. Therefore, the inhibitory action of K^+ channel openers on Ca^{2+} influx by the agonist seems to result from deactivation of L-type Ca^{2+} channels by hyperpolarization of the plasma membrane [6], as is the case of the KCl depolarization-induced Ca^{2+} influx.

Effects of Specific K^+ Channel Openers on Changes in $[Ca^{2+}]_i$, Force, and IP_3 Production Induced by U46619

It has been clear that levcromakalim, cromakalim, and Ki4032 are more specific K^+ channel openers than pinacidil, nicorandil, and KRN2391. The inhibitory mechanism of the specific opening of K^+ channels on agonist contraction was examined further [13]. U46619 produced an increase in $[Ca^{2+}]_i$ in a biphasic (phasic and tonic) manner. In the presence of cromakalim or Ki4032, $[Ca^{2+}]_i$ was reduced below the basal level. Cromakalim and Ki4032 almost abolished the increases in $[Ca^{2+}]_i$ and force in both phases induced by U46619. In the absence of $[Ca^{2+}]_o$ (0Ca-PSS), U46619 produced a transient increase in $[Ca^{2+}]_i$ and force of contraction; the latter was followed by a sustaining small force.

The tonic increase in $[Ca^{2+}]_i$ induced by U46619 is abolished in 0Ca-PSS. Because there was no Ca^{2+} to influx, the transient increases in $[Ca^{2+}]_i$ resulted from Ca^{2+} released from intracellular stores. When the preparation was perfused with 0Ca-PSS containing cromakalim or Ki4032, $[Ca^{2+}]_i$ was reduced to almost the same level as in their absence. In the presence of cromakalim or Ki4032, transient increases in $[Ca^{2+}]_i$ and force induced by U46619 were almost abolished. The inhibitory effect of cromakalim or Ki4032 on Ca^{2+} release was counteracted by the perfusion of 0Ca-20K-PSS containing 1 mM ethyleneglycoltetraacetic acid (EGTA) and blocked by TBA (3 mM). TBA and 20K-PSS in themselves did not affect either $[Ca^{2+}]_i$ or U46619-induced Ca^{2+} release in the absence of $[Ca^{2+}]_o$. Cromakalim or Ki4032 did not affect caffeine-induced Ca^{2+} release and force of contraction. Furthermore, in the absence of $[Ca^{2+}]_o$, the serial application of caffeine after the application of U46619 produced Ca^{2+} release but suppressed the force of contraction. In the presence of cromakalim, the Ca^{2+} release induced by U46619 was inhibited but that by caffeine was not inhibited but rather increased [13].

Because K^+ channel openers seemed to inhibit the production of inositol 1,4,5-trisphosphate (IP_3) stimulated by U46619, we therefore examined the effect of cromakalim on U46619-induced IP_3 production. In canine or porcine coronary arteries, the U46619-induced IP_3 production was inhibited by cromakalim. The inhibitory effect was blocked by TBA or counteracted by depolarization by 20K-PSS. Thus, the inhibitory effects of cromakalim and Ki4032 on the U46619-induced Ca^{2+} release may be exclusively the result of their plasma membrane hyperpolarizing action. It has been shown that cromakalim inhibits contractions of the rat isolated mesenteric bed induced by noradrenaline but not caffeine in 0Ca-PSS [31]. Thus, it is difficult to assume that K^+ channel openers act directly on the Ca^{2+} stores for Ca^{2+} to be depleted.

It is conceivable instead that hyperpolarization of the plasma membrane may inhibit the phosphatidylinositol turnover to result in a reduction of IP_3 or that hyperpolarization of plasma membrane produced by K^+ channel openers may affect intracellular Ca^{2+} stores and suppress the activity of only IP_3-induced Ca^{2+} release channels. We have shown that, in canine or porcine coronary arteries, the U46619-induced IP_3 production was inhibited by cromakalim [13,32]. This result coincides with the reports that levcromakalim inhibited noradrenaline-induced IP_3 synthesis and glibenclamide prevented the inhibitory actions [33]. Thus, it becomes obvious that there is a signaling pathway to relate membrane hyperpolarization with the membrane-associated enzyme activity, i.e., phospholipase C.

Hyperpolarization and Reduction of Ca^{2+} Sensitivity Induced by K^+ Channel Openers

Figure 2a shows the concentration–response curves for levcromakalim and KRN2391 to reduce the Ca^{2+} sensitivity in canine coronary artery [10,14]. The effects of KRN2391 were examined in the presence or absence of glibenclamide ($10^{-5}M$). Levcromakalim and KRN2391 reduced the Ca^{2+} sensitivity in a concentration-dependent manner. Although the effects of both drugs were blocked by glibenclamide, some glibenclamide-resistant component of KRN2391 remained. The reduction of $[K^+]_o$ produced a more prominent inhibition of the force of contraction than of $[Ca^{2+}]_i$ compared with relaxation by decreasing $[Ca^{2+}]_o$ in 30K-PSS [10,16].

Figure 2b shows the relationship between membrane potential and the reduction of Ca^{2+} sensitivity in the relaxations by levcomakalim or KRN2391 with plasma membrane hyperpolarization and the reduction of $[K^+]_o$ with repolarization [10,14]. We

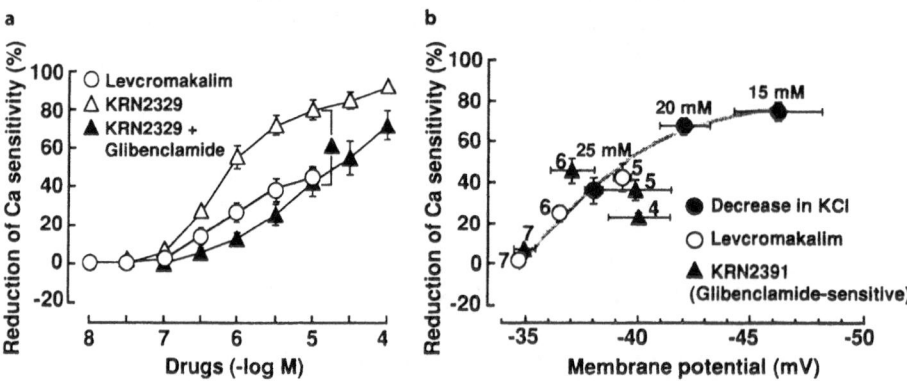

FIG. 2a,b. Concentration–response curves for levcromakalim and KRN2391 to reduce the Ca^{2+} sensitivity of contractile elements in 30 mM KCl-PSS. Influence of glibenclamide ($10^{-5}M$) on the concentration–response curve for KRN2391 is also shown. Relationship between membrane potential and reduction of the Ca^{2+} sensitivity of contractile elements in relaxation by levcomakalim or KRN2391 with plasma membrane hyperpolarization and the reduction of $[K^+]_o$ with repolarization from 30 mM KCl-PSS are shown. (Data adapted and modified from [10,14])

analyzed the glibenclamide-sensitive component in the effect of KRN2391 because KRN2391 is known to relax the coronary artery as an N–K hybrid [12,21]. The relationship between membrane repolarization and the reduction of Ca^{2+} sensitivity was very similar to that between hyperpolarization by levcromakalim or KRN2391 and the reduction, except that at $10^{-4} M$ KRN2391.

Comparison of Relaxations Produced by Repolarization, Removal of Extracellular Ca^{2+}, and Verapamil

Figure 3 shows the steady-state relationship between $[Ca^{2+}]_i$ and force during the inhibition of contraction obtained by reducing $[K^+]_o$ stepwise from 90 to 5 mM in 2.5 mM $CaCl_2$-PSS (2.5Ca-PSS) or by reducing $[Ca^{2+}]_o$ stepwise from 2.5 to 0.03 mM in 90K-PSS or the application of the Ca^{2+} channel blocker verapamil (10^{-7}–$10^{-5} M$) in 90K-2.5Ca-PSS in canine coronary artery loaded with fura-2. Even at the same $[Ca^{2+}]_i$ levels, the force generated by the muscle maintained depolarization by 90K-PSS was larger than that repolarized and activated by lower $[K^+]_o$. It has recently been shown that IP_3-induced Ca^{2+} release via activation of muscarinic receptors by acetylcholine is increased or decreased by depolarization or hyperpolarization, respectively, in voltage-clamped guinea pig coronary myocytes [34]. Even in the absence of acetylcholine, the formation of IP_3 may be stimulated by membrane depolarization [34]. Thus, Ca^{2+} sensitization by depolarization may be involved in the activation of protein kinase C as a result of the activation of phospholipase C, which activity may be controlled under the influence of membrane potential (Fig. 4).

We have reported that the activation of protein kinase C by phorbol 12,13-dibutyrate apparently increases the Ca^{2+} sensitivity of contractile elements [35,36]. There is also a report that a hyperpolarization-activated K^+ efflux appears to directly regulate adenylyl cyclase activity in *Paramecium* [37], and the membrane potential controlled by K^+ channels regulates the posttranscriptional synthesis and release of proteins such as tumor necrosis factor in macrophages [38]. Thus, the regulatory mechanisms of enzyme activity by the membrane potential may exist not only in smooth muscle cells but also in various cells. Furthermore, enzymes and ion channels can no longer be treated as separate and nonoverlapping groups of proteins [39].

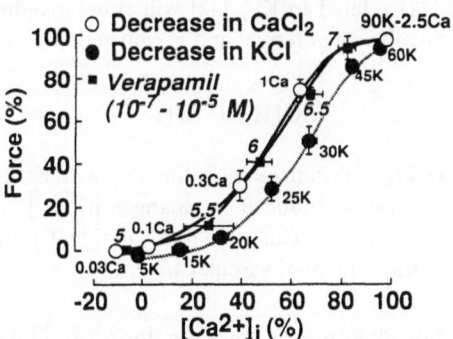

FIG. 3. $[Ca^{2+}]_i$–Force relation curves of the stepwise reduction of $[K^-]_o$ from 90 to 5 mM in 2.5 mM $CaCl_2$-PSS (2.5Ca-PSS) and the stepwise reduction of $[Ca^{2+}]_o$ from 2.5 to 0.03 mM in 90 mM KCl and in the presence of verapamil [10^{-7}–$10^{-5} M$; *italic number*, $-\log(M)$] in 90K-2.5Ca-PSS in canine coronary artery loaded with fura-2. (Data adapted and modified from [15,21])

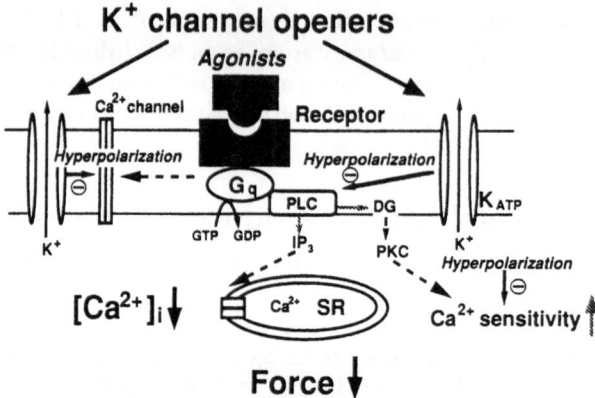

FIG. 4. Hyperpolarization–relaxation coupling in vascular smooth muscle. This concept comes from elucidation of the inhibitory mechanisms of hyperpolarization induced by K+ channel openers on the Ca²+ movements and force of contraction produced by either the stimulation of thromboxane A₂ receptors or depolarization with high KCl. The vasoconstrictor mechanisms of various agonists including thromboxane A₂ analogues have been proposed: that they release Ca²+ from intracellular stores, increase transmembrane Ca²+ influx, and increase Ca²+ sensitivity of contractile elements through coupling to the G protein [3–5]. When the plasma membrane is hyperpolarized by K+ channel openers, voltage-dependent L-type Ca²+ channels are deactivated and the influx of Ca²+ is decreased, as with KCl-induced Ca²+ influx. Hyperpolarization of the plasma membrane also has another inhibitory effect on the membrane-associated enzyme activity of phospholipase C [13,33,34]. The inositol 1,4,5-triphosphate (IP₃) production and IP₃-induced Ca²+ release from intracellular stores, which is related to the stimulation of the agonist receptors, are inhibited by the hyperpolarization of the plasma membrane by K+ channel openers

When one molecule exhibits both functions, the potential cross-regulation between channel activity and enzyme activity within the same molecule offers many intriguing possibilities for the integration of different cellular function. In line with such consideration, the β-subunits of voltage-gated K+ channels have been shown to belong to an NAD(P)H-dependent oxidoreductase superfamily [40].

Elucidation of the molecular structures of the β-subunits and high-affinity sulfonylurea receptor [41] related to K_{ATP} [42] will show insight into the signaling mechanisms between membrane potential and various enzyme activities.

Conclusion

Hyperpolarization by various substances, including that with K+ channel openers, and depolarization or repolarization induced by changes in $[K^-]_o$ modulates the Ca²+ sensitivity of contractile elements. This new facet of signal transduction therefore should be considered in the control of vascular tone.

Acknowledgments. We thank Professor Emeritus Norio Taira for his support and his insight concerning the importance of K+ channel openers on vascular tone regulation. This work was supported in part by a Grant-in-Aid for Scientific Research (Nos. 07457020, 07557329) from the Ministry of Education, Science, Sport and Culture, Japan.

References

1. Cook NS, Quast U (1990) Potassium channel pharmacology. In: Cook NS (ed) Potassium channels: structure, classification, function and therapeutic potential. Horwood, Chester, pp 181–255
2. Daut J, Standen NB, Nelson MT (1994) The role of the membrane potential of coronary endothelial and smooth muscle cells in the regulation of coronary blood flow. J Cardiovasc Electrophysiol 5:154–181
3. Nelson MT, Patlak JB, Worley JF, Standen NB (1990) Calcium channels, potassium channels, and voltage dependence of arterial smooth muscle tone. Am J Physiol 259:C3–C18
4. Kamm KE, Stull JT (1989) Regulation of smooth muscle contractile elements by second messengers. Annu Rev Physiol 51:299–313
5. Somlyo AP, Somlyo AV (1994) Signal transduction and regulation in smooth muscle. Nature 372:231–236
6. Yamagishi T, Yanagisawa T, Taira N (1992) Ca^{2+} influx induced by an agonist U46619 is inhibited by hyperpolarization induced by a K^+ channel opener, cromakalim, in canine coronary artery. Jpn J Pharmacol 59:291–299
7. Cook NS, Weir SW, Danzeisen MC (1988) Anti-vasoconstrictor effects of the K^+ channel opener cromakalim on the rabbit aorta—comparison with the calcium antagonist isradipine. Br J Pharmacol 95:741–752
8. Quast U, Guillon JM, Cavero I (1994) Cellular pharmacology of potassium channel openers in vascular smooth muscle. Cardiovasc Res 28:805–810
9. Bray KM, Weston AH, Duty S, Newgreen DT, Longmore J, Edwards G, Brown TJ (1991) Differences between the effects of cromakalim and nifedipine on agonist-induced responses in rabbit aorta. Br J Pharmcol 102:337–344
10. Okada Y, Yanagisawa T, Taira N (1993) BRL-38227 (levcromakalim)-induced hyperpolarization reduces the sensitivity of contractile elements to Ca^{2+} in canine coronary artery. Naunyn-Schmiedeberg's Arch Pharmacol 347:438–444
11. Yanagisawa T, Teshigawara T, Taira N (1990) Cytoplasmic calcium and the relaxation of canine coronary arterial smooth muscle produced by cromakalim, pinacidil and nicorandil. Br J Pharmacol 101:157–165
12. Okada Y, Yanagisawa T, Taira N (1991) An analysis of the nitrate-like and K^+ channel opening actions of KRN2391 in canine coronary arterial smooth muscle. Br J Pharmacol 104:829–838
13. Yamagishi T, Yanagisawa T, Taira N (1992) K^+ channel openers, cromakalim and Ki4032, inhibit agonist-induced Ca^{2+} release in canine coronary artery. Naunyn-Schmiedeberg's Arch Pharmacol 346:691–700
14. Okada Y, Yanagisawa T, Yamagishi T, Taira N (1993) K^+ channel opening action and KRN2391-induced reduction of Ca^{2+} sensitivity of arterial smooth muscle. Arch Intern Pharmacodyn Ther 326:33–51
15. Yanagisawa T, Kawada M, Taira N (1989) Nitroglycerin relaxes canine coronary arterial smooth muscle without reducing intracellular Ca^{2+} concentrations measured with fura-2. Br J Pharmacol 98:469–482
16. Yanagisawa T, Okada Y (1994) KCl depolarization increases Ca^{2+} sensitivity of contractile elements in coronary arterial smooth muscle. Am J Physiol 267:H614–H621
17. Satoh K, Yamada H, Yoneyama F, Taira N (1991) The groun at C2 of N-ethyl-nicotinamide determines the vasodilator potencies and mechanisms of action of nicorandil and its congeners in canine coronary arteries. Naunyn-Schmiedeberg's Arch Pharmacol 344:589–595
18. Endoh M, Taira N (1983) Relationship between relaxation and cyclic GMP formation caused by nicorandil in canine mesenteric artery. Naunyn-Schmiedeberg's Arch Pharmacol 322:319–321
19. Jinno Y, Kasai H, Ohta H, Nishikori K, Fukushima H, Ogawa N (1992) Contribution of cyclic GMP formation to KRN2391-induced relaxation in porcine coronary artery. Br J Pharmacol 106:906–909

20. Taira N (1989) Nicorandil as a hybrid between nitrates and potassium channel activators. Am J Cardiol 63:18J–24J
21. Yanagisawa T, Okada Y (1993) The structure-activity relationship of KRN2391 as an N–K hybrid. Cardiovasc Drug Rev 11:94–115
22. Edwards G, Weston AH (1990) Structure-activity relationships of K$^+$ channel openers. Trends Pharmacol Sci 11:417–422
23. Moncada S, Vane JR (1978) Unstable metabolites of arachidonic acid and their role in haemostasis and thrombosis. Br Med Bull 34:129–135
24. Tymkewycz PM, Jones RL, Wilson NH, Marr CG (1991) Heterogeneity of thromboxane A$_2$ (TP-) receptors: evidence from antagonist but not agonist potency measurements. Br J Pharmacol 102:607–614
25. Hirata M, Hayashi Y, Ushikubi F, Yokota Y, Kageyama R, Nakanishi S, Naromiya S (1991) Cloning and expression of cDNA for a human thromboxane A$_2$ receptor. Nature 349:617–620
26. Toda N (1982) Mechanism of action of carbocyclic thromboxane A$_2$ and its interaction with prostaglandin I$_2$ and verapamil in isolated arteries. Circ Res 51:675–682
27. Mori T, Yanagisawa T, Taira N (1990) Histamine increases vascular tone and intracellular calcium level using both intracellular and extracellular calcium in porcine coronary arteries. Jpn J Pharmacol 52:263–271
28. Okada Y, Yanagisawa T, Taira N (1992) KCl-depolarization potentiates the Ca^{2+} sensitization by endothelin-1 in canine coronary. Jpn J Pharmacol 60:403–405
29. Sperelakis N (1979) Origin of cardiac resting potential. In: Berne RM (ed) The handbook of physiology. Section 2: The cardiovascular system, vol 1. American Physiological Society, Baltimore, pp 187–267
30. Tseng G-N, Tseng-Crank J (1992) Differential effects of elevating [K]$_o$ on three transient outward potassium channels: dependence on channel inactivation mechanisms. Circ Res 71:657–672
31. Quast U, Baumlin Y (1991) Cromakalim inhibits contractions of the rat isolated mesenteric bed induced by noradrenaline but not caffeine in Ca^{2+}-free medium: evidence for interference with receptor-mediated Ca^{2+} mobilization. Eur J Pharmacol 200:239–249
32. Yamagishi T, Yanagisawa T, Taira N (1992) Activation of phospholipase C by the agonist U46619 is inhibited by cromakalim-induced hyperpolarization in porcine coronary artery. Biochem Biophys Res Commun 187:1517–1522
33. Ito S, Kajikuri J, Itoh T, Kuriyama H (1991) Effects of lemakalim on changes in Ca^{2+} concentration and mechanical activity induced by noradrenaline in the rabbit mesenteric artery. Br J Pharmacol 104:227–233
34. Ganitkevich VY, Isenberg G (1993) Membrane potential modulates inositol 1,4,5-trisphosphate-mediated Ca^{2+} transients in guinea-pig coronary myocytes. J Physiol (Lond) 470:35–44
35. Mori T, Yanagisawa T, Taira N (1990) Phorbol 12,13-dibutyrate increases vascular tone but has a dual action on intracellular calcium levels in porcine coronary arteries. Naunyn-Schmiedeberg's Arch Pharmacol 341:251–255
36. Kageyama M, Mori T, Yanagisawa T, Taira N (1991) Is staurosporine a specific inhibitor of protein kinase C in intact porcine coronary arteries? J Pharmacol Exp Ther 259:1019–1026
37. Schultz JE, Klumpp S, Benz R, Schürhoff-Goeters WJC, Schmid A (1992) Regulation of adenylyl cyclase from *Paramecium* by an intrinsic potassium conductance. Science 255:600–603
38. Haslberger A, Romanin C, Koerber R (1992) Membrane potential modulates release of tumor necrosis factor in lipopolysaccharide-stimulated mouse macrophages. Mol Biol Cell 3:451–460
39. Jan LY, Jan YN (1992) Tracing the roots of ion channels. Cell 69:715–718
40. McCormack T, McCormack K (1994) Shaker K$^+$ channel β subunits belong to an NAD(P)H-dependent oxidoreductase superfamily. Cell 79:1133–1135

41. Aguilar-Bryan L, Nicols CG, Wechsler SW, Clement IV JP, Boyd III AE, Gonzales G, Herrera-Sosa H, Nguy K, Bryan J, Nelson DA (1995) Cloning of the β cell high-affinity sulfonylurea receptor: a regulation of insulin secretion. Science 268:423–426
42. Inagaki N, Gonoi T, Clement JP IV, Namba N, Inazawa J, Gonzalez G, Aguilar-Bryan L, Seino S, Bryan J (1995) Reconstitution of IKATP: an inward rectifier subunit plus the sulfonylurea receptor. Science 270:1166–1170

Two Calcium Compartments in Vascular Smooth Muscle

Hideaki Karaki[1], Fujio Abe[2], Minori Mitsui-Saito[1],
Satoshi Kitajima[1], Ken-ichi Harada[1], Masatoshi Hori[1],
Koichi Sato[1], Hiroshi Ozaki[1], and Masao Endoh[2]

Summary. In vascular smooth muscle cell, we suggest the presence of two Ca^{2+} compartments. The first is the "contractile" compartment which regulates cytoplasmic Ca^{2+}-dependent mechanisms such as myosin light chain kinase (or contraction) and other enzymes. Ca^{2+} in this compartment increases to a level that is not so high, so that aequorin in this compartment is consumed only slowly. Most of the fura-2 signal represents Ca^{2+} in this compartment. The second compartment is the "non-contractile" Ca^{2+} compartment, which may be located in close vicinity to the plasma membrane and the sarcoplasmic reticulum (SR) and is segregated from the "contractile" compartment by a diffusion barrier. This barrier is so tight that the aequorin molecules diffuse only slowly between these two compartments. Ca^{2+} in this compartment increases so strongly that the aequorin is rapidly consumed. This compartment is detected more sensitively by aequorin than by fura-2 because Ca^{2+} concentration here is higher than that in the "contractile" compartment although the size of this compartment is smaller. Ca^{2+} in this compartment is taken up by the SR; it is not able to activate the contractile elements because this compartment does not contain contractile elements; it may regulate membrane Ca^{2+}-dependent mechanisms such as ion channels, ion pumps, and certain enzymes. Agonists may increase the Ca^{2+} level in these compartments mainly by Ca^{2+} influx and partly by Ca^{2+} release, whereas high K^+ increases Ca^{2+} exclusively by Ca^{2+} influx.

Key words. Smooth muscle—Cytosolic calcium—Calcium compartment—Calcium sensitivity—Calcium distribution

Introduction

It has been widely accepted that an increase in the cytosolic Ca^{2+} level ($[Ca^{2+}]_i$) in smooth muscle activates myosin light chain kinase (MLCK), which phosphorylates myosin light chain (MLC) and in turn activates the interaction between thick and thin filaments. Based on this phosphorylation theory, $[Ca^{2+}]_i$ is considered to be the only

[1] Department of Veterinary Pharmacology, Graduate School of Agriculture and Life Sciences, University of Tokyo, Bunkyo-ku, Tokyo 113, Japan
[2] Department of Pharmacology, Yamagata University School of Medicine, Yamagata 990-23, Japan

195

regulator of contraction. Recent observations, however, have revealed a dissociation between $[Ca^{2+}]_i$ and muscle tension. A part of this dissociation is explained by the presence of an additional regulatory mechanism that modulates the Ca^{2+} sensitivity of contractile elements [1]. It has also been suggested that the distribution of Ca^{2+} in cytoplasm is not uniform and that there is a Ca^{2+} compartment that is not coupled to contraction [2]. The major emphasis of this review will be on our recent findings on the Ca^{2+} compartments in vascular smooth muscle.

Ca^{2+} Influx and Contraction

In smooth muscle, there are two sources that supply Ca^{2+} to cytoplasm [3]. Opening of Ca^{2+} channels permits Ca^{2+} entry to induce a sustained increase in $[Ca^{2+}]_i$ and sustained contraction. In contrast, Ca^{2+} released from the sarcoplasmic reticulum (SR) increases $[Ca^{2+}]_i$ transiently to induce transient contraction. In the rat aorta loaded with a fluorescent Ca^{2+} indicator, fura-2, high-K^+, and norepinephrine (NE) induce a sustained increase in $[Ca^{2+}]_i$ [4], as shown in Fig. 1. The NE-induced increase is due to initial transient Ca^{2+} release followed by sustained Ca^{2+} influx because only the sustained increase in $[Ca^{2+}]_i$ was abolished in the Ca^{2+}-free solution (see Fig. 5) or in the presence of a Ca^{2+}-channel blocker, verapamil [5]. Comparing the increase in $[Ca^{2+}]_i$ and contraction, it is evident that the rate of increase in contraction is slower than that of $[Ca^{2+}]_i$ and that the maximally effective concentration of KCl induced a smaller contraction than NE, although $[Ca^{2+}]_i$ stimulated by KCl was greater than that stimulated by NE [4]. Other receptor agonists, such as prostaglandin $F_{2\alpha}$ [6], endothelin-1 [6,7], and a phorbol ester, 12-deoxyphorbol 13-isobutyrate (DPB) [8], also induced greater contraction than KCl at a given $[Ca^{2+}]_i$. These results are not due to artifacts of $[Ca^{2+}]_i$ measurement because these agonists also augmented the Ca^{2+}-induced contraction in permeabilized smooth muscle in which the Ca^{2+} concentration was clamped by a Ca^{2+} buffer.

Figure 2 shows the relationship among $[Ca^{2+}]_i$, MLC phosphorylation, and contraction in the presence of high K^+, NE, prostaglandin $F_{2\alpha}$, endothelin-1, and phorbol ester [6,8]. It is shown that although these agonists and phorbol ester increased $[Ca^{2+}]_i$ to levels lower than that due to high K^+, MLC phosphorylation and contraction were greater than that due to high K^+. These results suggest that receptor agonists increase

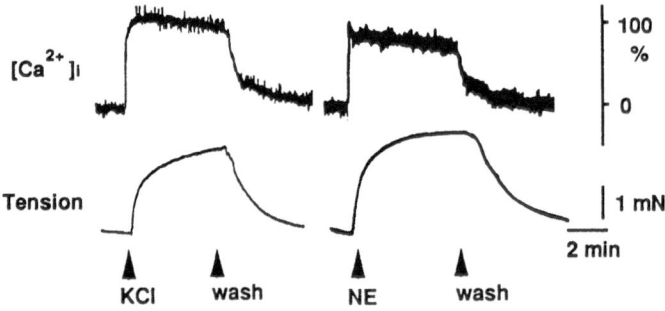

FIG. 1. Effects of 1 μM norepinephrine (*NE*) and 72.7 mM KCl (high K^+) in fura-2-loaded rat aorta. *[Ca²⁺]ᵢ*, fura-2-Ca^{2+} signal as indicated by the relative fluorescence ratio

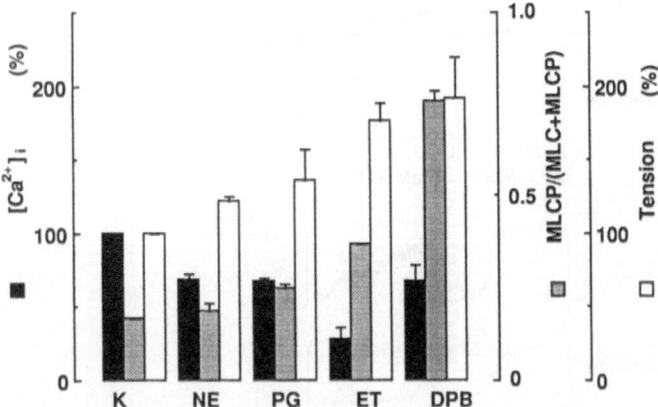

FIG. 2. Effects of maximally effective concentrations of KCl (72.7 mM), NE (1 μM), prostaglandin $F_{2\alpha}$ (*PG*; 10 μM), endothelin-1 (*ET*; 30 nM) and 12-deoxypholbol 13-isobutyrate (*DPB*; 1 μM) on $[Ca^{2+}]_i$, myosin light chain (*MLC*) phosphorylation, and contraction in the rat aorta measured 20 min after the addition of stimulant

Ca^{2+} sensitivity of MLC phosphorylation and that different agonists change Ca^{2+} sensitivity to different degrees. In addition, these agonists seem to activate the regulation mechanism that is not dependent on MLC phosphorylation [1,2,6,8].

Another type of dissociation was found using ATP and its analogues. ATP (Fig. 3a), α,β-methylene ATP, and ATPγS induced a transient large increase in $[Ca^{2+}]_i$ in the rat aorta. However, these agonists induced only a small transient contraction [9]. Thus, increase in $[Ca^{2+}]_i$ due to ATP, α,β-methylene ATP, and ATPγS is coupled only weakly to contraction. A similar dissociation was found in bovine trachea and guinea pig ileum stimulated with ATP (Fig. 3a). In the rabbit mesenteric artery and guinea pig vas deferens, however, the ATP-induced increase in $[Ca^{2+}]_i$ was followed by contraction and there seemed to be no dissociation between $[Ca^{2+}]_i$ and contraction (Fig. 3b). In contrast, high K^+-induced sustained increase in $[Ca^{2+}]_i$ was not coupled to contraction in vas deferens. These results suggest the tissue-dependent difference in the coupling between the sustained increase in $[Ca^{2+}]_i$ and contraction.

Caffeine also induced a large transient increase followed by a small sustained increase in $[Ca^{2+}]_i$ (Fig. 4). However, caffeine induced only transient contraction followed by relaxation below the resting tone [10]. This result suggests that the sustained increase in $[Ca^{2+}]_i$ due to caffeine is not coupled to contraction.

Ca²⁺ Release and Contraction

In Ca^{2+}-free solution, receptor agonists release SR Ca^{2+} through IP_3-sensitive Ca^{2+} channels [3]. As shown in Fig. 5, NE [4], prostaglandin $F_{2\alpha}$ [11] and endothelin-1 [7] induced a transient increase in $[Ca^{2+}]_i$ in Ca^{2+}-free solution. However, a transient increase in $[Ca^{2+}]_i$ due to Ca^{2+} release induced by prostaglandin $F_{2\alpha}$ or endothelin-1 was followed, if at all, by only a small contraction. Although the NE-induced transient increase in $[Ca^{2+}]_i$ was followed by transient contraction, the $[Ca^{2+}]_i$-tension relationship indicated that the peak level of contraction was smaller than the sustained contraction induced by high K^+ at a given $[Ca^{2+}]_i$. After the transient increase in $[Ca^{2+}]_i$

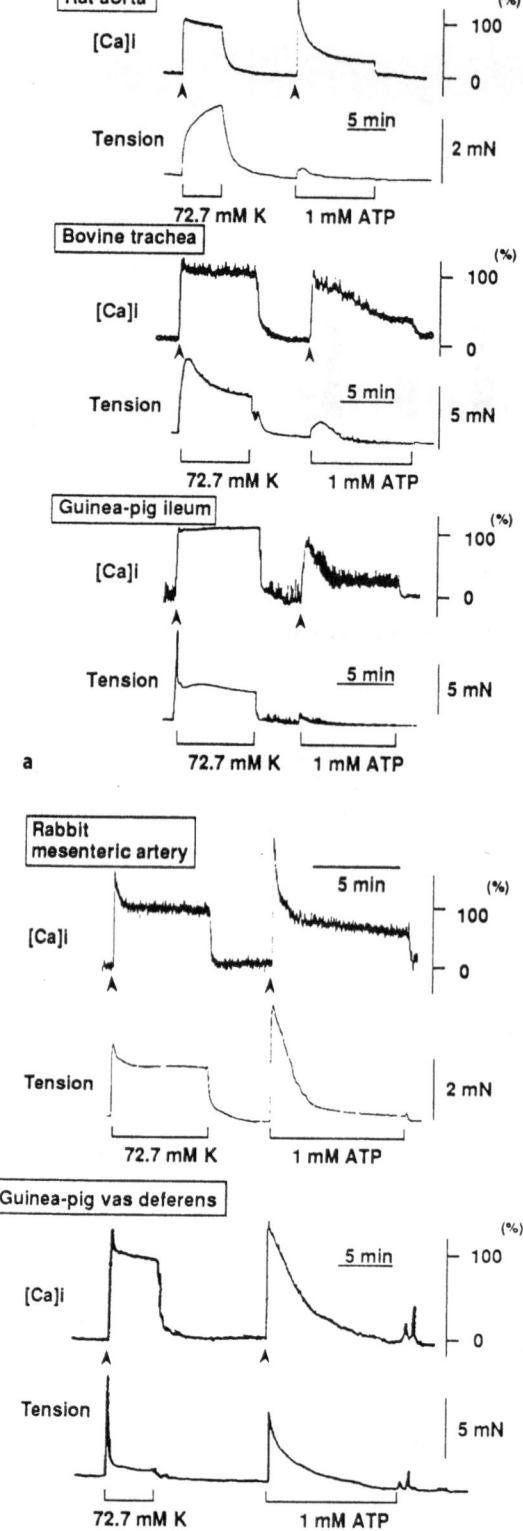

FIG. 3. Effects of 72.7 mM KCl and 1 mM ATP on $[Ca^{2+}]_i$ and contraction in a rat aorta, bovine trachea, and guinea pig ileum, and b rabbit mesenteric artery and guinea pig vas deferens

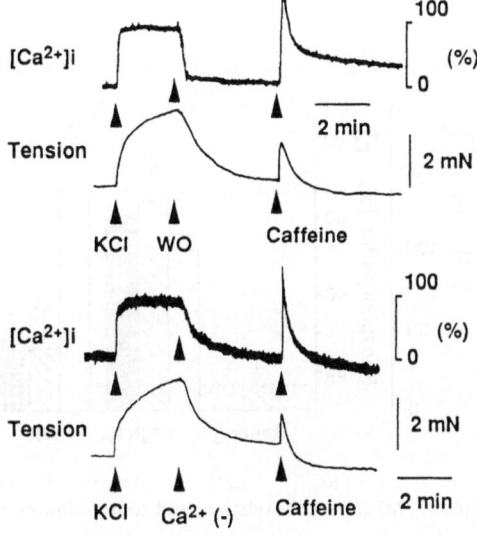

FIG. 4. Effects of high K+ and caffeine on [Ca²⁺]ᵢ and contraction in the presence (*upper*) and in the absence (*lower*) of external Ca²⁺ in the rat aorta

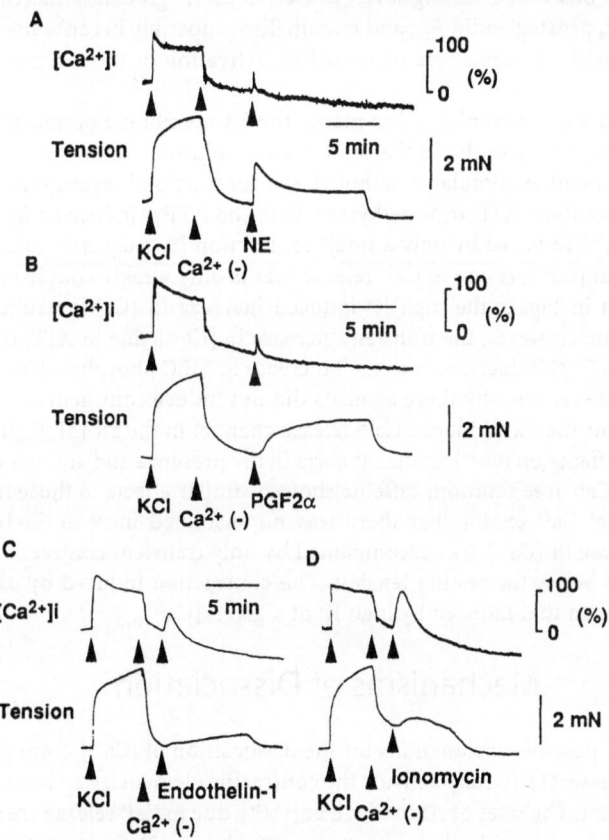

FIG. 5. Effects of A NE (1 μM), B prostaglandin F₂α (*PGF2α*; 10 μM), C endothelin-1 (30 nM), and D ionomycin (3 μM) on [Ca²⁺]ᵢ and contraction in the rat aorta in Ca²⁺-free solution. After stimulation with high K⁺, the muscle strip was washed with a normal K⁺ and Ca²⁻-free solution (*Ca²⁺(−)*) and then the stimulant was added

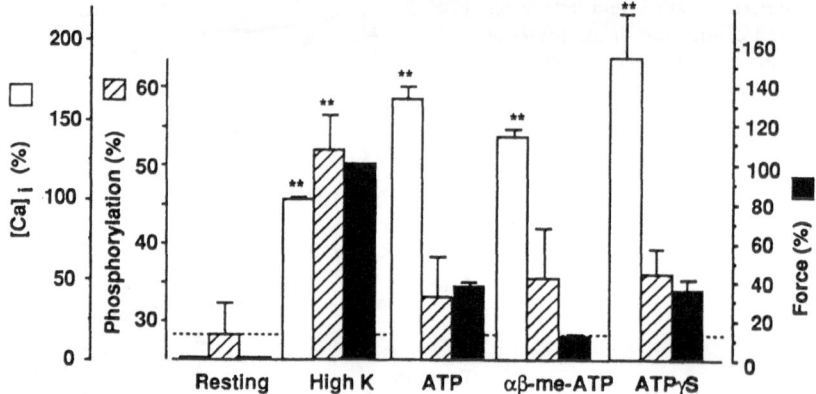

FIG. 6. Effects of KCl (72.7 mM), ATP (1 mM), α,β-methylene ATP (1 mM), and ATPγS (1 mM) on [Ca²⁺]ᵢ, MLC phosphorylation, and contraction in the rat aorta measured at the peak [Ca²⁺]ᵢ

returned to or below the resting level, muscle tension gradually increased in the presence of NE, prostaglandin $F_{2\alpha}$, and endothelin-1, possibly because the Ca^{2+} sensitivity of contractile elements was increased by activation of the receptor-G protein system [1].

Ionomycin is a Ca^{2+} ionophore that makes the SR membrane permeable and thus releases Ca^{2+}. Figure 5 also shows that, in Ca^{2+}-free solution, ionomycin releases Ca^{2+} more slowly than other stimulants, although the contraction is again very small [10].

In Ca^{2+}-free solution, ATP, α,β-methylene ATP, and ATPγS induced only a transient increase in $[Ca^{2+}]_i$ followed by only a small contraction [9], suggesting that the transient increase in $[Ca^{2+}]_i$ is due to Ca^{2+} release that is only weakly coupled to contraction. As shown in Fig. 6, the high K^+-induced increase in $[Ca^{2+}]_i$ resulted in MLC phosphorylation. However, the transient increase in $[Ca^{2+}]_i$ due to ATP, α,β-methylene ATP, and ATPγS induced only a small increase in MLC phosphorylation, and this seemed to be the reason why these agonists did not induce contraction.

Caffeine opens the Ca^{2+}-induced Ca^{2+}-release channel in the SR [3]. Figure 4 shows the effects of caffeine on $[Ca^{2+}]_i$ in the rat aorta in the presence and absence of external Ca^{2+} [4,10]. In Ca^{2+}-free solution, caffeine showed similar effects to those in the presence of external Ca^{2+} except that there was no sustained increase in $[Ca^{2+}]_i$. The transient increase in $[Ca^{2+}]_i$ was accompanied by only transient contraction followed by a relaxation below the resting tension. The contraction induced by caffeine was much smaller than that induced by high K^+ at a given $[Ca^{2+}]_i$.

Mechanisms of Dissociation

There are three possible explanations for the dissociation of $[Ca^{2+}]_i$ from contraction during Ca^{2+} release: (1) To fully activate the contractile elements, Ca^{2+} has to reach the central cytoplasm. The rates of rise and fall of $[Ca^{2+}]_i$ due to Ca^{2+} release are so fast that Ca^{2+} does not spread evenly throughout the cytoplasm. (2) Certain stimulants decreased the Ca^{2+} sensitivity of the contractile elements during Ca^{2+} release. (3) There are two Ca^{2+} compartments in cytoplasm: one coupled to contraction and the second not coupled to contraction. Some stimulants may increase Ca^{2+} in either of these compartments, whereas others may increase Ca^{2+} in both of these compartments.

Rates of Rise and Fall of the Ca²⁺ Transient

Soon after the opening of the SR Ca^{2+} channel, the Ca^{2+} concentration near the SR may become higher than the average cytoplasmic Ca^{2+} concentration. Then, Ca^{2+} diffuses slowly to the cytoplasm and gradually reaches an equilibrium. At the same time, Ca^{2+} is taken up by the SR again and extruded from the cell by the Ca^{2+} pump and the Na^+/Ca^{2+} exchange. The peak fura-2 signal may represent the peak Ca^{2+} concentration near the SR, whereas the peak Ca^{2+} concentration in central cytoplasm, which is much lower than that near the SR, may be attained after the peak fura-2 signal. This may be the reason why the peak contraction is lower than that predicted from the peak fura-2 signal. Such a dissociation may generally occur irrespective of the types of stimulants. Although NE, prostaglandin $F_{2\alpha}$, endothelin-1, and ATP analogues induced a similar increase in $[Ca^{2+}]_i$ due to Ca^{2+} release, these stimulants induced different magnitudes of contraction, suggesting that an additional explanation is necessary.

It is also probable that the rate of rise of $[Ca^{2+}]_i$ may determine the peak contraction because the slow Ca^{2+} release due to ionomycin induced only a small contraction. Furthermore, the rate of increase in $[Ca^{2+}]_i$ due to endothelin-1 was slower than that due to NE, and the transient contraction induced by endothelin-1 was smaller than that induced by NE. However, although ATP and its analogues induced a rapid increase in $[Ca^{2+}]_i$ the contraction was still small. These results suggest that although the rate of increase in $[Ca^{2+}]_i$ may affect the rate of increase in contraction, it does not seem to determine the peak level of contraction.

Decrease in Ca²⁺ Sensitivity

It has been shown that caffeine decreases Ca^{2+} sensitivity by directly inhibiting MLCK and the actin-myosin interaction [12]. This may be the reason why the caffeine-induced large transient increase in $[Ca^{2+}]_i$ was coupled only to a small transient contraction and why the caffeine-induced sustained increase in $[Ca^{2+}]_i$ was not coupled to contraction. To determine if other stimulants that release Ca^{2+} from SR also somehow decreased the Ca^{2+} sensitivity of contractile elements, stimulants were added during the sustained contraction induced by high K^+. As shown in Fig. 7, caffeine transiently augmented and then inhibited the contractions induced by high K^+. Caffeine showed similar dual effects when added during the NE-induced sustained contraction. These results suggest that although caffeine exerts both a contractile and a relaxant effect simultaneously, the onset of the relaxant effect is not rapid enough to completely inhibit the onset of contraction and, as a result, a small, initial transient contraction may be induced. In contrast to the effect of caffeine, NE, endothelin-1, prostaglandin $F_{2\alpha}$, ATP and its analogues, and ionomycin did not inhibit, but rather augmented, high-K^+-induced contraction when added during the high-K^+-induced sustained contraction. These results suggest that these stimulants, except for caffeine, may not decrease the Ca^{2+} sensitivity of the contractile elements.

Increase in Ca²⁺ Sensitivity

Another possibility is that an increase in $[Ca^{2+}]_i$ in the central cytoplasm following Ca^{2+} release (which may not be precisely determined by fura-2 because the signal of this Ca^{2+} indicator represents the average Ca^{2+} concentration in the entire cytoplasm) is not high enough to induce contraction by itself; transient contraction is induced only when the Ca^{2+} sensitivity of the contractile element is increased simultaneously with

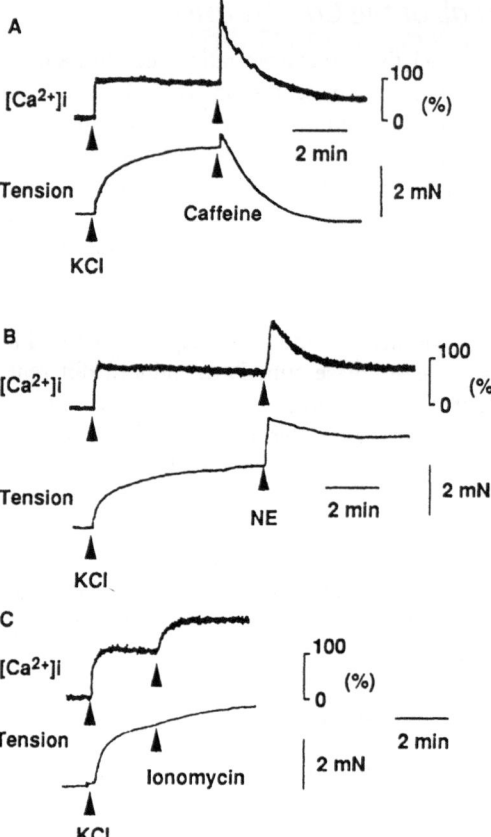

FIG. 7. Effects of A 20 mM caffeine, B 1 μM NE, and C 1 μM ionomycin on $[Ca^{2+}]_i$ and contraction in the rat aorta stimulated with 72.7 mM KCl

the small increase in $[Ca^{2+}]_i$. Although endothelin-1 and prostaglandin $F_{2\alpha}$ increase Ca^{2+} sensitivity, the onset of activation of this mechanism is slow and Ca^{2+} sensitivity increased only after Ca^{2+} release. In contrast, NE increases Ca^{2+} sensitivity quite rapidly and, thus, the transient increase in $[Ca^{2+}]_i$ due to NE is coupled to contraction.

In Ca^{2+}-free solution, these agonists induce sustained contraction without changing $[Ca^{2+}]_i$. This contraction is considered to be due to an increase in Ca^{2+} sensitivity [1,6]. Since the rate of increase in sustained contraction induced by NE was faster than that induced by endothelin-1 and prostaglandin $F_{2\alpha}$, NE seems to increase Ca^{2+} sensitivity more rapidly than endothelin-1 and prostaglandin $F_{2\alpha}$. Furthermore, ATP that did not increase the Ca^{2+} sensitivity did not induce contraction. These results seem to support the idea that Ca^{2+} sensitization is necessary to couple Ca^{2+} release with contraction. However, caffeine that did not increase Ca^{2+} sensitivity induced greater transient contraction than that induced by endothelin-1, prostaglandin $F_{2\alpha}$, or ATP. This discrepancy may indicate that Ca^{2+} sensitization is not necessary for transient contraction. Alternatively, caffeine may have increased $[Ca^{2+}]_i$ in the central cytoplasm strongly enough to induce contraction without Ca^{2+} sensitization because the caffeine-induced transient increase in $[Ca^{2+}]_i$ was larger than that induced by other stimulants. Further examination is necessary to evaluate this possibility.

Ca^{2+} Compartments

Subsequent to the opening of the plasma membrane Ca^{2+} channel, external Ca^{2+} at a concentration of more than 10^4 times the $[Ca^{2+}]_i$ enters the cell, establishing a large Ca^{2+} gradient between the submembrane area and the central cytoplasm. This change may be detected as a rapid and large increase in the fura-2 signal. During continuous Ca^{2+} influx (the smooth muscle Ca^{2+} channel is not completely inactivated because of the presence of window current [13]), equilibrium is reached and the Ca^{2+} in cytoplasm may spread more homogeneously. The sustained increase in $[Ca^{2+}]_i$ during continuous stimulation may represent this state. This may be the reason why the rate of rise of contraction is slower than the rate of rise of $[Ca^{2+}]_i$ measured with fura-2. The magnitude of sustained contraction is determined by the sustained $[Ca^{2+}]_i$. However, the sustained increase in $[Ca^{2+}]_i$ induced by ATP and its analogues, which is due to Ca^{2+} influx, was not coupled to contraction. Furthermore, ATP and its analogues did not increase MLC phosphorylation during a sustained increase in $[Ca^{2+}]_i$. Since these stimulants do not seem to decrease the Ca^{2+} sensitivity of the contractile elements, these findings suggest the existence of a Ca^{2+} compartment that is not coupled to contraction. This "noncontractile" compartment, which does not contain MLCK or contractile proteins, may be segregated from the "contractile" compartment that contains contractile elements.

Detection of $[Ca^{2+}]_i$ by Aequorin

To measure $[Ca^{2+}]_i$ simultaneously with contraction, a photoprotein, aequorin [14], and the fluorescent Ca^{2+} indicators such as fura-2 and indo-1 [15] are widely used. However, the results obtained with these two types of Ca^{2+} indicators are not always consistent. It has been shown that the intensity of aequorin luminescence correlates with the 2.5 power of Ca^{2+} concentration [14], whereas the fluorescence of fura-2 analogues changes as a linear function of Ca^{2+} concentration [15]. Therefore, if the Ca^{2+} level in a small compartment of the cell becomes higher than the rest of the cell, the aequorin signal becomes higher than the fura-2 signal obtained from the same cell, and this may at least partly be responsible for the difference in Ca^{2+} signals obtained with these two types of Ca^{2+} indicators, as has been suggested [2].

If we assume the presence of a "noncontractile" Ca^{2+} compartment that is small in size but achieves high $[Ca^{2+}]_i$, the question arises whether fura-2 can detect this compartment. For simplicity, it is assumed that the volume of the "noncontractile" compartment is 0.1% of the total cytoplasm, the resting $[Ca^{2+}]_i$ in both of these compartments is 100 nM, the peak $[Ca^{2+}]_i$ in the "noncontractile" compartment is 100 000 nM, or 100 μM, and the peak $[Ca^{2+}]_i$ in the "contractile" compartment is 500 nM. Taking the fura-2 signal in resting muscle as 1, it increases to 3 when only the "noncontractile" compartment is filled, to 5 when only the "contractile" compartment is filled, and to 7 when both of these compartments are filled with Ca^{2+}. If aequorin is used as an indicator, the resting aequorin signal of 1 increases to 65 when only the "noncontractile" compartment is filled, to 5 when only the "contractile" compartment is filled, and to 65 when both of these compartments are filled. Thus, aequorin is a better indicator for the localized high-Ca^{2+} concentration although fura-2 can also detect it. This unique property of aequorin is suitable for the detection of a high-Ca^{2+} compartment in the cell.

Differences Between the Aequorin Signal
and the Fura-2 Signal

In the ferret portal vein, NE induced a sustained increase in the Ca^{2+} signal measured with a fura-2 analogue, fura-PE3, and sustained contraction. Repeated applications of NE induced reproducible contractions and fura-PE3 signals [16]. High K^+ also induced a sustained increase in the fura-PE3 signal followed by contraction. Repeated applications of high K^+ induced similar changes in both fura-PE3 signal and contraction.

Figure 8 shows the effects of repeated applications of NE on contraction and the aequorin signal. The aequorin signal due to NE is composed of an initial large and transient increase followed by a small sustained increase. In contrast, high K^+ induced a relatively sustained increase in the aequorin signal that is smaller than the transient signal but greater than the sustained signal induced by NE. It was also found that the transient increase in aequorin signal in response to the second application of NE was only 26%, and the third aequorin signal was 20% of the first signal. In contrast, the second application of NE induced a contraction that was slightly greater than that induced by the first application. The small sustained increase in aequorin signal did not change with repeated applications of NE. After a 13-h resting period, the transient aequorin signal in response to NE recovered. However, the transient aequorin signal did not recover after a 3-h resting period (data not shown).

Similarly, the aequorin signal due to the second application of high K^+ was 56% of the first signal, and repeated stimulation did not induce a further decrease. Again, the contraction induced by the second application of high K^+ was greater than that induced by the first application. After a 13-h resting period, the aequorin signal in response to high K^+ recovered almost completely.

Since contraction, the fura-2 signal, and the sustained aequorin signal did not decline with repeated stimulation, the decrease in transient aequorin signal does not reflect reduced activation. One possible explanation is that the signal declines because of the decrease in active aequorin molecules. Aequorin is consumed by binding to Ca^{2+} [14], which suggests that NE induced a large increase in Ca^{2+} in a small cytosolic compartment, that aequorin in this compartment was rapidly consumed during the first application of NE, and that the increase in Ca^{2+} in this compartment induced by the second application of NE was not detectable by aequorin. Because aequorin is not

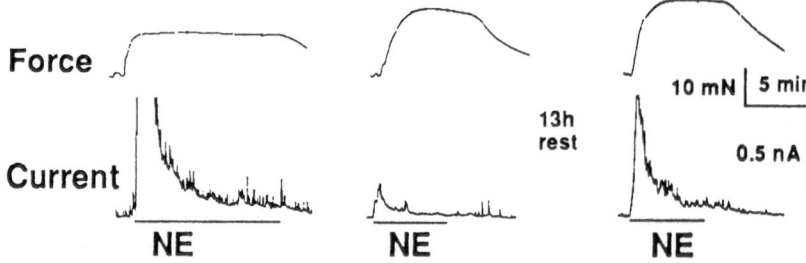

FIG. 8. Effects of repeated applications of 10μM NE on the aequorin signal (as indicated by current) and contraction in the ferret portal vein. NE was added five times and only the first and the fifth signals are shown. After the fifth stimulation, the muscle was unstimulated for a 13-h rest period and then stimulants were applied again

synthesized in the cell in our in vitro system [17], recovery of the aequorin signal may have resulted from the diffusion of aequorin from the area surrounding this compartment. The complete recovery of the aequorin signal took much longer than 3 h, suggesting that this compartment is isolated from the surrounding area by a diffusion barrier. Such a diffusion barrier may also help to keep a high Ca^{2+} concentration in this compartment.

These results also suggest that the NE-induced transient aequorin signal represents the Ca^{2+} compartment that is not directly coupled to smooth muscle contraction (the "noncontractile" Ca^{2+} compartment). The transient aequorin signal may be due to a large increase in Ca^{2+} in the small "noncontractile" compartment. In contrast, the sustained increase in the aequorin signal and the large portion of fura-2 signal may represent the "contractile" Ca^{2+} compartment, as suggested previously [2].

Although high K^+ induced a relatively sustained increase in the aequorin signal, the signal due to the second application of high K^+ was smaller than that induced by the first application. It was also observed that the aequorin signal recovered after a long resting period. These results suggest that high K^+ increases Ca^{2+} in both the "contractile" and "noncontractile" compartments. Since NE and high K^+ showed a cross-tachyphylactic effect on the aequorin signal, these two stimulants may share the ability to increase Ca^{2+} in the same "noncontractile" compartment.

Distribution of Ca^{2+} Indicators

There is evidence that fura-2 and aequorin are distributed unevenly in the cytoplasm. Fura-2 may be accumulated in organelles such as the SR and mitochondria and represent $[Ca^{2+}]_i$ in these compartments [18]. However, the release of SR Ca^{2+} increased rather than decreased the fura-2 signal. In addition, mitochondrial inhibitors such as KCN and hypoxia (that may decrease mitochondrial Ca^{2+}) did not decrease but rather increased $[Ca^{2+}]_i$ (unpublished observation). These results indicate that the fura-2 signal reflects neither the SR Ca^{2+} nor the mitochondrial Ca^{2+}. Even if the distribution of the indicators is not completely homogeneous, the existence of "contractile" and "noncontractile" compartments cannot be denied. Furthermore, the "noncontractile" compartment does not represent Ca^{2+} in the SR or mitochondria. However, the relative magnitude of these compartments, estimated by these indicators, could be affected by the inhomogeneity in distribution of the indicators.

Other Evidence for Ca^{2+} Compartments

Recently, it has been suggested that in smooth muscle cells there is a high-Ca^{2+} compartment in restricted diffusion spaces between the plasma membrane and intracellular organelles [19–22]. Van Breemen et al. [20] proposed that the superficial SR is able to take up entering Ca^{2+} (via the superficial buffer barrier), to amplify the Ca^{2+} signal by Ca^{2+}-induced Ca^{2+} release, and to unload Ca^{2+} to the extracellular space. They also discovered the restricted subplasmalemmal space that is separated from myoplasm. It has also been suggested that there is a Ca^{2+} compartment in cardiac cells located at the inner sarcolemmal leaflet anionic phospholipid that maintains a high concentration of Ca^{2+} for a short period of time [23].

Measuring $[Ca^{2+}]_i$ using aequorin, it has been shown that isoproterenol and forskolin increase the aequorin signal and simultaneously induce relaxation [24,25].

Measuring $[Ca^{2+}]_i$ with fura-2-2, on the other hand, these relaxants did not increase, but rather decreased $[Ca^{2+}]_i$ [26–28]. From these results, it has been proposed that the increase in cyclic adenosine monophosphate (cAMP) may open the Ca^{2+} channel, induce a localized increase in $[Ca^{2+}]_i$, activate the K^+ channel, hyperpolarize the membrane, inhibit the voltage-dependent Ca channel, decrease contractile $[Ca^{2+}]_i$, and inhibit contraction [2]. This possibility was supported by the findings that, in strongly depolarized smooth muscle in which the K^+ channel opening does not induce a hyperpolarization, isoproterenol and forskolin induced a slight increase in $[Ca^{2+}]_i$ measured with fura-2 (our unpublished observation).

Electrophysiological studies have suggested that Ca^{2+} influx activates Ca^{2+} release from the SR by the Ca^{2+}-induced Ca^{2+} release mechanism, and that the increase in $[Ca^{2+}]_i$ activates K^+ channels [29,30]. Interestingly, the time course of activation of the K^+ channel is much faster than that for the peak fura-2 signal [31; Y. Imaizumi, personal communication, 1995]. In addition, an activator of SR Ca^{2+} release, 9-methyl 7-bromoeudistomin D, activated the K^+ channel without inducing contraction [32]. These results support the existence of a "contractile" and "noncontractile" Ca^{2+} compartment and that Ca^{2+} in the "noncontractile" compartment regulates K^+ channel activity.

Ca²⁺ Movements and Ca²⁺ Compartments

Since NE releases Ca^{2+} from the SR, the transient aequorin signal (representing an increase in "noncontractile" Ca^{2+}) may be due to Ca^{2+} release. In a Ca^{2+}-free solution, NE induced a transient increase in aequorin signal that was much smaller than that obtained in the presence of external Ca^{2+}. This change was followed by a small transient contraction. After repriming by incubation with a solution containing Ca^{2+}, the muscle strip was incubated with Ca^{2+}-free solution and NE was applied again. The second application of NE induced a slightly (but not statistically significant) smaller aequorin signal although the third application induced a smaller transient signal than the first signal. In contrast, the second and third applications of NE induced that were contractions almost similar to that induced by the first stimulation. These results suggest that NE releases Ca^{2+} from its storage site and supplies Ca^{2+} to the "contractile" compartment. Ca^{2+} may also be supplied to the "noncontractile" compartment although its concentration is not high enough to consume aequorin rapidly.

After the addition of Ca^{2+} to the medium, application of NE induced a large transient increase in aequorin signal, although the second application induced only a small increase. These results suggest that the NE-induced large transient increase in aequorin signal observed in the presence of external Ca^{2+} is mainly due to Ca^{2+} influx and only partly due to Ca^{2+} release. Since not only high K^+ but also NE opens the voltage-dependent Ca^{2+} channel in vascular smooth muscle cells [4,5], the increase in Ca^{2+} in the "noncontractile" compartment may be due to Ca^{2+} influx through the voltage-dependent Ca^{2+} channel. NE-induced Ca^{2+} release and activation of the verapamil-insensitive Ca^{2+} entry [5] may also supply Ca^{2+} not only to the "contractile" compartment but also to the "noncontractile" compartment. Since ATP activates the verapamil-insensitive Ca^{2+} entry that is not coupled to contraction [9], this pathway may supply Ca^{2+} mainly to the "noncontractile" compartment.

In the rat aorta, in contrast, NE induced a large increase in $[Ca^{2+}]_i$ in Ca^{2+}-free solution. This difference may represent the difference in functional development of the SR between these tissues.

SR and the Ca^{2+} Compartment

To determine the relationship between the SR and the "noncontractile" Ca^{2+} compartment, the effects of the SR Ca^{2+} pump inhibitor, cyclopiazonic acid (CPA), and an inhibitor of Ca^{2+}-induced Ca^{2+} release, ryanodine, were examined [33]. In Ca^{2+}-free solution, high K^+ was ineffective. In contrast, NE induced a transient aequorin signal and a small contraction, both of which were strongly inhibited by CPA or ryanodine, suggesting that SR Ca^{2+} release is responsible for these changes.

In the presence of external Ca^{2+}, however, unexpected results were obtained. CPA enhanced the aequorin signal induced by NE and high K^+ without changing the contraction. On the other hand, ryanodine changed neither the aequorin signal nor contraction. Combined application of CPA and ryanodine again enhanced only the aequorin signal without changing contraction.

These results indicate that (1) SR Ca^{2+} release contributes only to the initial transient contraction induced by NE but not to the sustained contraction induced by NE or high K^+; (2) SR Ca^{2+} uptake does not contribute to decreased "contractile" Ca^{2+} and, therefore, contraction; (3) SR Ca^{2+} uptake decreases "noncontractile" Ca^{2+}; and (4) the "noncontractile" Ca^{2+} component is located adjacent to the SR Ca^{2+} pump.

Conclusions

From these results, we conclude that there are two Ca^{2+} compartments in vascular smooth muscle cytoplasm (Fig. 9). The first is the "contractile" compartment. Ca^{2+} in this compartment regulates cytoplasmic Ca^{2+}-dependent mechanisms such as MLCK (or contraction) and other enzymes. Agonists increase the Ca^{2+} concentration in this compartment by both Ca^{2+} influx and Ca^{2+} release, whereas high K^+ supplies Ca^{2+} solely by Ca^{2+} influx. Ca^{2+} in this compartment increases to a level which is not as high, so that the aequorin in this compartment is consumed only slowly. Most of the fura-2 signal represents Ca^{2+} in this compartment.

The second compartment is the "noncontractile" compartment. This compartment may be located in close vicinity to both the plasma membrane and the SR, which is segregated from the other cytoplasmic region ("contractile" compartment) by a diffusion barrier. This barrier is so tight that the aequorin molecules diffuse only slowly between these two compartments. Ca^{2+} in this compartment increases so strongly that the aequorin in this compartment is rapidly consumed. This compartment is detected more sensitively by aequorin than by fura-2, possibly because it is very small. Agonists may increase the Ca^{2+} level in this compartment mainly by Ca^{2+} influx and partly by Ca^{2+} release, whereas high K^+ increases Ca^{2+} exclusively by Ca^{2+} influx. Ca^{2+} in this compartment is not able to activate the contractile elements because this compartment does not contain contractile elements but rather regulates membrane Ca^{2+}-dependent mechanisms such as ion channels, ion pumps, and enzymes. Ca^{2+} in this compartment is taken up by the SR.

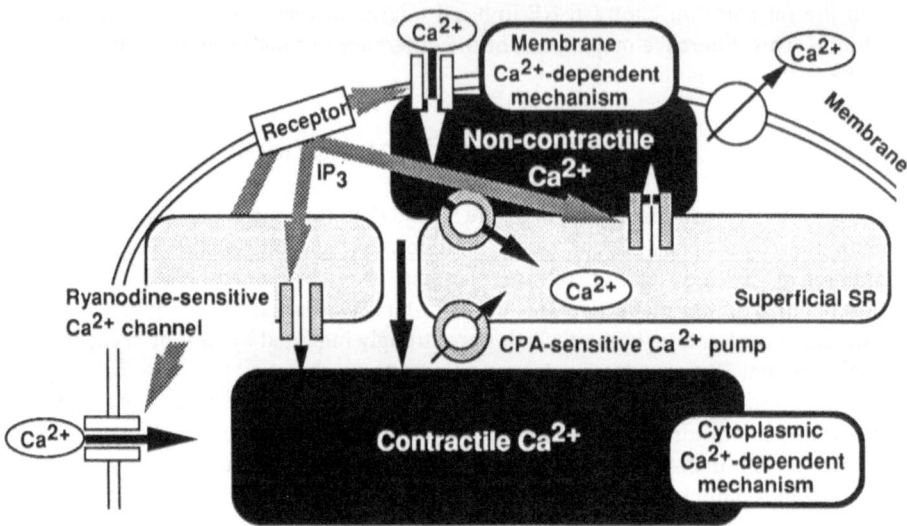

FIG. 9. Model of two Ca compartments in vascular smooth muscle. *SR*, sarcoplasmic reticulum

We also speculate that there may be a special coupling between the receptor and the SR so that stimulation of one type of receptor releases Ca^{2+} to increase "noncontractile" Ca^{2+}, whereas stimulation of another type of receptor releases Ca^{2+} to increase both "contractile" and "noncontractile" Ca^{2+}. There may be similar coupling between receptor and plasma membrane Ca^{2+} channels so that stimulation of ATP receptor opens the Ca^{2+} channel (or Ca^{2+}-permeable non-selective cation channel) that selectively fills the "noncontractile" compartment. Thus, the Ca^{2+} concentrations in these two compartments may be regulated independently.

Dissociation of $[Ca^{2+}]_i$ from contraction may thus be explained by the existence of two Ca^{2+} compartments. Additionally, some stimulants such as caffeine also decrease the Ca^{2+} sensitivity of the contractile elements to dissociate a sustained increase in $[Ca^{2+}]_i$ from contraction.

Acknowledgments. We are grateful to Dr. Yuji Imaizumi for his helpful suggestions. Original work for this study was supported by a Grant-in-Aid for Scientific Research from the Ministry of Education, Science and Culture of Japan.

References

1. Karaki H (1995) Regulation of smooth muscle: Phosphorylation-dependent and independent mechanisms. In: Kohama K, Saida K (eds) Smooth muscle contraction. Japan Sci Soc Press/Karger, Basel, pp 3–13
2. Karaki H (1989) Ca^{2+} localization and sensitivity in vascular smooth muscle. Trends Pharmacol Sci 10:322–325
3. Karaki H, Weiss GB (1988) Calcium release in smooth muscle. Life Sci 42:111–122
4. Sato K, Ozaki H, Karaki H (1988) Changes in cytosolic calcium level in vascular smooth muscle strips measured simultaneously with contraction using fluorescent calcium indicator fura 2. J Pharmacol Exp Ther 246:294–300

5. Karaki H, Sarto K, Ozaki H (1991) Different effects of verapamil on cytosolic Ca^{2+} and muscle tension in vascular smooth muscle. Jpn J Pharmacol 55:35–42

6. Hori M, Sato K, Sakata K, Ozaki H, Takano-Ohmuro H, Tsuchiya T, Sugi H, Kato I, Karaki H (1992) Receptor agonists induce myosin phosphorylation-dependent and phosphorylation-independent contractions in vascular smooth muscle. J Pharmacol Exp Ther 261:506–512

7. Sakata K, Ozaki H, Kwon SC, Karaki H (1989) Effects of endothelin on the mechanical activity and cytosolic calcium levels of various types of smooth muscle. Br J Pharmacol 98:483–492

8. Sato K, Hori M, Ozaki H, Takano-Ohmuro H, Tsuchiya T, Sugi H, Karaki H (1992) Myosin phosphorylation-independent contraction induced by phorbol ester in vascular smooth muscle. J Pharmacol Exp Ther 261:497–505

9. Kitajima S, Ozaki H, Karaki H (1993) The effects of ATP and $\alpha\beta$-methylene-ATP on cytosolic Ca^{2+} level and force in isolated rat aorta. Br J Pharmacol 110:263–268

10. Sato K, Ozaki H, Karaki H (1988) Multiple effects of caffeine on contraction and cytosolic free Ca^{2+} levels in vascular smooth muscle of rat aorta. Naunyn Schmiedebergs Arch Pharmacol 338:443–448

11. Ozaki H, Ohyama T, Sato K, Karaki H (1990) Ca^{2+}-dependent and independent mechanisms of sustained contraction in vascular smooth muscle of rat aorta. Jpn J Pharmacol 52:509–512

12. Ozaki H, Kasasi H, Hori M, Sato K, Ishihara H, Karaki H (1990) Direct inhibition of chicken gizzard smooth muscle contractile apparatus by caffeine. Naunyn Schmiedebergs Arch Pharmacol 341:262–267

13. Imaizumi Y, Muraki K, Takeda M, Watanabe M (1989) Measurments and simulation of noninactivating Ca current in smooth muscle cells. Am J Physiol 256:C880–C885

14. Blinks JR, Mattingly PH, Jewell BR, van Leeuwen M, Harrer GC, Allen DG (1978) Practical aspects of the use of aequorin as calcium indicator: assay, preparation, microinjection and interpretation of signals. Methods Enzymol 57:292–328

15. Grynkiewicz G, Poenie M, Tsien RY (1985) A new generation of Ca^{2+} indicators with greatly improved fluorescent properties. J Biol Chem 260:3444–3450

16. Abe F, Mitsui-Saito M, Karaki H, Endoh M (1995) Calcium compartments in vascular smooth muscle cells as detected by aequorin signal. Br J Pharmacol 116:3000–3004

17. Shimonura O, Johnson FH (1975) Regeneration of the photoprotein aequorin. Nature 256:236–238

18. Williams DA, Forgarty KE, Tsien RY, Fay SF (1985) Calcium gradients in single smooth muscle cells revealed by the digital imaging microscope using fura-2. Nature 318:558–561

19. Chen Q, van Breemen C (1993) The superficial buffer barrier in venous smooth muscle: sarcoplasmic reticulum refilling and unloading. Br J Pharmacol 109:336–343

20. Van Breemen C, Chen Q, Laher I (1995) Superficial buffer barrier function of smooth muscle sarcoplasmic reticulum. Trends Pharmacol Sci 16:98–105

21. Etter EF, Kuhn MA, Fay SF (1994) Detection of changes in near-membrane Ca^{2+} concentration using a novel membrane-associated Ca^{2+} indicator. J Biol Chem 269:10141–10149

22. Kargacin G (1994) Calcium signaling in restricted diffusion space. Biophys J 67:262–272

23. Langer GA (1994) Myocardial calcium compartmentation. Trends Cardiovasc Med 4:103–109

24. Morgan JP, Morgan KG (1984) Alterations of cytoplasmic ionized calcium levels in smooth muscle by vasodilators in the ferret. J Physiol (Lond) 357:539–551

25. Takuwa Y, Takuwa N, Rasmussen H (1988) The effects of isoproterenol on intracellular calcium concentration. J Biol Chem 263:762–768

26. Abe A, Karaki H (1989) Inhibitory effects of forskolin on cytosolic Ca^{2+} level and contraction in vascular smooth muscle. J Pharmacol Exp Ther 249:895–900

27. Abe A, Karaki H (1992) Mechanisms underlying the inhibitory effect of dibutyryl cyclic AMP in vascular smooth muscle. Eur J Pharmacol 211:305–311

28. Kwon SC, Ozaki H, Hori M, Karaki H (1993) Isoproterenol changes the relationship between cytosolic Ca^{2+} and contraction in guinea pig taenia caecum. Jpn J Pharmacol 61:57–64

29. Kitamura K, Sakai T, Kajioka S, Kuriyama H (1989) Activation of the Ca^{2+}-dependent K^+ channel by Ca^{2+} released from the sarcoplasmic reticulum of mammalian smooth muscle. Biomed Biochim Acta 48:S364–369

30. Suzuki M, Muraki K, Imaizumi Y, Watanabe M (1992) Cyclopiazonic acid, an inhibitor of the sarcoplasmic reticulum Ca^{2+} pump, reduces Ca^{2+}-dependent K^+ currents in guinea-pig smooth muscle cells. Br J Pharmacol 107:134–140

31. Sturek M, Kunda K, Hu Q (1992) Sarcoplasmic reticulum buffering of myoplasmic calcium in bovine coronary artery smooth muscle. J Physiol (Lond) 451:25–48

32. Imaizumi Y, Henmi H, Uyama Y, Watanabe M, Ohizumi Y (1993) Effects of 9-methyl-7-bromoeudistomin D (MBED), a powerful Ca^{2+} releaser, on smooth muscles of the guinea pig. Ann N Y Acad Sci 707:546–549

33. Abe F, Karaki H, Endoh M (1995) Possible role of SR in regulation of cytosolic Ca^{2+} in ferret portal vein. Jpn J Pharmacol 67[Suppl I]:175P

Nerve-Derived Nitric Oxide (NO) in the Regulation of Cerebrovascular Function

Noboru Toda and Tomio Okamura

Summary. We discovered nonadrenergic, noncholinergic vasodilator innervation in canine cerebral arteries 20 years ago by functional studies with nicotine and have continuously been studying to clarify the mechanism underlying neurogenic relaxation in primate and subprimate mammals. Cerebroarterial relaxations induced by nerve stimulation via electrical pulses and nicotine are endothelium-independent and are abolished by oxyhemoglobin, methylene blue, and nitric oxide (NO) synthase inhibitors of L-enantiomers; the inhibition caused by the enzyme inhibitors is reversed by L-arginine. Neurogenic relaxation is dependent on extracellular Ca^{2+} and calmodulin. NO_x is liberated during nerve stimulation, which also increases the content of cyclic guanosine monophosphate (cGMP) in the endothelium-denuded tissue. There are nerve fibers containing NO synthase-immunoreactivity or reduced nicotinamide adenine dinucleotide phosphate (NADPH) diaphorase in canine cerebral arteries. Damage of the pterygopalatine ganglion abolishes the response to nerve stimulation and perivascular innervation. We hypothesized that NO liberated from the vasodilator nerve acts as a neurotransmitter in cerebral arteries. NO derived from the nerve as well as the endothelium is expected to play a crucial role in the regulation of cerebrovascular tone and regional blood flow in the brain.

Key words: Vasodilator nerve—Nitric oxide (NO)—Neurotransmitter—NO synthase inhibitor—Cerebral arteries

Introduction

Autonomic efferent innervation in vasculature plays an important role in the regulation of vascular resistance, blood flow, and systemic blood pressure. Histological studies have demonstrated nerve fibers and bundles containing norepinephrine, acetylcholinesterase, ATP, and polypeptides such as substance P, calcitonin gene-related peptide (CGRP), and vasoactive intestinal polypeptide (VIP) in the walls of blood vessels [1-3]; however, the functional role of neurogenic mediators has not always been elucidated, except for norepinephrine from the adrenergic nerve. Vasoconstriction by adrenergic nerve stimulation is mediated via α_1 adrenoceptors

Department of Pharmacology, Shiga University of Medical Sciences, Seta, Ohtsu 520-21, Japan

activated by the amine in most vasculatures, whereas vasodilatation is caused via β_1 receptor subtypes in coronary arteries of experimental mammals [4]. Neurogenic vasoconstriction differs in regions of vasculature; arteries in the gastrointestinal tract, kidney, skin, skeletal muscle, for instance, respond to nerve stimulation with an evident constriction, whereas cerebral arteries constrict only slightly in response to adrenergic nerve stimulation. This is true in experimental animals in vivo and in isolated arteries. In particular, cerebral arteries isolated from dogs, Japanese monkeys, cows, and humans do not contract in response to perivascular nerve stimulation by electrical pulses and nicotine [5] but relax when partially contracted by prostaglandin $F_{2\alpha}$ or serotonin [6–8]. The relaxation is not reduced by β-adrenoceptor antagonists. Therefore, adrenergic neural regulation of cerebral arterial tone is, if any thing, minimal.

In the present chapter, an attempt is made to review briefly the functional characteristics of vasodilator nerves innervating the canine cerebral artery, with special reference to nitric oxide (NO).

Mechanical Response

Nonadrenergic, noncholinergic vasodilator innervation was first discovered in canine cerebral arteries in response to nicotine [6]. Endogenous substances that relax isolated cerebral arteries include ATP, substance P, VIP, and CGRP. There are networks of nerve fibers containing these substances in the vascular wall. Therefore, attention was directed to these substances, which may act as neurotransmitters in the vasodilator nerve. Our studies have proved that aminophylline in doses sufficient to suppress ATP-induced relaxation does not reduce neurally induced relaxation [8], and that endothelium denudation abolished the substance P-induced relaxation, whereas relaxations caused by nerve stimulation are not influenced [9]. The possible involvement of ATP and substance P in the response is thus excluded. Relaxations caused by VIP [8] and CGRP [10] are easily diminished by repeated applications. Neurally induced relaxations do not differ in cerebral arterial strips under control conditions and in those made unresponsive to these peptides (Fig. 1) [11], suggesting that VIP and CGRP can also be ruled out from neurotransmitter candidates. Similar results were also obtained in monkey and bovine cerebral arteries. However, in feline cerebral arteries, relaxations induced by nicotine were partially reduced when tachyphylaxis to CGRP developed. CGRP may participate partially in the relaxation induced by nerve stimulation. Saito et al. [12] also reported the involvement of CGRP in the same mammals; however, they did not perceive other mechanisms, such as NO, underlying the relaxation.

Vasodilatation of canine cerebral arteries elicited by transmural electrical stimulation (Fig. 2, upper tracing) or nicotine (Fig. 3) is abolished by treatment with NO synthase inhibitors, such as N^G-monomethyl-L-arginine (L-NMMA) and N^G-nitro-L-arginine (L-NA), but the D-enantiomers are without effect [9,10,13–15]. The inhibitory effect is reversed by L-, but not D-, arginine. L-Arginine applied to control media does not potentiate the response to nerve stimulation; however, the effect of NO synthase inhibitors is prevented by treatment with high concentrations of L-arginine (Fig. 2, lower tracing). Oxyhemoglobin and methylene blue also abolish neurogenic relaxation [16,17], in addition to the response to exogenously applied NO. Endothelium denudation does not influence the response to nerve stimulation.

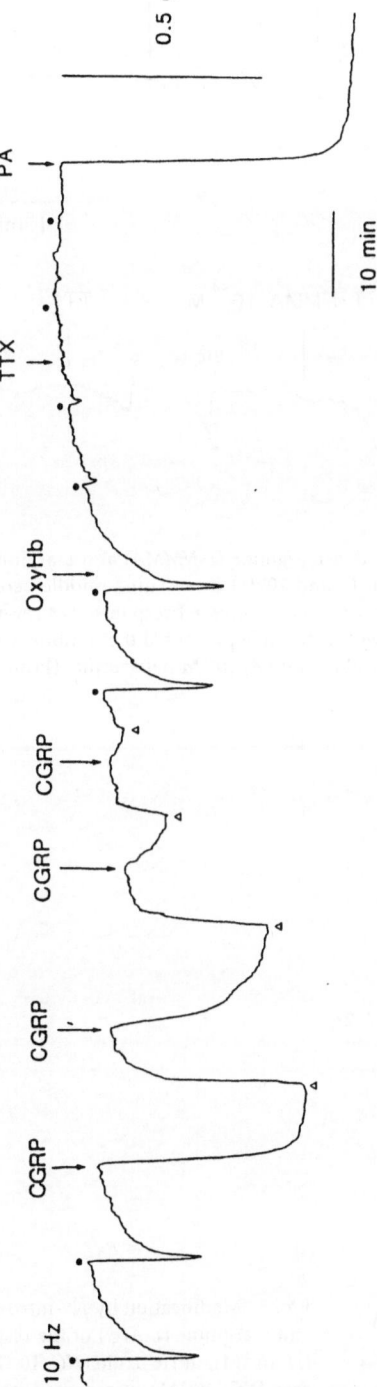

FIG. 1. Comparisons of the response to transmural electrical stimulation (10 Hz for 20 s) under control conditions and after development of tachyphylaxis to calcitonin gene-related peptide (*CGRP*) (10^{-8} M $\times$ 4) in a bovine basilar arterial strip partially contracted by prostaglandin $F_{2\alpha}$. The response was not reduced in the strip made almost unresponsive to CGRP but was markedly suppressed by oxyhemoglobin (*OxyHb*, 1.6×10^{-6} M) and abolished by tetrodotoxin (*TTX*, 3×10^{-7} M). *PA*, 10^{-4} M papaverine, which produces maximal relaxation. (From [11] with permission)

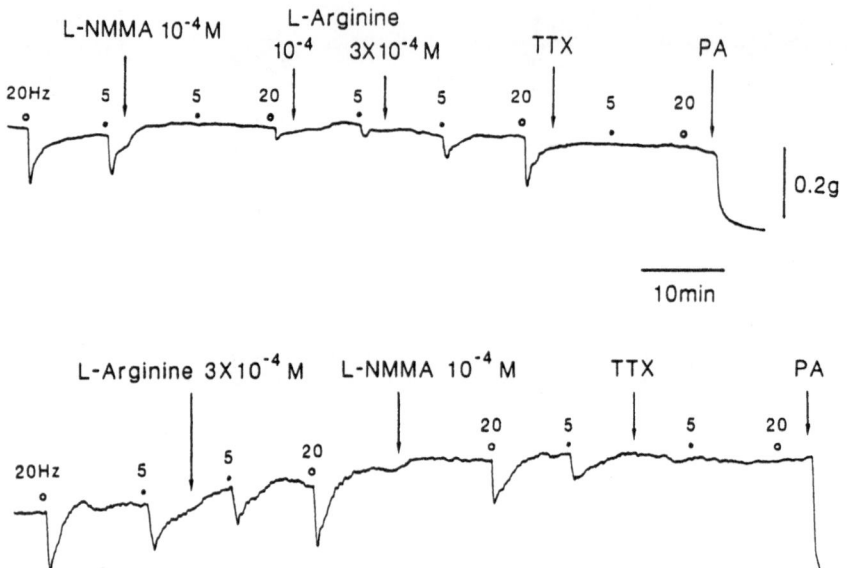

FIG. 2. Modification by N^G-monomethyl-L-arginine (L-NMMA) and L-arginine of the response to transmural electrical stimulation (5 and 20 Hz) in a canine middle cerebral arterial strip partially contracted by prostaglandin $F_{2\alpha}$. The depressed response was reversed by L-arginine (*upper tracing*), and pretreatment with L-arginine prevented the inhibitory effect of L-NMMA (*lower tracing*). TTX, 3×10^{-7} M tetrodotoxin; PA, 10^{-4} M papaverine. (From [14] with permission)

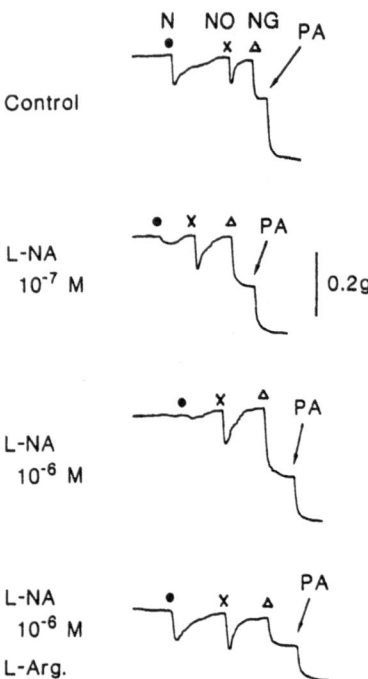

FIG. 3. Modification by N^G-nitro-L-arginine (L-NA) and L-arginine (L-Arg.) of the responses to nicotine (N, 10^{-4} M), nitric oxide (NO, 10^{-7} M), and nitroglycerin (NG, 10^{-8} M) in a canine basilar arterial strip partially contracted by prostaglandin $F_{2\alpha}$. L-NA suppressed only the response to nicotine in a dose-related manner. PA, 10^{-4} M papaverine

Release of NO_x and Content of cGMP

In superfused cerebral arterial strips denuded of the endothelium, the content of NO_x in the superfusate was colorimetrically measured. As compared with the value under control conditions, electrical or chemical stimulation of perivascular nerves markedly increased the NO_x content. Treatment with tetrodotoxin (for electrical stimulation) or hexamethonium (for nicotine) abolished the effects of nerve stimulation [14]. The results with nicotine are summarized in Fig. 4, left. On the other hand, the content of cyclic guanosine monophosphate (cGMP) in deendothelialized tissues increased in response to transmural electrical stimulation and nicotine (Fig. 4, right), and this effect was abolished by treatment with tetrodotoxin and hexamethonium, respectively [9,14]. These findings suggest that NO released during nerve stimulation activates guanylate cyclase and increases the synthesis of cGMP. The fact that the response to nerve stimulation is abolished by methylene blue, a soluble guanylate cyclase inhibitor, support this hypothesis.

Histological Study

Histochemical study has demonstrated the presence of perivascular nerve fibers and bundles containing NO synthase immunoreactivity and reduced nicotinamide adenine dinucleotide phosphate (NADPH) diaphorase in rat [18], canine [19], bovine (unpublished data), monkey [20], and human cerebral arteries [21]. The results in a section of the canine middle cerebral artery are shown in Fig. 5. It has been reported that NO synthase is identical to NADPH diaphorase in neurons [22]. These nerves are

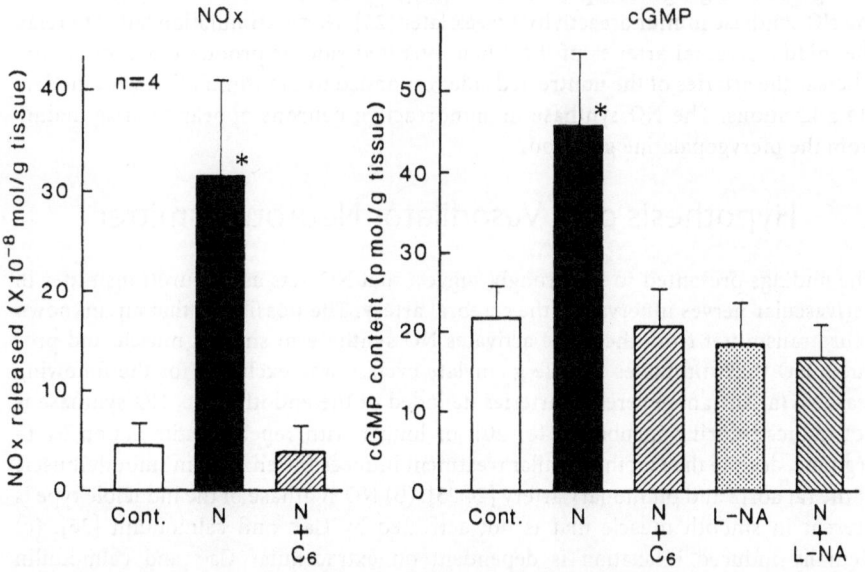

FIG. 4. NO_x content in bathing media containing endothelium-denuded canine cerebral arterial strips ($n = 6$) before (*Cont.*) and after treatment with nicotine (N, 10^{-4} M) and nicotine plus hexamethonium (C_6, 10^{-5} M) (*left*), and cyclic guanosine monophosphate (*cGMP*) content in the strips before and after treatment (*right*) [9,14]. L-*NA*, N^G-nitro-L-arginine (10^{-5} M)

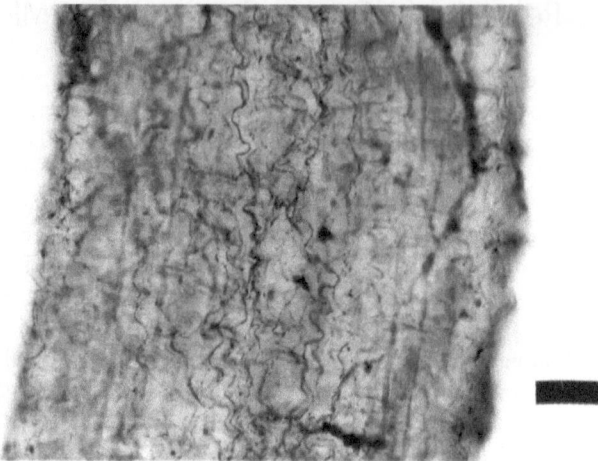

FIG. 5. Perivascular nerve fibers and bundles containing NO synthase immunoreactivity in a whole-mount preparation of the canine middle cerebral artery. Bar = 50 μm

expected to have the ability to synthesize and liberate NO. NO synthase coexists with VIP and cholinesterase in the pterygopalatine and otic ganglia in rats which supply neurons to cerebral arteries.

Denervation Study

In anesthetized dogs, injections of absolute ethanol in the vicinity of the pterygopalatine ganglion degenerated the ganglion and perivascular nerves containing NO synthase immunoreactivity 1 week later [23]. Nerve stimulation failed to relax the middle cerebral arteries of the ethanol-treated side or produced a contraction, whereas the arteries of the nontreated side responded to the stimulation with moderate relaxations. The NO synthase-immunoreactive neurons appear to arise mainly from the pterygopalatine ganglion.

Hypothesis on a Vasodilator Neurotransmitter

The findings presented so far strongly suggest that NO acts as a neurotransmitter in perivascular nerves innervating the cerebral artery. The possibility that an unknown neurotransmitter from the nerve activates NO synthase in smooth muscle and produces NO that stimulates soluble guanylate cyclase was excluded for the following reasons: (a) In canine cerebral arteries denuded of the endothelium, NO synthase is not induced during incubation for 20h or longer with repeated stimulation by L-arginine, despite the fact that similar treatment induces the enzyme in smooth muscle of the rat aorta and pulmonary artery [24,25]. (b) NO synthase of the inducible type is present in smooth muscle that is not activated by Ca^{2+} and calmodulin [26]. (c) Neurally induced relaxation is dependent on extracellular Ca^{2+} and calmodulin [27,28]. (d) The presence of NO synthase has been histochemically demonstrated in perivascular nerve and endothelium but not in smooth muscle [19].

Our hypothesis on the mechanism underlying neurogenic vasodilatation in cere-

FIG. 6. Hypothetical scheme of nitroxidergic innervation in canine cerebral arteries. *L-Arg.*, L-arginine; *L-Citru.*, L-citrulline; *RNO*, NO analog that liberates NO intracellularly

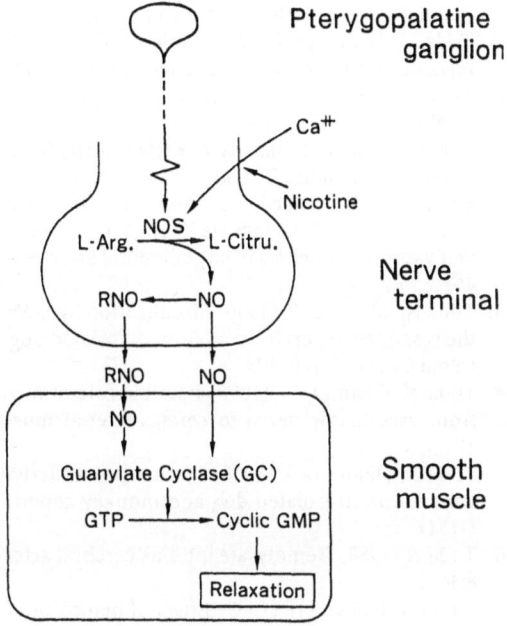

bral arteries is summarized in Fig. 6. NO synthase in nerve terminals is activated by Ca^{2+} introduced from external fluid by electrical or chemical stimulation. NO synthesized from L-arginine by the catalysis of this enzyme is liberated from the nerve as a neurotransmitter and activates soluble guanylate cyclase in smooth muscle. The perivascular nerve originates mainly from the pterygopalatine ganglion. In addition to canine cerebral arteries introduced in this chapter, human, Japanese monkey, bovine, pig, and feline cerebral arteries may possibly be innervated by NO-mediated (nitroxidergic; [29]) nerves. In these primate and subprimate mammals, NO derived from both the nerve and the endothelium appear to play important roles in the regulation of cerebral arterial tone and vascular resistance, thus controlling blood supply to vital brain areas.

References

1. Kobayashi S, Tsukahara S, Sugita K, Nagata T (1981) Adrenergic and cholinergic innervation of rat cerebral arteries. Histochemistry 70:129–138
2. Owman C (1990) Peptidergic vasodilator nerves in the peripheral circulation and in the vascular beds of the heart and brain. Blood Vessels 27:73–93
3. Suzuki N, Hardebo JE, Kahrstron J, Owman C (1990) Neuropeptide Y co-exists with vasoactive intestinal polypeptide and acetylcholine in parasympathetic cerebrovascular nerves originating in the sphenopalatine, otic and internal carotid ganglia of the rat. Neuroscience 36:507–519
4. Toda N, Okamura T (1990) Beta adrenoceptor subtype in isolated human, monkey and dog epicardial coronary arteries. J Pharmacol Exp Ther 253:518–524
5. Toda N, Fujita Y (1937) Responsiveness of isolated cerebral and peripheral arteries to serotonin, norepinephrine, and transmural electrical stimulation. Circ Res 33:98–104
6. Toda N (1975) Nicotine-induced relaxation in isolated canine cerebral arteries. J Pharmacol Exp Ther 193:376–384
7. Toda N (1981) Non-adrenergic, non-cholinergic innervation in monkey and human cerebral arteries. Br J Pharmacol 72:281–283
8. Toda N (1982) Relaxant responses to transmural stimulation and nicotine of dog and

monkey cerebral arteries. Am J Physiol 243:H145–H153

9. Toda N, Okamura T (1991) Role of nitric oxide in neurally induced cerebroarterial relaxation. J Pharmacol Exp Ther 258:1027–1032

10. Toda N, Okamura T (1991) Suppression by N^G-monomethyl-L-arginine of cerebroarterial response to nonadrenergic, noncholinergic vasodilator nerve stimulation. J Cardiovasc Pharmacol 17[Suppl III]:S234–S237

11. Ayajiki K, Okamura T, Toda N (1993) Nitric oxide mediates, and acetylcholine modulates, neurally induced relaxation of bovine cerebral arteries. Neuroscience 54:819–825

12. Saito A, Masaki T, Uchiyama Y, Lee TJF, Goto K (1989) Calcitonin gene-related peptide and vasodilator nerves in large cerebral arteries of cats. J Pharmacol Exp Ther 248:455–462

13. Toda N, Okamura T (1990) Modification by L-N^G-monomethyl arginine (L-NMMA) of the response to nerve stimulation in isolated dog mesenteric and cerebral arteries. Jpn J Pharmacol 52:170–173

14. Toda N, Okamura T (1990) Possible role of nitric oxide in transmitting information from vasodilator nerve to cerebroarterial muscle. Biochem Biophys Res Commun 170:308–313

15. Toda N, Okamura T (1990) Mechanism underlying the response to vasodilator nerve stimulation in isolated dog and monkey cerebral arteries. Am J Physiol 259:H1511–H1517

16. Toda N (1988) Hemolysate inhibits cerebral artery relaxation. J Cereb Blood Flow Met 8:46–53

17. Linnik MD, Lee TJF (1989) Effect of hemogloin on neurogenic responses and cholinergic parameters in porcine cerebral arteries. J Cereb Blood Flow Met 9:219–225

18. Bredt DS, Hwang PM, Snyder SH (1990) Localization of nitric oxide synthase indicating a neural role for nitric oxide. Nature 347:768–770

19. Yoshida K, Okamura T, Kimura H, Bredt DS, Snyder SH, Toda N (1993) Nitric oxide synthase-immunoreactive nerve fibers in dog cerebral and peripheral arteries. Brain Res 629:67–72

20. Yoshida K, Okamura T, Toda N (1994) Histological and functional studies on the nitroxidergic nerve innervating monkey cerebral, mesenteric and temporal arteries. Jpn J Pharmacol 65:351–359

21. Nozaki K, Moskowitz MA, Maynard KI, Koketsu N, Dawson TM, Bredt DS, Snyder SH (1993) Possible origins and distribution of immunoreactive nitric oxide synthase-containing nerve fibers in cerebral arteries. J Cereb Blood Flow Met 13:70–79

22. Dawson TM, Bredt DS, Fotuhi M, Hwang PM, Snyder SH (1991) Nitric oxide synthase and neuronal NADPH diaphorase are identical in brain and peripehral tissues. Proc Natl Acad Sci USA 88:7797–7801

23. Toda N, Ayajiki K, Yoshida K, Kimura H, Okamura T (1993) Impairment by damage of the pterygopalatine ganglion of nitroxidergic vasodilator nerve function in canine cerebral and retinal arteries. Circ Res 72:206–213

24. Wood KS, Buga GM, Byns RE, Ignarro LJ (1990) Vascular smooth muscle-derived relaxing factor (MDRF) and its close similarity to nitric oxide. Biochem Biophys Res Commun 170:80–88

25. Moritoki H, Ueda H, Yamamoto T, Hisayama T, Takeuchi S (1991) L-Arginine induces relaxation of rat aorta possibly through non-endothelial nitric oxide formation. Br J Pharmacol 102:841–846

26. Busse R, Mulsch A (1990) Induction of nitric oxide synthase by cytokines in vascular smooth muscle cells. FEBS Lett 275:87–90

27. Toda N, Okamura T (1992) Different susceptibility of vasodilator nerve, endothelium and smooth muscle functions to Ca^{++} antagonists in cerebral arteries. J Pharmacol Exp Ther 261:234–239

28. Okamura T, Toda N (1994) Inhibition by calmodulin antagonists of the neurogenic relaxation in cerebral arteries. Eur J Pharmacol 256:79–83

29. Toda N, Okamura T (1992) Regulation by nitroxidergic nerve of arterial tone. News Physiol Sci 7:148–152

Part 3

Mechanisms of Cardiac Regulation

Temporal Modulation of the Preferred Ca²⁺ Influx Pathway: A Novel Effect of β-Agonists on the Heart

MARTIN MORAD, JING FAN, and YAROSLAV SHUBA

Summary. The Na^+-Ca^{2+} exchanger and the Ca^{2+} channel are two major sarcolemmal Ca^{2+}-transporting proteins of cardiac myocytes. While the Ca^{2+} channel is effectively regulated by protein kinase A (PKA)-dependent phosphorylation, no enzymatic regulation of the exchanger protein has yet been identified. Here we report that isoproterenol regulates the Na^+-Ca^{2+} exchanger of the frog ventricular myocytes by activation of the β-receptor adenylate-cyclase cyclic adenosine monophosphate (cAMP)-dependent pathway. A β-blocker, propranalol, blocks the isoproterenol effect while forskolin, cAMP, and theophylline mimic the isoproterenol effect on $I_{Na\text{-}Ca}$ independently of $[Ca^{2+}]_i$, providing a molecular mechanism for the relaxant effect of the hormone. The regulation of the Ca^{2+} channel and the exchanger proteins by a common mechanism may provide for the simultaneous enhancement of Ca^{2+} current at the onset of the action potential followed by suppression of Ca^{2+} influx via the exchanger later in depolarization. Such a unique hormonally induced shift in the preferred pathways of Ca^{2+} transport may have evolved together with ultrastructural modification of the sarcoplasmic reticulum (SR) to accommodate the evolutionary and developmental needs of cellular Ca^{2+} metabolism.

Key words. Relaxant effect of β-adrenergics—Na^+-Ca^{2+} exchanger—Frog heart—Phosphorylation by PKA—Ca^{2+} transport in heart

Cellular Mechanisms Underlying the Relaxant Effect of Catecholamines

Adrenergic β-agonists are known to enhance the force of cardiac contraction and accelerate the rate of its relaxation. A number of interrelated molecular mechanisms appear to be responsible for these two distinct properties of catecholamines. For instance, while the increase in the force of contraction results from enhanced Ca^{2+} current and Ca^{2+} release [1–4], the phosphorylation of phospholamban and the subse-

Department of Pharmacology, Georgetown University School of Medicine, Washington, DC 20007, USA, and Mt. Desert Island Biological Laboratory, Salisbury Cove, ME 04672, USA

quent stimulation of the Ca²⁺ pump [5–7], in addition to decreased myofilament Ca²⁺ sensitivity [8–10], mediate the relaxant properties of β-agonists. Similarly, the finding the catecholamines suppress KCl-induced contractures in ventricular strips [11–13] is thought to be mediated by the catecholamine-induced stimulation of the sarcoplasmic reticulum (SR) Ca²⁺ pump under conditions where the sarcolemmal Ca²⁺ channels are fully inactivated following the first 30–60 s of exposure to 100 mM of KCl. Thus, in the mammalian heart the adrenaline-induced increase in intracellular Ca²⁺ during the twitch is handled by enhancement of Ca²⁺ reuptake by the SR, resulting in an increase in the fraction of Ca²⁺ recirculating to the release stores.

Quite similar to the mammalian myocardium, the frog heart also exhibits all the functional characteristics associated with the β-agonist response, i.e., an enhanced Ca²⁺ current producing an increase in the force of contraction, acceleration of the rate of relaxation, and suppression of KCl-induced contractures [13–16]. In light of recent reports suggesting the absence of both Ca-ATPase mRNA [17] and physiologically releasable Ca²⁺ stores [18–21] in the frog heart, the similarity in the β-agonist relaxant effects in mammalian and amphibian hearts would be somewhat surprising and unexpected if the relaxant response of the β-agonist were mediated solely by the cyclic adenosine monophosphate (cAMP)-dependent protein kinase A (PKA) phosphorylation of the phospholamban protein [5–7]. The possibility that the Na⁺-Ca²⁺ exchanger contributes significantly to the sequestration of Ca²⁺ in the frog heart was suggested from early findings that voltage-dependence of tension had a large sigmoid component inconsistent with voltage-dependence of I_{Ca} but consistent with that of the Na⁺-Ca²⁺ exchanger [19,20]. Further, the rate of relaxation of frog myocardium was markedly suppressed (from about 100 ms to 4.5 s) when Na⁺ was omitted from the extracellular solutions [16], and in such solutions, catecholamines failed to accelerate the rate of relaxation of contraction or suppress KCl-induced contractures [16]. These early findings suggest a possible involvement of the Na⁺-Ca²⁺ exchanger in mediating the β-agonist relaxant effect in the frog ventricular myocardium.

In this report, we have examined the possible effects of β-agonists on Ca²⁺ transport by the exchanger in frog ventricular myocytes. Our findings suggest that isoproterenol may inhibit Ca²⁺ transport by the exchanger by activating the adenylate cyclase-cAMP-dependent phosphorylation pathway, providing a molecular mechanism for catecholamine-induced suppression of KCl-induced contractures [13–16] and uncoupling of the duration of contraction from the action potential [13,15]. Thus, by simultaneously enhancing the Ca²⁺ current and suppressing the Na⁺-Ca²⁺ exchanger, β-agonists appear to shift the balance of Ca²⁺ transport from the exchanger to the Ca²⁺ channel during the plateau of the action potential. The large enhancement of I_{Ca} by isoproterenol results in rapid activation of contraction at the onset of the action potential but is followed by a rapid fall in tension in the later phases of the plateau where the exchanger is the dominant Ca²⁺ transporter. This subtle shift in Ca²⁺ transport mechanisms may provide the molecular mechanism by which hearts lacking well-developed SR can meet the cardiovascular challenges requiring a rapid rate of development of contraction and relaxation during the fight-or-flight response.

Method

Frog ventricular myocytes were enzymatically isolated [22] and whole-cell-clamped using 2–5 MΩ patch pipettes [23]. A Dagan 9000 patch clamp amplifier (Dagan, Minneapolis, MN, USA) was used to voltage-clamp the isolated myocytes. The data were collected, stored, and analyzed on a PC using pCLAMP 5.51 (Axon, CA, USA) and Origin (Microcal, MA, USA) software. The length of the myocyte and its shortening were monitored using a video monitor. The intracellular dialyzing solutions were designed to contain high K^+ (with tetraethylammonium (TEA) and Cs^+ as K^+ channel blockers) and 10 to 20 mM Na^+ to measure I_{Na-Ca} at physiological potentials. To block delayed outward rectifier K^+ channels, 10 mM intracellular TEA was included in the pipette dialyzing solutions. We avoided using complete replacement of intracellular K^+ with Cs^+ or TEA to prevent possible unexpected effects of these cations. The low-Ca^{2+} buffer internal solution contained (in mM): KCl 40, K-aspartate 60, TEA-Cl 10, NaCl 10 (or 20), Mg-ATP 5, hydroxyethylpiperazine ethanesulfonic acid (HEPES) 10, 1,2-bis (2-Aminophenoxylethane-N,N,N',N'-tetraacetic acid (BAPTA) 0.1, egtazic acid (EGTA) 0.2, pH 7.2. High-Ca^{2+} buffer solution had the same basic composition except that it was supplemented with 9 mM EGTA and 6.16 or 7.27 mM $CaCl_2$ to obtain a free Ca^{2+} concentration of 200 nM or 400 nM, respectively [24]. External Ringer's solution used to record the Na^+-Ca^{2+} exchanger current contained (in mM): NaCl 110, KCl 5.4, $CaCl_2$ 2, $MgCl_2$ 1, glucose 10, HEPES 10, pH 7.2. External solutions were supplemented with 10 μM nifedipine to block Ca^{2+} channels and 0.1 mM $BaCl_2$ and 5 mM CsCl to block inwardly rectifying K^+ channels. β-Agonists and substances affecting the adenylate cyclase/cAMP/PKA cascade were added to external solutions in appropriate concentrations. Ni^{2+} in concentrations of 3–5 mM was used in external solutions to block I_{Na-Ca}. Alternate switching between various external solutions was accomplished rapidly (<50 ms) using an electronically controlled multibarrel puffing system [25]. Myocytes dialyzed with high-Ca^{2+} buffer solutions failed to contract in response to depolarizing pulses while the low-buffered myocytes contracted regularly in response to Ca^{2+} influx via the Ca^{2+} channel and the Na^+-Ca^{2+} exchanger. Irrespective of the conditions used, we failed to identify a cAMP-dependent Cl^+ current [26–27] in frog ventricular myocytes.

Activation of Na^+-Ca^{2+} Exchanger Current

Two procedures were used to measure the exchanger current in frog ventricular myocytes. In one procedure, the inward and outward components of exchanger current were measured by a clamp pulse from −80 to +20 mV with variable durations, in a contracting ventricular myocyte in which I_K and I_{Ca} were blocked. As the duration of the clamp pulse was prolonged, the outward current decayed slowly and the tail currents accompanying the repolarization of membrane to −80 mV were enhanced. Both the slowly decaying outward current and the accompanying contractions as well as the repolarizing tail currents were blocked by 5 mM Ni^{2+}. Subtraction of current envelopes obtained in the presence and absence of Ni^{2+} revealed the exchanger component of the membrane current (Fig. 1A) [28,29].

Figure 1B illustrates the time course and magnitude of Ca^{2+} influx quantified from the envelope of I_{Na-Ca} (Fig. 1A). The traces of I_{Na-Ca} envelopes were digitally integrated to provide an estimate of the total charge transferred with time. Using 3Na:1Ca exchanger stoichiometry and length (220 μm) and diameter (8 μm) of a typical frog cardiomyocyte having an average membrane capacity of 55 pF, the total charge was then recalculated into the Ca^{2+} concentration. Depending on the magnitude of the I_{Na-Ca} elicited by depolarization, the threshold for myocyte shortening could be reached at various pulse durations. Generally, the longer depolarizations generated

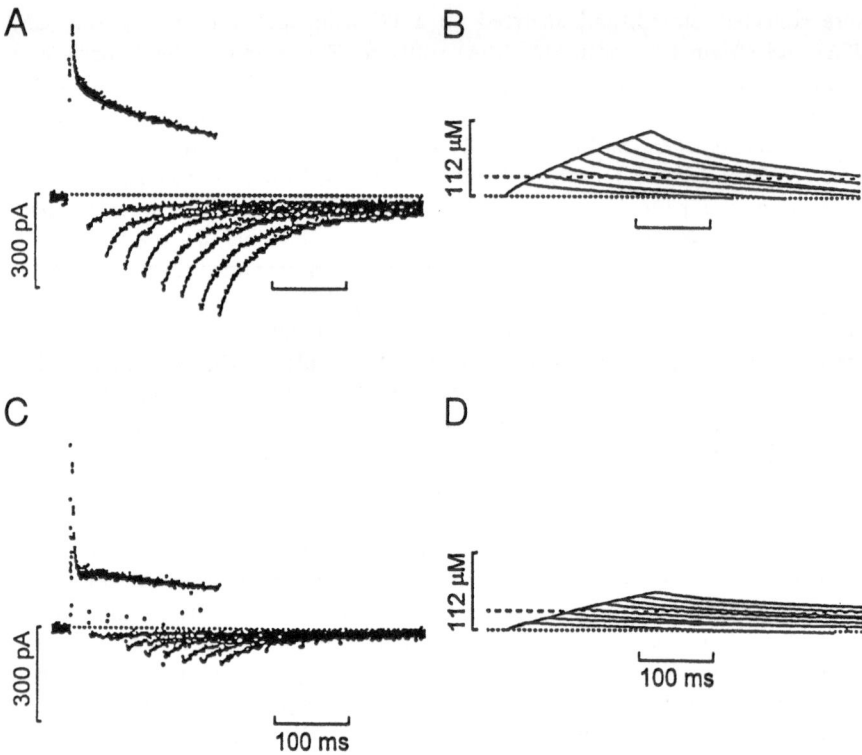

FIG. 1A–D. The effect of isoproterenol (ISO) on $I_{Na\text{-}Ca}$ in frog ventricular myocytes dialyzed with low-Ca^{2+}-buffer internal solution. **A,C** Superimposed traces of $I_{Na\text{-}Ca}$ in control (**A**) and in the presence of 5 µM ISO-containing solutions (**C**) obtained by subtraction of 5 mM Ni^{2+}-resistant component of current. Control external solution contained Ca^{2+}- and K$^+$-channel inhibitors (nifedipine and Ba^{2+}). Voltage-clamp pulses from −80 to +20 mV were applied in increasing duration from 25 to 200 ms in 25-ms increments. **B,D** Calculated time courses of hypothetical increase in [Ca^{2+}]$_i$ in control (**B**) and in the presence of 5 µM ISO (**D**). *Dashed line* indicates the threshold of video-monitored cell shortening. Note that while 50 ms depolarizing pulses were sufficient to produce cell shortening in constrol solutions, pulses in excess of 150 ms were required to raise [Ca^{2+}]$_i$ sufficiently to induce cell shortening in the presence of ISO (room temperature; cell capacity 59 pF; [Ca^{2+}]$_o$ = 2.0 mM; [Na$^+$]$_i$ = 20 mM). (Modified from [29a])

the stronger contractions. The dashed line of Fig. 1B represents the threshold of video-monitored cell shortening. Quantification of Ca^{2+} influx suggested that calcium concentrations in excess of 100 to 200 µM could be transported by the exchanger. Detectable myocyte shortening was observed with the influx of about 25–30 µM Ca^{2+}. The second procedure to measure $I_{Na\text{-}Ca}$ and its voltage-dependence was to employ a depolarizing pulse to potentials positive to +20 mV, activating $I_{Na\text{-}Ca}$ followed by ramp pulse to −120 mV (Fig. 2A). The magnitude and speed of the ramp pulse varied from cell to cell based on the extent of the activation of $I_{Na\text{-}Ca}$. Ni^{2+}-blockable current ($I_{Na\text{-}Ca}$) often showed a reversal potential (E_{rev}) around −27 ± 4.8 mV ($n = 5$) suggesting an E_{Ca} of +80.1 mV ([Ca]$_o$ = 2.0 mM) and providing for an effective [Ca]$_i$ of 4.3 µM following a 200-ms depolarizing pulse to +20 mV ([Na]$_i$ = 20 mM, [Na]$_o$ = 110 mM).

The density of the exchanger current (8.0 pA/pF at +20 mV) in frog ventricular myocyte often approximated the values obtained for basal I_{Ca} (5–8 pA/pF) [30], suggesting that, depending on membrane potential, the exchanger may generate equivalent Ca^{2+} influx to that produced by the Ca^{2+} channel. Considering the larger surface to volume ratio of frog versus mammalian ventricular myocytes and the lack of significant intracellular Ca^{2+} release pools in the frog ventricle [18–21], these findings suggest that the exchanger may contribute significantly to the elevation of cytosolic Ca^{2+} during the plateau phase of the frog ventricular action potential.

Modulation of Exchanger Activity by Catecholamines

Figure 1A,C compares the envelope $I_{Na\text{-}Ca}$ (Ni-subtracted currents) in the presence and absence of isoproterenol (ISO): 5 μM ISO suppressed both the outward and inward exchanger currents, and increased the duration of depolarizing pulse required for the threshold of contraction (Fig. 1C,D). Figure 2 illustrates the effect of 5 μM ISO on $I_{Na\text{-}Ca}$ in minimally Ca^{2+}-buffered, contracting ventricular myocytes. Rapid application of ISO slowly suppressed $I_{Na\text{-}Ca}$ by 40%–80% but did not alter its kinetics significantly (Fig. 2A,B). In the presence of isoproterenol, 5 mM Ni^{2+} rapidly and reversibly suppressed the residual exchanger current. The isoproterenol-induced inhibition of $I_{Na\text{-}Ca}$ was accompanied by a significant shift −19.6 ± 2.8 ($n = 5$) in the reversal potential of $I_{Na\text{-}Ca}$ toward more negative potentials (Fig. 2C), and a marked suppression of cell shortening (Fig. 1), suggesting a significant reduction of Ca^{2+} influx and $[Ca^{2+}]_i$.

The slow kinetics of suppression of $I_{Na\text{-}Ca}$ by isoproterenol is consistent with the activation of a second messenger signaling pathway. This effect was most likely mediated by the binding of the hormone to the β-receptor and the activation of the adenylate cyclase cAMP-dependent signaling pathway. Supportive data for this idea was obtained from the finding where: (1) β-blocker propranalol blocked the isoproterenol effect; (2) direct activation of adenylate cyclase by 10 μM forskolin, the application of 10–100 μM 8-Br-cAMP (a membrane-permeable cAMP analog), or theophylline [(1 mM), a phosphodiestrase inhibitor], mimicked the isoproterenol effects (i.e., suppressed $I_{Na\text{-}Ca}$ and cell shortening); (3) the effect of isoproterenol on $I_{Na\text{-}Ca}$ was attenuated by preexposure of myocytes to cAMP, while theophylline further potentiated the isoproterenol-suppressive effect; (4) inclusion of 2 mM guanosine diphosphate (GDP)-β-S in the pipette solution significantly attenuated but did not completely block the isoproterenol effect ($n = 5$); and (5) 1–10 μM okadaic acid (a phosphatase inhibitor) strongly suppressed $I_{Na\text{-}Ca}$ and further enhanced the isoproterenol effect when added together. These findings suggest that the isoproterenol effect on $I_{Na\text{-}Ca}$ is mediated primarily through the activation of the adenylate cyclase cAMP-dependent signaling pathway, resulting most likely from the phosphorylation of the exchanger protein.

The isoproterenol inhibition of $I_{Na\text{-}Ca}$ could be partly reversed by rapid elevation of $[Ca^{2+}]_o$ (Fig. 2A,B) ($n = 4$) or by depolarizing the membrane to more positive potentials. These experiments suggest that the inhibiting effect of isoproterenol is modulatory and reversible, since in the presence of isoproterenol using either more positive potentials or elevating the extracellular Ca^{2+} counteracted the inhibitory effects of the hormone on $I_{Na\text{-}Ca}$.

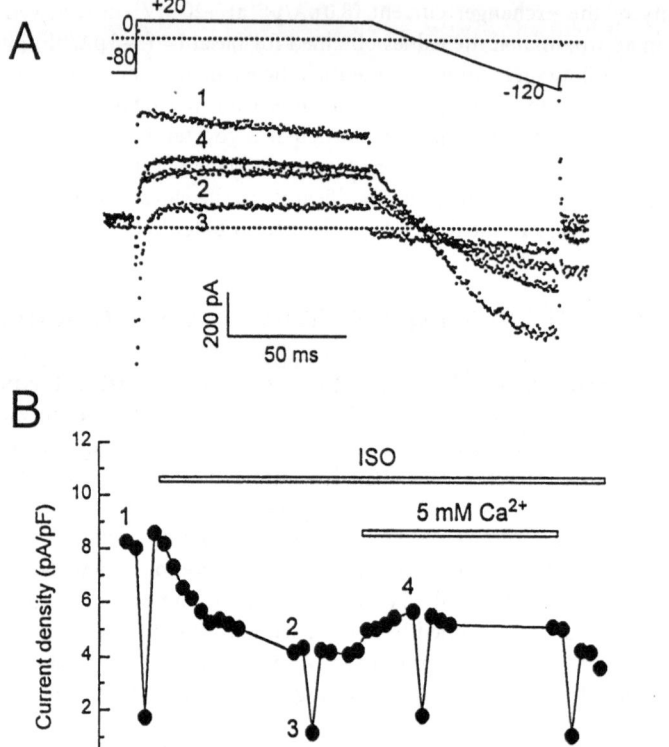

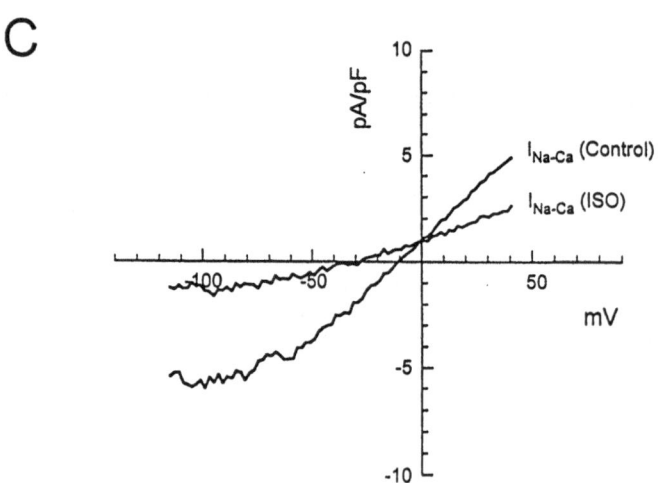

Discussion

Our results describe a novel property of β-agonists in frog ventricular myocytes and provide a possible molecular mechanism for previously observed intriguing findings in intact ventricular strips that β-agonists, while potentiating the phasic component of tension (twitch), suppress the KCl- or voltage clamp-induced maintained (tonic) component of tension [15,16]. Since activation of I_{Ca} produces the initial rapid influx of Ca^{2+} within 5–20 ms of depolarization, while the slower influx of Ca^{2+} via the Na^+-Ca^{2+} exchanger occurs during the later phase of the plateau, the simultaneous strong enhancement of I_{Ca} and suppression of I_{Na-Ca} during adrenergic stimulation may provide not only for the enhancement of rate of twitch but also for the later rapid fall of tension following the inactivation of I_{Ca}. Such differential, temporal modulation of Ca^{2+} influx may have both developmental and evolutionary significance for hormonal regulation of cellular Ca^{2+} metabolism. It should be pointed out that in the neonatal mammalian heart, where SR is poorly developed and the E-C coupling processes are similar to those in the amphibian heart [21,31,32], β-agonists similarly enhance the twitch and suppress KCl-induced contractures [11,12] consistent with their enhancement of I_{Ca} and suppression of I_{Na-Ca} described above.

Although there are no reports in support of the modulation of adult mammalian cardiac exchanger by phosphorylation, there are reports on ATP-dependent enhancement of Na^+-Ca^{2+} exchanger in the squid giant axon through kinase phosphorylation [37] as well as possible regulatory effects of ATP on the adult mammalian cardiac exchanger mediated via an aminophospholipid translocase [33]. In the adult mammalian cardiac cells, β-agonists were unable to suppress the exchanger in a manner similar to that in the frog ventricular myocytes (unpublished observations, Fan, Shuba, and Morad, 1995; [34]). The absence of such β-agonist-mediated modulation of the exchanger is consistent with the development of the SR Ca^{2+} pump and its regulation by PKA-mediated phosphorylation of phospholamban. Irrespective of the effects of β-agonists in the mammalian heart, it appears that in the frog heart the "relaxant" effect of catecholamines is in part mediated by the suppression of Ca^{2+} influx via the exchanger, through the β-receptor-adenylate cyclase-cAMP-dependent pathway. Our findings, therefore, imply that Na^+-Ca^{2+} exchanger protein or a molecule closely associated with it may be regulated by phosphorylation in the frog heart. The functional data, presented here on the frog heart exchanger, suggest that the exchanger protein contains a novel cAMP-dependent regulatory site. We have partially

---

FIG. 2A–C. The effect of isoproterenol (ISO) on I_{Na-Ca} in frog ventricular myocytes dialyzed with low-Ca^{2+}-buffer internal solution. A Ramp voltage-clamp protocol and corresponding original currents obtained in control external solution (1), after application of 5 µM of ISO (2), after addition of 5 mM of Ni^{2+} in the presence of ISO (3), and after washout of Ni^{2+} and elevation of the external Ca^{2+} concentration from 2 to 5 mM in the presence of ISO (4). B Time course of changes of the maximal outward current density at +40 mV in response to voltage-clamp pulses shown in A delivered at a frequency of 0.2 Hz during experimental interventions marked by *horizontal bars*; downward deflections of current density (e.g., 3) indicate rapid test applications and washout of 5 mM of Ni^{2+}; *numbers along the experimental points* mark traces shown in A. C Voltage-dependence of I_{Na-Ca} in control and ISO-containing solutions. I-Vs for control I_{Na-Ca} and I_{Na-Ca} in the presence of ISO were constructed from ramp records after subtraction of Ni^{2+}-resistant current shown in A (room temperature; cell capacity 62 pF; $[Ca^{2+}]_o = 2.0$ mM; $[Na^+]_i = 20$ mM). (Modified from [29a])

cloned the frog heart Na^+-Ca^{2+} exchanger from a frog heart cDNA library and have found a nine-amino-acid insertion, not present in the previously reported isoforms of the Na^+-Ca^{2+} exchanger, containing a putative nucleotide binding domain [35]. Since the possible PKA-dependent phosphorylation site (RKAVS) found in the mammalian exchanger between amino acids 385–389 [36] is also present in the frog heart exchanger, it is possible that the presence of the two domains on the exchanger may be essential in allowing the phosphorylation to proceed.

Acknowledgments. The author thanks Dr. Kathryn Sandberg for providing the frog cDNA library. This work was supported by grants from the National Institutes of Health (NIH) (R01-HL16152-22) and the American Heart Association (AHA), Maine Affiliate.

References

1. Reuter H (1983) Calcium channel modulation by neurotransmitters, enzymes, and drugs. Nature 301:569–574
2. Kameyama M, Hofmann F, Trautwein W (1985) On the mechanism of β-adrenergic regulation of the Ca^{2+} channel in the guinea pig heart. Pflugers Arch 405:285–293
3. Spurgeon MD, Baartz G, Raffaeli S, Hansford R, Talo A, Lakatta E, Capogrossi MD (1990) Simultaneous measurement of Ca^{2+} contraction and potential in cardiac myocytes. Am J Physiol 258:H574–H586
4. Callewaert G, Cleemann L, Morad M (1988) Epinephrine enhances Ca^{2+} current-regulated Ca^{2+} release and Ca^{2+} reuptake in rat ventricular myocytes. Proc Natl Acad Sci USA 85:2009–2013
5. Lindeman JP, Jones LR, Hathaway DR, Henry BG, Watanabe AM (1983) β-adrenergic stimulation of phospholamban phosphorylation and Ca^{2+}-ATPase activity in guinea pig ventricles. J Biol Chem 258:464–471
6. Wegener AD, Simmerman HKB, Lindemann JP, Jones LR (1989) Phospholamban phosphorylation in intact ventricles. J Biol Chem 264:11468–11474
7. Sham JSK, Jones LR, Morad M (1991) Phospholamban mediates the relaxant effect of β-adrenergic agonists in mammalian ventricular myocytes. Am J Physiol 261:H1344–H1349
8. McClellan GB, Winegrad S (1978) Cyclic nucleotide regulation of contractile proteins in mammalian cardiac muscle. J Gen Physiol 72:737–764
9. Endoh M, Blinks JR (1988) Action of sympathomimetic amines on the Ca^{2+} transients and contraction of rabbit myocardium: reciprocal changes in myofibrillar responsiveness to Ca^{2+} mediated through α- and β-adrenoreceptors. Circ Res 62:247–265
10. McIvor ME, Orchard CH, Lakatta EG (1988) Dissociation of change in apparent myofibrillar Ca^{2+} sensitivity and twitch relaxation induced by adrenergic and cholinergic stimulation in isolated ferret cardiac muscle. J Gen Physiol 92:509–529
11. Morad M (1969) Contracture and catecholamines in mammalian myocardium. Science 166:505–506
12. Morad M, Rollett EL (1972) Relaxing effects of catecholamines on mammalian heart. J Physiol (Lond) 224:537–558
13. Kavaler F, Morad M (1966) Paradoxical effects of epinephrine on excitation-contraction coupling in cardiac muscle. Circ Res 18:492–501
14. Morad M, Weiss J, Cleemann L (1978) The inotropic action of adrenaline on cardiac muscle: does it relax or potentiate tension? Eur J Cardiol 7:53–62
15. Morad M, Sanders C, Weiss J (1981) The inotropic actions of adrenaline on frog ventricular muscle: relaxing versus potentiating effects. J Physiol (Lond) 311:585–604
16. Morad M (1982) Ionic mechanisms mediating the inotropic and relaxant effects of adrenaline on the heart muscle. In: Riemersma RA, Oliver MF (eds) Catecholamines in the non-ischemic and ischemic myocardium. Elsevier, Amsterdam, pp 113–135

17. Vilsen B, Andersen JP (1992) Deduced amino acid sequence and E_1-E_2 equilibrium of the sarcoplasmic reticulum Ca^{2+}-ATPase of frog skeletal muscle: comparison with the Ca^{2+}-ATPase of rabbit fast twitch muscle. FEBS Lett 306:213–218

18. Page SG, Niedergerke R (1972) Structures of physiological interest in the frog heart ventricle. J Cell Sci 11:179–203

19. Morad M, Orkand, RK (1971) Excitation-contraction coupling in frog ventricle: evidence from voltage-clamp studies. J Physiol (Lond) 219:167–189

20. Klitzner T, Morad M (1983) Excitation-contraction coupling in frog ventricle: possible Ca^{2+} transport mechanisms. Pflugers Arch 398:274–283

21. Fabiato A, Fabiato F (1978) Calcium-induced release of calcium from the sarcoplasmic reticulum of skinned cells from adult human, dog, cat, rabbit, rat, and frog hearts and from fetal and newborn rat ventricles. Ann NY Acad Sci 307:491–522

22. Mitra R, Morad M (1985) A uniform enzymatic method for dissociation of myocytes from hearts and stomachs of vertebrates. Am J Physiol 249:H1056–H1060

23. Hamill OP, Marty A, Neher E, Sakman B, Sigworth FJ (1981) Improved patch-clamp technique for high-resolution current recording from cell and cell-free membrane patches. Pflugers Arch 391:85–100

24. Fabiato A, Fabiato F (1988) Computer program for calculating total from specified free or free turn specified total ionic concentrations in aqueous solutions containing multiple metals and ligands. Methods Enzymol 157:378–417

25. Cleemann L, Morad M (1991) Analysis of role of Ca^{2+} channel in cardiac excitation-contraction coupling: evidence from simultaneous measurements of intracellular Ca^{2+} contraction and Ca^{2+} current. J Physiol (Lond) 432:283–312

26. Harvey RD, Hume JR (1989) Autonomic regulation of a chloride current in heart. Science 244:983–985

27. Bahinski A, Nairn AC, Greengard P, Gadsby DC (1989) Chloride conductance regulated by cyclic AMP-dependent protein kinase in cardiac myocytes. Nature 340:718–721

28. Beuckelmann RJ, Wier WG (1989) Sodium-calcium exchange in guinea pig cardiac cells: exchange current and changes in intracellular Ca^{2+}. J Physiol (Lond) 414:499–520

29. Nabauer M, Morad M (1992) Modulation of contraction by intracellular Na^+ via Na^+-Ca^{2+} exchange in single shark (*Squalus acanthias*) ventricular myocytes. J Physiol (Lond) 457:627–637

29a. Fan, Shuba, Morad (1996) Proc Natl Acad Sci (in press)

30. Parsons TD, Hartzell HC (1993) Regulation of Ca^{2+} current in frog ventricular cardiomyocytes by guanosine 5'-triphosphate analogues and isoproterenol. J Gen Physiol 102:525–549

31. Morad M, Goldman YE (1973) Excitation-contraction coupling in heart muscle: membrane control of development of tension. Prog Biophys Mol Biol 27:257–313

32. Maylie JG (1982) Excitation-contraction coupling in neonatal and adult myocardium of cat. Am J Physiol 242:H834–H843

33. Hilgemann DW, Collins A (1992) Mechanism of cardiac Na^+-Ca^{2+} exchange current stimulation by Mg ATP: possible involvement of aminophospholipid translocase. J Physiol (Lond) 454:59–80

34. Main MJ, Cannell MB (1995) Effects of β-adrenergic stimulation on the Na^+-K^+ pump and Na^+-Ca^{2+} exchanger in isolated guinea-pig ventricular myocytes. J Physiol (Lond) 483:12P

35. Iwata T, Kraev A, Morad M, Carafoli E (1995) Cloning of the cDNA of the frog heart sarcolemmal Na^+-Ca^{2+} exchanger. Biophys J 68:A136

36. Nicoll D, Bongoni S, Philipson KD (1990) Molecular cloning and functional expression of the cardiac sarcolemmal Na^+-Ca^{2+} exchanger. Science 250:562–565

37. DiPolo R, Beauge L (1993) Effects of some metal-ATP complexes on Na^+-Ca^{2+} exchange in internally dialysed squid axons. J Physiol (Lond) 462:71–86

Interaction of the L-Type Calcium Channel with Calcium Channel Blockers

Franz Hofmann, Norbert Klugbauer, Lubica Lacinová,
Claudia Seisenberger, Angela Schuster, and Andrea Welling

Summary. The contribution of the primary structure and the β subunit to the block of the L-type α_{1C} calcium channel was studied. The α_{1C-a} and the α_{1C-b} subunits were truncated at aa 1733 and 1728, respectively, and were expressed stably in human embryonic kidney (HEK) 293 cells (α_{1C-at} and α_{1C-bt} cell line). The β_3 subunit was coexpressed stably with the α_{1C-a} subunit in Chinese hamster ovary (CHO) cells. The block of barium currents was tested under a variety of conditions. Nisoldipine blocked the α_{1C-bt} channel at lower concentrations than the α_{1C-at} channel. This finding confirms previous results with the full-length α_{1C-a} and α_{1C-b} channel. Coexpression of the β_3 subunit did not significantly affect the IC_{50} value for the isradipine block determined at a holding potential (HP) of −80 or −40 mV. In contrast, the IC_{50} value for the gallopamil block was three times lower in the $\alpha_{1C-a}\beta_3$-expressing CHO cell line than in the α_{1C-a}-expressing CHO cell line. These results show that the sensitivity of channel block depends not only on the drug-binding site but also on the membrane potential, the primary channel structure, and the presence of other subunits.

Key words. Calcium channel—Heart—Vascular smooth muscle—Stable cell line—HEK 293 cells

Introduction

The contraction of cardiac, vascular, and nonvascular smooth muscle depends on the release of calcium from intracellular stores and its influx from the extracellular space. A large proportion of extracellular calcium enters these cells through voltage-dependent L-type calcium channels. These channels are the therapeutic targets of a large class of drugs, namely the calcium channel blockers or calcium antagonists. Until 10 years ago, the biochemical targets of the calcium channel blockers were poorly defined. Since then, the molecular structure of these channels has been elucidated.

Calcium channels are multimeric protein complexes composed of up to four different proteins, namely the α_1, α_2/δ and β subunits (for references see [1]). The α_1

Institute of Pharmacology and Toxicology, Technische Universität München, D-80802 München, Germany

subunit is the principal subunit and contains the voltage-dependent channel pore, whereas the other proteins are auxiliary subunits with modulatory functions. The α_1 and the β subunit are encoded by at least six and four distinct genes, respectively. Each gene gives rise to several splice variants. The α_1 subunits of the heart and smooth muscle are the splice variants of the class C gene [2–4]. The cDNAs of the α_{1C-a} (cardiac) and α_{1C-b} (smooth muscle) subunits, which have been expressed singly or in combination with other subunits in Chinese hamster ovary (CHO) and human embryonic kidney (HEK) cells [5–9] induce regular voltage-dependent L-type calcium currents which are blocked by the calcium channel blockers. In addition to these, photoaffinity labeling studies [10–12] have suggested that the α_{1C} subunit is the major target for the known calcium channel blockers such as dihydropyridines (DHP), phenylalkylamines (PAA), and benzothiazepines.

In-depth investigations have shown that, at lower concentrations, many of the calcium channel blockers block the L-type calcium channels of vascular smooth muscle rather than those of the ventricular muscle. The basis for this apparent selectivity has been solved partially. One factor contributing to this tissue selectivity is the resting membrane potential, which is more positive in vascular than in cardiac muscle. Many of the calcium channel blockers interact in a voltage-dependent manner with high affinity with the inactivated channel [13,14]. It is therefore likely that the higher membrane potential of the smooth muscle contributes significantly to the tissue selectivity of some calcium antagonists. However, studies of the expressed channels showed that nisoldipine blocked barium currents through the smooth muscle α_{1C-b} channel more readily than through the cardiac α_{1C-a} subunit at the same membrane [15]. This finding suggested that the higher affinity of the DHPs for smooth rather than for cardiac muscle calcium channels is based partially on structural differences between the cardiac and smooth muscle channel.

Northern blot analysis and immunological studies suggested that the α_{1C} subunit is complexed with at least two other subunits, the β and α_2/δ proteins. These additional subunits have modulatory effects on voltage-dependence, kinetics of activation and inactivation, and sensitivity to regulatory mechanisms such as phosphorylation [7, 15–19]. Moreover, it was shown that the β subunit also affected the sensitivity of the channel against some but not all calcium channel blockers [20,21]. We have now used a number of different stable cell lines including some which express the α_{1C-a} or α_{1C-b} subunit truncated at the carboxy-terminal [22] to study in some detail the interaction between the calcium channel blockers and the cloned and expressed L-type calcium channel.

Materials and Methods

Cell Transfection and Culture

CHO cells were stably transfected with the recombinant plasmid pKNHα1/2a, yielding cell line CHOCa1 [7]. The plasmid contains the entire protein coding region of the rabbit cardiac α_{1C-a} subunits [3]. The construction of the expression plasmid pKNHβ3K carrying the complete protein coding region of the calcium channel β subunit type 3 (β_3), the 1.5 kb Asp718 fragment of pBH23 [23] including the consensus sequence for the initiation of translation in vertebrates, was blunted and inserted into pKNH in the same orientation with respect to the adenovirus late promoter yield pKNHα3K (for further details see [15]). CHOCa1 cells [7] expressing the α_{1C-a} subunit were cotransfected with 10 µg pKNHβK and 0.2 µg pSV2-His by electroporation, yielding the stable cell line CHOCa1β3. The coexpression of the β₃ subunit was verified by immunoblots with a specific antibody against the β₃ subunit [24]. The deletion mutants of the cardiac $\alpha_{1C\text{-}at}$ (t stands for truncated) and the smooth muscle $\alpha_{1C\text{-}bt}$ subunit were truncated at amino acid (aa) 1733 and aa 1728 (first deleted amino acid). The deletion mutants were constructed by the polymerase chain reaction (PCR) protocol of Wei et al. [22] using the plasmids pcDNA3HK1 and pcDNA3LK1 [9]. From several positive cell clones, H-L2 (smooth muscle) stably expressing the truncated $\alpha_{1C\text{-}bt}$ subunit and H-H8 (cardiac) stably expressing the truncated $\alpha_{1C\text{-}a}$ subunit were used for further experiments.

Measurements of Calcium Transients in Human Embryonic Kidney (HEK) 293 Cells

The intracellular calcium concentration ($[Ca^{2+}]_i$) was monitored by the dual wavelength method using the calcium-sensitive indicator fura-2 as previously described [25]. The cells were loaded for 1 h with 1 µM fura-2-AM at 37°C. Cover slips were then washed with the NaCl/hydroxyethylpiperazine ethanesulfonic acid (HEPES)-buffer (140 mM NaCl, 6.6 mM KCl, 1.18 mM MgSO₄, 2 mM CaCl₂, 10 mM Glucose, 5 mM HEPES pH 7.4) and superfused with this buffer at 37°C. The calcium-free NaCl/HEPES buffer contained 2 mM ethylene glycol-bis-(β-aminoethyl ether)-N,N,N',N'-tetraacetic acid (EGTA) but no added calcium. The $[Ca^{2+}]_i$ was calculated according to Grynkiewicz et al. [26]. Changes in $[Ca^{2+}]_i$ were initiated by superfusion of an individual cell with the depolarization buffer (NaCl/HEPES buffer containing 66 mM KCl and 80 mM NaCl). The depolarization buffer was applied by a micropipette located directly above the cell and operated by air pressure (Lorenz MPCU-3, Göttingen, Germany). Mibefradil was applied at the indicated concentration in the NaCl/HEPES buffer at least 1 min before the cell was depolarized by potassium.

Electrophysiological Recording

Ion currents were recorded under whole-cell patch clamp conditions [27] using an EPC-9 amplifier (HEKA Elektronik, Lambrecht, Germany). A standard program package provided by HEKA Elektronik was used for data acquisition and for compensation of the pipette and membrane capacitance. The patch pipettes pulled from borosilicate glass capillaries had resistances of 2 to 2.5 MΩ when filled with the intracellular solution. The membrane capacitance of individual cells ranged from 10 to 25 pF. The series resistance ranged from 2.5 to 10 MΩ and was compensated up to 40%. The leak current component was obtained by hyperpolarizing voltage steps from the holding potential (HP) and the multiplied current was subtracted on-line from the recorded trace. The barium currents (I_{Ba}) were elicited by 20- or 40-ms deporalization pulses to +20 or +30 mV from a HP of −80 mV. The steady-state inactivating curves were measured at 0.04 Hz using 5-s conditioning pulses, followed by a 10-ms return to the HP of −80 mV, followed by a 150-ms test pulse to +30 mV. The external solution consisted of (in mM): NaCl 82, tetraethylammonium chloride (TEA-Cl) 20, BaCl₂ 30, CsCl 5, MgCl₂ EGTA 0.1, HEPES 5, glucose 10, pH 7.4 (NaOH). The pipette solution contained in mM: CsCl 102, TEA-Cl 10, EGTA 10, MgCl₂ 1, NaATP 3, HEPES 5, pH 7.4 (CsOH). The stock solutions (10 mM) of mibefradil was prepared in bidistilled water. The stock solutions of gallopamil and isradipine were prepared in ethanol, stored at −20°C, and diluted to the required concentration in the extracellular solution. They were always used within 1 day. If not mentioned otherwise, all values are means ± S.E.M. with the number of cells in brackets. The significance of difference between two sets of observations was evaluated by Student's t-test.

Drugs and Reagents

Gallopamil was kindly provided by Knoll, Ludwigshafen, Germany. (±) Isradipine was from Sandoz, Nürnberg, Germany. Mibefradil, Ro 40-5967 ((1S,2S)-2-(2-[[3-(2-benzimidazolyl)propyl] methyl-amino]ethyl)-6-fluoro-1,2,3,4-tetrahydro-1-isopropyl-2-naphthylmethoxyacetate dihydrochloride) was kindly provided by Drs. Clozel and Osterrieder from Hoffmann-La Roche, Basel, Switzerland. All other chemicals were of the highest purity available.

Results

Basal Properties of the Truncated a_{1C} Subunits

Previously it was reported that deletion of part of the carboxy-terminal amino acids of the α_{1C} subunit increased the ionic current when the truncated α_{1C} subunit was expressed transiently in *Xenopus laevis* oocytes together with the β and α_2/δ subunit [22]. Both splice variants of the α_{1C} subunit were truncated at amino acid 1733 (α_{1C-at}) and 1728 (α_{1C-bt}) and stable cell lines were established in HEK 293 cells. From several positive clones, two cell lines were established, the H-L2 cell line expressing the α_{1C-bt} subunits (t stands for truncated) and the H-H8 cell line expressing the α_{1C-at} subunit. The I_{Ba} of these cell lines were not different from CHO cell lines expressing the full length construct [15,21]. I_{Ba} started at membrane potentials positive to −30 mV, was maximal between +20 and +30 mV, and reversed at +75 mV (Fig. 1). The maximal I_{Ba} density was 12 and 26 pA/pF for the α_{1C-at} and α_{1C-bt} expressing cell line, respectively. Steady-state inactivation curves were very similar for both cell lines. The membrane potentials at which the channels inactivated half-maximally were −8 and −9 mV and were not different from previously established values [20,21]. These results indicated that the new cell lines, which expressed only the truncated α_{1C} subunit, had basic barium currents which were very similar to those obtained with the full-length clones.

Measurement of $[Ca^{2+}]_i$ Transients

We tested if the newly established cell lines could be used to study $[Ca^{2+}]_i$ transients. Nontransfected and transfected cells were loaded with fura 2-AM. Potassium depolarization of a (66 mM K$^+$ extracellular) nontransfected cell never induced a change in the intracellular $[Ca^{2+}]_i$. In contrast, the change of the extracellular potassium concentration from 6 to 66 mM induced a $[Ca^{2+}]_i$ transient (Fig. 2). Repeated depolarization resulted in similar $[Ca^{2+}]_i$ transients, suggesting that the calcium channel could be opened repeatedly without inactivation. Potassium depolarization increased peak $[Ca^{2+}]_i$ from 107 ± 15 nM to 476 ± 124 nM ($n = 14$). The potassium-induced $[Ca^{2+}]_i$ transients were suppressed when calcium was omitted from the extracellular solution or when the channel was blocked by the calcium channel blocker mibefradil (Fig. 2). Half-maximal inhibition was observed at 1.7 ± 0.2 μM mibefradil. This IC$_{50}$ value is almost identical with that obtained in electrophysiological experiments [20,21]. These

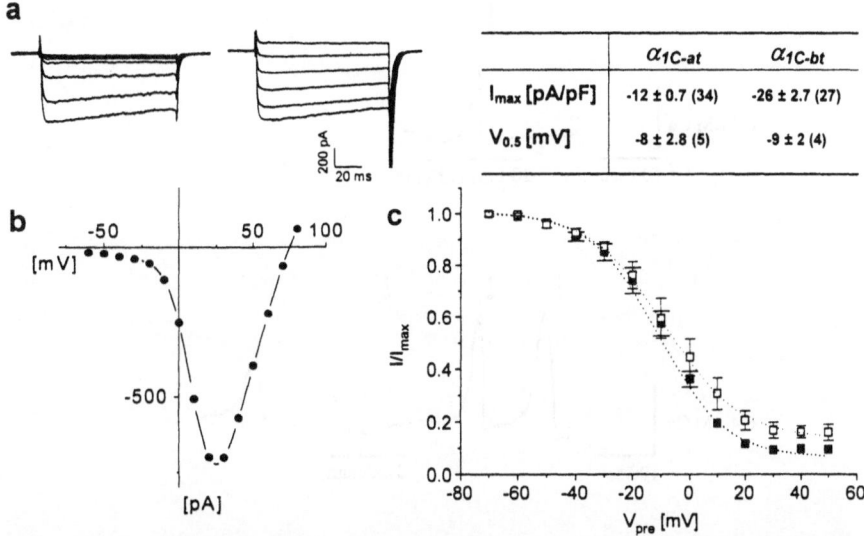

FIG. 1a–c. Characterization of the truncated smooth muscle calcium channel expressed stably in human embryonic kidney (HEK) 293 cells. **a** Individual barium current traces elicited by pulses from −80 to −60 through +70 mV in an α_{1C-bt} cell. **b** The corresponding current voltage relation. **c** The steady-state inactivation curve of α_{1C-at} (*open squares*) and α_{1C-at} (*solid squares*) cells. Each point is the mean ± SEM of four to five experiments. The curve was fitted by a Boltzmann equation. *Inset upper right*, I_{max} and $V_{0.5}$ values for both cell lines

findings suggested the truncated α_{1C} subunit cell lines may be good model cell lines to screen for L-type calcium channel blockers.

Interaction of the Channels with Nisoldipine

Several dihydropyridines were tested in the fura-2 experiments as calcium channel blockers. However, these experiments were inconclusive since the compounds absorbed light at the same wavelength as fura-2 and/or were destroyed by the ultraviolet light. We therefore used regular electrophysiological methods to test the effect of some dihydropyridines. Nisoldipine was used since we reported previously [15] that this compound blocked the α_{1C-b} (smooth muscle) channel at lower concentrations than the α_{1C-a} (heart) channel. This finding was surprising since the putative binding sites for DHPs are identical in both clones. These binding sites have been localized to the pore region of repeat I, III, and IV of the skeletal muscle calcium channel [10–12]. It is possible that truncation of the α_1 subunit abolished the differential DHP sensitivity of the cardiac and smooth muscle α_{1C} subunit. A shift of the HP from −80 mV to −40 mV decreased I_{Ba} by about 26% in both cell lines in the absence of nisoldipine (Fig. 3). A shift of the HP from −80 mV to −40 mV in the presence of 1 nM nisoldipine reduced further I_{Ba} in both cell lines (Fig. 3). The α_{1C-at} cell channel was unblocked almost completely when the HP was returned to −80 mV, whereas the α_{1C-bt} cell channel recovered only partially from the block. The differing extent of block was still obvious when these experiments were repeated in the presence of 10 nM nisoldipine. These results suggested that both truncated channel subunits were blocked in voltage-dependent manner by nisoldipine.

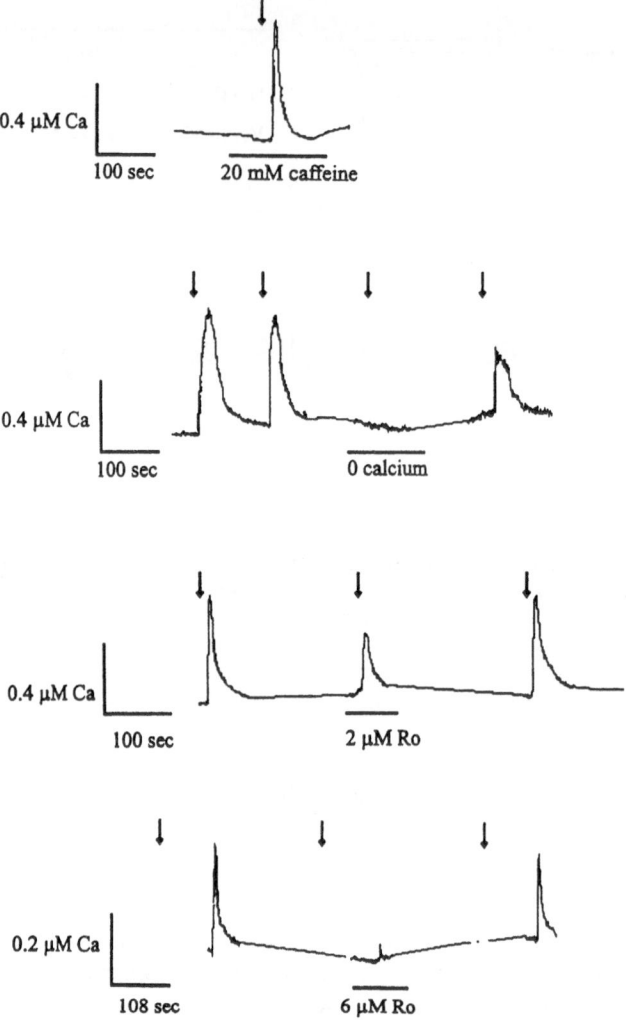

FIG. 2. [Ca²⁺]ᵢ transients are blocked by mibefradil. Four cells expressing the truncated α1$_{C\text{-bt}}$ subunit (smooth muscle; *upper two panels*) or the truncated $\alpha_{1C\text{-at}}$ subunit (cardiac muscle; *lower two panels*) were loaded with 1 µM fura-2. The [Ca²⁺]ᵢ transients were recorded as described in "Methods." The extracellular [K⁺] was increased to 66 mM for 30 s at the *arrows*. Note that removal of extracellular calcium repressed the [Ca²⁺]ᵢ transient, whereas emptying of intracellular stores by caffeine had no effect. [Ca²⁺]ᵢ transients were also suppressed transiently by superfusion with the channel blocker mibefradil. Fluorescent light was recorded only during the time indicated by the *darker line*

The truncated smooth muscle $\alpha_{1C\text{-bt}}$ subunit was more sensitive to the nisoldipine block than the cardiac $\alpha_{1C\text{-at}}$ subunit. Inspection of the block's time course suggested that the onset of block at HP −40 mV was faster in the $\alpha_{1C\text{-bt}}$ cell than in the $\alpha_{1C\text{-at}}$ cell at 1 and 10 nM nisoldipine (Fig. 4). Statistical analysis of the on-rates at 10 nM nisoldipine yielded values of 26 ± 5.3 (6) and 10 ± 1.0 (7) for the $\alpha_{1C\text{-at}}$ and $\alpha_{1C\text{-bt}}$ cells, respectively. These values are significantly different at $P < 0.01$. The second remarkable difference between both channels was that the recovery from block was quite

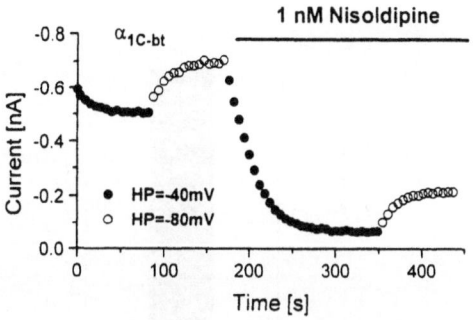

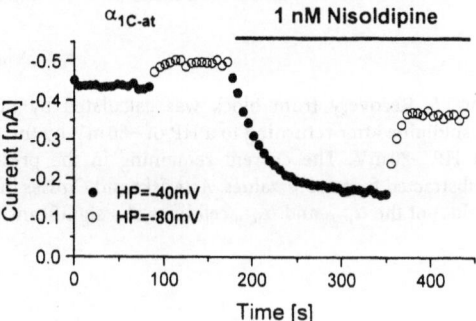

FIG. 3. Nisoldipine blocks I_{Ba} of an $\alpha_{1C\text{-bt}}$ (*top*) and $\alpha_{1C\text{-at}}$ (*bottom*) cell. Panels show the time course of the I_{Ba} elicited from a HP of −80 mV (*open circles*) or −40 mV (*solid circles*). The time of nisoldipine application is indicated by the *line*. Pulse length was 40 ms and the depolarization frequency was 0.2 Hz

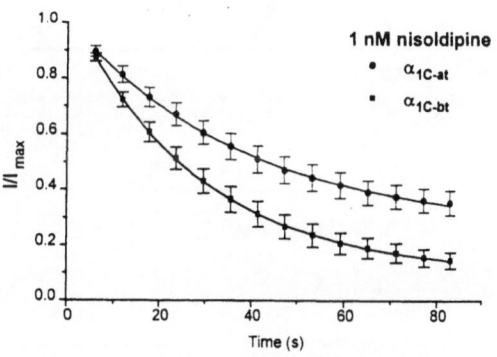

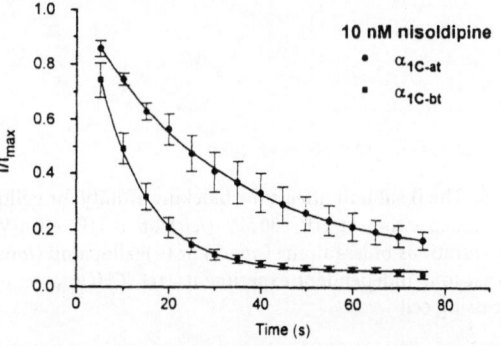

FIG. 4. The time course of channel block after shifting the HP from −80 to −40 mV in the presence of 1 nM (*top*) and 10 nM (*bottom*) nisoldipine is faster in $\alpha_{1C\text{-bt}}$ (*solid squares*) than in $\alpha_{1C\text{-at}}$ (*solid circles*) cells. The number of experiments was 8 and 5 for $\alpha_{1C\text{-bt}}$ and $\alpha_{1C\text{-at}}$ cells, respectively. The spline curves are the monoexponential fits

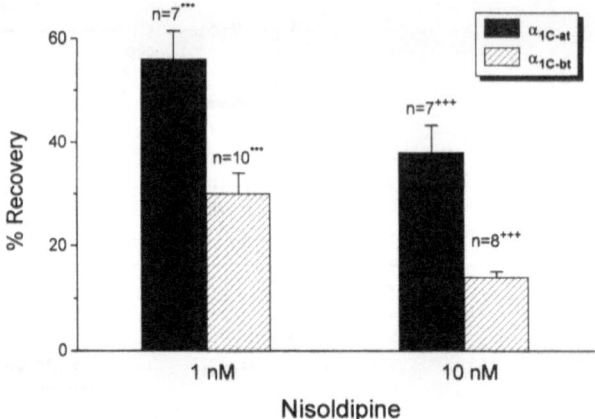

FIG. 5. Recovery from block was calculated by dividing maximal I_{Ba} in the presence of nisoldipine after returning to a HP of −80 mV by the maximal I_{Ba} in the absence of nisoldipine at HP −80 mV. The current remaining in the presence of nisoldipine at HP −40 mV was substracted from both values. *Asterisks* and *Crosses* indicate a statistical difference between the values of the $\alpha_{1C\text{-bt}}$ and $\alpha_{1C\text{-at}}$ cell lines at a significance level of $P < 0.001$

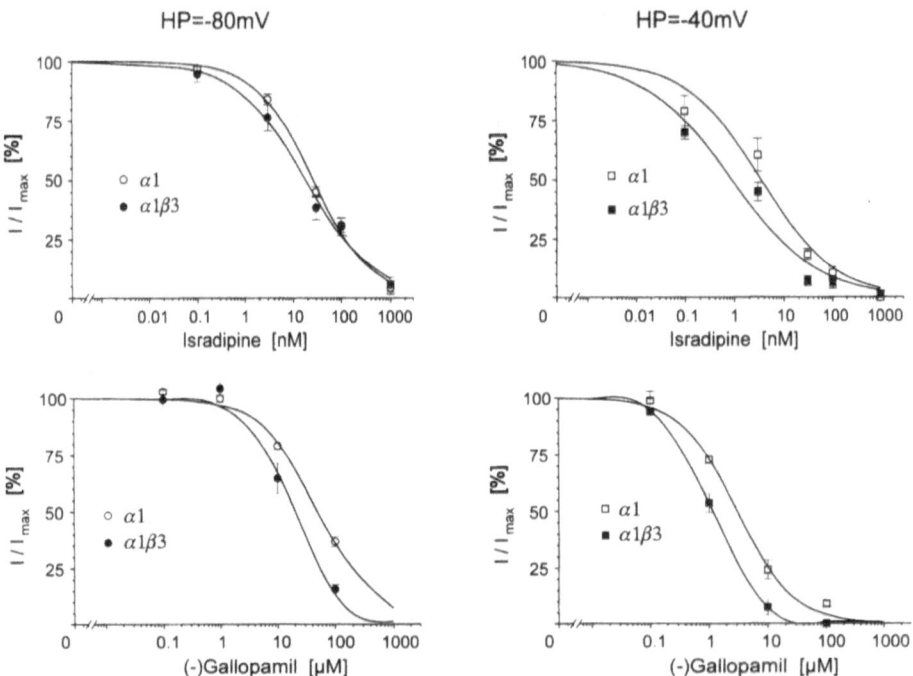

FIG. 6. The β subunit affects the blocking affinity for gallopamil but not for isradipine. I_{Ba} was determined either at HP −80 MV (*left*) or at HP −40 mV (*right*) in the presence of various concentrations of isradipine (*upper*) or (−)gallopamil (*lower*). Each *point* is the mean ± SEM of at least four independent experiments. α1, CHOα$_{1C\text{-a}}$ expressing cell; α1β3, CHOα$_{1C\text{-a}}$ and β$_3$ expressing cell

different (Fig. 5). Statistical analysis of these values indicated the difference in the recovery from block was significant at $P < 0.001$. These results agree with those published by Welling and coworkers [15] and strongly support the hypotheses that (a) the primary structure of the α_{1C} subunit contributes significantly to the affinity of nisoldipine block and (b) the differing DHP sensitivity is not modified by truncation of the α_{1C} subunit.

The β Subunit Affects the Affinity for Calcium Channel Block

The experiments described so far have indicated that the primary structure of the α_{1C} subunit contributed to the affinity of the subunit for certain DHPs. Other experiments [21] have pointed to the possibility that the β subunit might also affect the sensitivity of the channel for blocking drugs. This possibility was investigated using two CHO cell lines, one which expressed only the $\alpha_{1C\text{-}a}$ subunit and a second expressing the $\alpha_{1C\text{-}a}$ and the β_3 subunit. Isradipine, a DHP, and gallopamil, a PAA, were used to test this possibility since it is believed that DHPs bind to the channel from the extracellular space [28] whereas PAAs bind from the cytosolic side of the channel [29]. The β subunits bind to the channel from the cytosolic side. Both drugs were tested at the two HPs of −80 mV and −40 mV since it has been suggested that these drugs bind to the inactivated state of the channel with higher affinity than to the other states. It was expected that the drugs should block the current at lower concentrations at a HP of −40 mV than at −80 mV. As expected, both compounds blocked the channel in both cell lines voltage-dependently (Fig. 6). A shift in the HP from −80 mV to −40 mV decreased the IC_{50} value tenfold (isradipine) or 20-fold (gallopamil). The IC_{50} values for isradipine obtained with the CHOα_1 and CHO$\alpha_1\beta_3$ cell line were identical. However, the IC_{50} values obtained with gallopamil differed significantly between the CHOα_1 cell line and the CHO$\alpha_1\beta_3$ cell line. Coexpression of the β_3 subunit decreased the IC_{50} values threefold at both HPs, suggesting that the β_3 subunit affected the affinity of the channel for PAAs but not for DHPs.

Discussion

The experiments described in this chapter support the notion that a variety of factors affect the affinity of the L-type calcium channel for various calcium channel blockers. The established factors are:

1. The structure of the drug-binding sites as defined by photoaffinity labeling [10–12] and site-directed mutagenesis [30]. Site-directed mutagenesis showed that mutations of the primary structure close to the binding site identified by Regulla and coworkers [10] abolished the high-affinity block of the channel by isradipine (Schuster et al., unpublished).
2. The state of the channel. The affinity of the channel for calcium blockers increases with increasing membrane depolarization, indicating that calcium channel blockers bind with high affinity to the inactivated state.
3. The primary structure of the α_{1C} subunit. The results of this study confirm and extend that of a previous study [15], which showed that the two splice variants of the α_{1C} gene are differentially sensitive towards nisoldipine block. The smooth muscle $\alpha_{1C\text{-}bt}$ subunit was already blocked tonically at a HP of −80 mV (not shown)

suggesting that nisoldipine also interacted with the rested or closed state of the channel. The truncated smooth muscle channel did recovery poorly from inactivation upon returning the HP to −80 mV. This study supports the notion that the different sensitivity does not depend on the particular cell line used for transfection since the different sensitiviy was observed in CHO and HEK 293 cells. In addition, the different sensitivity has been observed now with two different constructs, i.e., the full-length and the carboxy-terminal-truncated α_{1C} subunits. The reproducibility of the difference indicates (a) that the carboxy-terminal part of the α_{1C} subunit does not affect the channel block by nisoldipine, although its deletion increased ionic current [22] and (b) that some structural features of the α_{1C} subunits, which apparently are not directly involved in high-affinity binding of DHPs [10–12], significantly affect the sensitivity of channel block.

4. The coexpression of the β subunit. The β_3 subunit decreased the IC_{50} value for gallopamil but not that for isradipine. This differential effect is in line with the hypothesis that the PAAs bind to the intracellular side of the channel [29].

In conclusion, these experiments show that a number of factors affect the affinity of the L-type calcium channel for calcium channel blockers. Presumably they do so by changing the tertiary structure of the α_1 subunit to allow high-affinity binding of the calcium channel blockers.

Acknowledgments. This work was made possible by grants from SET, Fond der chemischen Industrie, and Deutsche Forschungsgemeinschaft.

References

1. Hofmann F, Biel M, Flockerzi V (1994) Molecular basis for Ca^{2+} channel diversity. Annu Rev Neurosci 17:399–418
2. Mikami A, Imoto K, Tanabe T, Niidome T, Mori Y, Takeshima H, Narumiya S, Numa S (1989) Primary structure and functional expression of the cardiac dihydropyridine-sensitive calcium channel. Nature 340:230–233
3. Biel M, Ruth P, Bosse E, Hullin R, Stühmer P, Flockerzi V, Hofmann F (1990) Primary structure and functional expression of high voltage activated calcium channel from rabbit lung. FEBS Lett 269:409–412
4. Koch WJ, Ellinor PT, Schwartz A (1990) cDNA cloning of a dihydropyridine-sensitive calcium channel from rat aorta. J Biol Chem 265:17786–17791
5. Bosse E, Bottlender R, Kleppisch T, Hescheler J, Welling A, Hofmann F, Flockerzi V (1992) Stable and functional expression of the calcium channel α_1 subunit from smooth muscle in somatic cell lines. EMBO J 11:2033–2038
6. Yoshida A, Takahashi M, Nishimura S, Takeshima H, Kokubun S (1992) Cyclic AMP-dependent phosphorylation and regulation of the cardiac dihydropyridine-sensitive Ca channel. FEBS Lett 309:343–349
7. Welling A, Bosse E, Cavalié A, Bottlender R, Ludwig A, Nastainczyk W, Flockerzi V, Hofmann F (1993) Stable coexpression of calcium channel α_1, and β and α_2/δ subunits in a somatic cell line. J Physiol 471:749–765
8. Perez-Reyes E, Yuan W, Wei X, Bers DM (1994) Regulation of the cloned L-type cardiac calcium channel by cyclic-AMP-dependent protein kinase. FEBS Lett 342:119–123
9. Zong X, Schreieck J, Mehrke G, Welling A, Schuster A, Bosse E, Flockerzi V, Hofmann F (1995) On the regulation of the expressed L-type calcium channel by cAMP-dependent protein kinase. Pflugers Arch 430:340–347

10. Regulla S, Schneider T, Nastainczyk W, Meyer HE, Hofmann F (1991) Identification of the site of interaction of the dihydropyridine channel blockers nitrendipine and azidopine with the calcium channel α_1 subunit. EMBO J 10:45–49
11. Striessnig J, Murphy BJ, Catterall WA (1991) Dihydropyridine receptor of L-type Ca^{2+} channels: Identification of binding domains for [^{3}H](+)-PN200-110 and [^{3}H]azidopine within the α_1 subunit. Proc Natl Acad Sci USA 88:10769–10773
12. Kalász H, Watanabe T, Yabana H, Itagaki K, Naito K, Nakayama H, Schwartz A, Vaghy PL (1993) Indentification of 1,4-dihydropyridine binding domains within the primary structure of the α_1 subunit of the skeletal muscle L-type calcium channel. FEBS Lett 331:177–181
13. Bean BP (1984) Nitrendipine block of cardiac calcium channels: High-affinity binding to the inactivated state. Proc Natl Acad USA 81:6388–6392
14. Sanguinetti MC, Kass RS (1984) Voltage-dependent block of calcium channel current in calf cardiac Purkinje fiber by dihydropyridine calcium channel antagonists. Circ Res 55:336–348
15. Welling A, Kwan YW, Bosse E, Flockerzi V, Hofmann F, Kass RS (1993) Subunit-dependent modulation of recombinant L-type calcium channels: molecular basis for dihydropyridine tissue selectivity. Circ Res 73:974–980
16. Singer D, Biel M, Lotan I, Flockerzi V, Hofmann F, Dascal N (1991) Roles of the subunits of calcium channel in its expression and function. Science 253:1553–1557
17. Neely A, Wei X, Olcese R, Birnbaumer L, Stefani E (1993) Potentiation by the β subunit of the ratio of the ionic current to the charge movement in the cardiac calcium channel. Science 262:575–578
18. Olcese R, Qin N, Schneider T, Neely A, Wei X, Stefani E, Birnbaumer L (1994) The amino terminus of a calcium channel β subunit sets rates of channel inactivation independently of the subunit's effect on activation. Neuron 13:1433–1438
19. Haase H, Karczewski P, Beckert R, Krause EG (1993) Phosphorylation of the L-type calcium channel β subunit is involved in β-adrenergic signal transduction in canine myocardium. FEBS Lett 335:217–222
20. Welling A, Lacinova L, Donatin K, Ludwig A, Bosse E, Flockerzi V, Hofmann F (1995) Expression of the L-type calcium channel with two different β subunits and its modulation by Ro 40-5967. Pflugers Arch 429:400–411
21. Lacinová L, Welling A, Bosse E, Ruth P, Flockerzi V, Hofmann F (1995) Interaction of Ro 40-5967 with the stable expressed α_1 subunit of the cardiac L-type calcium channel. J Exp Pharmacol Ther 274:54–63
22. Wei X, Neely A, Lacerda AE, Olcese R, Stefani E, Perez-Reyes E, Birnbaumer L (1994) Modification of Ca^{2+} channel activity by deletions at the carboxyl terminus of the cardiac α_1 subunit. J Biol Chem 269:1635–1640
23. Hullin R, Singer-Lahat D, Freihel M, Biel M, Dascal N, Hofmann F, Flockerzi V (1992) Calcium channel β subunit heterogeneity: Functional expression of the cloned cDNA from heart, aorta and brain EMBO J 11:885–890
24. Ludwig A, Bosse E, Brandt W, Flockerzi V, Hofmann F (1994) Production of specific antibodies against the β_2 and β_3 subunit of the high voltage activated calcium channel. Naunyn Schmiedebergs Arch Pharmacol 349:R 40
25. Ruth P, Wang G-X, Boekhoff I, May B, Pfeifer A, Penner R, Korth M, Breer H, Hofmann F (1993) Transfected cGMP dependent protein kinase suppresses calcium transients by inhibition of inositol 1,4,5 triphosphate production. Proc Natl Acad Sci USA 90:2623–2627
26. Grynkiewicz G, Poenie M, Tsien RY (1985) A new generation of Ca^{2+} indicators with greatly improved fluorescence properties. J Biol Chem 260:3440–3450
27. Hamill OP, Marty E, Neher E, Sakmann B, Sigworth FJ (1981) Improved patch-clamp techniques for high-resolution current recording from cells and cell-free membrane patches. Pflugers Arch 391:85–100
28. Kwan YW, Bangalore R, Lakitsh M, Glossmann H, Kass RS (1995) Inhibition of cardiac L-type calcium channels by quartenary amlodipine: Implication for

pharmacokinetics and access to dihydropyridine binding site. J Mol Cell Cardiol 27:253–256

29. Hescheler J, Pelzer D, Trube G, Trautwein W (1982) Does the organic calcium channel blocker D600 act from inside or outside of the cardiac cell membrane. Pflugers Arch 393:287–291

30. Tang S, Yatani A, Bahinski A, Mori Y, Schwartz A (1993) Molecular localization of regions in the L-type calcium channel critical for dihydropyridine action. Neuron 11:1013–1021

Modulation of Single Cardiac L-Type Ca²⁺ Channels by Phosphorylation and a Dihydropyridine Ca²⁺ Agonist

RIKUO OCHI[1], LI HONGYU[1], and TAKESHI NAKAMURA[2]

Summary. Single-channel studies have shown that protein kinase A-dependent phosphorylation of cardiac L-type Ca²⁺ channels definitely increases the channel availability, thereby increasing the macroscopic Ca²⁺ current. We investigated whether the open probability during nonblank sweeps (Po) of such channels was increased by phosphorylation-mediated mode 2 activity in the presence and absence of a 1,4-dihydropyridine (DHP) Ca²⁺ agonist. Single-channel currents were recorded using the cell-attached patch clamp technique from guinea pig isolated ventricular myocytes with Ba²⁺ as the charge carrier. In 18 (control) and 13 (test) patches. 10^{-5} M isoproterenol (ISO) increased the mean current of the total sweeps 3-fold, availability 2.1-fold, Po from 0.12 to 0.17, mean open time from 0.72 to 0.87 ms, and the percentage of sweeps with mean open times longer than 3 ms from 0.19% to 0.68%. Neither the Po increase nor mean open time prolongation was due to mode 2 activity. In the presence of 10^{-7} or 10^{-6} M BAY K 8644, the Po of seven patches was 0.26 and the mean open time was 2.88 ms, which were increased by ISO (10^{-6} M) to 0.44 and 4.13 ms, respectively. Therefore, phosphorylation of cardiac L-type Ca²⁺ channels by β-adrenergic stimulation promoted mode 2 activity in the presence but not in the absence of a DHP Ca²⁺ agonist.

Key words. L-Type Ca²⁺ channel—β-Adrenergic stimulation—Phosphorylation—BAY K 8644—Cardiac myocyte

Introduction

L-Type Ca²⁺ channels, which are the main voltage-gated Ca²⁺ channels in cardiac muscle, are regulated by various neurotrnsmitters, hormones, autacoids, and drugs [1]. The mechanisms responsible for their regulation or modulation are classified into two categories: (1) phosphorylation of the channel by protein kinases and (2) direct binding of the drug to the channel. Protein kinase A (PKA)-mediated phosphorylation, represented by enhancement of the L-type current by β-adrenergic agonists [2–5], prevails in various physiological and pathophysiological processes that regulate

[1] Department of Physiology, Juntendo University, School of Medicine, Hongo, Bunkyo-ku, Tokyo 113, Japan
[2] Laboratory of Cellular Neurobiology, School of Life Science, Tokyo University of Pharmacy and Life Science, Tokyo 192-03, Japan

cardiac L-type channels. Acetylcholine [6,7] and adenosine [8–10] antagonize β-adrenoceptor agonist-induced activation of adenylate cyclase, resulting in inhibition of the L-type current. In addition to cyclic adenosine monophosphate (cAMP)-dependent regulation , nitric oxide (NO) has been shown to depress the L-type current via activation of cyclic guanosine monophesphate (cGMP)-dependent protein kinase G (PKG) [11,12]. Moreover, an increase in the intracellular concentration of Ca^{2+} augments the L-type current via calmodulin kinase activation [13]. In contrast to these physiological regulatory processes that proceed sequentially via multiple enzymatic reactions. 1,4-dihydropyridine (DHP) Ca^{2+} antagonists and agonists modulate L-type channels by binding to them directly. According to the modes hypothesis [14], DHP Ca^{2+} antagonists inhibit the L-type current by switching the mode of the L-type channel from normal (mode 1) to blank mode (mode 0). Single-channel recordings demonstrated that nitrendipine enhanced nonrandom occurrences of blank sweeps [15]. Conversely, DHP Ca^{2+} agonists switched the mode to a state with long openings (mode 2), thereby increasing the L-type current [2,14,16,17, but see 18]. Analysis of single-channel currents has shown that isoproterenol (ISO), a β-adrenoceptor agonist, at a low physiological concentration (10^{-7}M), increases the availability of the L-type channel (ratio of nonblank to total sweeps, Ps) accompanied by a small change in the open probability during nonblank sweeps (Po) [4]. However, higher concentrations of β-adrenoceptor agonists with a phosphodiesterase inhibitor, high concentrations of cAMP analogues [19], and high concentrations of okadaic acid [20], an inhibitor of phosphatases 1 and 2A, increase Po by inducing mode 2 openings. As the $α_1$-subunit, the major subunit of the L-type channel, possesses a multiple consensus sequence for PKA [21], it has been proposed that extensive phosphorylation produces made 2 sweeps, which result in an increase in Po [19,20]. Although the increase in L-type channel Ps [4] was almost large enough to explain the magnitude of the increase in the macroscopic L-type current in response to β-adrenoceptor stimulation, i.e., two- to fourfold in mammalian cardiac muscles [3], the Po increase could induce a proportionally much greater increase in the L-type current. Therefore, the mechanism responsible for regulating Po should be clarified. We used very high concentrations of ISO to investigate the effect of extensive phosphorylation on the L-type channel. In addition, we studied the influence of phosphorylation on the efficacy of the DHP Ca^{2+} agonist BAY K 8644 in producing long openings.

Methods and Definitions

Single Ca^{2+} channel currents were recorded from ventricular myocytes isolated enzymatically from guinea pigs using the cell-attached patch clamp technique [22]. The pipette solution contained (in mM): 100 $BaCl_2$, 5 2-[4-(2-hydroxyethyl)-1-piperazinyl ethanesulfonic acid (HEPES), and 0.03 tetrodotoxin; its pH was adjusted to 7.4 with tris(hydroxymethyl)-aminomethane. The cells were superfused with a high-K aspartate solution containing (in mM): 140 K aspartate, 1 $MgCl_2$, 1 O,O'-bis(2-aminoethyl) ethyleneglycol-N,N,N'-N'-tetraacetic acid (EGTA), 10 glucose, and 5 HEPES; its pH was adjusted to 7.4 with KOH. Isoproterenol was added to the superfusate and BAY K 8644 was added either to the superfusate or the pipette solution. The single-channel currents were filtered by a Bessel filter (96 dB/decade) with a cutoff frequency of 1 or 1.5 kHz. All the data were obtained from patches containing only one functionally active L-type channel. At least 500 depolarization steps, each with a duration of

100 ms, were applied at 2 Hz in the presence of each test solution. The experiments were conducted at room temperature (25°C). Statistical analyses were performed using Student's t-test for non-paired samples, with differences at $P < 0.05$ being considered significant. The whole-cell Ca current (I_{Ca}) was determined from the number of functional channels in the cell membrane (N), channel availability (Ps, ratio of current-containing to total sweeps), open probability for the total current-containing sweeps (Po) and unitary current amplitude (i_{Ca}) using the formula $I_{Ca} = N \cdot Ps \cdot Po \cdot i_{Ca}$. Using the open probability for the total duration of depolarization (Po*), including blank sweeps (Po* = Ps · Po), $I_{Ca} = N \cdot Po* \cdot i_{Ca}$.

Results

Effects of High Concentrations of Isoproterenol

To establish whether the ISO-induced changes of the single L-type Ca²⁺ channel current were concentration-dependent, the reagent was added to the superfusate cumulatively from low (10^{-9} M) to high (10^{-4} M) concentrations. Figures 1–3 show the results of a typical experiment. Fig. 1 shows 13 consecutive sweeps together with the mean currents from 500 or 1000 sweeps in the presence of each test solution. The mean current clearly increased in response to 10^{-8} M ISO and reached its maximal amplitude in the presence of 10^{-6} M. Increasing the concentration of ISO to 10^{-5} and 10^{-4} M did not result in further appreciable changes in the mean current. The efffect of ISO was gradually reduced by washing it out. Single Ba²⁺ currents occurred in bursts, the kinetics of which did not appear to be affected much by ISO. However, ISO reduced the number of blank seeeps (increased Ps). Long openings, a criterion for mode 2 activity, occurred in the control during the 8th sweep and in the presence of 10^{-7} and 10^{-6} M ISO during the 5th and 12th sweeps, respectively. Figure 2 shows the sweep-by-sweep changes of Po plotted sequentially versus the number of depolarizations up to 500. Isoprenaline reduced the number of nonrandomly appearing blank sweeps. The Po for the current-containing sweeps was variable, i.e., about 0.2 in the control; it increased from about 0.1 during the initial half and about 0.3 in the latter half of the depolarization procedure in the presence of 10^{-8} M ISO and was about 0.3 during the initial 300 sweeps in the presence of 10^{-6} M ISO. However, high-Po sweeps with a Po larger than 0.5 occurred rarely and sporadically.

The mean open time of each sweep (tm) was plotted versus the number of depolarizations (Fig. 3). The tm value was about 1 ms in the majority of nonblank sweeps and was affected little by ISO. Sweeps with a long tm occurred occasionally and those with tm longer than 3 ms are indicated by solid circles. Such long-tm sweeps occurred most often in the presence of 10^{-5} M ISO, but they did not occur consecutively as they did in the presence of a Ca²⁺ agonist. Therefore, the increase in the mean current, which is proportional to Po*, can be explained by the increase in Ps shown in the experiment illustrated in Figs. 1–3.

Figure 4 summarizes the dependence of Po*, Po, and Ps on the ISO concentration. The test potential was either 0 or 10 mV and the holding potential was −80 mV. The number of patches was 18 in the control experiment and 10 to 14 in the presence of ISO, except 10^{-9} M, when it was 6. The mean values ± SD were plotted versus the ISO concentration. In the control experiment, Po* was 0.042 ± 0.040, Po was 0.12 ± 0.07, and Ps was 0.36 ± 0.18. The control Po* was considerably lower than 1, indicating that the control L-type current could be enhanced as much as 20-fold as the result of an

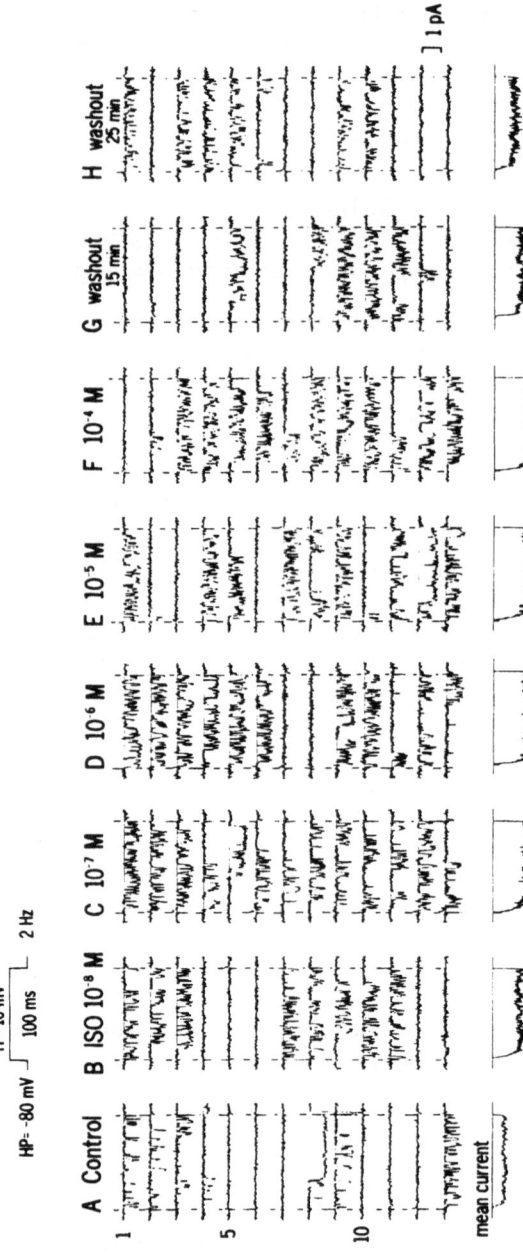

FIG. 1. Effects of high concentrations of isoproterenol (ISO) on single Ca²⁺ channel currents. The currents were recorded from a cell-attached patch using a 100-mM Ba²⁺-containing pipette, and repetitive 100 ms depolarization steps at 2 Hz were applied. Thirteen consecutive traces and the mean current obtained from 500 or 1000 sweeps in the presence of each solution are shown. The integrals of the mean current [proportional to the open probability for the total duration of depolarization (Po*)] normalized by the control value in B to H were: 2.24, 2.89, 2.93, 3.00, 2.93, 3.20, 2.12, and 1.57. The ratio of nonblank to total sweeps (Ps) values in A to H were: 0.30, 0.69, 0.71, 0.70, 0.73, 0.75, 0.46, and 0.53, respectively. HP, holding potential; TP, test potential

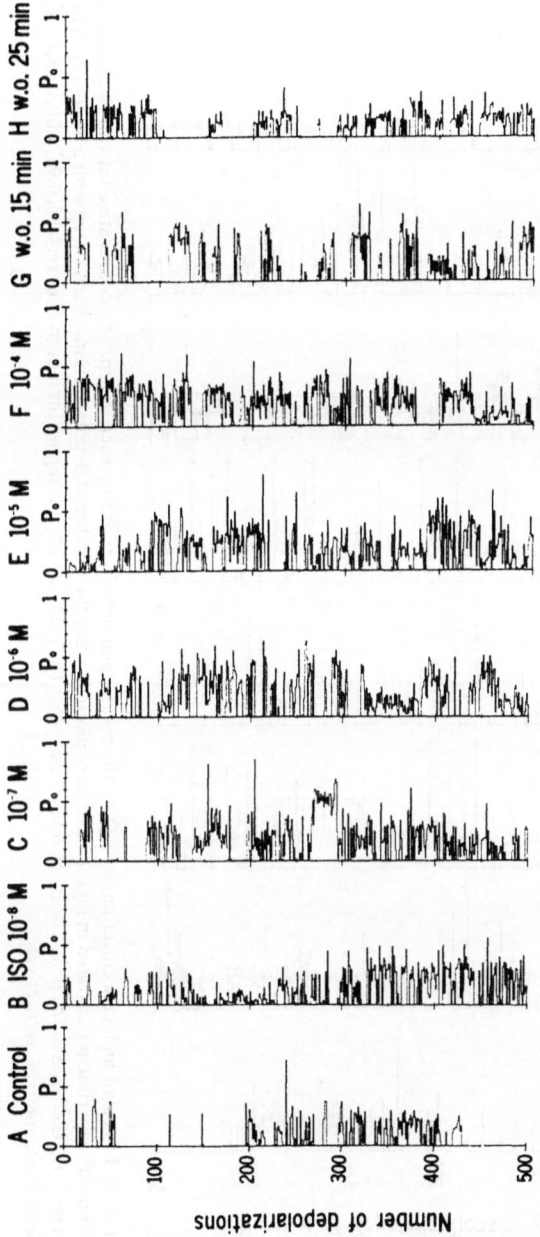

FIG. 2. Effects of high concentrations of ISO on the open probability (Po) during each sweep. The consecutive Po values obtained from the experiment illustrated in Fig. 1 plotted against the number of depolarizations are shown. The mean Po value of the current-containing sweeps in A to H were: 0.17, 0.17, 0.21, 0.22, 0.21, 0.22, 0.24, and 0.16, respectively. w.o., washout of ISO

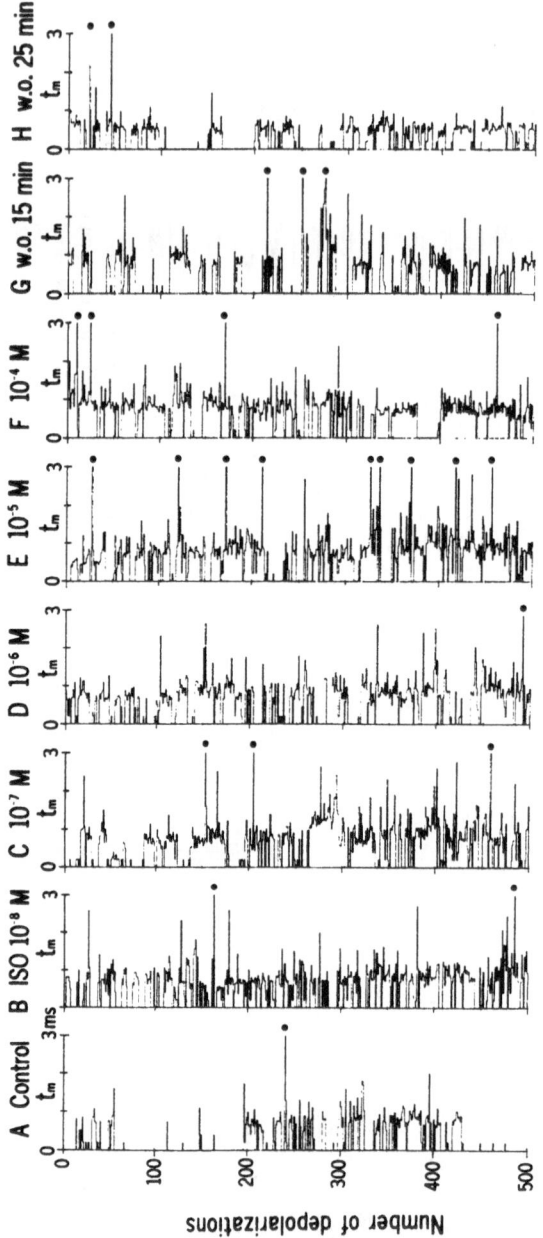

FIG. 3. Effects of high concentrations of ISO on the mean open time (*tm*) during each sweep. The consecutive tm values obtained from the experiment illustrated in Figs. 1 and 2 were plotted versus the number of depolarizations. Each sweep with a tm longer than 3 ms is marked by a *solid circle*. The mean open time values (*ms*) obtained by averaging tm in *A* to *H* were: 0.88, 0.94, 1.00, 0.93, 0.94, 0.89, 0.92, and 0.59, respectively

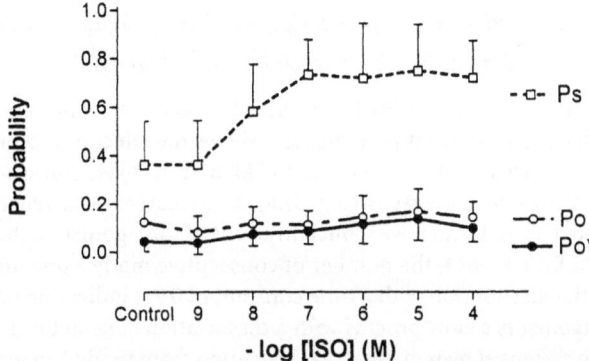

FIG. 4. Dependence of Ps, Po, and Po* on isoproterenol concentrations. Mean values ± SD of Ps (availability), Po (open probability during the current-containing sweeps), and Po* (= Ps · Po) from 18 patches are plotted versus ISO concentration. In comparison with the control values, Ps, Po*, and Po increased significantly in the presence of ISO in excess of 10^{-8}, 10^{-7}, and at 10^{-5} M, respectively. Note that Po, and consequently Po*, can be enhanced considerably by appropriate stimulation

increase in Po*. The respective mean values normalized by the control values in the presence of 10^{-9}, 10^{-8}, 10^{-7}, 10^{-6}, 10^{-5}, and 10^{-4} M ISO were Po*: 0.87, 1.72, 1.97, 2.67, 3.19, and 2.25; Po: 0.65, 0.94, 0.89, 1.17, 1.36, and 1.14 and Ps: 1, 1.60, 2.02, 1.98, 2.06, and 1.99. Therefore, Po* increased over twofold in the presence of ISO over 10^{-6} M. The Po* increases paralleled those of Ps, which increased twofold in the presence of ISO over 10^{-7} M. The Po change varied as the ISO concentration increased. However, it was necessary for Po to increase by 10%–20% in the presence of over 10^{-6} M ISO to increase Po* by 2.25- to 3.19-fold; in the presence of such a concentration, Ps increased twofold. The influence of extensive phosphorylation on the open time was evaluated by determining its influence on tm. After averaging the open times obtained from all the openings in each experiment, the tm ± SE values were 0.72 ± 0.10 ms in the control experiment and 0.72 ± 0.12, 0.72 ± 0.13, 0.79 ± 0.16, 0.78 ± 0.10, 0.87 ± 0.17 and 0.88 ± 0.19 ms in the presence of 10^{-9}, 10^{-8}, 10^{-7}, 10^{-6}, 10^{-5}, and 10^{-4} M ISO, respectively. The small increase in tm from 0.72 to 0.87 ms in the presence of 10^{-5} M ISO is sufficient to account for the increase in Po. Assuming that different gating patterns are distinguishable on a sweep-to-sweep basis, as they are with the slow state-transitions related to availability, the contribution of mode 2 openings to the increase in tm was evaluated by counting the number of sweeps with a long tm. In a large number of sweeps (ranging from 5710 to 12830), the percentage of sweeps with a tm longer than 3 ms was 0.19% in the control experiment and 0.24%, 0.33%, 0.21%, 0.68%, and 0.80% in the presence of 10^{-8}, 10^{-7}, 10^{-6}, 10^{-5}, and 10^{-4} M ISO, respectively. Therefore, this percentage was higher with 10^{-5} and 10^{-4} M ISO. However, these increases were too small to explain the increase in tm obtained from the total openings. As from Po of 0.12 and tm of 0.72 ms, the mean number of openings per sweep would be 17. Then, even if the open time of long-tm sweeps was 100 ms, as the increase in the percentage of long-tm sweeps with 10^{-4} M ISO was 0.61%, mean open time would only be expected to increase by 0.04 ms, far less than the actual increase in tm from 0.72 to 0.88 ms. Therefore, a sudden transition to the long open-time mode, like that which occurs in the presence of a DHP Ca²⁺ agonist, is not the major factor responsible for the increase in Po induced by high concentrations of ISO [23].

Increased Mode 2 Openings by Phosphorylation in the Presence of a DHP Ca^{2+} Agonist

By inducing mode 2 sweeps, 1,4-dihydropyridine Ca^{2+} agonists, represented by BAY K 8674, increase the L-type current [14]. Figure 5 shows the effect of ISO on the agonist action of BAY K 8644. In the presence of 10^{-6} M BAY K 8644, consecutive mode 2 sweeps occurred from 5 to 7 sweeps (Fig. 5Aa). Consecutive occurrences of mode 2 sweeps were also detected with lower concentrations of this agonist. In the presence of 2.10^{-8} and 10^{-7} M BAY K 8644, the number of consecutive mode 2 openings showed a single exponential distribution with a time constant of 0.7 s, indicating that the dissociation of this agonist is a slow process with a dissociation constant of $1.5 s^{-1}$. During the 9th and 10th sweeps shown in Fig. 5 Aa, transition from mode 1 to mode 2 sweeps occurred during the initial depolarization phase, suggesting that the binding of BAY K 8644 to the L-type channel is facilitated by depolarization. The addition of 10^{-6} M ISO in the presence of this Ca^{2+} agonist reduced the number of blank sweeps (mode 0) and increased Ps from 0.23 to 0.47. However, the mean current was increased mode by ISO than expected from the increase in Ps. The sequential plot of Po versus the number of depolarizations indicates that the large-Po sweeps corresponding to mode 2 sweeps occurred in the presence of BAY K 8644 with and without ISO, and that the mode 2 sweeps occurred more frequently with both agents than with BAY K 8644 alone (Fig. 5B), as reported previously [1].

Figure 6 summarizes the effect of ISO on Po during individual sweeps in the absence and presence of BAY K 8644. A further series of 15 experiments (not illustrated in Fig. 4) was carried out in which the control Po was 0.068, which was increased slightly to 0.087 by 10^{-7} M ISO (Fig. 6A,B). Clearly, high-Po sweeps occurred rarely in the absence of a Ca^{2+} agonist. In the presence of BAY K 8644, the distribution of Po became bimodal and another family of sweeps with a peak near Po = 1 appeared. In the presence of 10^{-7} or 10^{-6} M BAY K 8644 the Po value of 7 patches was 0.262 (mean from 5011 current-containing sweeps) (Fig. 6C). The addition of 10^{-6} M ISO increased the number of high-Po sweeps, resulting in a marked increase in Po to 0.440 (from 4756 sweeps). In the experiments in the presence of BAY K 8644 shown in Fig. 6C and D, tm was 2.88 ms ($n = 18210$) in the absence of 10^{-6} M ISO and 4.13 ms ($n = 33230$) in its presence. Therefore, the ISO-induced increase in Po in the presence of BAY K 8644 was due mainly to prolongation of the open time, i.e., enhancement of mode 2 activity.

Discussion

Single-channel studies have shown that β-adrenergic stimulation increases the open-state probability for the total duration of depolarization (Po*) of the L-type channel and thereby increases the macroscopic cardiac L-type current [1,2,5]. A similar mechanism is responsible for the cAMP-mediated increase in the L-type current of human atrial myocytes in the presence of 5-hydroxytryptamine [24]. The parameter Po* is determined by the availability (Ps) and open probability of current-containing sweeps (Po). β-Adrenoceptor agonists increase Ps, which was demonstrated by the slow-state transitions due to nonrandom occurrences of blank and nonblank sweeps [4,25]. The present study confirmed that an increase in Ps is the predominant factor that governs increases in Po*. In comparison with the control value of 0.36, Ps increased by 100% in response to ISO as in a previous study, whereas Po increased only by 10%–20% even in the presence of 10^{-5} and 10^{-4} M ISO. However, although

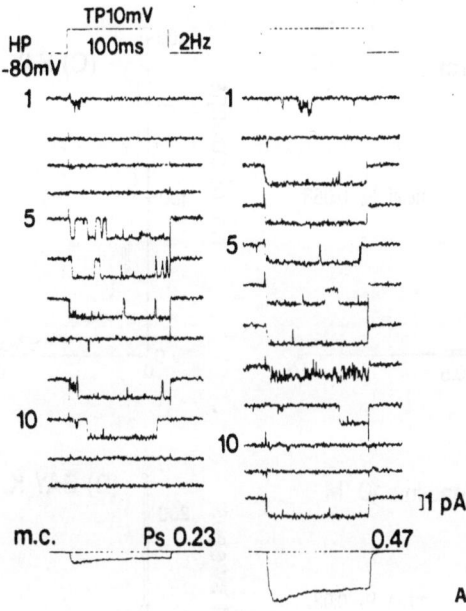

(a) BAY K 10⁻⁶M   (b) BAY+ISO 10⁻⁶M

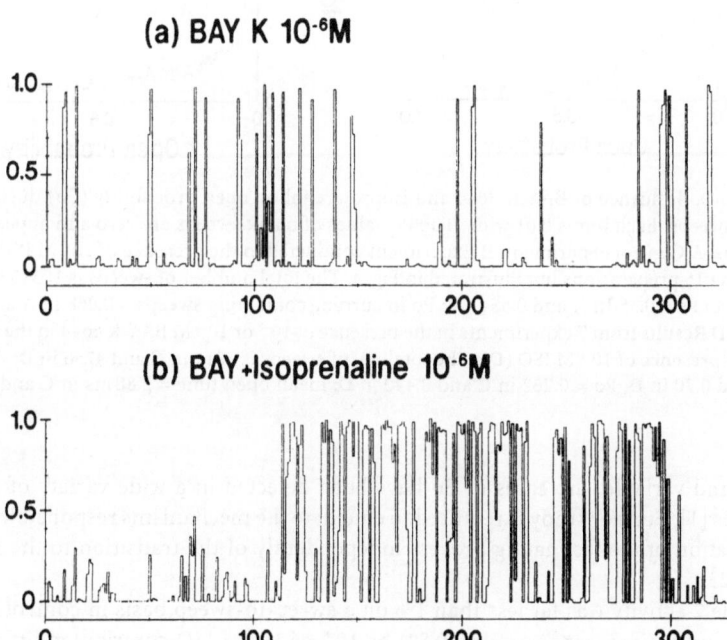

FIG. 5A,B. Effect of isoproterenol on single-channel currents in the presence of BAY K 8644. A Specimen records and mean current (*m.c.*) from 1000 (*a*) and 900 (*b*) sweeps. Note the mean current was increased by ISO more than the increase expected as a result of the increase in Ps. B Sequential plots of Po versus the number of depolarizations. *HP*, holding potential; *TP*, test potential

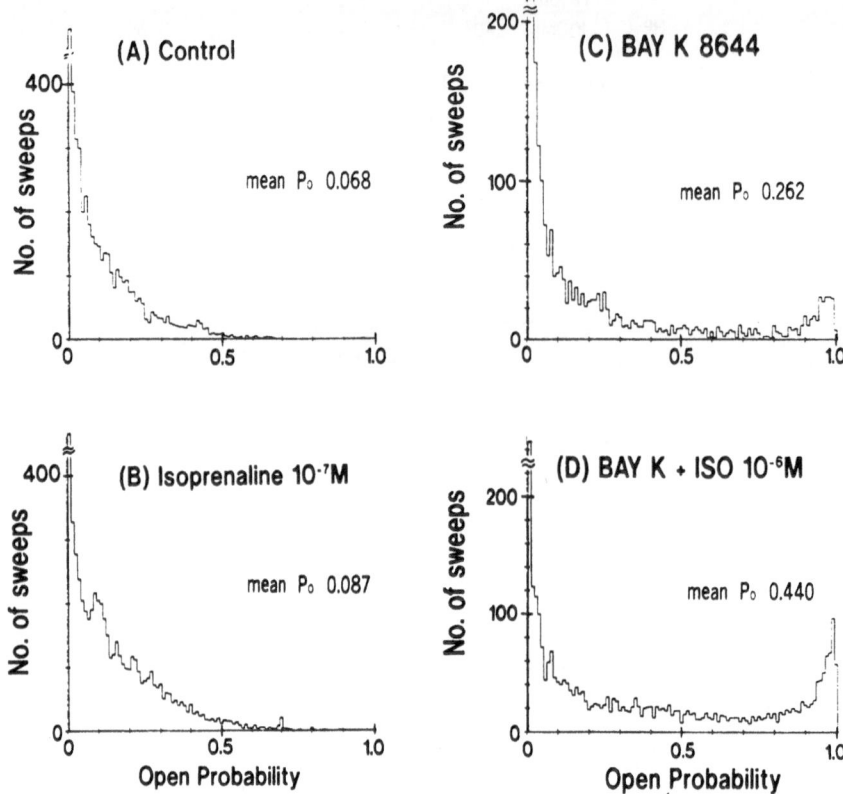

FIG. 6A–D. Influence of BAY K 8644 and isoproterenol on open probability (Po) during individual sweeps. Each bin is 0.01 wide. The Po values of blank sweeps are zero and appear in the first bins. A Control experiment. B Experiment conducted in the presence of 10^{-7} M ISO carried out using 15 preparations not illustrated in Fig. 4. The total number of sweeps is 10315 in A and 9038 in B; Ps = 0.35 In A and 0.55 in B; Po in current-containing sweeps = 0.068 in A and 0.087 in B. C, D Results from 7 experiments in the presence of 10^{-7} or 10^{-6} M BAY K 8644 in the absence (C) and presence of 10^{-6} M ISO (D). The total no. of sweeps is 5011 in C and 4756 in D; Ps = 0.47 in C and 0.70 in D; Po = 0.262 in C and 0.440 in D; mean open time = 2.88 ms in C and 4.13 ms in D

small and variable, increases in Po have been detected in a wide variety of cardiac muscles [1]. Further study is required to elucidate the mechanisms responsible for the modulation of the fast gating process independently of the transition to the mode 2 state [23].

Mode 2 activity was far less than 1% on a sweep-to-sweep basis in control experiments and its increase to around 0.8% by 10^{-5} or 10^{-4} M ISO contributed little to the ISO-induced increase in Po of guinea pig isolated ventricular cells superfused with Ca^{2+}-free high K^+ solution. Hitherto, mode 2 activity has been induced in the absence of a Ca^{2+} agonist by 2.10^{-6} M ISO with 2.10^{-5} M isobutylmethylxanthine, 4 mM 8-Br-cAMP [19], and 10^{-5}-$7.5.10^{-4}$ M okadaic acid [20]. As demonstrated by the high-Po values of 0.26 in the absence of ISO and 0.44 in its presence observed with BAY K 8644-treated myocytes, marked increases in Po are evoked by mode 2 openings. Mode 2 activity can be an important mechanism that increases the L-type current under some circumstances. The effect of PKA-mediated activation on mode 2 activity may be modulated by the intracellular Ca^{2+} concentration via activation of other kinases. Moreover, in view of the modulation of DHP Ca^{2+} agonist action by β-adrenoceptor stimulation we observed, we speculate that the binding of intrinsic agonist-like messengers to DHP receptors produced under as yet unidentified conditions is facilitated by phosphorylation, which induces mode 2 activity of single cardiace L-type channels of guinea pig ventricular muscle.

Acknowledgment. This work was supported by Grants-in-Aid for Scientific Research from the Japanese Ministry of Education, Science and Culture.

References

1. McDonald TF, Pelzer S, Trautwein W, Pelzer DJ (1994) Regulation and modulation of calcium channels in cardiac, skeletal, and smooth muscle cells. Physiol Rev 74:365–507
2. Tsien RW, Bean BP, Hess P, Lansman JB, Nilius B, Nowycky MC (1986) Mechanism of calcium channel modulation by β-adrenergic agents and dihydropyridine calcium agonists. J Mol Cell Cardiol 18:691–710
3. Kameyama M, Hofmann F, Trautwein W (1985) On the mechanism of β-adrenergic regulation of the Ca channel in the guinea pig heart. Pflügers Arch 405:285–293
4. Ochi R, Kawashima Y (1990) Modulation of slow gating process of calcium channels by isoprenaline in guinea pig ventricular cells. J Physiol (Lond) 424:187–204
5. Ochi R (1993) Single-channel mechanism of β-adrenergic enhancement of cardiac L-type calcium current. Jpn J Physiol 43:571–584
6. Ochi R (1981) Decrease in calcium conductance by acetylcholine in mammalian ventricular muscle. In: Ohnishi ST, Endo M (eds) The mechanism of gated calcium transport across biological membranes. Academic, New York, pp 79–86
7. Hescheler J, Kameyama M, Trautwein W (1986) On the mechanism of muscarinic inhibition of the cardiac Ca current. Pflügers Arch 407:182–189
8. Belardinelli L, Isenberg G (1983) Actions of adenosine and isoproterenol on isolated mammalian ventricular myocytes. Circ Res 53:287–297
9. Kato M, Yamaguchi H, Ochi R (1990) Mechanism of adenosine-induced inhibition of calcium current in guinea pig ventricular cells. Circ Res 67:1134–1141
10. Jahnel U, Nawrath H, Ochi R (1992) Adrenoceptor-mediated effects on calcium channel currents are antagonized by 5'-(N-ethyl)-carboxamide-adenosine in guinea pig atrial cells. Naunyn Schmiedebergs Arch Pharmacol 345:564–569
11. Mery PF, Lohmann SM, Walter U, Fischmeister R (1991) Ca^{2+} current is regulated by cyclic GMP-dependent protein kinase in mammalian cardiac myocytes. Proc Natl Sci 88:1197–1201
12. Wahler GM, Dollinger S (1995) Nitric oxide donor SIN-1 inhibits mammalian cardiac calcium current through cGMP-dependent protein kinase. Am J Physiol 268:C45–C54
13. Anderson ME, Braun AP, Schulman H, Premack BA (1994) Multifunctional Ca^{2+} calmodulin-dependent protein kinase mediates Ca^{2+}-induced enhancement of the L-type Ca^{2+} current in rabbit ventricular myocytes. Circ Res 75:854–861
14. Hess P, Lansman JB, Tsien RW (1984) Different modes of Ca channel gating behaviour favoured by dihydropyridine Ca agonists and antagonists. Nature 31:538–544
15. Kawashima Y, Ochi R (1988) Voltage-dependent decrease in the availability of single calcium channels by nitrendipine in guinea-pig ventricular cells. J Physiol (Lond) 402:219–235
16. Ochi R, Hino N, Niimi Y (1984) Prolongation of calcium channel open time by the dihydropyridine derivative BAY K 8644 in cardiac myocytes. Proc Jpn Acad 60:153–1567
17. Kokubun S, Reuter H (1984) Dihydropyridine derivatives prolong the open state of Ca channels in cultured cardiac cells. Proc Natl Acad Sci USA 81:4824–4827

18. Lacerda AE, Brown AM (1989) Nonmodal gating of cardiac calcium channels as revealed by dihydropyridines. J Gen Physiol 93:1243–1273
19. Yue DT, Herzig S, Marban E (1990) β-adrenergic stimulation of calcium channels occurs by potentiation of high-activity gating mode. Proc Natl Acad Sci USA 87:753–757
20. Ono K, Fozzard HA (1993) Two phosphatase sites on the Ca^{2+} channel affecting different kinetic functions. J Physiol (Lond) 470:73–84
21. Mikami A, Imoto K, Tanabe T, Niidome T, Mori Y, Takeshima H, Narumiya S, Numa S (1989) Primary structure and functional expression of the cardiac dihydropyridine-sensitive calcium channel. Nature 340:230–233
22. Hamill OP, Marty A, Neher E, Sakmann B, Sigworth FJ (1981) Improved patch clamp techniques for high resolution current recording from cells and cell-free membrane patches. Pflügers Arch 391:85–100
23. Hirano Y, Suzuki K, Yamawake N, Hiraoka M (1994) Multiple kinetic effects of β-adrenergic stimulation on single cardiac L-type Ca channels. Am J Physiol 266:C1714–C1721
24. Jahnel U, Nawrath H, Rupp J, Ochi R (1993) L-type calcium channel activity in human atrial myocytes as influenced by 5-HT. Naunyn Schmiedebergs Arch Pharmacol 348:396–402
25. Herzig S, Patil P, Neumann J, Staschen C-M, Yue D (1993) Mechanisms of β-adrenergic stimulation of cardiac Ca^{2+} channels revealed by discrete-time Markov analysis of slow gating. Biophys J 65:1599–1612

Molecular Mechanism by Which the Cardiac SR Ca Pump is Regulated

MICHIHIKO TADA and TOSHIHIKO TOYOFUKU

Summary. Cardiac Ca ATPase (SERCA2) regulates intracellular Ca levels by pumping Ca into the sarcoplasmic reticulum (SR). The Ca ATPase activity of cardiac SR is regulated through protein kinase-catalyzed phosphorylation of phospholamban, which is expressed in cardiac myocytes and in slow skeletal and smooth muscles. Phospholamban is observed as a homopentamer, formed from subunits of 6080 Da. Cyclic adenosine monophosphate (cAMP)-dependent protein kinase (PKA)- and Ca/calmodulin-dependent protein kinase-catalyzed phosphorylation residues (Ser 16 and Thr 17) are located in the N-terminal cytoplasmic domain, whereas the C-terminal 22 residues are extremely hydrophobic and are considered to be embedded in the membrane. Phospholamban functions as an inhibitory cofactor for Ca ATPase through a direct protein-protein interaction. PKA-catalyzed phosphorylation of Ser 16 resulted in the dissociation of phospholamban from Ca ATPase, thus augmenting the ATPase activity. To define the molecular mode of interaction between two proteins, interaction sites have been identified by using biochemical and molecular biological techniques. Six residues of SERCA2, Lys-Asp-Asp-Lys-Pro-Val402, were found to be important for interaction with phospholamban. On the other hand, the hydrophilic cytoplasmic portion of phospholamban contains potential binding sites with SERCA2, while the hydrophobic transmembrane portion is also required for the fully functional interaction. Molecular interaction between two proteins therefore appears to occur in a dual mode.

Key words. Ca ATPase—Calcium—Cardiac sarcoplasmic reticulum—cAMP-dependent protein kinase—Phospholamban

Introduction

The level of intracellular Ca has a crucial role in the biological events inside the cell. In muscle cells, depolarization of the sarcolemmal membrane (SL) opens the dihydropyridine-sensitive Ca channel. The Ca ion, which enters the cell through the channel, triggers Ca release from the sarcoplasmic reticulum (SR) through the Ca release channel (ryanodine receptor), leading to muscle contraction. Ca ATPase in

Department of Medicine and Pathophysiology, Osaka University, School of Medicine, Suita, Osaka 565, Japan

the SR transports cytoplasmic Ca into the SR lumen to reduce the intracellular Ca concentration, resulting in muscle relaxation. In cardiac muscle cells, Ca uptake by cardiac Ca ATPase (SERCA2) is regulated by another SR protein, termed phospholamban. Phospholamban is expressed in cardiac, slow-twitch skeletal, and smooth muscle, and is colocalized with SERCA2 [1,2]. Under β-adrenergic stimulation, phospholamban is phosphorylated by cyclic adenosine monophosphate (cAMP)-dependent protein kinase, resulting in the stimulation the Ca-dependent ATPase activity of the Ca pump. This process can account for the positive inotropic effects of β-adrenergic stimulation on the heart. This article reviews several features of the phospholamban-Ca ATPase system, leading to the important notion that a protein-protein interaction between these SR proteins can modulate Ca signaling in cardiac muscle, resulting in control of myocardial contractility.

Effects of Phospholamban Phosphorylation on the Reaction Sequence of SR Ca ATPase

It has been demonstrated that cAMP-dependent phosphorylation of phospholamban enhances Ca uptake and Ca-dependent ATPase activity by the cardiac SR [3,4]. Since the Ca transport cycle of Ca ATPase contains a series of kinetic steps, it was of great interest to identify which steps of the Ca transport cycle are regulated by phospholamban.

Kinetic studies indicate a complex series of intermediate reaction steps in the Ca ATPase reaction cycle that involve the sequential formation and degradation of phosphorylated intermediates (EP) [5]. During the transport cycle, the ATPase enzyme undergoes distinct conformational changes. The enzyme can exist in two different conformational states, E_1 and E_2, which exhibit different affinities for Ca [6]. The E_1 form has a high affinity for Ca, and the E_2 form has a low affinity. The phosphorylated intermediate EP was also shown to exhibit two comparable forms, E_1P and E_2P. In the physiological state, Ca ATPase translocates Ca according to the reaction sequence shown by the equation in Fig. 1 [7], where i and o refer to the inside- and outside-oriented configuration of the SR membrane, respectively. In this reac-

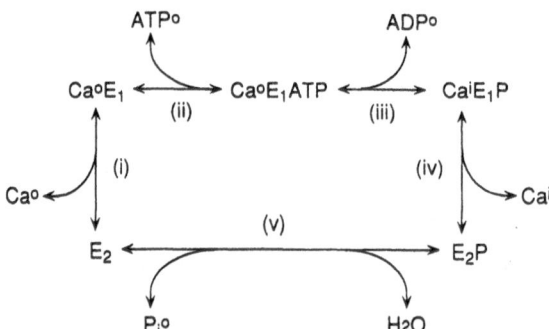

FIG. 1. Reaction sequence according to which Ca ATPase translocates Ca. i, inside-oriented and o, outside-oriented configuration of the sarcoplasmic reticulum (SR) membrane; steps (i) and (iv), rate-limiting steps

tion, conversions of E_2 to E_1 and E_1P to E_2P (steps (i) and (iv)) are the rate-limiting steps [7].

Phosphorylation of phospholamban enhances ATPase activity and Ca uptake activity by increasing the Ca affinity of Ca ATPase [3,4]. This activation of the ATPase reaction is due to the acceleration of the enzyme reaction turnover [8,9]. Presteady-state kinetic studies have revealed that the two rate-limiting steps, steps (i) and (iv), are accelerated by phospholamban phosphorylation [10,11]. These correspond to the conformational transition steps of the ATPase enzyme, suggesting that phospholamban exerts its action by regulating the cation-induced conformational change of the ATPase molecule.

Molecular Structure of Phospholamban

Phospholamban has been demonstrated to exist as an oligomer in either native or purified form. Even in the presence of a strong detergent such as sodium dodecyl sulfate (SDS), the phospholamban protein still remained an oligomer at a temperature below 50°C, and became a monomer in a temperature-dependent manner [12]. The molecular weight of phospholamban oligomer was 27 kDa, and that of monomer was 6 kDa, based on the mobility on SDS-polyacrylamide gel of Laemmli's system. By phosphorylation of cardiac SR, the mobility of phospholamban was decreased on SDS polyacrylamide gels. The pattern of temperature-dependent and phosphorylation-dependent mobility shift suggested that phospholamban is a pentamer composed of five identical monomers [13]. The application of a low-angle laser light scattering technique showed that the molecular weight of phospholamban oligomer is 30 400 Da, indicating that phospholamban is a pentamer [14].

Purification of canine phospholamban [15,16] and its cDNA sequencing [17-19] have revealed its molecular structure. The amino acid sequence of phospholamban, deduced from the nucleotide sequence, is 52 amino acids long, which corresponds to the calculated molecular weight of 6080 Da [17,19]. Fig. 2 shows that the amino acid sequences of phospholamban deduced from the cDNA nucleotide sequence are well conserved among several species, including humans [2,19-22]. Since phospholamban is encoded by only one gene which is located on human chromosome 6 [20], the oligomer should be composed of five identical monomers (homopentamer).

Hydropathy plots have suggested that this peptide is an amphipathic peptide; the NH$_2$-terminal half (Met1 to Asn 30, named domain I) is hydrophilic, whereas the COOH-terminal half (Leu 31 to Leu 52, named domain II) is extremely hydrophobic. As shown in Fig. 3, domain I is exposed at the cytoplasmic surface, whereas domain II is embedded within the SR membrane [23]. Analysis of the predicted secondary

```
Human     MEKVQYLTRSAIRRASTIEMPQQARQKLQNLFINFCLILICLLLICIIVMLL
Rabbit    *E****L****I*******MPQ****N**N**I*******************
Dog       *D****L****I*******MPQ****N**N**I*******************
Pig       *D****I****I*******MPQ****N**N**I*******************
Chicken   *E****I****L*******VNP****R**E**V*******************
```

FIG. 2. Comparison of amino acid sequences of phospholamban monomer in human, dog, pig, and chicken [4,19-22]. Residues are represented by the one-letter code. Identical residues among these five species except for the human sequence are shown as *asterisks*

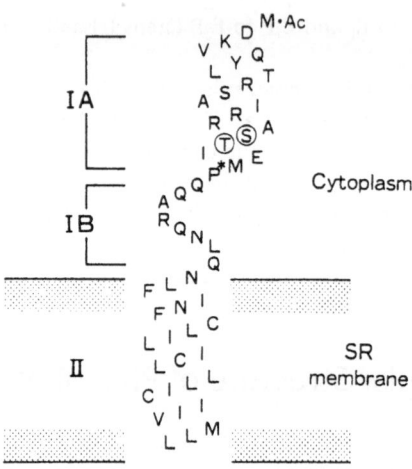

FIG. 3. Secondary structure of canine phospholamban monomer [23]. The two α-helices, domain IA and domain II, are connected by domain IB, which forms a random structure. Domain I is exposed at the cytoplasmic surface, whereas domain II is anchored in the sarcoplasmic reticulum (SR) membrane. The circled residues S and T represent Ser16 and Thr17, which are phosphorylated by cyclic adenosine monophosphate (cAMP)-dependent and Ca/calmodulin-dependent protein kinase, respectively. The asterisk indicates the helix-braking Pro21

structure indicated that this molecule is rich in alpha helix; two helices (domain IA and II) are connected by less structured domain IB. Secondary structure analysis using circular dichroism also supports this structural prediction [24].

Domain I contains specific phosphorylation sites; cAMP-dependent protein kinase phosphorylated Ser 16, and Ca/calmodulin-dependent protein kinase phosphorylated Thr17 [18,25]. Two Arg residues, Arg13 and 14, adjacent to the two phosphorylatable residues were proven to be essential for phosphorylation [25], in accordance with the consensus sequence for protein kinase substrate.

Domain II should contain the key amino acid for oligomeric organization, because the tryptic digestion product of phospholamban, which is devoid of the cytoplasmic portion, remained pentameric [13]. In the intramembrane domain, three Cys residues lie at every five residues (Cys 36, 41, and 46), suggesting that the neighboring domain II could form an oligomer by disulfide bonds between each Cys residues. By site-directed mutagenesis techniques [25], replacement of one or more of these Cys residues reduced the stability of phospholamban oligomer; the mutants dissociated to protomers at a lower temperature than did the wild-type oligomer (Fig. 4). In particular, Cys 41 is important in stabilizing the oligomeric structure. However, these Cys residues in the neighboring monomers could not form disulfide bonds for oligomer formation, because these Cys residues existed as free SH groups [18]. Instead, formation of hydrogen bonds between neighboring Cys residues is probably responsible for pentamer structure formation. The fact that the mutant in which Cys was replaced by Ala does exist as an oligomer at ambient temperature supports this idea. The size, hydrophobicity, and polarity of the side chain of Cys residues probably match the microenvironment, allowing the hydrophobic residues in neighboring helices to create optimal stabilizing forces in the SR membrane.

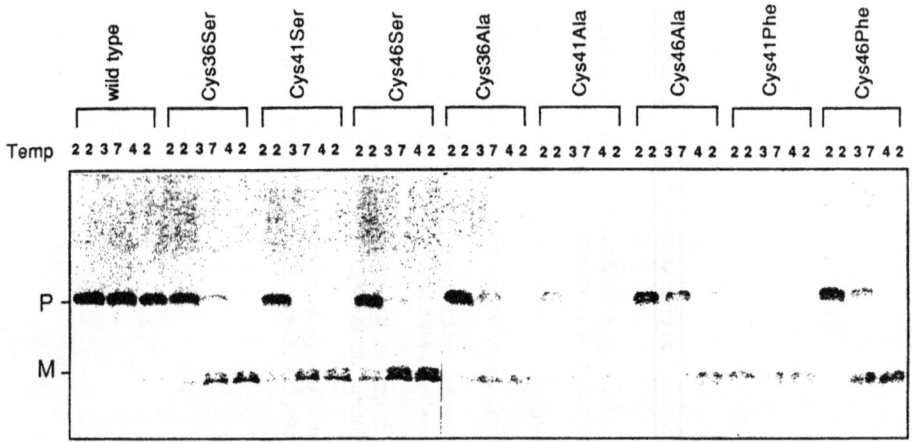

FIG. 4. Thermal stability of phospholamban mutated in transmembrane Cys [25] residues. The microsomal fraction from COS-1 cells transiently expressing phospholamban protein mutant in Cys residues was preincubated with sodium dodecyl sulfate-polyacrylamide gel electrophoresis (SDS-PAGE) loading buffer at 22°, 37°, and 42°C for 2 min and separated in 13.5% SDS-PAGE. They were immunoblotted with monoclonal antibody A1. *Temp*, preincubation temperature; *M*, monomeric; *P*, pentameric forms of phospholamban

Molecular Interaction Between SR Ca ATPase and Phospholamban

Phospholamban-Interacting Site of Ca ATPase

An experiment using a cross-linking agent demonstrated a direct interaction between the two SR proteins, Ca ATPase and phospholamban [26]. The Lys residue of purified phospholamban (Lys3) was conjugated with Denny-Jaffe cross-linking reagent. Light activation of conjugated phospholamban incubated with purified Ca ATPase from cardiac muscle resulted in the formation of a complex only when phospholamban was at the unphosphorylated state and the Ca ATPase was at the Ca-free state (E_2 conformation). The domain of the ATPase that interacts with phospholamban was identified by sequencing the photoaffinity-labeled peptide. This peptide, whose two Lys residues (Lys 397 and Lys 400) were labeled, was found to originate in a region that is just six amino acids on the COOH-terminal side of the phosphorylation domain (Fig. 5). The amino acid sequence in the phosphorylation site among cation-transporting ATPase shares a high degree of homology, whereas the putative phospholamban binding domain is present only in SR-type ATPase, especially SERCA1 and 2, but not SERCA3, neither in SR-type ATPase nor in other plasma membrane ATPases.

The functional significance of this sequence for phospholamban interaction is confirmed by the following studies: the in vitro coexpression system of two proteins in heterogeneous cells showed that phospholamban interacts with SERCA1 and SERCA2, but not SERCA3, and that chimeric Ca^{2+}-ATPase between SERCA2 and SERCA3 containing the phosphorylation and the nucleotide binding domains of SERCA2 interacts with phospholamban [27]; mutant Ca^{2+}-ATPase with replacement of amino acid residues in this sequence showed that six serial amino acid residues,

Phospholamban-binding peptide

		FILDKVDGETCSLNEFTITGSTYAPIGEVHKDDKPVKCHQTDGLVELATICALCNDSALDYNE	AKGVYEKVGWATE
Ca (SR)			
SERCA1	LGCTSVICSDKTGTLTTNQ	MSVCKMFIIDKVDGDFCSLNEFSITGSTYAPEGEVLKNDKPIRSGQFDGLVELATICALCNDSSLDYNE	TKGVYEKVGEATE
SERCA2	LGCTSVICSDKTGTLTTNQ	MSVCRMFIILDKVDGETCSLNEFTITGSTYAPIGEVHKDDKPVKCHQTDGLVELATICALCNDSALDYNE	AKGVYEKVGWATE
SERCA3	LGCTSVICSDKTGTLTTNQ	MSVCRMFVVAEAEAGACRLHEFTISGTTYTPEGEVRQGEQLVRCCQFDGLVELATICALCNDSSLDYNE	TKGVYEKVGEATE
Ca (PM)	MGNATAICSDKTGTLTMNR	MTVVQAYINEK HY KKVPEPEAT PPNILSYL VYGISVNCA YTSKILPPEK	EGGLPRHVGNKTE
Na/K	LGSTSTICSDKTGTLTQNQ	MTVAHMWFDNQIHEADTTENQ SGVSFDKTSATWLALSRIAGLCNRAVFQANQDNLPILKRAVAGDASE	
	LGSTSTICSDKTGTLTQNQ	MTVAHMWFDNQIHEADTTENQ SGISFDKTSLSWNALSRIAALCNRAVFQAGQDSVPILKISVAGDASE	
H	MSGVNMLCSDKTGTLTKNK	MEIQEQCFTFEEG NDLKSTLVLAALAAKWREPPRDALDTMVLGAADLDE	
	LAGVEILCSDKTGTLTKNK	LSLHEIYTVEGVD PDDLMLTAPLAASRKKKGLDAIDKAFLKSLKQYPKAK	
K	AGDVDLLLDKTGTITLGN	RQASEFIPAQGVD EKTLADAAQLASLADETPEGRSIVILAKQRFNLRER	
	ANDLDVIMLDKTGTLTQGN	FTVTGIELD EAYQEEEILKYIGALEAHANHPLAIGIM NYLKEK	

Phosphorylation Domain

Lys-Asp-Asp-Lys-Pro-Val402, in this sequence are especially important for the functional interaction [28]; and a synthetic peptide covering this sequence was able to compete for phospholamban with cardiac Ca^{2+}-ATPase [29]. The finding that the phospholamban-binding domain exists in close proximity to the active phosphorylation site of Ca ATPase (Asp 351) suggests that binding of phospholamban to this site could have significant effects on steps involving phosphorylation of Ca ATPase.

Ca^{2+} ATPase-Interacting Site of Phospholamban

Antiphospholamban monoclonal antibody A1, the epitope that was identified as a region involving Arg9, enhances the Ca uptake of cardiac SR vesicles [30–32]. The antibody activated the Ca uptake and ATPase activity by increasing the affinity for Ca. Phospholamban coexpressed with slow/cardiac Ca ATPase in heterogeneous cells diminished the affinity of the ATPase for Ca [33]. These results support the direct protein-protein interaction of two proteins.

Mutant phospholamban with replacement of amino acid residues in domain I showed that not only the positively and negatively charged side chain but also the hydrophobic side chain of amino acid residues in domain IA of phospholamban are involved in this interaction [33], which is summarized in Fig. 6A. On the basis of the predicted structural model of domain IA (Fig. 6B), charged amino acid residues are clustered on one side of an α-helical wheel, while hydrophobic residues are on the other side. As the hydrophobic interaction has been proposed to be a major factor in protein-protein interaction in general [34], this hydrophobic surface could possibly interact with a reciprocal hydrophobic surface on SERCA2. The hydrophilic surface was also found to contribute to the interaction by virtue of the appropriate formation of electrostatic contacts, which has been proposed previously [35,36]. Thus, if the cytoplasmic domain IA formed an amphiphatic α-helix, it could fit compactly into a complimentary pocket in its interaction with SERCA2, thereby accounting for the hydrophobic and electrostatic contributions to the interaction between two proteins. Together with evidence that a phospholamban-interacting site exists in the unique sequence near the phosphorylation site (Asp351) of Ca^{2+}-ATPase, the cytoplasmic part of phospholamban has been revealed to play an important role in the functional interaction with SERCA2.

FIG. 5. The amino acid sequence of the cross-linked peptides obtained from rabbit cardiac SR ATPase and from canine fast skeletal muscle SR ATPase is aligned with homologous regions in other sequences [26]. Phospholamban was conjugated with ^{125}I-labeled Denny-Jaffe reagent. Light activation of conjugated phospholamban incubated with purified ATPase resulted in the formation of a complex. The phospholamban-ATPase complex was cleaved at azo linkage sodium dithionite. This cleavage leaves the ^{125}I-label attached to the domain that interacts with phospholamban. The ATPase was then digested with CNBr and fractionated using reverse-phase high-performance liquid chromatography (HPLC) followed by ion exchange column chromatography. The ^{125}I-labeled peptides were sequenced. Two *arrows* indicate the lysine residues where the cross-linking reagent became bound. Each *horizontal line* represents the following ATPase sequences, from *top* to *bottom*: rabbit fast-twitch muscle SR Ca ATPase (*SERCA1*), rabbit slow-twitch/cardiac muscle SR Ca ATPase (*SERCA2*), rabbit organellar SR Ca ATPase (*SERCA3*), human plasma membrane Ca ATPase [*Ca(PM)*], sheep plasma membrane Na/K ATPase (*Na/K*), torpedo plasma membrane Na/K ATPase (*Na/K*), *Saccharomyces cerevisiae* H ATPase (*H*), *Escherichia coli* K ATPase (*K*), and *Streptococcus faecalis* K ATPase (*K*)

(A)   **(B)**

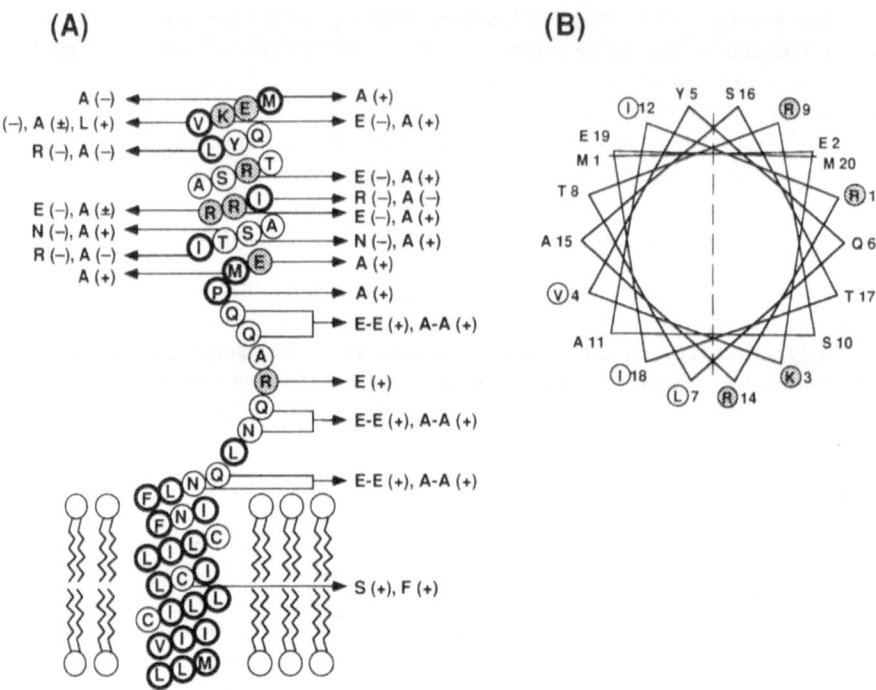

FIG. 6A,B. Structure and function of phospholamban. A Summary of phospholamban mutation [33]. Replacement of amino acid residues of phospholamban was performed by oligonucleotide-directed mutagenesis. Each mutant phospholamban cDNA was cotransfected with SERCA2 cDNA into heterogeneous cells, and microsomes were prepared from the transfected cells and used for the Ca-dependent Ca uptake assays. Effects of mutant phospholamban on Ca uptake of SERCA2 were compared with that of wild-type phospholamban. Mutant proteins with changes in charged and hydrophobic amino acids of E2 to I18 lost the function, whereas mutants with changes of E19 to N30, and C41 retained the function. B α-helical wheel analysis of NH$_2$-terminal residues (M1 to M20) of phospholamban. *Shaded circles*, charged amino acid; *open circles*, hydrophobic amino acid; (+), retention of phospholamban inhibitory effect; (−), loss of phospholamban inhibitory effect; (±) partial loss of phospholamban inhibitory effect

An experiment brought about by the reconstitution of synthesized phospholamban peptides and purified Ca^{2+}-ATPase addressed the new aspects of a protein-protein interaction between two proteins [37,38]. The peptide corresponding to 25 amino acid residues from the NH$_2$-terminus (Met 1 to Arg 25) inhibited Ca uptake, and this inhibition was diminished by phosphorylation of the peptide. Our recent experiments [38] have shown that the synthetic peptide corresponding to domain I of phospholamban (Met 1 to Asn 31) inhibits purified cardiac SR Ca ATPase activity in a dose-dependent manner, and this inhibition is diminished by phosphorylation of the peptide. However, the affinity of ATPase activity for Ca was not changed by these maneuvers (Fig. 7), suggesting that this peptide affected only the V_{max} of Ca ATPase activity. On the other hand, peptides containing domain II, the intramembrane portion of phospholamban, decreased the Ca affinity of ATPase, and phosphorylation of the peptide relieved this inhibitory effect (Fig. 8). These results are summarized in Table 1.

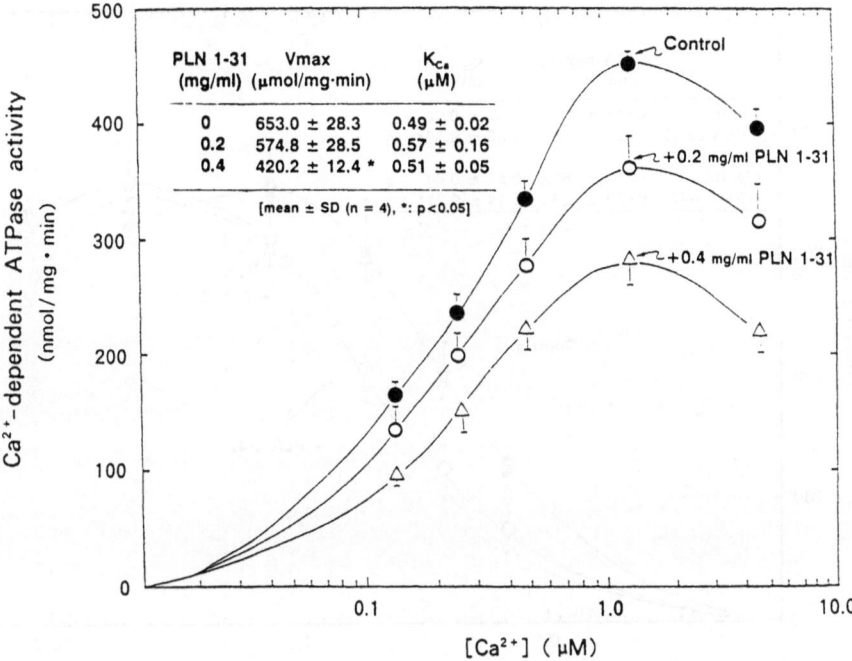

FIG. 7. Effects of the synthetic phospholamban peptide corresponding to the cytoplasmic portion (*PLN 1-31*) on purified Ca ATPase [38]. Purified Ca ATPase was preincubated with (*open circles, triangles*) or without (*solid circles*) PLN 1-31 at 25°C for 10 min; then the samples were subjected to the ATPase assay. The final concentration of purified ATPase in the assay medium was 40 µg of protein/ml and those of PLN 1-31 were 0.2 mg/ml (*open circles*) and 0.4 mg/ml (*triangles*). The results are the mean ± SD of four different experiments

TABLE 1. Effects of phospholamban peptides on reconstituted cardiac SR Ca pump ATPase activity.

Peptides	Molar ratio[a]	n	V_{max} (nmol/mg per min)	K_{Ca} (µM)
Control		4	653.0 ± 28.3	0.49 ± 0.02
+PLN 1-31	[330]	4	420.2 ± 12.4[b]	0.51 ± 0.05
Control		3	634.5 ± 112.4	0.52 ± 0.02
+PLN 28-47	[100]	3	657.7 ± 43.5	1.33 ± 0.30[b]
Control		4	627.8 ± 63.6	0.51 ± 0.04
+PLN 8-47	[100]	3	625.3 ± 51.8	1.18 ± 0.20[b]
+PLN 8-47-P	[100]	3	669.0 ± 68.4	0.72 ± 0.09

SR, sarcoplasmic reticulum; PLN 1-31, NH_2-terminal hydrophilic domain; PLN 28-47 and PLN 8-47, COOH-terminal hydrophobic sequence.
Data are expressed as mean ± SD. Data from [38].
[a] Between peptides and ATPase.
[b] $P < 0.05$ *vs* control by unpaired *t*-test.

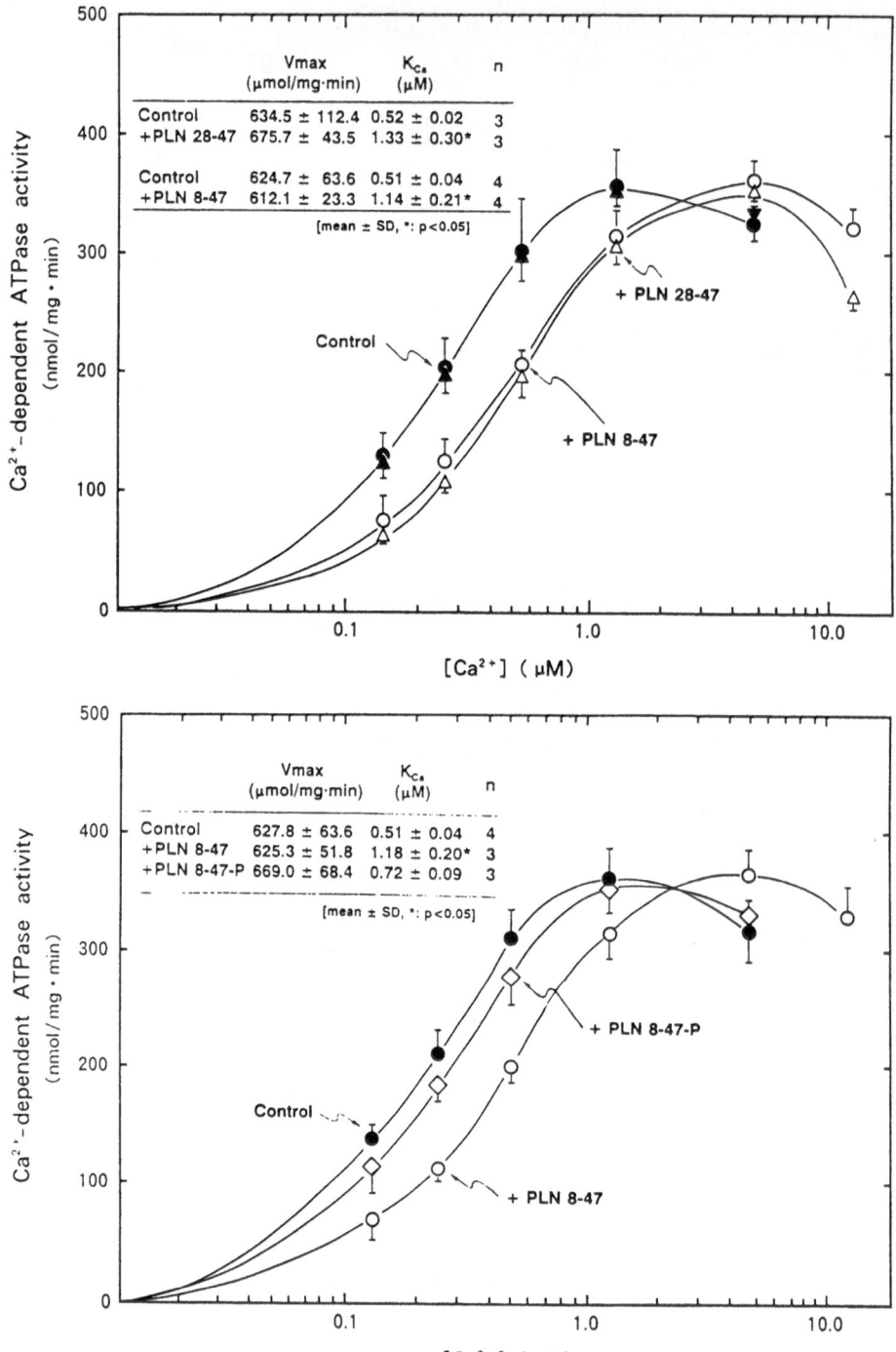

In these experiments, purified canine cardiac Ca ATPase in permeable vesicles of phospholipid was preincubated with synthetic partial phospholamban peptide corresponding to the NH_2-terminal hydrophilic domain (PLN 1–31) or was incorporated into liposomes with synthetic phospholamban peptides containing the COOH-terminal hydrophobic sequence (PLN 28–47, PLN 8–47) by the freeze-throw-sonication method before ATPase assay. For phosphorylation of PLN 8–47, liposomes containing the peptides were first phosphorylated by cAMP-dependent protein kinase. The phosphorylated vesicles were then collected by ultracentrifugation. V_{max} and K_{Ca} were determined from Ca-dependent profiles of ATPase activity using the double reciprocal plot of Lineweaver and Burk [38].

Our results indicated that, in terms of phospholamban-mediated regulation of Ca ATPase, not only the cytoplasmic domain but also the intramembrane portion of phospholamban are required. As the peptides devoid of NH_2-terminal 7 residues had no effect on the V_{max}, the residues responsible for the V_{max} effect could reside in the NH_2-terminal portion. The COOH-terminal intramembrane domain could contribute to the effects on Ca affinity.

Taking these kinetic and chemical properties into consideration, we might predict the mechanism of regulation of SR Ca ATPase by phospholamban. Domain I of unphosphorylated phospholamban may interact directly with the E_2 form of the ATPase to inhibit the conversion between E_2 and E_1. The interaction is diminished by phosphorylation of phospholamban. Changes in the electrostatic properties of the SR membrane on phospholamban phosphorylation may also contribute to the increased Ca affinity of ATPase. Domain II of phospholamban may not be a mere anchor, but may rather play an important role in the interaction between the two proteins in addition to domain I. It remains to be examined how transmembrane helices of Ca ATPase and domain II of phospholamban interact and how the signal of phosphorylation and dephosphorylation of domain I is transduced into the changes in the interaction between these intramembranous domains. Also intriguing is how the oligomeric structure of phospholamban contributes to the molecular interaction between the two proteins. Studies using synthetic phospholamban variants corresponding to the intramembrane portion or biologically synthesized mutants could give us more clues. Furthermore, mutations on key domain and other related regions of the two proteins may give us the ultimate answers.

FIG. 8. Effects of synthetic phospholamban peptides containing the intramembrane domain of phospholamban (*PLN 28–47* and *PLN 8–47*) on purified Ca ATPase [38]. **Top** Ca ATPase was reconstituted with PLN 28–47 (*open triangles*) or PLN 8–47 (*open circles*) at molar ratio 100 between the peptide and ATPase. Samples were then subjected to the ATPase assay. In the control experiments (*solid triangles* for PLN 28–47, *solid circles* for PLN 8–47), the reconstitution was carried out by fusing the ATPase-containing vesicles with liposomes that contained the same amounts of phosphatidyl choline as the peptide-containing vesicles. Results represent the mean ± SD of three different experiments. **Bottom** Ca ATPase was reconstituted with unphosphorylated (*open circles*) or phosphorylated (*diamonds*) PLN 8–47. In the control experiment (*solid circles*), the reconstitution was carried out by fusing the ATPase-containing vesicles with liposomes that contained the same amounts of phosphatidyl choline as the peptide-containing vesicles

References

1. Burk SE, Lytton J, MacLennan DH, Shull G (1989) cDNA cloning, functional expression, and mRNA tissue distribution of a third organellar Ca^{2+} pump. J Biol Chem 264:18561–18568
2. Fujii, J. Lytton J, Tada M, MacLennan DH (1988) Rabbit cardiac and slow-twitch muscle express the same phospholamban gene. FEBS Lett 227:51–55
3. Kirchberger MA, Tada M (1976) Effects of adenosine 3': 5'-monophosphate-dependent protein kinase on sarcoplasmic reticulum isolated from cardiac and slow and fast contracting skeletal muscles. J Biol Chem 251:725–729
4. Tada M, Kirchberger MA, Repke DI, Katz AM (1974) The stimulation of calcium transport in cardiac sarcoplasmic reticulum by adenosine 3': 5'-monophosphate-dependent protein-kinase J Biol Chem 249:6174–6180
5. Tada M, Yamamoto T, Tonomura Y (1978) Molecular mechanism of active calcium transport by sarcoplasmic reticulum. Physiol Rev 58:1–79
6. Tada M, Katz AM (1982) Phosphorylation of the sarcoplasmic reticulum and sarcolemma. Annu Rev Physiol 44:401–423
7. Tada M, Kadoma M, Inui M, Fujii J (1988) Regulation of Ca^{2+}-pump from cardiac sarcoplasmic reticulum. Methods Enzymol 157:107–153
8. Tada M, Ohmori F, Yamada M, Abe H (1979) Mechanism of the stimulation of Ca^{2+}-dependent ATPase of cardiac sarcoplasmic reticulum by adenosine 3': 5'-monophosphate-dependent protein kinase: role of the 22,000-dalton protein. J Biol Chem 254:319–326
9. Hicks MJ, Shigekawa M, Katz AM (1979) Mechanism by which cyclic adenosine 3': 5'-monophosphate-dependent protein kinase stimulates calcium transport in cardiac sarcoplasmic reticulum. Circ Res 44:384–391
10. Tada M, Yamada M, Ohmori F, Kuzuya T, Inui M, Abe H (1980) Transient state kinetic studies of Ca^{2+}-dependent ATPase and calcium transport by cardiac sarcoplasmic reticulum: effect of cyclic AMP-dependent protein kinase-catalyzed phosphorylation of phospholamban. J Biol Chem 255:1985–1992
11. Tada M, Yamada M, Kadoma M, Inui M, Ohmori F (1982) Calcium transport by cardiac sarcoplasmic reticulum and phosphorylation of phospholamban. Mol Cell Biochem 46:73–95
12. Le Peuch CJ, Haiech J, Demaille JG (1979) Concerted regulation of cardiac sarcoplasmic reticulum calcium transport by cyclic-adenosine-monophosphate-dependent and calcium-calmodulin-dependent phosphorylations. Biochemistry 18:5150–5157
13. Wegener AD, Simmerman HKB, Liepnieks J, Jones LR (1986) Proteolytic cleavage of phospholamban purified from canine cardiac sarcoplasmic reticulum vesicles: generation of a low resolution model of phospholamban structure. J Biol Chem 261:5154–5159
14. Watanabe Y, Kijima Y, Kadoma M, Tada M, Takagi T (1991) Molecular weight determination of phospholamban oligomer in the presence of sodium dodecyl sulfate: application of low-angle laser light scattering photometry. J Biochem 110:40–45
15. Inui M, Kadoma M, Tada M (1985) Purification and characterization of phospholamban from canine cardiac sarcoplasmic reticulum. J Biol Chem 257:10052–10062
16. Jones LR, Simmerman HKB, Wilson WW, Gurd FRN, Wegener AD (1985) Purification and characterization of phospholamban from canine cardiac sarcoplasmic reticulum. J Biol Chem 260:7721–7730
17. Fujii J, Kadoma M, Tada M, Toda H, Sakiyama F (1986) Characterization of structural unit of phospholamban by amino acid sequencing and electrophoretic analysis. Biochem Biophys Res Commun 138:1044–1050
18. Simmerman HKB, Collins JH, Theibert JL, Wegener AD, Jones LR (1986) Sequence analysis of phospholamban: identification of phosphorylation sites and two major structural domains. J Biol Chem 261:13333–13341

19. Fujii J, Ueno A, Kitano K, Tanaka S, Kadoma M, Tada M (1987) Complete complementary DNA-derived amino acid sequence of canine cardiac phospholamban. J Clin Invest 79:301–304

20. Fujii J, Zarain-Herzberg A, Willard HF, Tada M, MacLennan DH (1991) Structure of the rabbit phospholamban gene, cloning of the human cDNA, and assignment of the gene to human chromosome 6. J Biol Chem 266:11669–11675

21. Verboomen H, Wuytack F, Eggermont JA, De Jaegere S, Missiaen L, Raeymaekers L, Casteels R (1989) cDNA cloning and sequencing of phospholamban from pig stomach smooth muscle. Biochem J 262:353–356

22. Toyofuku T, Zak R (1991) Characterization of cDNA and genomic sequences encoding a chicken phospholamban. J Biol Chem 266:5375–5383

23. Tada M, Kadoma M (1989) Regulation of the Ca^{2+} pump ATPase by cAMP-dependent phosphorylation of phospholamban. Bioessays 10:157–163

24. Simmerman HKB, Lovelace DE, Jones LR (1989) Secondary structure of detergent-solubilized phospholamban, a phosphorylatable, oligomeric protein of cardiac sarcoplasmic reticulum. Biochim Biophys Acta 997:322–329

25. Fujii J, Maruyama K, Tada M, MacLennan DH (1989) Expression and site-specific mutagenesis of phospholamban: studies of residues involved in phosphorylation and pentamer formation. J Biol Chem 264:12950–12956

26. James P, Inui M, Tada M, Carafoli E (1989) Nature and site of phospholamban regulation of the Ca^{2+} pump of sarcoplasmic reticulum. Nature 342:90–92

27. Toyofuku T, Kurzydlowski K, Tada M, MacLennan DH (1993) Identification of regions in the Ca^{2+}-ATPase of sarcoplasmic reticulum that affect functional association with phospholamban. J Biol Chem 268:2809–2815

28. Toyofuku T, Kurzydlowski K, Tada M, MacLennan DH (1994) Amino acids Lys-Asp-Asp-Lys-Pro-Val402 in the Ca^{2+}-ATPase of cardiac sarcoplasmic reticulum are critical for functional association with phospholamban. J Biol Chem 269:22929–22932

29. Vorherr T, Chiesi M, Schwaller R, Carafoli E (1992) Regulation of the calcium ion pump of sarcoplasmic reticulum: reversible inhibition by phospholamban and by the calmodulin binding domain of the plasma membrane calcium ion pump. Biochemistry 31:371–376

30. Suzuki T, Wang JH (1986) Stimulation of bovine cardiac sarcoplasmic reticulum Ca^{2+} pump and blocking of phospholamban phosphorylation and dephosphorylation by a phospholamban monoclonal antibody. J Biol Chem 261:7018–7023

31. Morris GL, Cheng H-C, Colyer J, Wang JH (1991) Phospholamban regulation of cardiac sarcoplasmic reticulum $(Ca^{2+}-Mg^{2+})$-ATPase: mechanism of regulation and site of monoclonal antibody interaction. J Biol Chem 266:11270–11275

32. Kimura Y, Inui M, Kadoma M, Sasaki T, Tada M (1991) Effects of monoclonal antibody against phospholamban on calcium pump ATPase of cardiac sarcoplasmic reticulum. J Mol Cell Cardiol 23:1223–1230

33. Toyofuku T, Kurzydlowski K, Tada M, MacLennan DH (1994) Amino acids Glu2 to Ile18 in the cyoplasmic domain of phospholamban are essential for functional association with the Ca^{2+}-ATPase of sarcoplasmic reticulum. J Biol Chem 269:3088–3094

34. Chothia C, Janin J (1975) Principles of protein-protein recognition. Nature 256:705–708

35. Chiesi M, Schwaller R (1989) Involvement of electrostatic phenomena in phospholamban-induced stimulation of Ca uptake into cardiac sarcoplasmic reticulum. FEBS Lett 244:241–244

36. Xu Z-C, Kirchberger MA (1989) Modulation by polyelectrolytes of canine cardiac microsomal calcium uptake and the possible relationship to phospholamban. J Biol Chem 264:16644–16651

37. Kim HW, Steenaart NAE, Ferguson DG, Kranias EG (1990) Functional reconstitution of the cardiac sarcoplasmic reticulum Ca^{2+}-ATPase with phospholamban in phospholipid vesicles. J Biol Chem 265:1702–1709

38. Sasaki T, Inui M, Kimura T, Kuzuya T, Tada M (1992) Molecular mechanism of regulation of Ca^{2+} pump ATPase by phospholamban in cardiac sarcoplasmic reticulum. J Biol Chem 267:1674–1679

Mechanism of the Inotropic Action of Endothelin on the Ferret and Human Heart

Jessica Grossman, Thomas Hampton, Jianxun Wang, Zhihua Qiu, and James Morgan

Summary. Endothelin increases cardiac contractility by enhancing Ca^{2+} responsiveness with little or no increase in intracellular Ca^{2+}. The increased Ca^{2+} responsiveness caused by endothelin is due to cytoplasmic or membrane alterations mediated by the endothelin receptor-second messenger system. Presently, there are no clinically available drugs that increase inotropy by enhancing myocardial responsiveness to Ca^{2+}. Further delineation of the mechanisms by which endothelin enhances myocardial responsiveness to Ca^{2+} could lead to new pharmacological therapies for the acute and chronic treatment of patients with left ventricular systolic dysfunction.

Key words. Calcium indicators—Cardiac contractility—Myofilament calcium-responsiveness—Endothelin—human myocytes

Introduction

Evidence for Endocardial Regulation of Myocardial Function

The endocardial endothelium, the internal lining of the cardiac chamber, has been shown to modulate substantially the contraction of adjacent myocardium [1–5]. Selective removal of this endocardial endothelial layer modifies myocardial contraction in a typical manner, i.e., produces a decrease in the amplitude of contraction and an earlier onset of relaxation. This combination of actions is different from other inotropic interventions such as reduction or increase in extracellular calcium, changed frequency of stimulation, hypoxia, acidosis, or reduction of cyclic adenosine monophosphate (cAMP)-mediated effects, all of which are associated with a decrease in maximal unloaded shortening velocity (V_{max}) [6–10]. These effects of endocardial endothelium have been confirmed in myocardium from various species, including dog, cat, rabbit, rat, and ferret [1–5,11]. In addition, the presence or absence of the endocardial endothelial layer has been shown to modify greatly the effects of some circulating substances on myocardial contraction, such as angiotensin and α- and β-adrenergic agonists [4,11–14]. The mechanism by which the endocardial endothelial cells modulate myocardial function is still unknown, but the endocardium appears to

Harvard-Thorndike Laboratories, Beth Israel Hospital, Harvard Medical School, Boston, MA 02159, USA

play an important role in regulating cardiac function. The purpose of these experiments was to further delineate the cellular actions of endothelin and its potential for use as an inotropic agent in the failing human heart.

The cardiac actions of endothelin appear to be similar to those produced on vascular smooth muscle. Endothelin causes vasoconstriction by binding to receptors on vascular smooth muscle cells. Receptor binding activates phospholipase C, which increases levels of inositol 1,4,5-trisphosphate (IP_3), and diacylglycerol [15–17]. IP_3 increases intracellular Ca^{2+} by increasing sarcoplasmic reticular release of Ca^{2+} and by increasing Ca^{2+} entry into the cell (in this paper, Ca^{2+} refers to ionized calcium). The increased intracellular Ca^{2+} causes smooth muscle cell contraction.

However, unlike smooth muscle cells, the increase in cardiocyte contractility seems to occur with little or no increase in intracellular Ca^{2+}. In fura-2-loaded rat myocytes, Kramer et al. [18] found that endothelin increased contractility without increasing diastolic or systolic intracellular Ca^{2+} levels.

Methods and Results

Intact and detergent-skinned ferret papillary muscle preparations were used in these experiments. Also discussed are results obtained with isolated human myocytes. Calcium measurements were performed with the photoprotein aequorin in intact papillary muscles and with indo-1 in isolated myocytes. The details of these methods are described in the literature cited.

Evidence for Endocardial Regulation of Myocardial Function

Figure 1 shows the effects of the selective removal of endocardium on intracellular calcium (Ca^{2+}_i) and myocardial contraction. The selective removal of endocardium decreased the amplitude of contraction and induced an earlier onset of relaxation

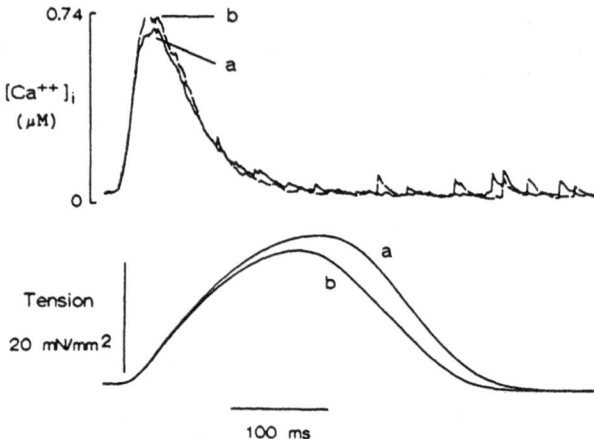

FIG. 1. Effect of the removal of endocardium on aequorin light signal and contraction in a ferret papillary muscle. *a*, control; *b*, removal of endocardium. Stimulation interval, 4 s; 30°C; 30 signals averaged. The resting $[Ca^{2+}]_i$ is 0.21 μM (the division in the y axis is not arithmetic because of the nonlinear relation between the aequorin signal and $[Ca^{2+}]$). (From [28] with permission)

without decreasing the Ca^{2+}_i level (Fig. 1). This phenomenon also occurred at steady-state force and Ca^{2+}_i (Fig. 2). These results suggest that intact endocardium enhances performance of the heart, probably by modulating the myofilament Ca^{2+}-responsiveness, consistent with results of other investigators [19,20].

Cellular Mechanism of Endocardial Effects on the Heart

We hypothesize that endothelin-1 is the major substance that mediates endocardium-induced myocardial actions. This hypothesis is strongly supported by experiments in which endothelin-1 specifically reversed the effects induced by the removal of endocardium (Fig. 3). In addition, the removal of endocardium decreased the myofilament Ca^{2+}-responsiveness (Fig. 4A), whereas endothelin-1 could reverse this effect by enhancing the myofilament Ca^{2+}-responsiveness (Fig. 4B). These results strongly suggest that intact endocardium modulates myocardial contractility by increasing the myofilament Ca^{2+}-responsiveness through endothelium-derived compounds, such as endothelin-1.

Evidence that Endocardial Substances Act Through Second Messenger Pathways

Most likely, endothelin exerts its myocardial actions through a receptor-second messenger pathway, because it did not exert any cardiac actions on saponin-skinned fibers in which the receptor-second messenger pathway was inoperative (Fig. 5). Figures 6 and 7 show that the direct effects of endothelin in skinned cardiac muscle preparations are to decrease sensitivity and efficacy, in marked contrast to the positive inotropic action observed in muscles with their sarcolemma intact.

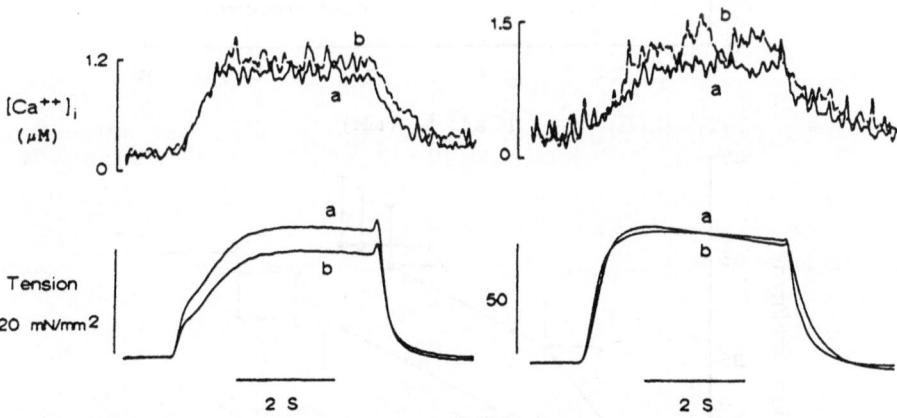

FIG. 2. Effects of the removal of endocardium on steady-state force and intracellular Ca^{2+} in muscles during tetanus (in the presence of $6\,\mu M$ ryanodine), 30°C, 12 Hz, 50 ms pulse duration, five signals averaged. *Left panel*, $[Ca^{2+}]_o = 4\,mM$. *Right panel*, $[Ca^{2+}]_o = 10\,mM$. The resting $[Ca^{2+}]_i$ is $0.25\,\mu M$ in the left panel and $0.30\,\mu M$ in the right panel (the division in the y axis is not arithmetic because of the nonlinear relation between the aequorin light and $[Ca^{2+}]$). Data for the left and right panels were from different muscles. *a*, control; *b*, after the removal of endocardium. (From [28] with permission)

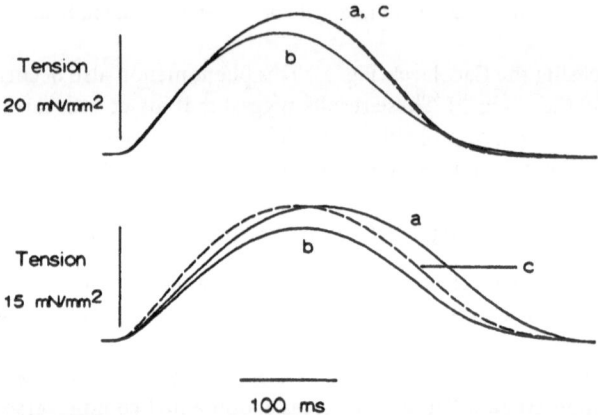

FIG. 3. Effects of endothelin-1 and Ca^{2+} on the contraction after the removal of endocardium. Stimulation interval, 4 s; 30°C. *Upper panel, a,* control; *b,* removal of endocardium; *c,* removal of endocardium plus 3×10^{-8} M endothelin-1. *Lower panel, a,* control; *b,* removal of endocardium; *c,* removal of endocardium plus ~0.5 mM $[Ca^{2+}]_o$. (From [28] with permission)

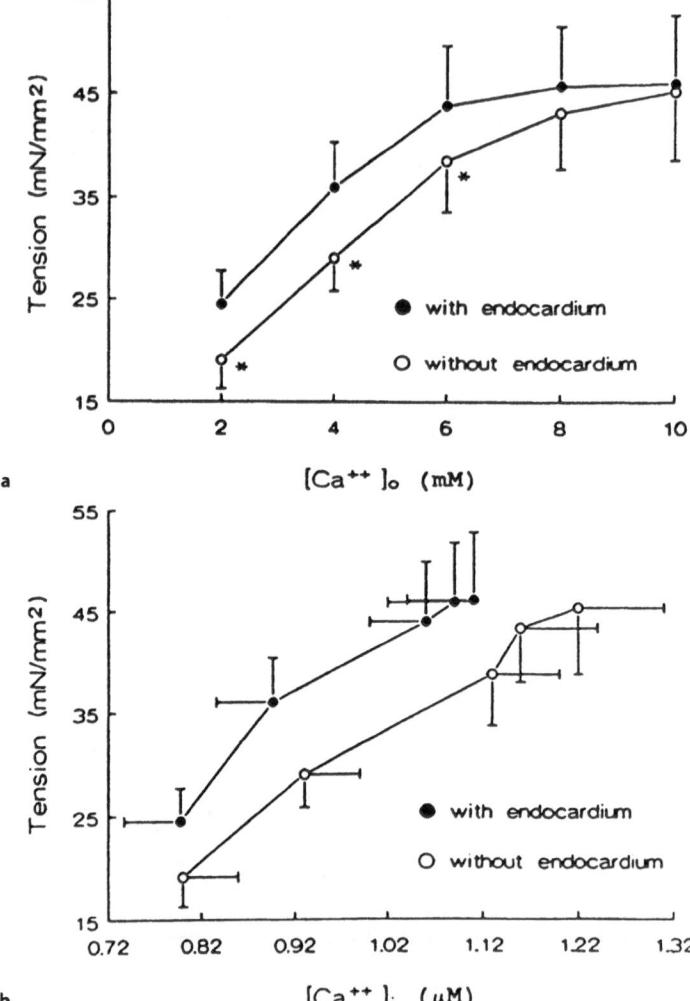

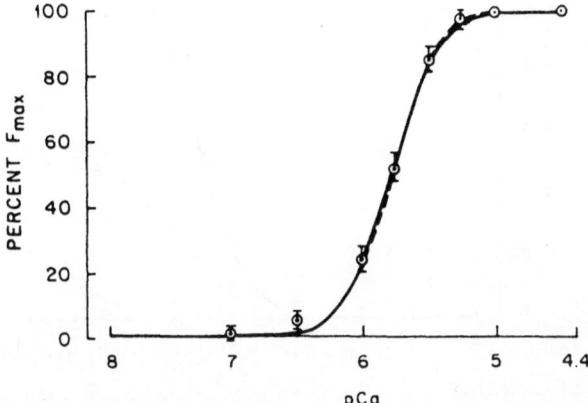

FIG. 5. Graph of force versus Ca²⁺ relation of skinned control muscles (*solid circles*) and of muscles pretreated with endothelin and then skinned (*open circles*). Force is plotted as percent of maximal force of each muscle. Data were fitted to a modified Hill equation. (From [27] with permission)

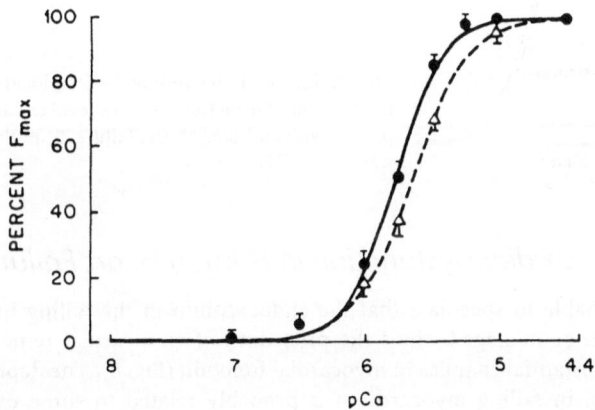

FIG. 6. Graph of force versus Ca²⁺ relation of skinned control muscles before (*circles*) and after the addition of endothelin to the Ca²⁺ buffers (*triangles*) (drug/buffer group). Force is plotted as percent of maximal force of each muscle. (From [27] with permission)

FIG. 4a,b. Graphs showing the effect of the removal of endocardium on Ca²⁺ and tension relation in ferret papillary muscles ($n = 6$). *Solid circles*, with endocardium; *open circles*, without endocardium. **a** $[Ca^{2+}]_o$-peak tension relation. *$P < 0.02$ (paired t test) versus the corresponding value of the control curve. **b** Peak $[Ca^{2+}]_i$-peak tension relation. SEM was shown in x axis data because the peak $[Ca^{2+}]_i$ and its increments by $[Ca^{2+}]_o$ were different from muscle to muscle. (From [28] with permission)

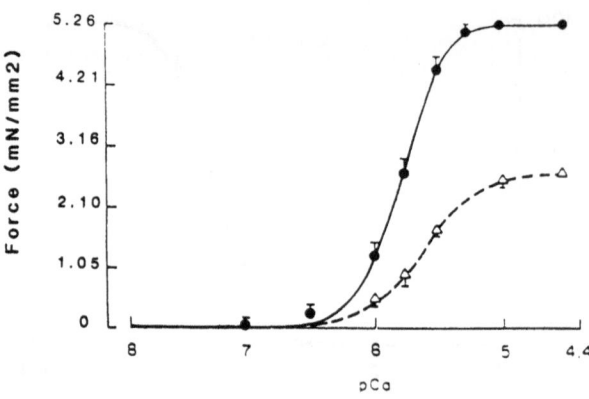

FIG. 7. Graph showing changes in Ca^{2+}-activated force in the presence and absence of endothelin. Units for force are millinewtons per mm^2 of muscle. Skinned control muscles before (*circles*) and after the addition of endothelin to the Ca^{2+} buffers (*triangles*) (drug/buffer group). (From [27] with permission)

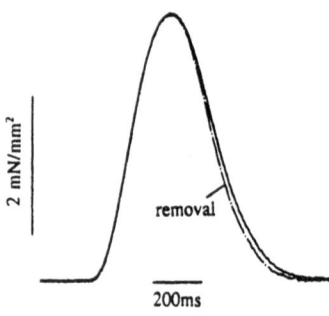

FIG. 8. Effect of the removal of endocardium on the myocardial contraction of a trabeculae carneae from a patient with end-stage heart failure. Stimulation interval was 4 s at 30°C

Endocardial Dysfunction in Human Heart Failure

It seems reasonable to speculate that the endocardium in the failing human heart is dysfunctional or damaged, since the procedure of endocardial removal did not produce any substantial changes in myocardial function (Fig. 8). The depressed myocardial function in failing myocardium is probably related to some extent to the endocardial dysfunction. Decreased endothelin receptor function might be another possibility that accounts for the depressed myocardial function, but this seems unlikely, because endothelin greatly enhances the amplitude of contraction of failing human cardiac myocytes loaded with the fluorescent Ca^{2+}-indicator, indo-1/AM (Fig. 9).

Discussion

Mechanism of Endocardial Effects on the Heart

It has been suggested that endocardium modulates myocardial function by releasing diffusible substances, such as endothelin-1 (a 21-residue bioactive peptide with receptors on cardiac myocytes) and endothelium-derived relaxant factor (EDRF). The experimental evidence includes (a) the negative inotropic effects of endocardial re-

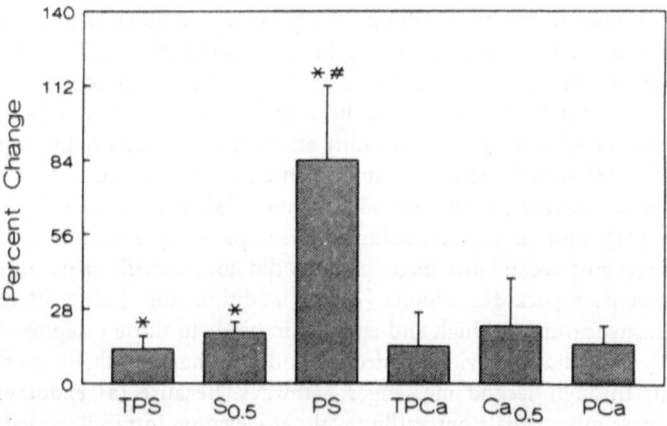

FIG. 9. Response of single cardiac myocytes from failing human heart to 10 nM ET-1. Values (means ± SEM) are the averaged data from eight myocytes isolated from four hearts. *TPS*, time to peak shortening; $S_{0.5}$, time to 50% decline of peak shortening; *PS*, peak shortening; *TPCa*, time to peak intracellular Ca^{2+}; $Ca_{0.5}$, time to 50% decline of peak intracellular Ca^{2+}; *PCa* peak intracellular Ca^{2+}; $Ca_{0.5}$, time to 50% decline of peak intracellular Ca^{2+}; *PCa*, peak intracellular Ca^{2+}. *P < 0.05 (paired t test) versus the values before ET-1, and #P < 0.05 (unpaired t-test) versus the value of peak intracellular Ca^{2+} (PCa) (eight myocytes for each of the six groups). (From [20a] with permission)

moval were reversed in bioassay experiments where an endocardium-denuded papillary muscle was exposed to the effluent from a column of cultured porcine endocardial endothelial cells on microcarrier beads [3]; (b) cultured porcine endocardial endothelial cells released an unstable humoral agent whose effects on an endothelium-denuded pig coronary artery were indistinguishable from EDRF [3]; and (c) the endothelium-derived substance, endothelin-1, specifically reversed the characteristic changes induced by the removal of endocardial endothelium [4]. It seems likely that endocardial endothelium regulates excitation-contraction coupling, and therefore the contractility of the heart, by releasing endogeneous substances.

A change in contractility can occur by three general mechanisms: (1) by altering the availability of activator calcium; (2) by affecting myofilament calcium responsiveness; and (3) by a combination of these two effects. Experiments have shown that the removal of endocardial endothelium decreased myofilament calcium responsiveness, and therefore contractility, probably due to the loss of substances (such as endothelin) released to the adjacent cardiac myocytes. This hypothesis was supported by the application of endothelin, which reversed the decreased myofilament calcium responsiveness and the other alterations of contraction induced by the removal of endocardial endothelium [4]. EDRF elevates the cellular level of cyclic guanosine monophosphate (cGMP), decreases the amplitude of contraction, and enhances relaxation [3,20]. Therefore, it seems likely that endothelin and EDRF modulate and balance the myocardial contraction-relaxation cycles.

Evidence that Endocardial Substances Act Through Second Messenger Pathways

In addition to calcium, the IP$_3$/DAG (inositol 1,4,5-trisphosphate/diacylglycerol) pathway, and cyclic nucleotide-mediated pathways appear to be important second messenger systems in the myocardium. It is generally accepted that the two major substances released from the endothelial cells are endothelin and EDRF, and that they exert their biological actions through one or more of these second messenger pathways. In isolated rat cardiac myocytes, the administraction of the protein kinase C (DAG pathway) inhibitor, H-7, significantly attenuated the positive inotropic effects of endothelin [18]; in isolated ferret papillary muscles, the administration of protein kinase C (PKC) activator, PMA, substantially modulated the myocardial actions of endothelin [21]; and in saponin-skinned ferret papillary muscles in which the endothelin receptor-second messenger pathway did not normally operate, endothelin did not exert its myocardial actions [22]. In addition, the density of endothelin receptors in myocardium is high and endothelin binds to those receptors with high affinity [23]. These lines of evidence strongly indicate that endothelin exerts its cardiac actions through second messenger pathways. Because (a) endothelin could greatly increase myocardial contractility without elevating intracellular calcium levels, and (b) endothelin-induced changes in contraction are different from those of cyclic nucleotide-mediated pathways, it is therefore reasonable to propose that the regulatory role of the endocardial substance on myocardial function occurs largely through an effect mediated by the IP_3/DAG pathway.

Several studies have demonstrated that endothelin is a positive inotropic agent in cardiac myocytes and isolated cardiac muscles. The inotropic effect of endothelin has been found to be long-lasting and difficult to wash out [19,20]. Kelly et al. [24] have demonstrated that the increased inotropy caused by endothelin is accompanied by little or no increase in intracellular Ca^{2+}. The increase in Ca^{2+} that does occur appears to be mediated by an increase in IP_3 which releases calcium from the sarcoplasmic reticulum (SR) [25]. Based on these results, it was concluded that endothelin increased Ca^{2+} responsiveness of the myocardium. However, it is difficult to assess true myofilament responsiveness to Ca^{2+} in intact, actively contracting muscles because of the complex interactions caused by the short duration of Ca^{2+} availability, the inhomogeneous distribution of the intracellular Ca^{2+}, and the limited precision of available techniques for quantifying intracellular Ca^{2+} concentration. Therefore, to determine if endothelin's positive inotropic effect is related to structural modifications of the myofilaments, we performed Ca^{2+} concentration-response curves on chemically skinned muscles [26]. Our results showed that endothelin, at a concentration of 100 nM, is a positive inotropic agent in isolated ferret right ventricular papillary muscles. This concentration of endothelin has been demonstrated to produce a maximal response in intact, isolated cardiac muscles [19,27]. Our results, however, indicate that the positive inotropic effects of endothelin are not mediated by alterations of Ca^{2+} binding to the myofilaments, i.e., actin, myosin, and troponin regulatory complex. Incubation of intact papillary muscles with endothelin for 2 h caused a sustained increase in contractility, but did not significantly alter either the pCa_{50}, the Hill coefficient, or the maximal Ca^{2+}-activated force (F_{max}) when the fibers were subsequently skinned.

When endothelin was added to Ca^{2+} buffer solutions and allowed to interact directly with skinned myofilaments, the pCa_{50} was increased, indicating a decrease in Ca^{2+} sensitivity. The Hill coefficient and F_{max} were also decreased [26]. Endothelin, therefore, is a direct Ca^{2+} desensitizer that decreases maximal force development. However, it is unlikely that endothelin, a 21-amino-acid peptide, could cross the intact cell membrane and bind to the myofilaments. When endothelin was present in the Ca^{2+} buffer solutions and exposed to the skinned muscles, it is possible that endothelin, through nonspecific binding, was able to interact directly with either actin, myosin, or the troponin complex, thus interfering with Ca^{2+} binding and myofilament contraction. It is likely that endothelin's effects of increased inotropy and enhanced Ca^{2+} responsiveness in intact, actively contracting muscles are receptor-mediated.

One of the receptor-mediated-second messenger pathways which could increase Ca^{2+} responsiveness is phospholipase C activation. Activation of phospholipase C increases production of diacylglycerol. Diacylglycerol in turn activates protein kinase C, which then phosphorylates specific intracellular substrates, including the sarcolemmal-bound Na^+-H^+ antiporter. Phosphorylation increases activity of the antiporter, increasing intracellular pH. Alkalosis is a known sensitizer of myofilaments to Ca^{2+}. Intracellular alkalosis in rat myocytes following endothelin administration has been demonstrated [18]. Using the proton selective fluorescent probe 2',7'-bis-(carboxyethyl)-5,6-carboxyfluorescein (BCECF), it was found that in isolated rat myocytes, endothelin at a concentration of 100 pM increased intracellular pH by 0.08 ± 0.02. When the Na^+-H^+ antiporter was inhibited with amiloride, or when inhibitors of protein kinase C were added, they observed that the inotropic response to endothelin was reduced, but not completely abolished. This decrease in inotropy was restored by intracellular alkalization with NH_4Cl [24]. Skinned muscle studies did not show an increase in Ca^{2+} responsiveness because the sarcolemma is disrupted and the cytoplasm and intracellular enzymes are washed away; the pH of the Ca^{2+} buffer solutions used to cause contraction and relaxation of the myofilaments is titrated to 7.10 and maintained via an effective buffering system. Therefore, if the increased Ca^{2+} responsiveness induced by endothelin is secondary to protein kinase C-mediated intracellular alkalosis, then myofilaments pre-exposed to endothelin and then skinned would fail to show any change in the pCa_{50}.

It should be noted that inhibition of intracellular alkalosis did not completely inhibit the positive inotropic effect of endothelin. Kelly et al. [24] found that prior treatment of rat myocytes with pertussis toxin abolished the positive inotropic effect of endothelin. Prior treatment with the β-agonist isoproterenol also markedly inhibited the positive inotropic effect. They theorized that both pertussis toxin and β-agonists caused uncoupling of pertussis toxin-sensitive G proteins from the endothelin receptor and that G proteins are thus a necessary link in the endothelin intracellular signalling pathway. Importantly, they found that pertussis toxin did not inhibit the increase in intracellular pH, implying that phospholipase C was still activated by endothelin [18].

With regard to EDRF, it is well known that EDRF causes vasodilating effects on smooth muscle cells by elevating the intracellular level of cGMP [28]. In cardiac muscle, increases in the intracellular cGMP level lead to a reduction in the amplitude of contraction and an earlier onset of relaxation [3]. Moreover, EDRF provided significant myocardial protection after ischemia and reperfusion [29]. These reports suggest that EDRF is involved in the regulation of myocardial contraction, but the details and mechanisms are unknown.

Endocardium and Abnormalities of Contractile Function in Cardiac Hypertrophy and Failure

Studies from different experimental models of cardiac hypertrophy and failure showed that, in most cases, (a) the amplitude of contraction was decreased, (b) the myofilament calcium responsiveness was decreased, and (c) the responses of the myocardium to isoproterenol and milrinone were decreased [30,31]. We speculate that the endocardial function has been damaged (or disturbed) in the severely hypertrophied and failing myocardium which is, to some extent, responsible for the depressed myocardial function. The following points support this hypothesis: first, the selective removal of endocardium decreases the myofilament Ca^{2+}-responsiveness, and similarly, the myofilament Ca^{2+}-responsiveness is decreased in the failing myocardium [30]. Second, the removal of endocardium decreases the responses of the myocardium to α-receptor agonists [13]; similarly, in failing myocardium, the myocardial responsiveness to α-receptor agonists was substantially decreased [11]. Third, our preliminary data showed that the procedure of endocardial endothelial removal did not alter the myocardial contraction of severely hypertrophied and failing myocardium, suggesting that the endocardium was already damaged or dysfunctional. The decreased myofilament calcium responsiveness in failing myocardium may be partially due to the reduced or diminished release of endothelin, because endothelin greatly enhances myofilament calcium responsiveness [18,22]. In addition, the prolonged contraction may be partially due to the reduced or diminished release of EDRF, since EDRF has the ability to enhance myocardial relaxation [3].

Endocardial Dysfunction in Human Heart Failure

Similar to the findings from experimental animal models, myocardial function was depressed in failing human myocardium, and we speculate that this may be related in part to functional damage of the endocardial endothelium. This speculation is supported by the following experimental evidence: first, the EDRF release from endothelial cells was greatly reduced in patients with chronic congestive heart failure [32]. Second, the removal of endocardium decreases the myofilament Ca^{2+}-responsiveness [4], and similarly, the myofilament Ca^{2+}-responsiveness was reduced in failing human myocardium [30]. Third, our preliminary data showed that the procedure of endocardial removal did not alter myocardial contraction in human failing myocardium, suggesting that the endocardium was already damaged or dysfunctional.

Taken together, these lines of evidence indicate that the loss of functional endocardium may be partially responsible for depressed myocardial function in failing myocardium.

Conclusion

In conclusion, endothelin increases inotropy in myocardial tissue by enhancing Ca^{2+} responsiveness with little or no increase in intracellular Ca^{2+}. The increased Ca^{2+} responsiveness caused by endothelin is not due to changes of Ca^{2+} binding mediated directly by myofilaments; rather, the increased Ca^{2+} responsiveness is due to cytoplasmic or membrane alterations mediated by the endothelin receptor-second messenger system. At present there are no clinically available drugs which increase inotropy by increasing myocardial responsiveness to Ca^{2+}; all available positive inotropic drugs act predominantly to increase intracellular Ca^{2+}, which can have deleterious side effects in patients with heart failure whose myocardium may exhibit abnormal intracellular Ca^{2+} handling [30]. Further delineation of the mechanisms by which endothelin enhances myocardial responsiveness to Ca^{2+} could lead to new pharmacological therapies for the acute and chronic treatment of patients with left ventricular systolic dysfunction.

Acknowledgments. These studies were supported in part by grants from the National Institutes of Health (HL31117, HL07374, DA05171) and a Grant-in-Aid from the American Heart Association to James P. Morgan.

References

1. Brutsaert DL, Meulemans AL, Sipido KR, Sys SU (1988) Effects of damaging the endocardial surface on the mechanical performance of isolated cardiac muscle. Circ Res 62:358–366
2. Ramaciotti C, Sharkey A, McClellan G, Winegrad S (1991) Endothelial cells regulate cardiac contractility. Proc Natl Acad Sci USA 4033–4036
3. Smith JA, Shah AM, Lewis MJ (1991) Factors released from endocardium of the ferret and pig modulate myocardial contraction. J Physiol (Lond) 439:1–14
4. Wang JX, Morgan JP (1991) Endocardial endothelium modulates myofilament Ca^{2+} responsiveness in aequorin-loaded ferret myocardium. Circ Res 70:754–760
5. Li K, Stewart DJ, Rouleau JL (1991) Myocardial contractile actions of endothelin-1 in rat and rabbit papillary muscles: Role of endocardial endothelium. Circ Res 69:301–312
6. Chappell S, Henderson A, Lewis MJ (1986) Characterization of the mechanical behavior of isolated papillary muscle preparations of the ferret. J Pharmacol Methods 15:35–49
7. Tyberg JV, Yeatman LA, Parmley WW, Urschal CW, Sonnenblick EH (1970) Effect of hypoxia on mechanics of cardiac contraction. Am J Physiol 218:1780–1788
8. Henderson AH, Brutsaert DL (1973) An analysis of the mechanical capabilities of heart muscle during hypoxia. Cardiovasc Res 7:763–776
9. Fry CH, Poole-Wilson PA (1981) Effects of acid-base changes on excitation-contraction coupling in guinea pig and rabbit cardiac ventricular muscle. J Physiol 313:141–160
10. Winegrad S (1984) Regulation of cardiac contractile proteins—correlation between physiology and biochemistry. Circ Res 55:565–574
11. Calderone A, Bouvier M, Li K, Juneau C, de Champlain J, Rouleau JL (1991) Dysfunction of the beta- and alpha-adrenergic systems in a model of congestive heart failure. The pacing-overdrive dog. Circ Res 69:332–343
12. Meulemans AL, Sipido KR, Sys SU, Brutsaet DL (1988) Atriopeptin III induces early relaxation of isolated papillary muscle. Circ Res 62:1171–1174
13. Meulemans AL, Andries LJ, Brutsaert DL (1990) Endocardial endothelium mediates positive inotropic response to α_1-adrenoceptor agonist in mammalian heart. J Mol Cell Cardiol 22:667–685
14. Meulemans AL, Andries LJ, Brutsaert DL (1990) Does endocardial endothelium mediate positive inotropic response to angiotensin I and angiotensin II? Circ Res 66:1591–1601
15. Yanagisawa M, Kurihara H, Kimura S, Tosnobe Y, Yobayashi M, Mitsui Y, Yuzaki Y, Goto K, Masaki T (1988) A novel potent vasoconstrictor peptide produced by endothelial cells. Nature 332:411–415
16. Lerman A, Hildebrand FL, Margulies KB, O'Murchu B, Perrella MA, Heublein DM, Swab TR, Burnett JC (1990) Endothelin: a new cardiovascular regulatory peptide. Mayo Clin Proc 65:1441–1455
17. Simonson MS, Dunn MJ (1990) Cellular signalling by peptides of the endothelin gene family. FASEB J 4:2989–3000
18. Krämer BK, Smith TW, Kelly RA (1991) Endothelin and increased contractility in adult rat ventricular myocytes: Role of intracellular alkalosis by activation of the protein kinase C-dependent Na^+-H^+ exchanger. Circ Res 68:269–279

19. Moravec CS, Reynolds EE, Stewart RW, Bond M (1989) Endothelin is a positive inotropic agent in human and rat heart in vitro. Biochem Biophys Res Commun 159:14–18

20. Ishikawa R, Yanagisawa M, Kimura S, Goto K, Masaki T (1988) Positive inotropic action of novel vasoconstrictor peptide endothelin on guinea pig atria. Am J Physiol 255:H970–H973

20a. Qiu Z, Wang J, Perreault CL, Meuse AJ, Grossman W, Morgan JP (1992) Effects of endothelin on intrarellular Ca^{2+} and contractility in singular ventricular myocytes from the ferret and human. Eur J Pharmacol 214:293–296

21. Wang JX, Morgan JP (1992) Role of endothelin in the regulation of intracellular Ca^{2+} and contractility in ferret myocardium. Biophys J 61:A164

22. Wang JX, Paik G, Morgan JP (1991) Endothelin 1 enhances myofilament Ca^{2+} responsiveness in aequorin-loaded ferret myocardium. Circ Res 69:582–589

23. Gu XH, Casley DJ, Nayler WG (1989) Identification of specific high affinity binding sites for ^{125}I-labelled endothelin in rat cardiac membranes. J Mol Cell Cardiol 21:S4

24. Kelly RA, Eid H, Krämer BK, O'Neill M, Liang BT, Reers M, Smith TW (1990) Endothelin enhances the contractile responsiveness of adult rat ventricle myocytes to Ca^{2+} by a pertussis toxin-sensitive pathway. J Clin Invest 86:1164–1171

25. Wang J, Flemal K, Morgan JP (1993) Endothelin-1 enhances cross-bridge function of ferret myocardium: role of second messengers. Am J Physiol 265:H2168–H2174

26. Paik GY, Wang JX, Perreault CL, Morgan JP (1994) Endothelin-1 does not alter Ca^{2+} responsiveness in saponin-skinned ferret papillary msucles. Eur J Pharmacol 264:437–443

27. Wang J, Paik GY, Morgan JP (1991) Endothelin-1 enhances myofilaments Ca^{2+} responsiveness in aequorin-loaded ferret myocardium. Circ Res 69:582–589

28. Rapoport RM, Murad F (1983) Agonist-induced endothelium-dependent relaxation in rat thoracic aorta may be mediated through cGMP. Circ Res 52:352–357

29. Johnson G, Tsao PS, Lefer AM (1991) Cardioprotective effects of authentic nitric oxide in myocardial ischemia with reperfusion. Cirt Care Med 19:244–252

30. Perreault CL, Meuse AJ, Bentivegina LA, Morgan JP (1990) Abnormal intracellular calcium handling in acute and chronic heart failure: Role in systolic and diastolic dysfunction. Eur Heart J II:8–21

31. Feldman MD, Copelas L, Gwathmey JK, Phillips P, Warren SE, Schoen FJ, Grossman W, Morgan JP (1987) Deficient productin of cyclic AMP: Pharmacologic evidence of an important cauase of contractile dysfunction in patients with end-stage heart failure. Circulation 75:331–339

32. Drexler H, Hayoz D, Munzel T, Hornig B, Just H, Brunner H, Zelis R (1992) Endothelial function in chronic congestive heart failure. Am J Cardiol 69:1596–1610

33. Finkel MS, Oddis CV, Jacob TD, Watkins SC, Hattler BG, Simmons RL (1992) Negative inotropic effects of cytokines on the heart mediated by nitric oxide. Science 257:387–389

Physiological Significance of the Change in the Ca²⁺ Sensitivity of the Contractile Elements in Cardiac Muscle

KIMIAKI KOMUKAI and SATOSHI KURIHARA

Summary. Recent development in methods to measure intracellular Ca^{2+} concentration ($[Ca^{2+}]_i$) using Ca^{2+} indicators has brought about clarification of the temporal relation between a change in $[Ca^{2+}]_i$ and contraction. Intracellular Ca^{2+} increases immediately after stimulation and exponentially decays after reaching its peak (Ca^{2+} transient). Tension starts to rise following an increase in $[Ca^{2+}]_i$. Several factors are considered to be involved in the decay of the Ca^{2+} transient. Ca^{2+} removal by the sarcoplasmic reticulum (SR) and Na-Ca exchanger is primarily responsible for the decay of Ca^{2+} transient. However, a change in the affinity of troponin-C for Ca^{2+}, a major intracellular Ca^{2+} binding protein, influences the decay of $[Ca^{2+}]_i$. The affinity of troponin-C for Ca^{2+} is altered by a change in developed tension and this intrinsic regulation of the affinity of troponin-C for Ca^{2+} is important for understanding the molecular mechanism of tension development under physiological and pathophysiological conditions in mammalian cardiac muscles.

Key words. Cardiac muscle—Ca^{2+}—Contraction

Introduction

The contraction of cardiac muscle, as regulated by Ca^{2+}, is essentially the same as that of skeletal muscle [1]. However, the number of Ca^{2+} binding sites of Ca^{2+} in cardiac troponin-C is different from that in skeletal troponin-C: there are two high-affinity sites and one low-affinity site in cardiac troponin-C, and two high-affinity sites and two low-affinity sites in skeletal troponin-C [2]. The steady-state relationship between the Ca^{2+} concentration ($[Ca^{2+}]$) and tension in cardiac muscle has been studied using skinned preparations which can be directly activated by Ca^{2+} [3]. However, the development of methods to measure the transient change in the intracellular Ca^{2+} concentration ($[Ca^{2+}]_i$) with contraction provides information regarding the regulatory mechanisms of Ca^{2+} during contraction in cardiac muscles. In this short review, we will discuss the regulation of cardiac muscle contraction by $[Ca^{2+}]_i$ and the physiological significance of the change in the affinity of troponin-C for Ca^{2+} in cardiac muscle contraction.

Department of Physiology, Jikei University of School of Medicine, Minato-ku, Tokyo 105, Japan

Relation Between Ca²⁺ Concentration and Contraction in Skinned Cardiac Preparations at Different Muscle Lengths

Skinned preparations of cardiac muscles treated with a detergent can be directly activated with Ca^{2+}, facilitating study of the relation between $[Ca^{2+}]$ and tension (pCa-tension relation) at steady state. The pCa-tension relation in cardiac muscle is influenced by muscle length; stretching the preparation shifts the pCa-tension relation to the left and increases the Ca^{2+} sensitivity of the contractile elements [4]. The dependence of tension development on muscle length in cardiac muscle is more prominent than in skeletal muscle [5]. In skeletal muscle fibers, the length–tension relation at different $[Ca^{2+}]$ used for activation is essentially the same [6]. Therefore, a geometrical factor (overlap of actin and myosin filaments) is important for the determination of the length-dependence of tension development. However, the length–tension relation in skinned cardiac muscle differs at different $[Ca^{2+}]$ for activation, and the ascending limb of the length–tension relation at a higher $[Ca^{2+}]$ nearly reaches that of skeletal muscle fiber [5,7]. Similarly, the length–tension relation in intact mammalian cardiac muscle, which was measured using twitch contraction, is influenced by the extracellular Ca^{2+} concentration ($[Ca^{2+}]_o$) [8]. Therefore, these results suggest that $[Ca^{2+}]$ for the activation of contraction is a factor which determines the length-dependent change in developed tension in cardiac muscles. The direct comparison of the length–tension relation in skeletal and cardiac muscle in intact preparations is not straightforward, because the length–tension relation in intact cardiac muscle is measured using twitch contraction while the relation in intact skeletal muscle is measured using tetanic contraction. Since tension in tetanic contraction is sustained and the contractile apparatus is fully activated by Ca^{2+} during stimulation, the length–tension relation in skeletal muscle represents the relation at steady state. However, tension in twitch contraction is transient and the contractile apparatus is not sufficiently equilibrated with Ca^{2+}.

Measurement of Intracellular Ca²⁺ Transient in Cardiac Muscles

Various types of intracellular Ca^{2+} indicators are now available for the measurement of intracellular Ca^{2+} transient. Fluorescent Ca^{2+} indicators are favorable for Ca^{2+} transient measurement in single myocytes and multicellular preparations, as they give a large Ca^{2+} signal. Further, the acetoxymethyl form of these indicators is easily introduced into the cells. However, the fluorescent Ca^{2+} indicators of the acetoxymethyl form permeate the membrane of intracellular organella as well as the cell membrane, and are converted to acid form in the organella. Therefore, the change in Ca^{2+} concentration within the organella is contaminated with the changes in the fluorescent signals of the Ca^{2+} indicators [9], and thus these indicators are disadvantageous for the measurement of myoplasmic Ca^{2+} concentration. Injection of the acid form of fluorescent dyes is a reliable method for the introduction of the dyes into cells. However, it was suggested that the injected dyes bind to intracellular soluble proteins, altering the affinity of the dyes for Ca^{2+} [10]. In addition, movement of the preparation influences the fluorescent signals. Thus, quantitative measurement using the fluorescent Ca^{2+} indicators with contraction is not easy. The fluorescent Ca^{2+} indicators which are conjugated with a large molecule (such as dextran) might be better for the quantitative measurement of $[Ca^{2+}]_i$ [11], although the injection of the dyes might be more difficult than for nonconjugated dyes.

The Ca^{2+} sensitive photoprotein aequorin, with a relatively high molecular weight (21 000 Da), might pose problems similar to those of fluorescent dyes with regard to the quantification of $[Ca^{2+}]_i$ [12]. However, aequorin does not penetrate into intracellular organella and the aequorin light signal reflects the myoplasmic Ca^{2+} concentration change. The advantages of aequorin are that the Ca^{2+} signal of aequorin is not influenced by movement of the preparation, and that simultaneous measurement of Ca^{2+} signals and contractions is feasible.

Relation Between Ca²⁺ Transient and Tension in Mammalian Cardiac Muscle

The Ca^{2+} signal rises immediately after the start of the action potential, and tension starts to increase following the increase in Ca^{2+} signal. The Ca^{2+} signal decays during the rising phase of tension development. When $[Ca^{2+}]_i$ increases, Ca^{2+} is bound to the regulatory site of troponin-C, and the time course of troponin-Ca complex is just behind the change in $[Ca^{2+}]_i$ [13]. In addition to Ca^{2+} binding to troponin-C, Ca^{2+} is also bound to calmodulin, another Ca^{2+}-binding protein [14]. The concentrations of troponin-C at the regulatory site and calmodulin are 70 μM and 50 μM, respectively. The peak of the Ca^{2+} transient measured using various types of Ca^{2+} indicators is about 1–1.5 μM, although some uncertainties regarding the absolute value of $[Ca^{2+}]_i$ exist [15–17]. Therefore, most of Ca^{2+} increased in the myoplasm is bound to Ca^{2+}-binding proteins and the increase in free Ca^{2+} is a small fraction of the total Ca^{2+} delivered to the myoplasm; the main source of Ca^{2+} is the released Ca^{2+} from the sarcoplasmic reticulum (SR), and the Ca^{2+} current is considered to be a trigger for the Ca^{2+} release from the SR [3,17]. Therefore, a part of the decay of the Ca^{2+} transient reflects Ca^{2+} binding to troponin-C. Thus, the change in the affinity of troponin-C for Ca^{2+} is considered to influence $[Ca^{2+}]_i$.

Changes in the Affinity of Troponin-C for Ca²⁺

Effects of Length Change on the Ca²⁺ Transient in Twitch

Tension development of cardiac muscle is profoundly influenced by muscle length [5]. Allen and Kurihara [18] measured intracellular Ca^{2+} transient at different muscle lengths and found that the decay of the Ca^{2+} transient is shortened at a longer muscle length without an accompanying change in the peak. They also observed a transient increase in $[Ca^{2+}]_i$ (extra-Ca^{2+}) during the falling phase of the Ca^{2+} transient when the muscle length was quickly changed from a longer to a shorter length [18]. Similar results have been reported elsewhere [19,20]. However, a quick release applied to the preparations treated with 2,3-butanedione monoxime (BDM) does not produce the extra-Ca^{2+} [21] (Fig. 1). These results indicate that the extra-Ca^{2+} in response to a quick release is induced by a change in tension rather than by the change in length.

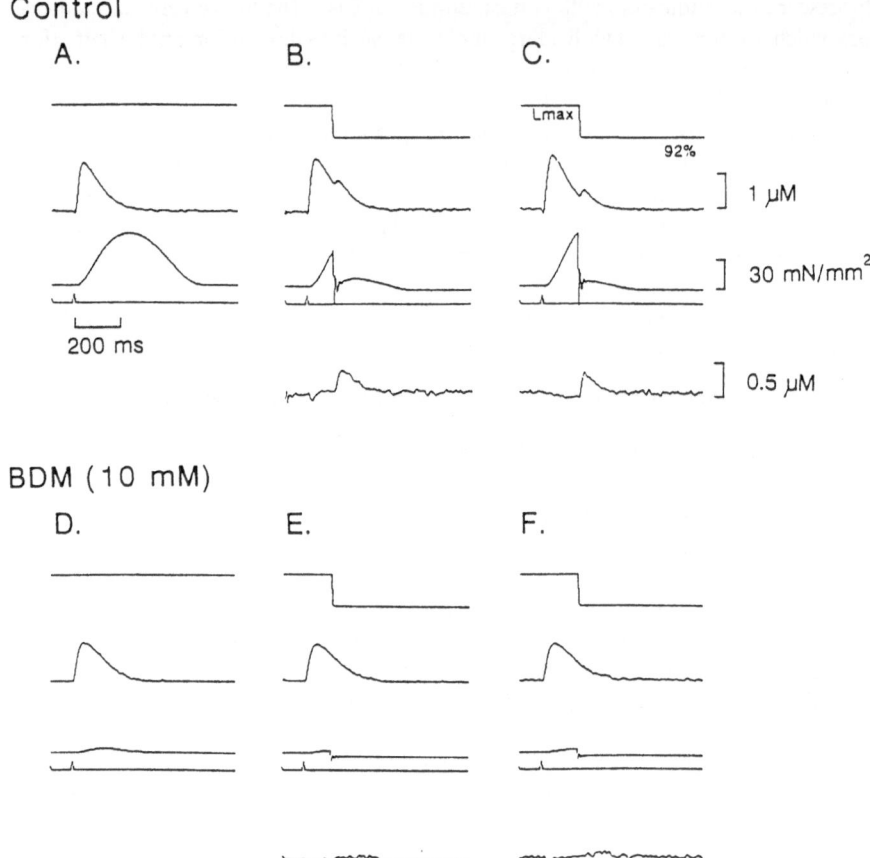

FIG. 1A–F. Effects of muscle length change from L_{max} to 92% L_{max} on the aequorin-injected ferret papillary muscle in the presence or absence of 2,3-butanedione monoxime (*BDM*). In A–F, traces (from *top* to *bottom*) show muscle length, Ca^{2+} transient, tension, stimulus, and extra-Ca^{2+}. The aequorin light signal was converted to $[Ca^{2+}]_i$. Extra-Ca^{2+} is the difference in Ca^{2+} transients measured at L_{max} and when the muscle length was altered. In the presence of BDM (10 mM), tension was suppressed and the extra-Ca^{2+} in response to the length change was not observed. (Komukai and Kurihara, unpublished data)

Effect of Length Change in Tetanized Preparation

Cardiac muscle can be tetanized using ryanodine and repetitive stimulation [22]. Tetanization is advantageous compared to twitch contraction for the measurement of the relation between $[Ca^{2+}]_i$ and tension at quasi-steady state in intact preparations. With altered muscle lengths, Saeki et al. [23] measured the change in $[Ca^{2+}]_i$ in tetanized ferret papillary muscle which was injected with aequorin (Fig. 2). They observed a sharp rise in $[Ca^{2+}]_i$ in response to quick release of muscle, which was followed by an exponential decay. In response to the release, tension was suddenly decreased and then redeveloped. The time course of the decay of the increased Ca^{2+} corresponded with that of the redeveloped tension. Restoration of the muscle length

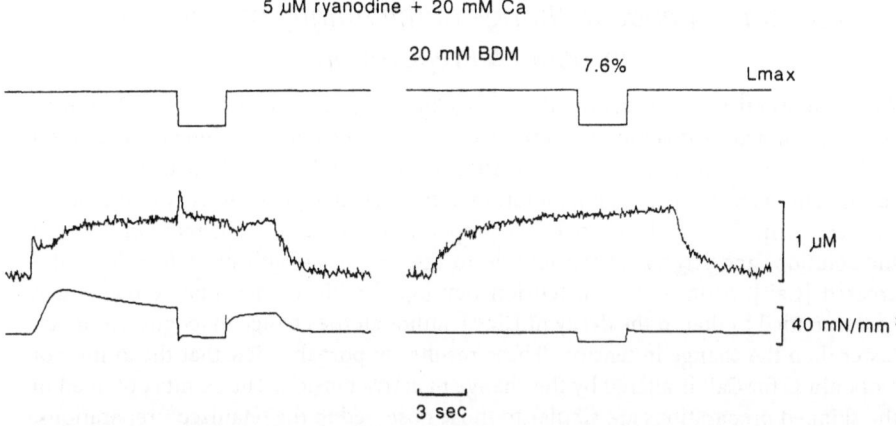

FIG. 2. Change in $[Ca^{2+}]_i$ and tension in response to length change in tetanized preparation. The preparation was treated with ryanodine $(5\,\mu M)$ and 20 mM $[Ca^{2+}]_o$. Repetitive stimulation (40 ms duration, 10 Hz) produced tetanic contraction. The length change from L_{max} to 92.4% L_{max} (*top trace*) transiently increased $[Ca^{2+}]_i$ (*middle trace*) and then suddenly decreased tension (*bottom trace*). Stretching the muscle to L_{max} restored tension and transiently decreased $[Ca^{2+}]_i$ (*left panel*). These changes were inhibited in the presence of 20 mM BDM. $[Ca^{2+}]_i$ was converted from the original record of the aequorin light signal by Saeki et al. [23]

to the original level before the release produced a short-lived tension change, but a transient change in $[Ca^{2+}]_i$ appearing in the release was not detected. The short-lived increase in tension was followed by a slow increase in active tension (delayed activation), and $[Ca^{2+}]_i$ decayed in accordance with the delayed activation. The time courses of the redeveloped tension and the decay of $[Ca^{2+}]_i$ were quite similar. In twitch contraction, $[Ca^{2+}]_i$ transiently changes and troponin-C is not sufficiently equilibrated with $[Ca^{2+}]_i$. However, in tetanic contraction, the Ca^{2+} binding site of troponin-C is equilibrated with Ca^{2+} and is almost saturated when the muscle is tetanized at 20 mM $[Ca^{2+}]_o$. Thus, the tension developed at 20 mM $[Ca^{2+}]_o$ is the maximal level. The change in $[Ca^{2+}]_i$ in response to mechanical perturbations is considered to be induced by a transient change in active tension, not in passive tension, because the changes in $[Ca^{2+}]_i$ and tension are in phase. Our hypothesis is that this transient change in active tension is the trigger for the change in $[Ca^{2+}]_i$. The origin of the extra-Ca^{2+} is the troponin-Ca complex and the alteration of the affinity of troponin-C for Ca^{2+} produces the extra-Ca^{2+}. Since the cross-bridge attachment is directly related to tension development, the tension-dependent change in $[Ca^{2+}]_i$ (extra-Ca^{2+}) implies that the affinity of troponin-C for Ca^{2+} is influenced by the change in the cross-bridge attachment. No significant change in $[Ca^{2+}]_i$ is observed in the short-lived transient increase in tension when the muscle is stretched to the length before the release. The short-lived transient tension might be due to the forcibly detached cross-bridges; strain was not applied to the cross-bridges. Thus, the affinity of troponin-C was not altered. A similar tension-dependent change in $[Ca^{2+}]_i$ was reported in aequorin-injected barnacle muscles; the strain on the cross-bridges was suggested to be important for the change in the affinity of troponin-C for Ca^{2+} [24].

Tension-Dependent Change of the Affinity of Troponin-C in Skinned Preparations

Allen and Kentish [25] measured the change in $[Ca^{2+}]$ in the solution when Triton X-treated, skinned cardiac muscle is released. They activated the skinned preparation with a small concentration of Ca^{2+} and applied a quick release to the activated preparation. The change in $[Ca^{2+}]$ in the solution induced by the quick release was measured with aequorin. The quick release of the preparation produced an increase in $[Ca^{2+}]$ in the solution, and stretching the muscle to the original length prior to release decreased $[Ca^{2+}]$. With a stretch, tension developed with a slow time course which corresponded to that of the decay of $[Ca^{2+}]$, although the change in length was much faster than the change in tension. These results support the view that the affinity of troponin-C for Ca^{2+} is altered by the change in active tension. The results obtained in the skinned preparations are similar to those observed in the tetanized preparations, although the transient increase in $[Ca^{2+}]$ appeared at the beginning of quick release is not observed in skinned preparations [23]. The reason for the difference in $[Ca^{2+}]$ change in the skinned and tetanized preparations is not clear at present. However, the Ca^{2+} buffering systems, including the Ca^{2+} regulation mechanisms in these two preparations, are different and this might explain the difference in changes in $[Ca^{2+}]$ at the beginning of quick release.

The change in the affinity of the contractile apparatus at different muscle lengths can be demonstrated by measuring $^{45}Ca^{2+}$ binding to the myofilaments [26]. More $^{45}Ca^{2+}$ binds to the contractile elements at a longer muscle length than at a shorter length. However, no increase in the $^{45}Ca^{2+}$ binding to the myofibril is observed at the longer muscle length when tension development is inhibited by vanadate [26]. Therefore, these results also support the view that more Ca^{2+} is bound to troponin-C if more tension is produced and that the affinity of troponin-C for Ca^{2+} is increased by the attachment of the cross-bridges.

Thus, mammalian cardiac muscle has an intrinsic control mechanism for regulating contraction. If $[Ca^{2+}]_i$ increases and Ca^{2+} is bound to troponin-C, the cross-bridges attach to thin filaments, thereby increasing the affinity of troponin-C for Ca^{2+}. Thus, more tension can be produced by cross-bridge attachment. When $[Ca^{2+}]_i$ is decreased, Ca^{2+} dissociates from troponin-C and the cross-bridges detach from the thin filaments. The detachment of the cross-bridges decreases the affinity of troponin-C for Ca^{2+} and relaxation is facilitated. The cross-bridge-dependent change in the affinity of troponin-C for Ca^{2+} might facilitate the contraction and relaxation cycle in cardiac muscles.

Physiological Significance of the Tension-Dependent Change in the Affinity of Troponin-C for Ca^{2+}

Relation Between Ca^{2+} Transient and Tension at different Muscle Lengths and at different $[Ca^{2+}]_o$

If Ca^{2+} transient and tension are measured at different lengths, the decay time of Ca^{2+} transient at a longer length is shorter than that at a shorter length. In addition, the relaxation time is prolonged at the longer length compared to the shorter length. If the muscle length is fixed at each length and the Ca^{2+} transient and tension are measured, the difference of the decay of the Ca^{2+} transients is small compared to the change in [Ca^{2+}]$_i$ induced by a quick muscle length change from a longer to a shorter length with the same amount (unpublished observation). Therefore, a transient change in tension (the transient change in the cross-bridge attachment) is more effective for the change in the affinity of troponin-C for Ca^{2+}. At a fixed length, the time course of tension development is slower than that with the change of tension induced by a quick release. If the tension change is slow, the tension-dependent change in the affinity of troponin-C for Ca^{2+} is slow. The increased [Ca^{2+}]$_i$ with a slow time course is quickly removed by intracellular Ca^{2+} regulation mechanisms, mainly by SR. In the presence of caffeine, which inhibits Ca^{2+} removal, the change in [Ca^{2+}]$_i$ is larger than that in the absence of caffeine when initial muscle length is shortened. Therefore, the speed of tension change and the rate of Ca^{2+} removal might be the critical factors in the determination of the change in [Ca^{2+}]$_i$ induced by length change.

Changes in Ca^{2+} Transient and Tension in β-Adrenoceptor Stimulation

Contraction of cardiac muscle is modulated by the neurotransmitters in the autonomic nervous system. Stimulation of the β-adrenoceptor shows various functional alterations, which are induced by the phosphorylation of target proteins of cyclic adenosine monophosphate (cAMP)-dependent protein kinase. The magnitude of contraction is increased and accompanied by a faster time course, thereby shortening the time to peak tension and the relaxation time [27,28,29]. These changes are partly due to the increased Ca^{2+} transient which accompanies the faster time course. The slightly faster time to peak of the Ca^{2+} transient is probably a factor related to the faster time to peak tension. However, the faster cross-bridge cycling rate may also be another factor explaining the faster time to peak tension [30]. For the initiation of relaxation, Ca^{2+} must dissociate from the binding site of troponin-C. Therefore, the removal of Ca^{2+} from the myoplasm is a prerequisite for the initiation of relaxation. However, the concentration dependence of the shortening of the decay time of Ca^{2+} differs from that of the relaxation time [29]. In addition, the recovery of the decay time of Ca^{2+} transient, which is induced by the removal of isoprenaline or by the addition of acetylcholine to the isoprenaline-treated preparation, does not accompany the restoration of the relaxation time [31]. Therefore, the rate of Ca^{2+} removal is not a rate-limiting step for determining the rate of relaxation, although the removal of Ca^{2+} from the myoplasm is a prerequisite for the initiation of relaxation.

The affinity of troponin-C for Ca^{2+} is another factor which influences the rate of relaxation. If the affinity of troponin-C for Ca^{2+} is decreased, Ca^{2+} dissociates from troponin-C at a faster rate and relaxation should be accelerated. In the isoprenaline-treated cardiac muscles, troponin-I is phosphorylated and the affinity of troponin-C for Ca^{2+} is decreased through the interaction between troponin-I and -C [32]. However, a higher concentration of isoprenaline is required for the decrease in Ca^{2+} sensitivity of the contractile elements compared to that required for the shortening of relaxation time [29]. The relaxation time is not significantly altered, even though the functions of both factors which accelerate relaxation (shortening of the decay time of Ca^{2+} and the decrease of the Ca^{2+} sensitivity of the contractile elements) are enhanced by isoprenaline. In addition to these factors, an increase in the peak tension probably influences the decay of Ca^{2+} transient and relaxation through the tension-dependent change in the affinity of troponin-C for Ca^{2+}. The increased tension increases the affinity of troponin-C for Ca^{2+}. This shortens the decay time of Ca^{2+} transient and prolongs the relaxation time. Therefore, three factors are related to the faster decay of Ca^{2+} transient: (1) faster Ca^{2+} uptake by the SR, (2) an increase in the Ca^{2+} sensitivity of the contractile elements induced by an increased tension, and (3) the decrease in the Ca^{2+} sensitivity induced by the phosphorylation of troponin-I. The third factor which prolongs the decay of Ca^{2+} transient antagonizes the function of the other two factors. Relaxation is also influenced by these factors, but it is facilitated by the faster Ca^{2+} uptake by the SR and a decrease in the Ca^{2+} sensitivity of the contractile elements. However, these effects are antagonized by a tension-dependent increase in the Ca^{2+} sensitivity. The relative contribution of these factors to the time courses of the Ca^{2+} transients and tension are still under investigation, and these effects might differ among different species [28,29].

Conclusion

A change in $[Ca^{2+}]_i$ is essential for contraction and relaxation in mammalian cardiac muscles. However, the change in the affinity of troponin-C, a major intracellular Ca^{2+} binding protein responsible for the regulation of contraction, profoundly influences contractile properties and $[Ca^{2+}]_i$. The affinity of troponin-C for Ca^{2+} is influenced by a change in the cross-bridge attachment and detachment. This mechanism functions in the physiological contraction–relaxation cycle. If the developed tension is altered under physiological and pathophysiological conditions, the involvement of this mechanism in the changes in the time courses of the Ca^{2+} transient and tension should be considered.

Acknowledgments. The work for this review was supported by a Grant-in-Aid for Scientific Research from the Ministry of Education, Science and Culture of Japan, by the Uehara Memorial Foundation, by the Sankyo Life Science Foundation, and by the Vehicle Racing Foundation. The authors thank Mrs. Mary Beth Sibuya for reading the manuscript. K. K. thanks Professor Tetsuo Okamura for his encouragement.

References

1. Ebashi S, Endo M (1968) Calcium ion and muscle contraction. Prog Biophys Mol Biol 18:123–183
2. Holroyde MJ, Robertson SP, Johnson JD, Solaro RJ, Potter JD (1980) The calcium and magnesium binding sites on cardiac troponin and their role in the regulation of myofibrillar adenosine triphosphate. J Biol Chem 255:11688–11693
3. Fabiato A (1982) Calcium release in skinned cardiac cells: Variations with species, tissues and development. Fed Proc 41:2238–2244
4. Hibberd MG, Jewell BR (1982) Calcium- and length-dependent force production in rat ventricular muscle. J Physiol (Lond) 329:527–540
5. Allen DG, Kentish JC (1985) The cellular basis of the length–tension relation in cardiac muscle. J Mol Cell Cardiol 17:821–840
6. Moss RL (1979) Sarcomere length–tension relations of frog skinned muscle fibres during activation at short length. J Physiol (Lond) 292:177–192
7. Fabiato A, Fabiato F (1975) Dependence of the contractile activation of skinned cardiac cells on the sarcomere length. Nature 256:54–56

8. Allen DG, Jewel BR, Murray JW (1974) The contribution of activation processes to the length–tension relation of cardiac muscle. Nature 248:606–607

9. Miyata H, Silverman HS, Sollot SJ, Lakatta EG, Stern MD, Hansford RG (1991) Measurement of mitochondrial free Ca^{2+} concentration in living single rat cardiac myocytes. Am J Physiol 261:H1123–H1134

10. Konishi M, Olson A, Hollingworth S, Baylor SM (1988) Myoplasmic binding of fura-2 investigated by steady-state fluorescence and absorbance measurements. Biophys J 54:1089–1104

11. Konishi M, Watanabe M (1994) Measurement of resting $[Ca^{2+}]_i$ in frog skeletal muscle fibers with fura-2 conjugated to dextran. Biophys J 66:A340

12. Blatter LA, Blinks JR (1991) Simultaneous measurement of Ca^{2+} in muscle with Ca^{2+} electrodes and aequorin. J Gen Physiol 98:1141–1160

13. Kurihara S (1994) Regulation of cardiac muscle contraction by intracellular Ca^{2+}. Jpn J Physiol 44:591–611

14. Cheung WY (1980) Calmodulin plays a pivotal role in cellular regulation. Science 207:19–27

15. Allen DG, Kurihara S (1980) Calcium transients in mammalian ventricular muscle. Eur Heart J 1[Suppl A]:1–15

16. Berlin JR, Konishi M (1993) Ca^{2+} transients in cardiac myocytes measured with high and low affinity Ca^{2+} indicators. Biophys J 65:1632–1647

17. Beuckelmann DJ, Wier WG (1988) Mechanism of release of calcium from sarcoplasmic reticulum of guinea pig cardiac cells. J Physiol (Lond) 405:233–255

18. Allen DG, Kurihara S (1982) The effects of muscle length on intracellular calcium transients in mammalian cardiac muscle. J Physiol (Lond) 327:79–94

19. Housmans PR, Lee NMK, Blinks JR (1983) Active shortening retards the decline of the intracellular calcium transient in mammalian heart muscle. Science 221:159–161

20. Backx PH, ter Keurs HEDJ (1993) Fluorescent properties of rat cardiac trabeculae microinjected with fura-2 salt. Am J Physiol 264:H1098–H1110

21. Kurihara S, Saeki Y, Hongo K, Tanaka E, Suda N (1990) Effect of length change on intracellular Ca transients in ferret ventricular muscles treated with 2,3-butanedione monoxime (BDM). Jpn J Physiol 40:915–920

22. Yue DT, Marban E, Wier WG (1986) Relationship between force and intracellular $[Ca^{2+}]$ in tetanized mammalian heart muscle. J Gen Physiol 87:223–242

23. Saeki Y, Kurihara S, Hongo K, Tanaka E (1993) Alterations in intracellular calcium and tension of activated ferret papillary muscles in response to step length changes. J Physiol (Lond) 463:291–306

24. Gordon AM, Ridgway EB (1990) Stretch of active muscle during the declining phase of the calcium transient produces biphasic change in calcium binding to the activating sites. J Gen Physiol 96:1013–1035

25. Allen DG, Kentish JC (1988) Calcium concentration in the myoplasm of skinned ferret ventricular muscle following changes in muscle length. J Physiol (Lond) 407:489–503

26. Hofmann PA, Fuchs F (1987) Effect of length and cross-bridge attachment on Ca^{2+} binding to cardiac troponin-C. Am J Physiol 253:C90–C96

27. Endoh M, Blinks JR (1988) Actions of sympathomimetic amines on the Ca^{2+} transients and contractions of rabbit myocardium: Reciprocal changes in myofibrillar responsiveness to Ca^{2-} mediated through α- and β-adrenoceptors. Circ Res 62:247–265

28. Kurihara S, Konishi M (1987) Effects of β-adrenoceptor stimulation on intracellular Ca transients and tension in rat ventricular muscle. Pflügers Arch 409:427–437

29. Okazaki O, Suda N, Hongo K, Konishi M, Kurihara S (1990) Modulation of Ca^{2+} transients and contractile properties by β-adrenoceptor stimulation in ferret ventricular muscles. J Physiol (Lond) 423:221–240

30. Hoh JFY, Rossmanith GH, Kwan LJ, Hamilton AM (1988) Adrenaline increases the rate of cycling of crossbridges in rat cardiac muscle as measured by pseudo-random binary noise-modulated perturbation analysis. Circ Res 62:452–461

31. Hongo K, Tanaka E, Kurihara S (1993) Alterations in contractile properties and Ca^{2+} transients by β- and muscarinic receptor stimulation in ferret myocardium. J Physiol (Lond) 461:167–184

32. Robertson SP, Johnson JD, Holroyde MJ, Kranias EG, Potter JD, Solaro RJ (1982) The effect of troponin-I phosphorylation on the Ca^{2+}-binding properties of the Ca^{2+}-regulatory site of bovine cardiac troponin. J Biol Chem 257:260–263

Uncoupling of the β_2-Adrenoceptor Effect on Ca^{2+} Regulation and cAMP in Cardiac Cells

RUI-PING XIAO and EDWARD G. LAKATTA

Summary. Studies in rat ventricular myocytes demonstrate that while both β_1-adrenergic receptor stimulation (β_1ARS) and β_2AR stimulation (β_2ARS) increase cyclic adenosine monophosphate (cAMP) to a similar extent, the effects of β_2ARS on cytosolic Ca^{2+} (Ca_i) transient and contraction are largely dissociated from the cAMP increase. In canine ventricular myocytes, β_2ARS augments the amplitude of I_{Ca}, Ca_i transient, and contraction without increasing cell cAMP. In rat cells, β_2ARS by zinterol (ZINT) or by isoproterenol in the presence of the selective β_1AR antagonist CGP 20712A increases contraction amplitude to about the same extent as β_1ARS by norepinephrine (NE). While β_1ARS has a potent effect to abbreviate the durations of the contraction and Ca_i transient, β_2ARS has only a minor relaxation effect in rat cells. β_2ARS does not result in phospholamban phosphorylation to the same extent in either rat or canine cells as does β_1ARS. In addition, β_1ARS, but not β_2ARS, increases the diastolic Ca^{2+} level and evokes spontaneous Ca_i oscillations. β_2ARS prolongs the action potential to a greater extent than does β_1ARS. β_1ARS and β_2ARS also differ in their effects on I_{Ca}: whereas both increase the peak I_{Ca} amplitude to a similar extent, only β_2ARS markedly prolongs the I_{Ca} inactivation time. A peptide inhibitor of protein kinase A abolishes β_1ARS, but only partially affects β_2ARS-induced increase in I_{Ca} in canine cells; the β_2AR effect to increase I_{Ca} is abolished by a G protein inhibitor, GDPβS. Additionally, the G_s-coupled β_2AR activates a pertussis toxin (PTX)-sensitive G protein pathway that leads to inhibition of its effects. This provides a mechanism to protect the heart from Ca^{2+} overload and arrhythmias during the response in stress.

Key words. β-Receptor subtypes—G proteins—Cytosolic calcium—Cardiac myocytes—Calcium current

Introduction

β-Adrenoceptor (βAR) stimulation (βARS) increases the rate and force of myocardial contraction and enables the heart to respond appropriately to increased peripheral demands. Evidence from radioligand binding and functional studies [1–5] indicates that β_1AR and β_2AR coexist in the hearts of various mammalian species, and that both

Laboratory of Cardiovascular Science, Gerontology Research Center, National Institute on Aging, National Institutes of Health, Baltimore, MD 21224, USA

$\beta_1 AR$ and $\beta_2 AR$ stimulation play a significant role in the regulation of inotropic or chronotropic activities of the heart [6–8]. Early studies have well established that both $\beta_1 AR$ and $\beta_2 AR$ subtype stimulation increase the activity of adenylate cyclase via an interaction with G_s in cardiac preparations from several species, and subsequently elevate the cell cyclic adenosine monophosphate (cAMP) concentration [9–13]. Although the intracellular signal transduction pathway for $\beta_1 AR$ stimulation distal to cAMP augmentation has been intensively studied, little information exists as to the specific mechanisms that couple $\beta_2 AR$ stimulation to its cellular responses. Specifically, it is not clear whether the functional effects of $\beta_2 AR$ stimulation on cardiac myocytes are mediated by cAMP-dependent mechanisms. Recent evidence for distinct actions of βAR subtype stimulation on the cytosolic I_{Ca}, Ca_i transient, twitch amplitude, cAMP production, and cAMP-dependent protein phosphorylation in single rat and dog ventricular myocytes has emerged, and will be summarized.

Results and Discussion

Distinct Effects of βAR Subtype Stimulation on Cardiac Excitation-Contraction Coupling in Single Rat Ventricular Myocytes

Figure 1 illustrates the representative effects of $\beta_1 AR$ and $\beta_2 AR$ stimulation on contraction and Ca_i transient in individual rat heart cells. Panel A, upper tracing, shows that $\beta_1 AR$ stimulation by norepinephrine (NE) [1,14,15] increases the electrically stimulated contraction amplitude and that this is reversed by CGP 20712A (CGP), the $\beta_1 AR$-specific antagonist [16,17]. Thus, NE exerts its positive inotropic effect almost exclusively through $\beta_1 AR$ stimulation in rat cardiac cells. It has previously been shown that the $\alpha_1 AR$ blocker, prazosin at $1\,\mu M$, as well as the $\beta_2 AR$ blocker, ICI 118,551 (ICI,

---

FIG. 1. A Representative effects of the β_1-adrenoceptor (AR) agonist norepinephrine (NE) on the simultaneously recorded Ca_i transient and contraction. The *upper tracing* is a continuous recording showing the effect of NE in augmenting the contraction amplitude. The *lower tracings* were obtained at the times indicated in the upper tracing and show the Ca_i transient and contraction for control conditions (tracing *a*), during exposure to NE at $10^{-7}\,M$ (tracing *b*) and the presence of NE plus CGP ($3 \times 10^{-7}\,M$), a β_1-adrenoreceptor inhibitor (tracing *c*). The *tracings on the right* are those of *a* and *b* normalized to their peaks and superimposed. B An example of the effect of the $\beta_2 AR$ agonist zinterol (ZINT) on the simultaneously recorded Ca_i transient and cell length. The *upper tracing* is a chart recording that shows the effect of ZINT ($10^{-5}\,M$) on twitch amplitude. The *lower tracings* were obtained at the times indicated in the upper tracing. Tracings *a–c* represent Ca_i transient and contraction under control conditions, when the effect of ZINT was stable, and following the addition of a selective β_2-adrenoreceptor blocker, ICI ($10^{-7}\,M$), respectively. The *tracings on the right* are those of the Ca_i transient and contraction prior to and following exposure to ZINT, normalized to their peak amplitude, and superimposed, to better show the effects of ZINT on the kinetics of Ca_i transient and twitch. Data from [13]. Single ventricular cardiac myocytes were isolated from 2- to 4-month-old rat hearts by a standard enzymatic technique [47]. For some studies, myocytes were loaded with the fluorescent Ca^{2+} probe indo-1 acetoxymethyl ester (indo-I AM, Molecular Probes, Eugene, OR, USA) at room temperature as previously described [47]. After indo-1 AM loading, cells were placed on the stage of a modified inverted microscope (model IM-35, Zeiss, Oberkohen, FRG) equipped for simultaneous recording of indo-1 fluorescence and cell length [47]

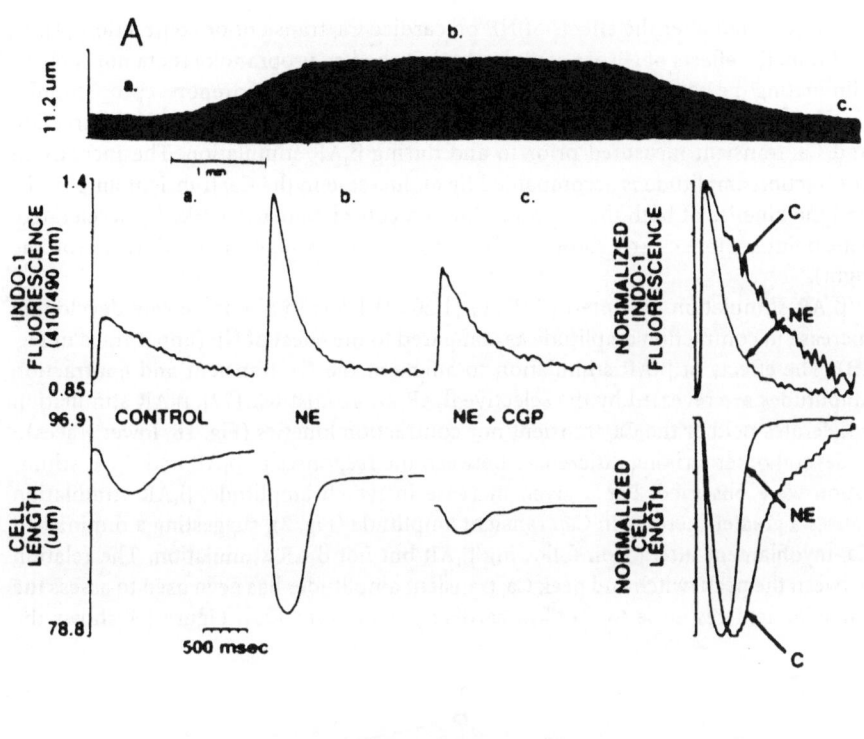

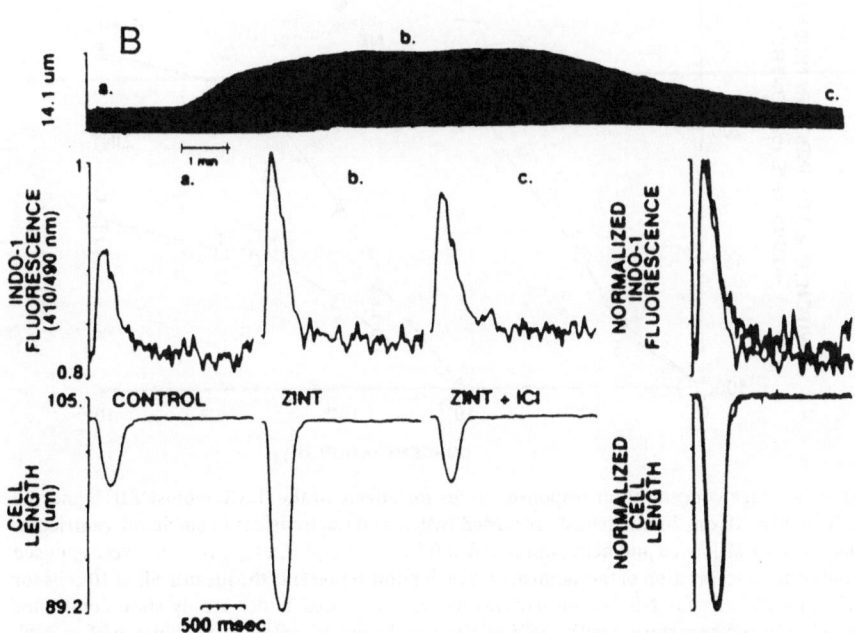

0.1 µM), do not alter the effects of NE on cardiac Ca_i transient or contraction [1]. In addition, the effects of NE are completely abolished by propranolol (data not shown), eliminating the possibility that the effects of NE occur via β_3-adrenoreceptor stimulation [18,19]. Figure 1A, lower traces, show the simultaneously recorded contraction and Ca_i transient measured prior to and during β_1AR stimulation. The increase in contraction amplitude is accompanied by an increase in the Ca_i transient amplitude, and the kinetics of both the Ca_i transient and contraction are markedly accelerated. This point is more clearly shown in the normalized and superimposed traces (on the right).

β_2AR stimulation by zinterol (ZINT) [1,20,21] leads to a more slowly developing increase in contraction amplitude as compared to the effect of NE (upper trace in Fig. 1B). The effects of β_2AR stimulation to augment the Ca_i transient and contraction amplitudes are reversed by the selective β_2AR antagonist ICI [22]. β_2AR stimulation accelerates neither the Ca_i transient nor contraction kinetics (Fig. 1B, lower traces).

Several other striking differences between the responses to β_1AR and β_2AR stimulation were observed. For a given increase in twitch amplitude, β_1AR stimulation causes a greater increase in Ca_i transient amplitude (Fig. 2), suggesting a diminished Ca_i-myofilament interaction following β_1AR but not β_2AR stimulation. The relation between the peak twitch and peak Ca_i transient amplitudes has been used to assess the "myofilament response to Ca^{2+}" in cardiac preparations [23]. Figure 3A shows the

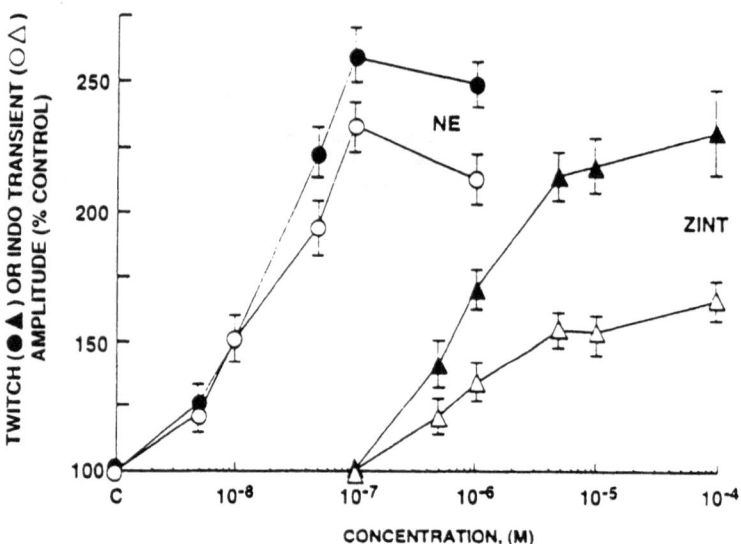

FIG. 2. Average concentration-response curves for effects of the β_2AR agonist ZINT and the β_1AR agonist NE on simultaneously recorded twitch and Ca_i transient in single rat ventricular cells, indo-1 AM-loaded and field-stimulated at 0.5 Hz in 1 mM $[Ca^{2+}]_o$. Myocytes were exposed to only one concentration of the agonist, and each point represents the mean ± SE of 10 cells for ZINT and 25 cells for NE. All measurements were obtained under steady-state conditions following 10 min superfusion with ZINT or NE. Results are expressed as percentage of control. Control values for ZINT cells (n = 50) are: twitch amplitude, 6.29 ± 0.26% of the resting cell length; the peak height of indo-1 fluorescence transient (the difference between systolic and diastolic levels of indo-1 fluorescence ratio), an index of the Ca_i transient, 0.208 ± 0.005. Control values for NE cells (n = 125) were: twitch amplitude, 6.36 ± 0.32% of the resting cell length; peak height of Ca^{2+}_i transient, 0.206 ± 0.005. Data from [1]

relation between changes of contraction amplitude and changes of the peak height of Ca_i transient measured during the negative staircase that ensues after stimulation of rat myocytes from rest (see Fig. 3A, inset). In Figure 3B, when the Ca_i-contraction relation after stimulation with the β_1AR agonist (NE) and β_2AR agonist (ZINT) are compared with that of the negative staircase (which represents the relation between the Ca_i transient and contraction in the absence of βAR stimulation), it is evident that this relation is markedly shifted to the right by NE; in contrast, it is not altered by ZINT. Thus, for a given level of Ca_i, twitch amplitude is lower in the presence of β_1AR than in the presence of β_2AR stimulation.

The average dose-response relations for the effects of βAR stimulation of the kinetics of the twitch and Ca_i transients are illustrated in Fig. 4. The maximal effect of NE in reducing the $t_{1/2}$ of the contraction was 35.6%; in reducing the $t_{1/2}$ of the Ca_i transient, it was 29.9%. In contrast, ZINT had only a slight effect on the kinetics of contraction. The maximal effect of ZINT in reducing the $t_{1/2}$ of contraction was 8.0%. On average, ZINT did not reduce the time course of the Ca_i transient. Figure 4 also clearly demonstrates that the small effect of ZINT on the twitch duration was not concentration-dependent, whereas the marked effects of NE monotonically increased with drug concentration. Note that, although the concentration ranges in Fig. 4 for ZINT and NE are different, their corresponding positive inotropic effects, as indexed by the increased contraction amplitudes, are comparable (compare with Fig. 2). Thus, for a given augmentation of the twitch amplitude, NE accelerated the kinetics of the contraction and Ca_i transient to a far greater extent.

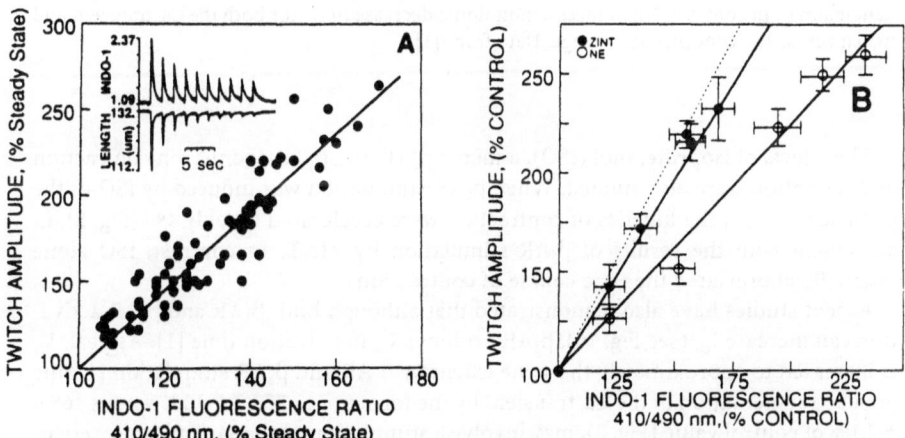

FIG. 3. A Graph showing the relation between changes in peak amplitude of the Ca_i transient and changes in twitch amplitude during the negative staircase after stimulation from rest (eight cells). The insert shows a representative example of a negative staircase after field stimulation at 0.5 Hz from rest of a rat ventricular cell loaded with the pentapotassium salt of indo-1 (indo-1/FA). B Graph showing the relation between the change in the peak amplitude of Ca_i transient and that of the twitch amplitude evoked by β_1AR or β_2AR stimulation (data from concentration response curves in Fig. 2). The relation obtained from the negative staircase in A (*dashed line* in B) represents the relation between the indo-1 fluorescence and contraction amplitudes in the absence of β-adrenoreceptor stimulation. This relation is markedly shifted rightward by NE but is not significantly shifted by ZINT. The slopes of the lines fitted to the NE and ZINT data are significantly different ($P < 0.05$, by analyses of covariance with test for homogeneity of slopes). Data from [1]

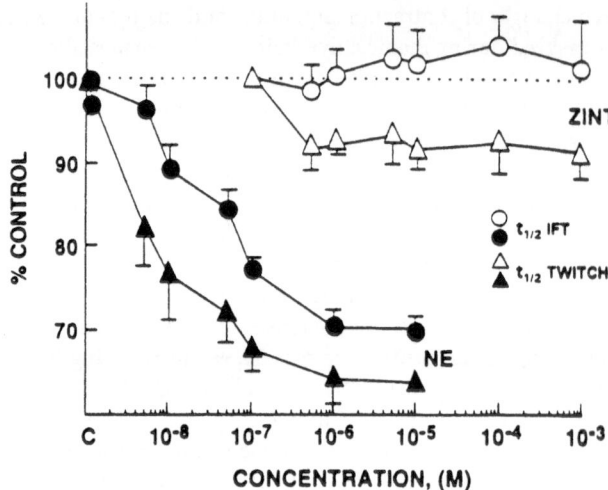

FIG. 4. Comparison of the average concentration-response relations for effects of β_1AR agonist NE or β_2AR agonist ZINT on the half-time ($t_{1/2}$) of the Ca_i transient (*circles*) and $t_{1/2}$ of the contraction (*triangles*) of isolated rat ventricular myocytes. Cells used to determine concentration response curves for ZINT and NE are the same as those depicted in Fig. 1. In control cells before ZINT ($n = 60$), $t_{1/2}$ of the Ca_i transient was 389.51 ± 8.00 ms, and $t_{1/2}$ of contraction was 488.6 ± 13.96 ms. In control cells for NE ($n = 150$), $t_{1/2}$ of the Ca_i transient was 396.89 ± 10.74 ms, and $t_{1/2}$ of contraction was 495.11 ± 22.30 ms. Note that ZINT does not reduce the duration of the Ca_i transient and has only a minor effect in decreasing the twitch duration, in no dose-dependent manner. In contrast, NE induces a monotonic decrease in $t_{1/2}$ for both the Ca_i transient and twitch across the concentration range. Data from [1]

The effects of isoproterenol (ISO), a mixed β_1AR and β_2AR agonist, on contraction and relaxation were also studied. When β_2AR stimulation was induced by ISO in the presence of CGP, the kinetics of contraction were accelerated by only 4% (Fig. 5), in agreement with the results of β_2AR stimulation by ZINT. In contrast, ISO alone markedly abbreviated the time course of contraction.

Recent studies have also demonstrated that although both β_1AR and β_2AR activation can increase I_{Ca} (see Fig. 16), β_2AR prolongs I_{Ca} inactivation time [1]. As peak I_{Ca} is increased to approximately the same extent by β_1AR and β_2AR stimulation [1], the greater augmentation of the Ca_i transient by the former, i.e., 233.3 ± 9.1% versus 168.0 ± 7.1% of control value (Fig. 2), may involve a stimulation of the sarcoplasmic reticulum (SR) pump or a direct action on the SR release channel by β_1AR stimulation, actions not apparently shared by β_2AR stimulation. In addition, different effects of β_1AR and β_2AR stimulation on Ca^{2+} metabolism are also indicated by the observation that only β_1AR, but not β_2AR stimulation increases resting $[Ca^{2+}]_i$ and the likelihood of Ca^{2+} oscillations to occur [1]. This observation is not trivial since spontaneous Ca^{2+} oscillations can activate depolarizing membrane currents, which may lead to a disturbance of the electrical behavior of the heart and lead to arrhythmia [24,25]. Recent studies in canine and sheep heart show that β_2AR stimulation is indeed less arrhythmogenic than is β_1AR stimulation [4,26]. The results described above may provide the cellular mechanism for the different arrhythmogenic actions of β_1AR versus β_2AR agonists.

FIG. 5. Average increases in twitch amplitude (percentage of control) and abbreviation of $t_{1/2}$ of contraction (percentage of control) induced by isoproterenol (ISO) (10^{-6} M) and ISO (10^{-6} M) in the presence of CGP (3×10^{-7}M) or ICI (10^{-7}M). Note that ISO alone markedly increases twitch amplitude and abbreviates contraction duration. In the presence of the β_1AR antagonist CGP, ISO still significantly increases twitch amplitude. However, the relaxation effect is abolished. In the presence of both β_1AR and β_2AR blockers (CGP +ICI), both the positive inotropic effect and relaxation effect of ISO are abolished

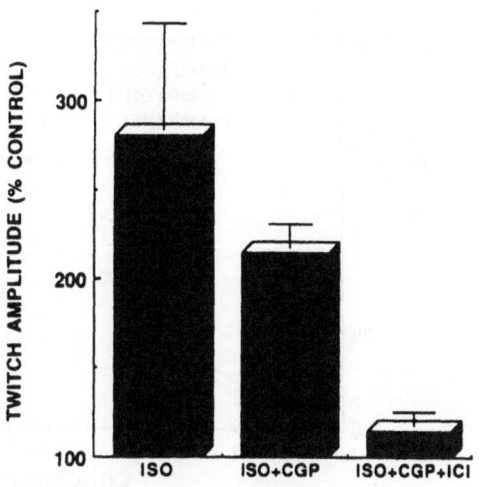

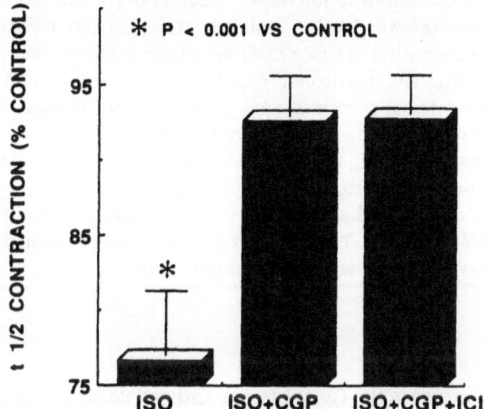

β_2AR-Stimulated Increase in cAMP is Dissociated from Its Effects on Ca^{2+} Hemostasis and Contraction in Rat Myocytes

Recent studies demonstrate that in rat cardiac myocytes, as in many other species, both β_2AR and β_1AR are coupled to adenylate cyclase and when stimulated, lead to an increase in the cellular cAMP level [9–13]. Figure 6 shows the dose-response relations of β_1AR and β_2AR stimulation to increase the steady levels of total and particulate cAMP content. Both NE and ZINT increase the total cellular cAMP content to about the same extent over the entire agonist concentration range used. The particulate cAMP is also increased by the β_1AR and β_2AR agonists. However, the maximal magnitude of the increase in the particulate cAMP by ZINT is only 50% of that by NE. These results suggest that βAR subtype stimulation increases cellular cAMP in different subcellular compartments.

Figure 7A compares the dose-response relation for total cellular cAMP production induced by β_1AR and β_2AR stimulation to the β_1AR and β_2AR stimulated increases in the Ca_i transient and contraction amplitudes. Note that the curves for the β_1AR effects

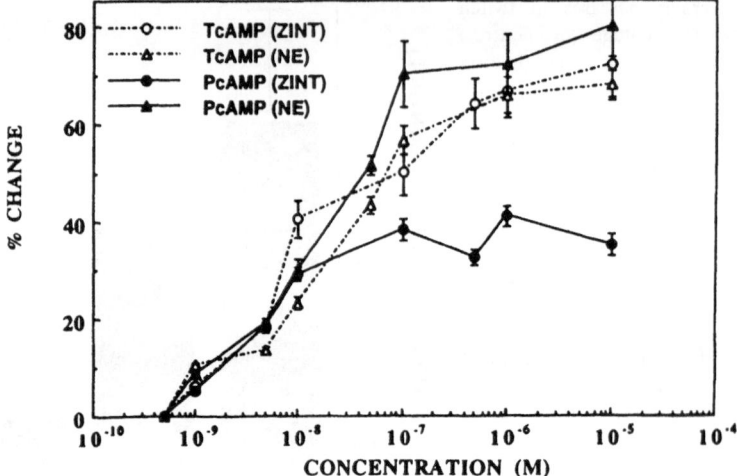

FIG. 6. Concentration response curves of NE and ZINT to increase cyclic adenosine monophosphate (cAMP) level in isolated rat ventricular myocytes. Cells were incubated with varying concentration of NE or ZINT for 10 min at room temperature (23°C) before subsequent analysis of total and particulate cAMP measurements (TcAMP and PcAMP, respectively). Data are presented as percent change (mean ± SE of 10-myocyte preparations for ZINT and 5-myocyte preparations for NE). The control value of the total cAMP content is 6.91 ± 0.71 pmol/mg of protein ($n = 12$), and the control value of the particulate cAMP content is 2.94 ± 0.39 pmol/mg of protein (approximately 43% of the total cAMP content) ($n = 12$). Data from [13]. Suspensions of adult rat cardiac myocytes were incubated for 10 min at 23°C with the indicated concentration of ZINT of NE. The cellular cAMP content of isolated myocytes was determined as described previously [28] with minor modifications

to increase the Ca_i transient and cell contraction amplitude overlap that for the β_1AR-stimulated increase in the total cellular cAMP. The EC_{50} of NE for the responses of the total cellular cAMP, Ca_i transient, and contraction are all comparable (1.99×10^{-8} M, 1.92×10^{-8} M, and 1.90×10^{-8} M, respectively). The most striking finding in Fig. 7A, however, is that while the major portion of the β_2AR agonist induced increase in cAMP occurs over concentrations ranging from 5×10^{-10} M to 10^{-7} M, this increase in cAMP is not accompanied by any detectable increase in the Ca_i transient amplitude or in contraction amplitude. Rather, the Ca_i transient and contraction amplitudes begin to increase only at those concentrations of the β_2AR agonist at which the cAMP production has already approached its maximum. Accordingly, the EC_{50} for ZINT to increase total cAMP (1.02×10^{-8} M) is about two orders of magnitude lower than that for the ZINT-induced increase in Ca_i transient and contraction amplitudes (9.06×10^{-7} M and 9.02×10^{-7} M, respectively). Thus the effects of β_2AR stimulation on Ca_i transient and contraction are dissociated from the β_2AR stimulation-induced increase in the total cellular cAMP content. Following β_1AR stimulation, the increase in the total cAMP also shows a close relationship with the abbreviation of the Ca_i transient and contraction (Fig. 7B), similar to the relationship with the Ca_i transient and contraction amplitude responses. In contrast, at no concentration does the β_2AR agonist accelerate the kinetics of the Ca_i transient, and only a slight acceleration of the kinetics of contraction (in a non-dose-dependent manner) occurs (Fig. 7).

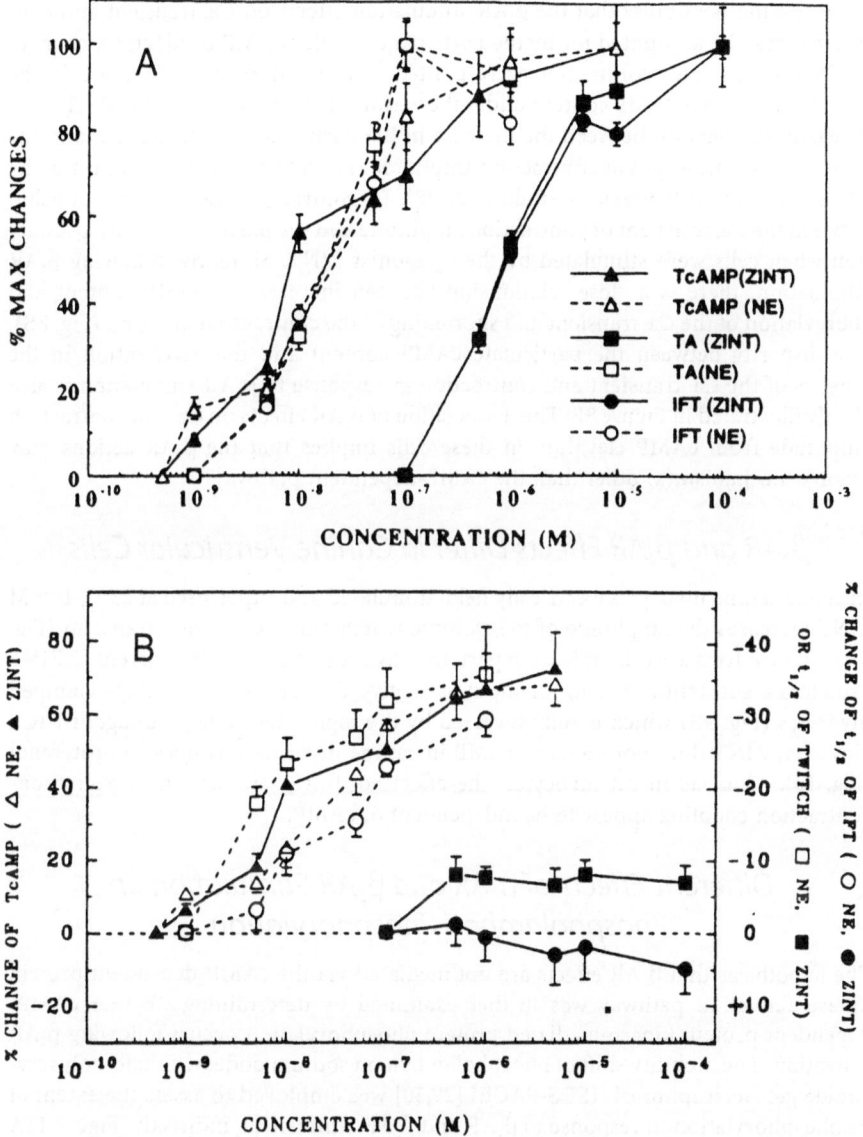

FIG. 7. A Concentration-response curves of the relative ZINT- and NE-induced increases in the total cAMP (*TcAMP*) and the Ca_i transient (*IFT*) or twitch amplitudes (*TA*). All values were determined 10 min after exposure to NE or ZINT ($n = 5$–10 for cAMP; $n = 10$–30 for IFT and TA measurements). Data are presented as percent of maximum change. Control value of the total cAMP content is 6.91 ± 0.71 pmol/mg of protein ($n = 12$). The maximum change of total cAMP is $78.3.0 \pm 4.1\%$ of control and $76.5 \pm 7.3\%$ of control for ZINT and NE, respectively. The maximum changes of contraction and Ca_i transient amplitudes induced by NE were $156.70 \pm 6.56\%$ and $123.10 \pm 5.20\%$ ($n = 25$), respectively. The maximum changes of contraction and Ca_i transient amplitudes induced by ZINT were $136.9 \pm 10.13\%$ and $74.39 \pm 5.25\%$, respectively. Data from [13]. B Concentration-response curves of the ZINT- and NE-induced increases in the total cAMP (*TcAMP*) and changes in the $t_{1/2}$ of the Ca_i transient (*IFT*) and twitch. Data are presented as percent change (mean $\pm$ SE, $n = 5$–10 for cAMP measurement, $n = 10$–30 for IFT $t_{1/2}$ and twitch $t_{1/2}$). Control values for the total cAMP is the same as in A. Twitch and Ca_i transient data are from cells in Fig. 4. Data from [13]

To test the possibility that the $\beta_2 AR$ stimulation effects on Ca_i transient and contraction may be accounted for by the particulate cellular cAMP production, changes in Ca_i transient and contraction were plotted as a function of the increase in the particulate cellular cAMP content under the various drug treatments (Fig. 8). There is a near-linear relation between the increase in the particulate cAMP content and the increase in Ca_i transient or contraction amplitude (Fig. 8A) during $\beta_1 AR$ activation by NE, consistent with previous studies [27,28]. In contrast, there is no relationship between the Ca_i transient or contraction amplitude and the particulate cAMP production when cells were stimulated by the β_2 agonist ZINT. Similarly, following $\beta_1 AR$ stimulation, there is a close relationship between increases in cAMP content and abbreviation of the Ca_i transient and shortening of the contraction duration (Fig. 8B). The disparity between the particulate cAMP content and the acceleration in the kinetics of the Ca_i transient and contraction in response to $\beta_2 AR$ stimulation is also clearly illustrated in Figure 8B. The dissociation of $\beta_2 AR$ effects on Ca_i and contraction amplitude from cAMP elevation in these cells implies that the $\beta_2 AR$ actions may involve mechanism(s) other than the cAMP-dependent pathway.

$\beta_2 AR$ and $\beta_1 AR$ Effects Differ in Canine Ventricular Cells

In single canine myocytes electrically field-stimulated and superfused at 23°C, 10^{-5} M ZINT increases the amplitude of the isotonic twitch and indo-1 ratio transient (Fig. 9A). These effects are due, at least in part, to activation of L-type Ca^{2+} current as ZINT produces a substantial rise in nifedipine-sensitive Ca^{2+} currents in voltage-clamped myocytes (Fig. 9B) which is fully reversed by the highly selective β_2-antagonist ICI. However, ZINT does not increase cAMP in canine myocytes, as does isoproterenol (Fig. 10). Thus, as in rat myocytes, the effects of $\beta_2 AR$ stimulation in excitation-contraction coupling appear to be independent of cAMP.

Different Effects of $\beta_1 AR$ and $\beta_2 AR$ Stimulation on Phospholamban Phosphorylation

The hypothesis that $\beta_2 AR$ effects are not mediated via the cAMP-dependent protein kinase activation pathway was further examined by determining whether cAMP-dependent protein kinase-mediated protein phosphorylation occurs following $\beta_2 AR$ activation. The mobility shift of phospholamban on sodium dodecyl sulfate-polyacrylamide gel electrophoresis (SDS-PAGE) [29,30] was employed to assess the extent of its phosphorylation in response to $\beta_1 AR$ and $\beta_2 AR$ stimulation indirectly. Figure 11A shows that $\beta_1 AR$ stimulation of myocytes by NE produces a large mobility shift in phospholamban on SDS-PAGE, with the formation of five discrete bands of decreasing mobility. The occurrence of several de novo bands following $\beta_1 AR$ stimulation has been reported previously with perfused guinea pig hearts, and correlated with phosphorylation of serine residue 16 of phospholamban by cAMP-dependent protein kinase [29]. $\beta_2 AR$ stimulation by ZINT, in contrast, is much less effective in inducing a mobility shift in phospholamban on SDS-PAGE. Only one or two new mobility forms are induced, corresponding to the bands with the least mobility shifts. Figure 11B shows that ISO, a mixed $\beta_1 AR$ and $\beta_2 AR$ agonist, also induces five distinct mobility states of phospholamban on SDS-PAGE, as does NE, again indicating different degrees of phosphorylation of the pentamer at serine 16 by cAMP-dependent protein kinase. Furthermore, when ISO is acting in the β_1 mode, i.e., in the presence of $\beta_2 AR$

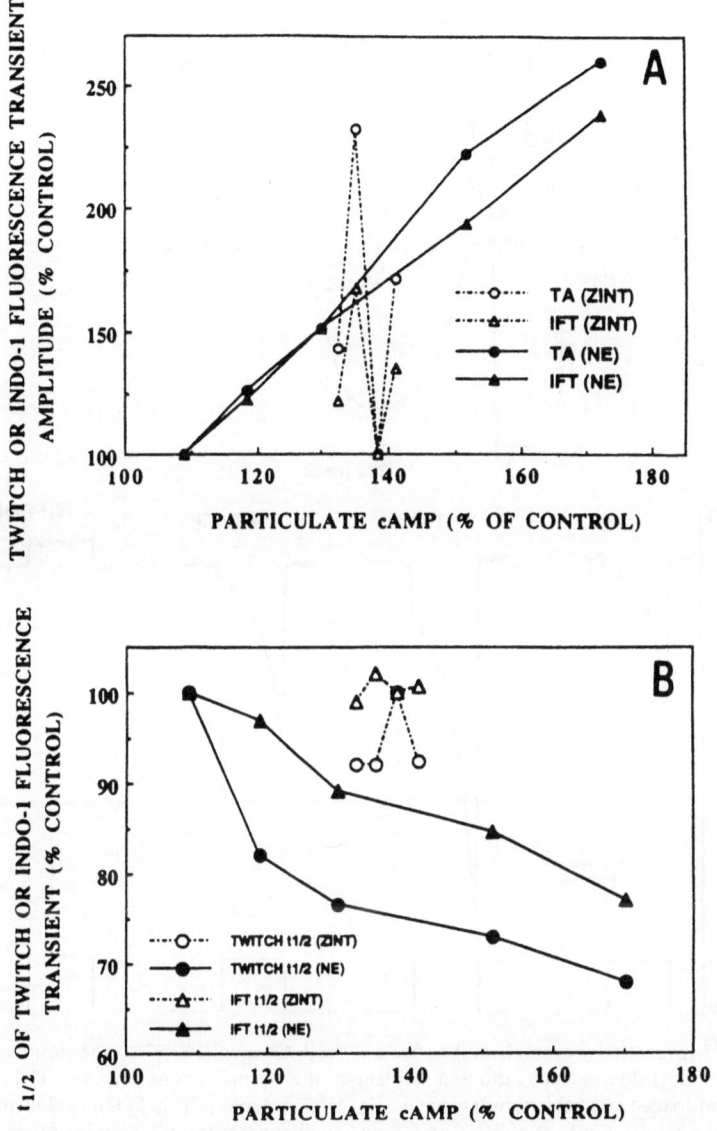

FIG. 8. **A** The increase in cell Ca_i transient amplitude (*IFT*) and contraction amplitude (*TA*) are plotted as a function of the particulate cellular cAMP (*PcAMP*) content following β_1AR and β_2AR stimulation. Data are presented as percentage of control values. The control values for particulate cAMP is the same as in Fig. 5, and the control values of IFT and TA are the same as in Fig. 7. Data from [13]. **B** The relationship between the changes in the particulate cAMP content and the changes in the IFT $t_{1/2}$ and twitch $t_{1/2}$. Data are presented as percentage of control. Control values for the total and the particulate cAMP are the same as in Fig. 6. In control cells before ZINT ($n = 60$), IFT $t_{1/2}$ was 389.51 ± 8.00 ms, and twitch $t_{1/2}$ was 488.6 ± 13.96 ms. In control cells for NE ($n = 70$), IFT $t_{1/2}$, and twitch $t_{1/2}$ were 396.89 ± 10.74 and 495.11 ± 22.3 ms, respectively. Data from [13]

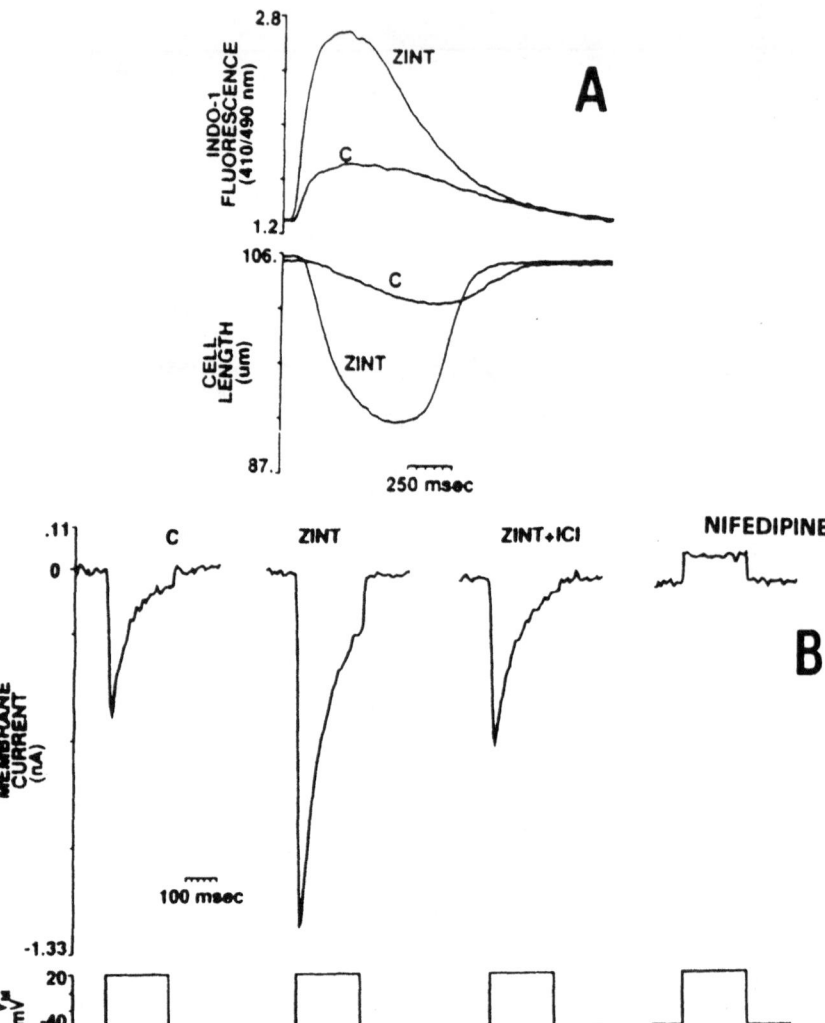

FIG. 9. **A** Representative example of the effects of the β_2AR agonist ZINT on the simultaneously recorded indo-1 fluorescence ratio and cell length of a normal canine myocyte. The cell was indo-1/AM-loaded and field-stimulated at 0.5 Hz, 23°C, in 1 mM $[Ca^{2+}]_o$. Seven canine myocytes gave similar results. **B** Effects of ZINT on L-type Ca^{2+} channel current in a canine myocyte. The increase in L-type Ca^{2+} current was abolished by ICI 118,551 (ICI) and the current itself was abolished by nifedipine. Traces are representative of those from five cells. Data from [36]

blocker, the same five new mobility forms of phospholamban are still observed. In contrast, there is only a single mobility form when ISO is acting in the β_2 mode, i.e., in the presence of β_1AR blocker. It has been shown previously that when ISO functions in the β_2 mode, it does not induce an acceleration in contraction kinetics in rat cardiac myocytes while it increases contraction amplitude [1]. Figure 11B also shows that blockade of both β_1 and β_2 receptors completely abolishes all ISO effects on phosphorylation of phospholamban. The distinct response of SR phospholamban phosphorylation to β_1AR and β_2AR activation in rat cells is in remarkable agreement with the functional observation that β_1AR but not β_2AR stimulation markedly accelerates the

FIG. 10. Effects of ZINT and ISO on cAMP content of canine myocytes. *Open squares,* ISO; *solid squares,* ZINT. All data are mean ± SEM for seven myocyte preparations in each group. None of the cAMP values for ZINT-treated cells were significantly different from their respective control values. Redrawn from [36]

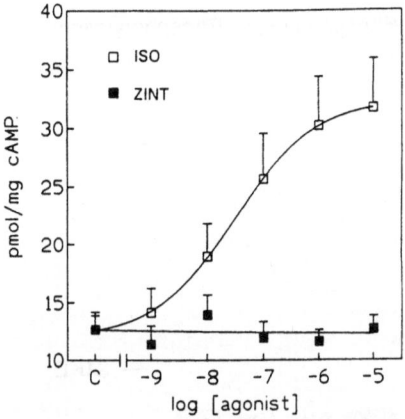

kinetics of Ca_i transient and contraction (Fig. 4). Since phosphorylation of phospholamban is associated with increased Ca^{2+} pumping into the SR [31] and by itself is sufficient to increase the rate of relaxation of the Ca_i transient [32], it appears that the failure of β_2AR stimulation to increase the rate of decay of the Ca_i transient and to accelerate relaxation in rat cells may well be a consequence of the inability of β_2AR stimulation to cause significant phosphorylation of phospholamban. These results, combined with those in Fig. 6, also indicate that the contributions of total cellular cAMP or the particulate cAMP to induce protein phosphorylation are not equivalent, when arising as a consequence of β_1AR and β_2AR stimulation.

Figure 11C shows that, as in rat myocytes, β_2AR stimulation by ZINT has no effect on phospholamban phosphorylation in dog myocytes. In contrast, ISO markedly increases phospholamban phosphorylation. During β_2AR stimulation in canine myocytes, what is the mechanism underlying the relaxation effect of β_2AR stimulation in the absence of an increase in cAMP and phospholamban phosphorylation?

Species-Dependent Differences in Effect of β_2AR Stimulation on Relaxation

As described above, in rat ventricular myocytes, while β_1AR stimulation markedly accelerates the Ca_i transient decline and contractile relaxation, β_2AR stimulation has only a minor relaxation effect. However, the effects of β_2AR stimulation on relaxation are species-dependent. In cat and sheep cardiac muscles, as in rat heart cells, β_1AR but not β_2AR stimulation significantly accelerates cardiac relaxation [33,34]. In contrast, in human and canine heart (Fig. 9A), β_2AR activation dramatically accelerates cardiac relaxation, as does β_1AR stimulation [8,35,36]. The mechanisms which underlie the species-dependent differences in β_2AR relaxation effect remain unclear. In rat cardiac ventricular myocytes, SR Ca^{2+}-ATPase is the dominant factor that determines the rate of decline of Ca_i transient and relaxation [37]. The acceleration of the Ca_i transient decline after β_1AR stimulation is thought to be due largely to cAMP-dependent phosphorylation of phospholamban, resulting in increased Ca^{2+} accumulation into this membrane system [31,32]. The reduced efficacy of β_2AR agonists in inducing phospholamban phosphorylation in rat heart cells provides a biochemical basis for the inability of β_2AR stimulation to accelerate Ca_i transient and contraction kinetics as

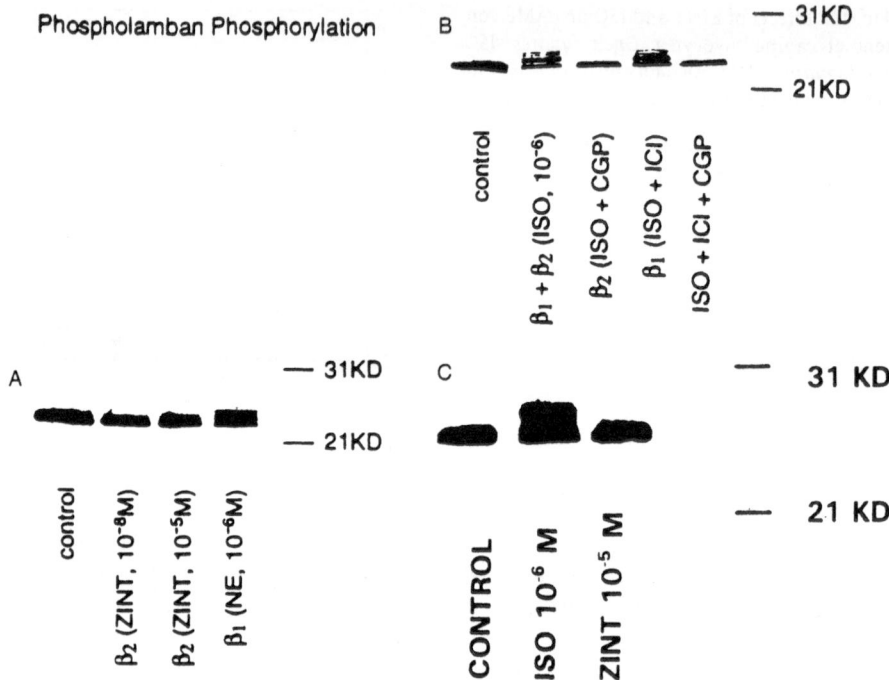

FIG. 11. Western blot of phospholamban in isolated rat (A,B) and canine (C) ventricular myocytes. Each cell suspension was exposed to drugs for 10 min at room temperature (23°C), then subjected to sodium dodecyl sulfate-polyacrylamide gel electrophoresis (SDS-PAGE) followed by Western blotting. The blot was incubated with phospholamban monoclonal antibody 3A1 at 1/500 dilution and developed colorimetrically. A Effects of NE on phospholamban phosphorylation indexed by mobility states of phospholamban on SDS-PAGE. In response to NE (10^{-6} M), five discrete mobility states representing different extents of phospholamban phosphorylation are resolved. B β_1- plus β_2-adrenergic stimulation induced by ISO or selective β_2- or β_1-adrenergic effects in the presence of selective β_1- or β_2-adrenergic blockers (CGP or ICI). Data in A, B from [13]. C Effects of mixed β_1- and β_2-adrenergic stimulation or β_2-adrenergic stimulation induced by ISO (10^{-6} M) and ZINT (10^{-5} M) on phospholamban phosphorylation. Data from [36]. The amount of phospholamban phosphorylation in suspensions of single myocytes was detected by its characteristic mobility shift on SDS-PAGE [13,29]. Then, 80 µg of protein were loaded per gel lane, and electrophoresis conducted on a 7%–18% polyacrylamide gradient gel according to Laemmli [48] until the tracking dye reached the bottom of the gel. Samples were transferred to nitrocellulose in 50 mM phosphate (pH 7.4) at 3 A for 90 min. The nitrocellulose sheet was blotted with bovine serum albumin, and then incubated with phospholamban monoclonal antibody 3A1 at a 1/500 dilution. Antibody binding was detected colorimetrically, using alkaline phosphatase-coupled protein A (Sigma Chemical, St. Louis, MO, USA) and bromochloroindolyl/nitro blue tetrazolium (Promega, Madison, WI, USA) [48]

compared to β_1AR stimulation. In other species, however, the SR mechanism is a less important determinant than it is in rat cells [37,38], and the β_2AR induced relaxation effect could be mediated in part by other mechanisms. In canine heart cells, since the β_2AR agonist ZINT has no effect on cellular cAMP production and phospholamban phosphorylation (Figure 11C) [35,36,39], the relaxation effect of β_2AR stimulation is not likely to be mediated by a cAMP-dependent mechanism, unless an increase in cAMP in an undetectable compartment is advocated.

Many Ca²⁺-dependent regulatory mechanisms are accelerated in response to the enhanced Ca$_i$ signalling. During βAR stimulation, [Ca²⁺]$_i$ is significantly elevated because of the greater I$_{Ca}$ influx and the enhanced Ca$_i$ transient. The [Ca²⁺]$_i$-dependence of the SR Ca²⁺ pump or on Ca²⁺ efflux via the Na⁺-Ca²⁺ exchanger, may play a role in the βAR-stimulated relaxation effect in some species and may account for β₂AR relaxation effects in canine cardiac cells. Thus, an increase in extracellular [Ca²⁺] accelerates the kinetics of Ca$_i$ transient and contraction in canine ventricular myocytes in a manner similar to the relaxation effect induced by βAR stimulation (Fig. 12). Also, in rat ventricular myocytes, an increase in bathing [Ca²⁺] from low (0.5mM) to higher (1.5mM) concentrations results in an acceleration of the Ca$_i$ transient decline and contractile relaxation by 24% and 34%, respectively [40]. However, a further increase of bathing [Ca²⁺] from a level of 1.5mM has no effects on the kinetics of Ca$_i$ transient and contraction while it does increase Ca$_i$ transient and contraction amplitudes [41]. The exact mechanisms of the species-dependent differences in effects of β₂AR stimulation on relaxation require further studies.

Pertussis Toxin Treatment Selectively Potentiates the Effects of β₂AR Stimulation

It has recently been shown that some cell surface membrane receptors can couple to both stimulatory and inhibitory G proteins [42–44]. Does β₂AR stimulation exert its effects by coupling to G proteins other than G$_s$? Pertussis toxin (PTX) has been employed to determine whether G$_i$ or G$_o$ could be involved in the β₂AR signal transduction pathway. In cells incubated with PTX (0.75μg/ml at 37°C for at least 3h), successful inactivation of inhibitory G protein (G$_i$/G$_o$) is verified by a loss of the ability

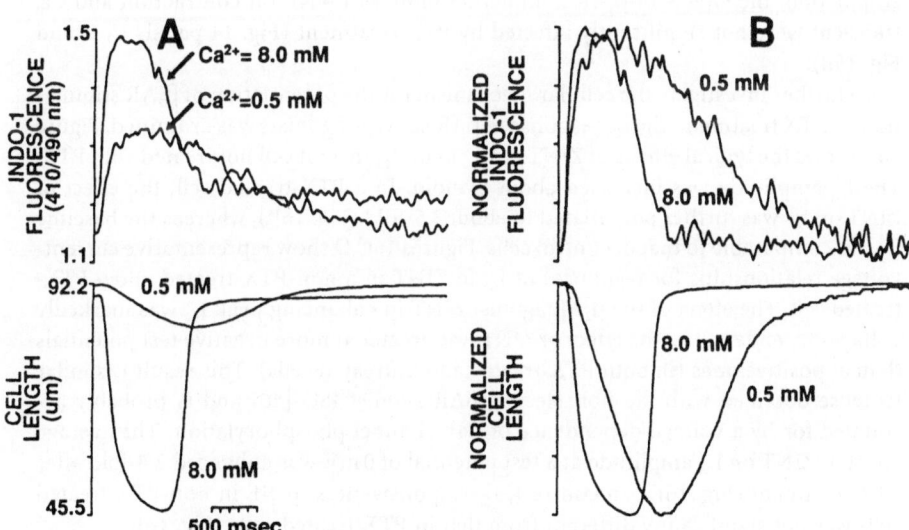

FIG. 12. Representative example of the effects of an increase in extracellular [Ca²⁺] (from 0.5 to 8.0mM) on the simultaneously recorded indo-1 fluorescence ratio and contraction in a canine ventricular myocyte. Note that high [Ca²⁺] not only increases the amplitudes of Ca$_i$ transient and contraction, but also markedly accelerates the decline of the Ca$_i$ transient and relaxation (A). This is better shown in the normalized traces (B). The cell was indo-1/AM loaded and field-stimulated at 0.5 Hz at 23°C

of adenosine to reverse the positive inotropic effect of $\beta_1 AR$ stimulation, since adenosine is generally thought to modulate βAR stimulation negatively via activating a PTX-sensitive G protein pathway. Figure 13 shows the representative effects of PTX treatment in abolishing the antagonistic effects of $10^{-6} M$ adenosine on βAR stimulation. In the absence of PTX treatment, the effects of NE ($10^{-7} M$) on Ca$_i$ transient and contraction amplitudes were completely inhibited by adenosine. In contrast, after PTX treatment the effects of NE were not affected by adenosine. Similar results were obtained when cells were stimulated by the $\beta_2 AR$ agonist ZINT rather than NE. In addition, the antagonistic effects of acetylcholine ($10^{-6} M$) on βAR stimulation in rat ventricular myocytes are also blocked by the same PTX pretreatment (not shown). Similar results are observed in canine myocytes.

Figure 14 illustrates the effect of PTX treatment on the responses of the Ca$_i$ transient and contraction to the $\beta_2 AR$ agonist ZINT. Panels A, B show representative examples of the maximum effects of ZINT ($10^{-5} M$) on the Ca$_i$ transient and contraction in a control cell and a PTX-treated cell, respectively. The effects of ZINT in increasing the Ca$_i$ transient and contraction amplitudes are enhanced by PTX. On average, PTX treatment enhanced the ZINT-induced increase in contraction amplitude about twofold (Fig. 14C). This effect was associated with an increase in the Ca$_i$ transient amplitude (Fig. 14D). Also, note that ZINT markedly accelerated the kinetics of the Ca$_i$ transient and contraction in the PTX-treated cells, as shown in the normalized and superimposed tracings in panel B. Spontaneous Ca$_i$ oscillations and contractile waves (not shown) were also frequently observed in PTX-treated cells but not in control cells during exposure to ZINT [45]. A similar potentiation effect of PTX treatment was observed when $\beta_2 AR$ stimulation was induced by ISO plus a $\beta_1 AR$ blocker (Fig. 15). In contrast to the marked effects of PTX in potentiating the cell responses to $\beta_2 AR$ stimulation, the effects of $\beta_1 AR$ stimulation induced by NE on contraction and Ca$_i$ transient were not significantly affected by PTX treatment (Fig. 14 panels C, D and Fig. 15B).

To further investigate the cellular mechanism for the potentiation of $\beta_2 AR$ stimulation by PTX treatment, the I_{Ca} response to βAR subtype agonists was examined. Figure 16A shows the typical effects of ZINT at $10^{-5} M$ on I_{Ca} in a rat cell not treated with PTX. The I_{Ca} amplitude was increased about twofold. In a PTX-treated cell, the effect of ZINT on I_{Ca} was further potentiated to about 3.5-fold (Fig. 16B), whereas the baseline I_{Ca} was comparable to that in control cells. Figures 16C,D show representative current-voltage relationships for responses of I_{Ca} to ZINT in a non-PTX-treated and a PTX-treated cell. The effect of the $\beta_2 AR$ agonist ZINT in enhancing peak I_{Ca} was markedly voltage-dependent, i.e., the effect of ZINT was greater at more negative test potentials than at positive ones (in both PTX-treated and untreated cells). This result is similar to those obtained with the nonselective βAR agonist ISO [46] and is probably accounted for by a voltage-dependence of Ca^{2+} channel phosphorylation. The average effect of ZINT on I_{Ca} amplitude at a test potential of $0 mV$ was enhanced 2.8-fold after PTX treatment (Fig. 16E). In contrast, I_{Ca} responsiveness to NE in non-PTX-treated cells was not significantly different from that in PTX-treated cells (Fig. 16E).

In addition to increasing the I_{Ca} amplitude, ZINT prolonged the I_{Ca} inactivation time in non-PTX-treated cells (from $16.9 \pm 1.3 ms$ to $25.0 \pm 1.8 ms$, $P < 0.01$, $n = 6$), [1]. However, in PTX-treated cells, the I_{Ca} decay time was not significantly altered by ZINT ($18.3 \pm 2.0 ms$ and $19.4 \pm 1.4 ms$, $n = 6$, before and after superfusion with ZINT, respectively).

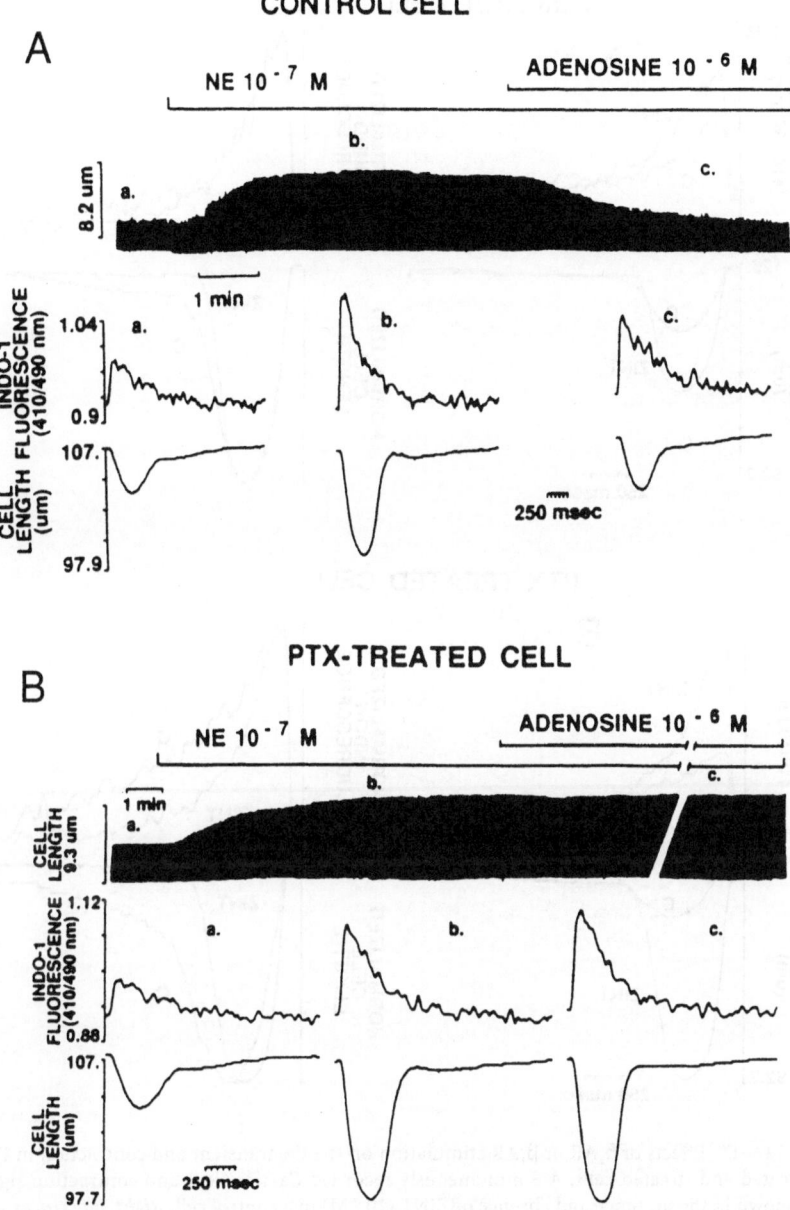

FIG. 13. Representative effects of adenosine (10^{-6} M) on the NE (10^{-7} M)-induced increases in Ca_i transient and contraction amplitudes. A Antagonistic effects of adenosine in a myocyte not treated with pertussis toxin (*PTX*). Continuous tracing at the *top*, chart recording of the cell contraction. An upward deflection indicates cell shortening. Traces *beneath* the continuous tracing, obtained at times indicated in the top tracing, show the simultaneously recorded Ca_i transient and contraction (plotted *downward*) before NE (*a*), after exposure to NE (*b*), and after adenosine addition (*c*). B Typical result obtained in a PTX-treated cell. The experimental conditions are the same as in A. Note that the effects of NE on Ca_i transient and contraction amplitudes are not affected by adenosine. Data from [45]

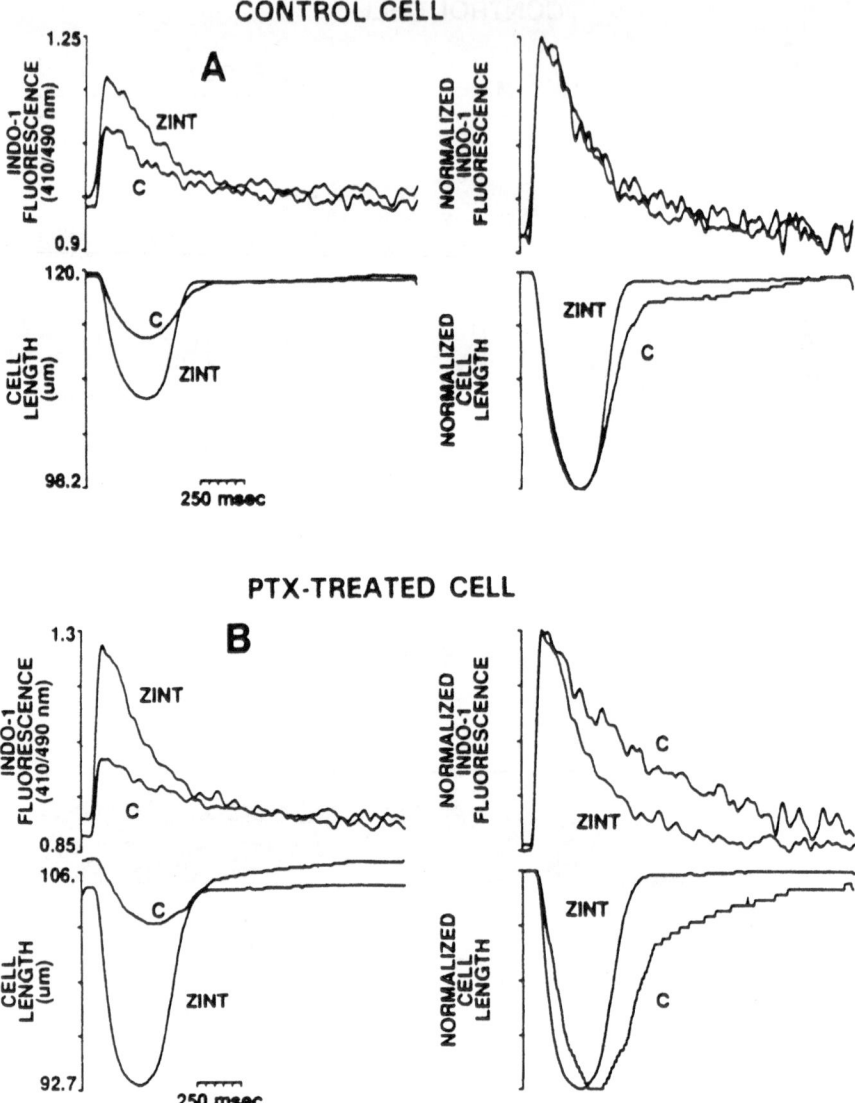

FIG. 14A–D. Effects of β_2AR or β_1AR stimulation on the Ca_i transient and contraction in PTX-untreated and -treated cells. A Simultaneously recorded Ca_i transient and contraction signals are shown in the presence and absence of ZINT (10^{-5} M) in a control cell. *Right-side traces* show the Ca_i transient and contraction normalized to their peaks. B Tracings as in A but in a PTX-treated cell. C Bar graph showing the average effects of ZINT and NE in increasing contraction amplitude in the PTX-untreated cells ($n = 15$ for ZINT and $n = 20$ for NE, *solid bars*) and PTX-treated cells ($n = 9$ for ZINT and $n = 10$ for NE, *open bars*). Data are presented as percentage of control. (*$P < 0.001$ vs PTX-untreated cells). D Effects of ZINT and NE on Ca_i transient amplitude in the absence and presence of PTX treatment. Data were obtained in those cells as in C and are presented as percentage of control. (*$P < 0.001$ vs PTX-untreated cells). Data from [45]

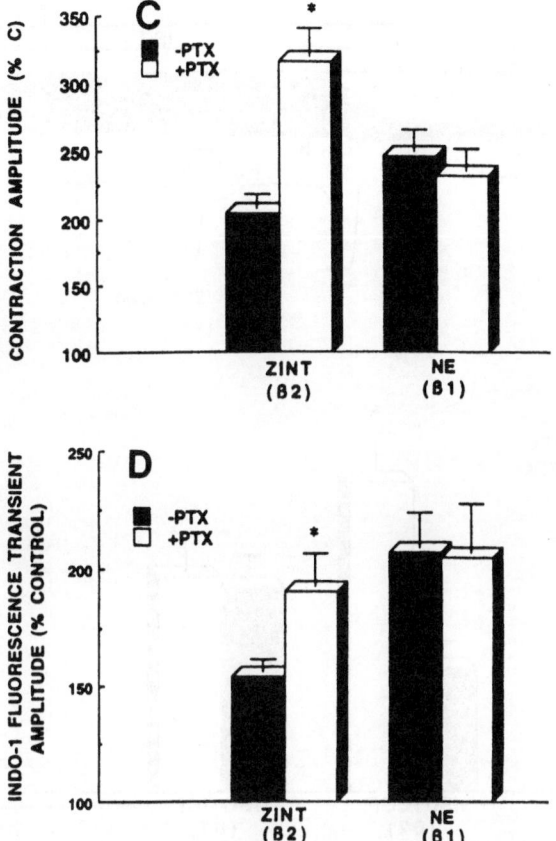

FIG. 14A–D. *Continued*

The potentiating effect of PTX was manifested not only as an increase in the maximum response but also as an increase in the sensitivity of cardiac myocyte response to β_2AR stimulation. Figure 17A illustrates that the dose-response curve for the effects of the selective β_2AR agonist ZINT on contraction amplitude was shifted markedly leftward and upward. The maximal increase in contraction amplitude after ZINT was enhanced from $201 \pm 23.0\%$ of the control in non-PTX-treated cells to $307 \pm 29.8\%$ of the control in treated cells. The EC_{50} was markedly decreased by PTX pretreatment, from about $1.0\,\mu M$ to $70\,nM$.

The dose-response curve of contraction amplitude to ZINT in PTX-treated cells superimposes that for the ZINT-induced increase in cAMP (Fig. 6). In addition, recent studies have shown that PTX does not alter the β_2AR dose response relation to increase cAMP (R.A. Altschuld et al., personal communication). Thus, in the absence of PTX, the dissociation of the positive inotropic effect of β_2AR stimulation from the β_2AR-stimulated increase in cAMP may be largely explained by the PTX-sensitive inhibitory pathway. In contrast to β_2AR stimulation, the dose-response curve for the β_1AR agonist NE effect in increasing contraction was not significantly altered by PTX treatment (Fig. 17B). Thus, only the effects of β_2AR stimulation, and not the effects of β_1AR stimulation, are significantly potentiated by PTX treatment. Results similar to those in rat cells were obtained in canine cells following PTX treatment.

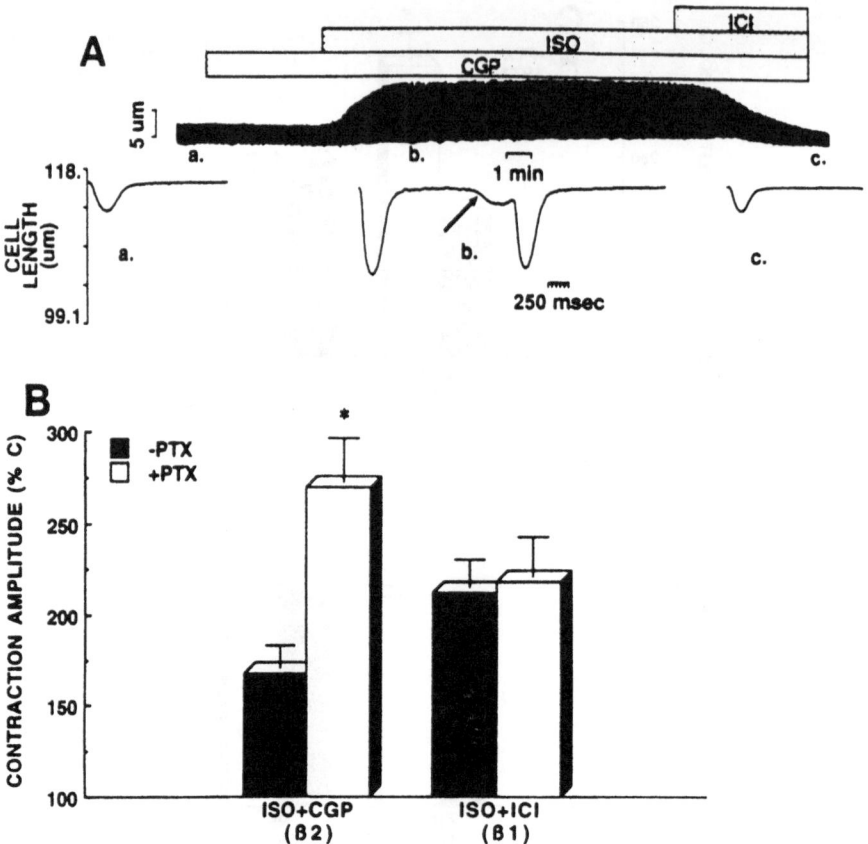

FIG. 15A,B. Effect of β₂AR stimulation by ISO (10^{-6} M) plus CGP (3×10^{-7} M) to increase contraction amplitude. A Representative result obtained in a PTX-treated cell. *Top*, continuous chart recording of cell contraction. Note that the effect of ISO plus CGP is blocked by the subsequent addition of the β₂AR blocker ICI (10^{-7} M). *Bottom*, contraction tracings obtained at the time points indicated, showing control (*a*), results obtained after addition of ISO with CGP (*b*), and the antagonistic effect of ICI (*c*). Note that the spontaneous contractile waves (*arrow*) that occur during β₂AR stimulation are also inhibited by ICI. B Average effect of ISO (10^{-6} M) in the presence of CGP (3×10^{-7} M) or ICI (10^{-7} M) on contraction amplitude in non-PTX-treated cells (*solid bars*) and in PTX-treated cells (*open bars*). Note that the effect of ISO acting in the β₂ mode (ISO plus CGP), but not in the β₁ mode (ISO plus ICI), is significantly enhanced by PTX treatment. *$P < 0.001$ *vs* non-PTX-treated cells ($n = 10$ for both groups). Data from [45]

The results in Figs. 14–17 suggest that β₂AR simultaneously couples to G_s and to the second, PTX-sensitive G protein. Thus, the simultaneous activation of an inhibitory signaling pathway by β₂AR stimulation might override or significantly modify the cAMP-dependent modulation on contraction and Ca_i transient in rat cells (Fig. 18). However, the PTX-sensitive G-protein coupling cannot explain the effects of β₂AR in augmenting I_{Ca} (Figs. 9B and 16), resulting in an augmentation of the Ca_i transient and contraction amplitude in either rat or canine cells. More recent studies (R.-P. Xiao et al., personal communication) in canine myocytes show that while the augmentation of I_{Ca} induced by the β₁AR agonist NE (10^{-7} M) is completely blocked by a specific peptide inhibitor of protein kinase A [pyruvate kinase isoenzyme (PKI), 50 μM in

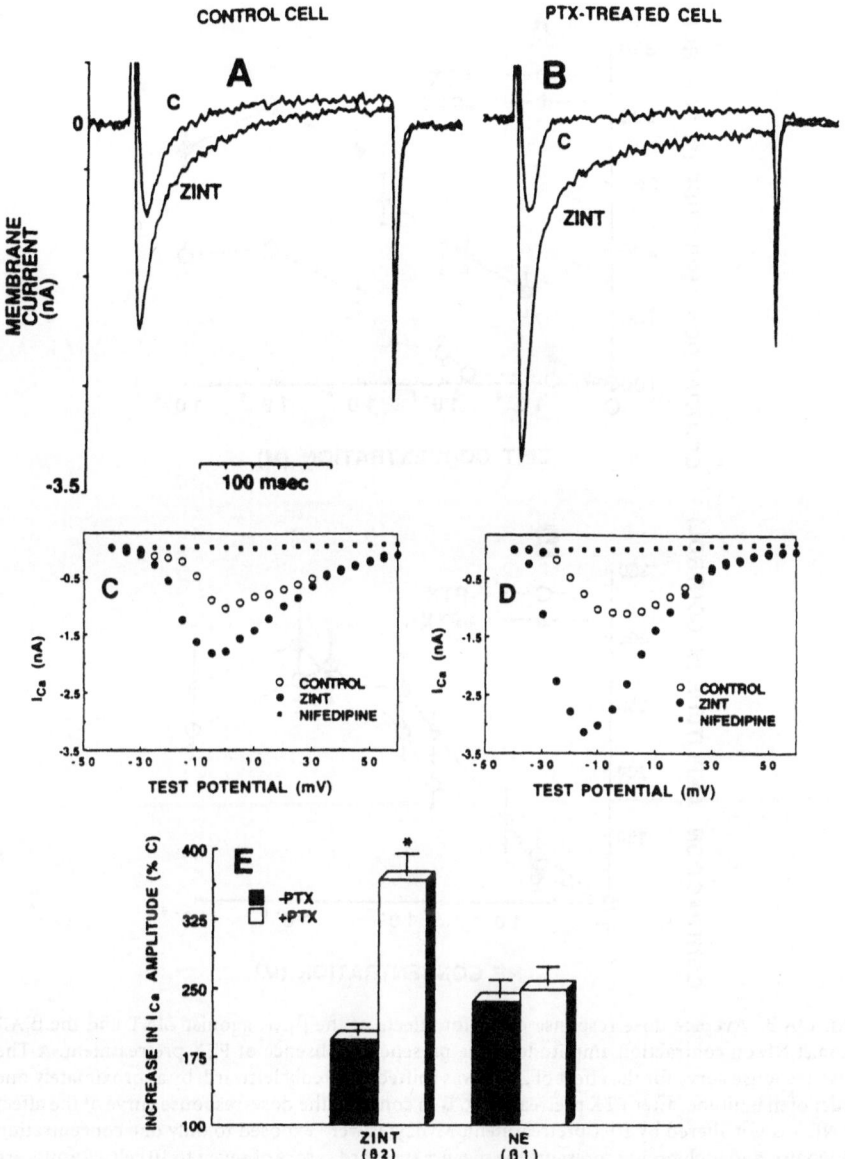

FIG. 16A–E. Effect of ZINT (10^{-5} M) on I_{Ca}. A Superimposed current tracings before (C) and after ZINT in a non-PTX treated cell. Currents were elicited by depolarizing test pulses from a holding potential of –40 to 0 mV for 200 ms at 0.5 Hz. B Same experiment as in A, except in a PTX-treated cell. Note that the augmentation of I_{Ca} induced by ZINT is enhanced, compared with that in the non-PTX-treated cell in A. C Current-voltage relations of I_{Ca} under control conditions, with ZINT, and with ZINT plus nifedipine (2 μM) in a cell that was not treated with PTX. The cell was depolarized from a holding potential of –40 mV to test potentials from –35 to +60 mV increments. D Current-voltage plots for PTX-treated cells, measured under the same experimental conditions as in C. E Average effects of ZINT (10^{-5} M) and NE (10^{-7} M) in increasing I_{Ca} amplitude at a test potential of 0 mV in the absence and presence of PTX treatment. *$P <$ 0.001 versus non-PTX-treated cells ($n = 6$ for both ZINT groups, $n = 4$ for both NE groups). Data from [45]

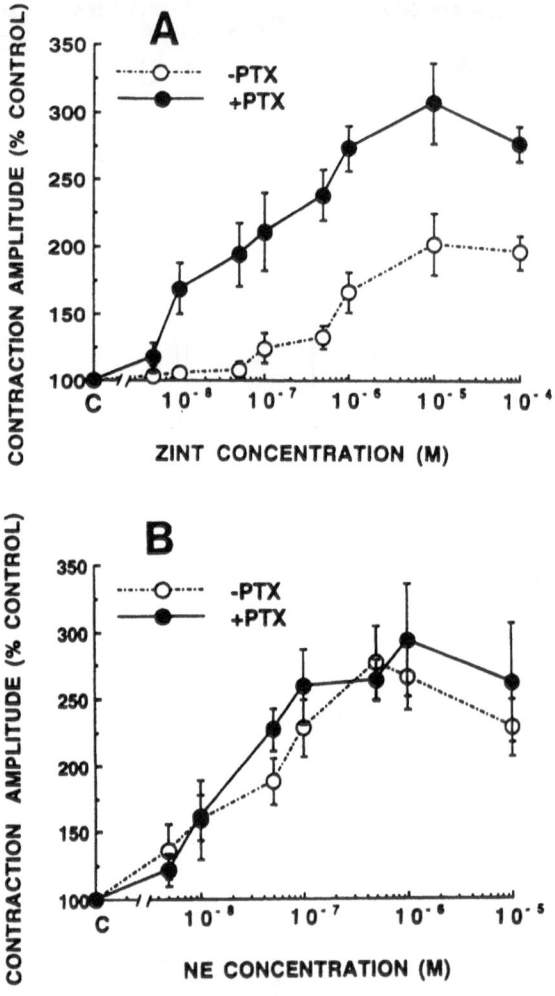

FIG. 17A,B. Average dose-response curve for effects of the β_2AR agonist ZINT and the β_1AR agonist NE on contraction amplitude in the presence or absence of PTX pretreatment. A The dose-response curve for the effect of ZINT was shifted markedly leftward, by approximately one order of magnitude, after PTX pretreatment. B In contrast, the dose-response curve of the effect of NE was not altered by PTX pretreatment. Myocytes were exposed to only one concentration of agonist, and each point represents the mean ± standard errors of seven to 10 cells. Results are expressed as percentage of the control value. Control values of contraction amplitude for ZINT experiments are 6.89 ± 0.31% and 6.86 ± 0.124% of the resting cell length for control cells (n = 62) and PTX-treated cells (n = 58), respectively. Control values of contraction amplitude for NE experiments are 6.93 ± 0.33% and 6.28% of the resting cell length for control cells (n = 50) and PTX-treated cells (n = 50), respectively. Data from [45]

pipette filling solution], the β_2AR-stimulated increase in I_{Ca} by ZINT (10^{-5} M) persists in the presence of PKI. While the increase in I_{Ca} induced by β_2AR stimulation cannot be completely blocked by PKI, a G-protein inhibitor, GDPβS (5 mM in pipette filling solution), completely abolishes the effect of β_2AR stimulation in increasing I_{Ca}. (The β_1AR stimulation-induced increase in I_{Ca} is also abolished, as expected on the basis of

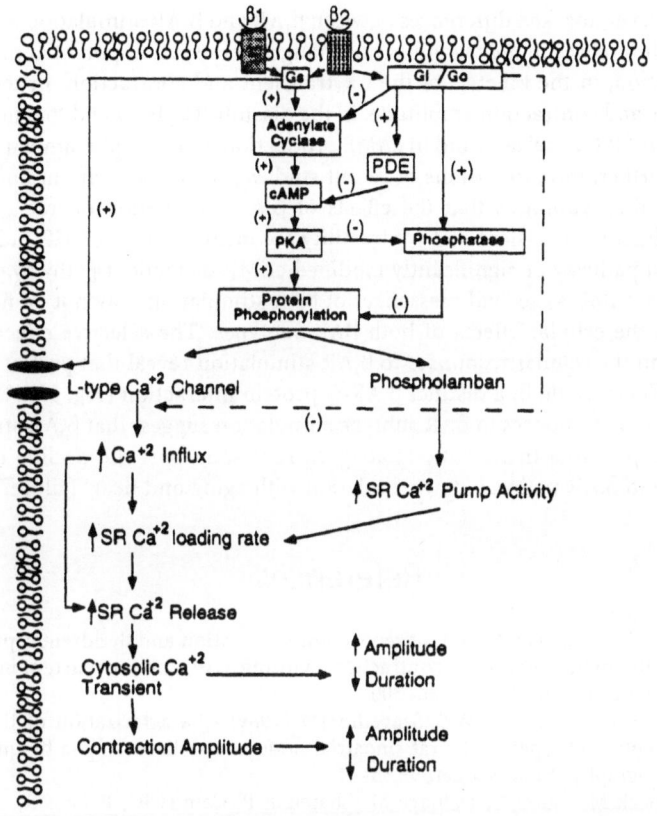

FIG. 18. A scheme depicting possible β_2AR signalling pathways in cardiac ventricular cells. In rat ventricular myocytes, the β_2AR, like the β_1AR, couples to G$_s$ and its stimulation leads to an activation of adenylyl cyclase and an increase in cyclic adenosine monophosphate (*cAMP*). However, the increased cAMP is largely dissociated from phospholamban phosphorylation and the increases in Ca$_i$ transient and contraction amplitudes after β_2AR stimulation. In canine myocytes, the cAMP signalling pathway is totally bypassed during β_2AR stimulation. We propose two hypotheses to explain the actions of β_2AR stimulation on cardiac I$_{Ca}$, Ca$_i$ transient and contraction. First, β_2AR stimulated G$_s$ could directly couple to L-type Ca^{2+} channels and increase I$_{Ca}$, subsequently increasing the Ca$_i$ transient and contraction in amplitude. Second, the cAMP signalling pathway may be significantly modified. β_2AR could simultaneously couple to multiple G proteins, such as G$_i$/G$_o$. These G proteins could activate phosphodiesterase (*PDE*) or phosphatase and offset the effect of cAMP. *PKA*, protein kinase A; *SR*, sarcoplasmic reticulum

a G$_s$ requirement for adenylyl cyclase activation.) Thus, the effect of β_1AR stimulation on I$_{Ca}$ in canine ventricular cells is due exclusively to cAMP-dependent protein phosphorylation, but the effect of β_2AR stimulation on I$_{Ca}$ may be mediated by non-cAMP-dependent G protein-coupled signaling pathway(s).

Conclusion

The results of recent studies clearly show that functional β_2ARs are present in rat and canine cardiac ventricular cells. Stimulation of these receptors produces a marked increase in contractility, which is equal in magnitude to that induced by β_1AR stimulation. However, marked differences between β_1AR and β_2AR stimulation are evident, including differences in the magnitude of changes in the action potential duration, in I_{Ca} inactivation, in the kinetics of the Ca_i transient and contraction, in the relation between Ca_i and contraction amplitude, in the diastolic Ca_i level and the induction of spontaneous SR Ca^{2+} release, and in cAMP production and phospholamban phosphorylation. Furthermore, the results of recent studies provide several lines of evidence supporting the hypothesis that the effects of β_2AR stimulation on rat and canine cardiac cellular Ca_i transient and contractility are mediated by a cAMP-independent biochemical pathway or significantly modified cAMP-dependent pathway. Thus, the "dogma" on cAMP as second messenger of βAR stimulation may not be necessarily true for all the cellular effects of both βAR subtypes. The selective effects of PTX treatment on the cellular responses to β_2AR stimulation reveal that part of the βAR-subtype differences lie in a distinct β_2AR-G protein interaction (Fig. 18). The differences in cardiac responses to βAR subtype stimulation suggest that β_2AR stimulation may offer a potential therapeutic strategy to reverse in part the decline in cardiac reserve due to β_1AR pathway downregulation with aging and heart failure.

References

1. Xiao R-P, Lakatta EG (1993) β_1-adrenoceptor stimulation and β_2-adrenoceptor stimulation differ in their effects on contraction, cytosolic Ca^{2+}, and Ca^{2+} current in single rat ventricular cells. Circ Res 73:286–300
2. Saito K, Torda T, Potter WZ, Saavedra JM (1989) Characterization of β_1- and β_2-adrenoceptor subtypes in the rat sinoatrial node and stellate ganglia by quantitative autoradiography. Neurosci Lett 96:35–41
3. Waelbroeck M, Taton G, Delhaye M, Chatelain P, Camus JC, Pochet R, Leclerc JL, DeSmet JM, Robberecht P, Christopher J (1983) The human heart beta-adrenergic receptors: II. Coupling of beta$_2$-adrenergic receptors with the adenylate cyclase system. Mol Pharmacol 24:174–182
4. Cerbai E, Masini I, Mugelli A (1990) Electrophysiological characterization of cardiac β_2-adrenoceptors in sheep Purkinje fibers. J Mol Cell Cardiol 22:859–870
5. Brodde O-E (1988) The functional importance of beta$_1$ and beta$_2$ adrenoceptors in the human heart. Am J Cardiol 62:24C–29C
6. Motomura S, Zerkowski H-R, Daul A, Brodde O-E (1990) On the physiologic role of beta-2 adrenoceptors in the human heart: in vitro and in vivo studies. Am Heart J 119:608–619
7. Ask JA, Stene-Larsen G, Helle KB, Resch F (1985) Functional β_1- and β_2-adrenoceptors in the human myocardium. Acta Physiol Scand 123:81–88
8. del Monte F, Kaumann AJ, Pool-Wilson PA, Wynne DG, Pepper J, Harding SE (1993) Coexistence of functioning β_1- and β_2-adrenoceptors in single myocytes from human ventricle. Circulation 88:845–863
9. Dohlman HG, Caron MG, Lefkowitz RL (1991) Model systems for the study of seven-transmembrane-segment receptors. Annu Rev Biochem 60:653–688
10. Strader CD, Sigal IS, Dixon RAF (1989) Structural basis of β-adrenergic receptor function. FASEB J 3:1825–1832
11. O'Dowd BF, Hantowich M, Regan JW, Leader WM, Caron MC, Lefkowitz RJ (1988) Site-directed mutagenesis of the cytoplasmic domains of the human β_2-adrenergic receptor. J Biol Chem 263:15985–15992
12. Frielle T, Daniel KW, Caron MG, Lefkowitz RJ (1988) Structural basis of β-adrenergic receptor subtype specificity studied with chimeric β_1/β_2-adrenergic receptors. Proc Natl Acad Sci USA 85:9494–9498
13. Xiao R-P, Hohl C, Altschuld R, Jones L, Livingston B, Ziman B, Tantini B, Lakatta EG

(1994) β₂-adrenergic receptor-stimulated increase in cAMP in rat heart cells is not coupled to changes in Ca^{2+} dynamics, contractility, or phospholamban phosphorylation. J Biol Chem 269:19151–19156

14. Lefkowitz RJ (1975) Heterogeneity of adenylate cyclase-coupled β-adrenergic receptors. Biochem Pharmacol 24:583–590

15. Lands AM, Arnold A, McAuliff JP, Ludeuena FP, Brown TG (1967) Differentiation of receptor systems activated by sympathomimetic amines. Nature 214:597–598

16. Ikezono K, Michel MC, Zerkowski H-R, Beckeringh JJ, Brodde O-E (1987) The role of cyclic AMP in the positive inotropic effect mediated by beta 1- and beta 2-adrenoceptors in isolated human right atrium. Naunyn Schmiedebergs Arch Pharmacol 335:561–566

17. Dooley DJ, Bittiger H, Reymann NC (1986) CGP 20712 A: a useful tool for quantitating β₁- and β₂-adrenoceptors. Eur J Pharmacol 130:137–139

18. Emorine LJ, Marullo S, Briend-Sutren M-M, Patey G, Tate K, Delavier-Klutchko C, Strosberg AD (1989) Molecular characterization of the human β₃-adrenergic receptor. Science 245:1118–1121

19. Kaumann AJ (1989) Is there a third hear β-adrenoceptor? Trends Pharmacol Sci 10:316–320

20. Bristow MR, Hershberger RE, Port JD, Minobe W, Rasmussen R (1989) β₁- and β₂-adrenergic receptor-mediated adenylate cyclase stimulation in nonfailing and failing human ventricular myocardium. Mol Pharmacol 35:295–303

21. Minneman KP, Hegstrand LR, Molinoff PB (1979) The pharmacological specificity of β₁- and β₂-adrenergic receptors in rat heart and lung in vitro. Mol Pharmacol 16:21–33

22. O'Donnell SR, Wanstall JC (1989) Evidence that ICI 118,551 is a potent, highly beta₂-selective adrenoceptor antagonist and can be used to characterize beta-adrenoceptor populations in tissues. Life Sci 27:671–677

23. Spurgeon HA, duBell WH, Stern MD, Ziman BD, Silverman HS, Capogrossi MC, Talo A, Lakatta EG (1992) Cytosolic calcium and myofilaments in single rat cardiac myocytes achieve a dynamic equilibrium during twitch relaxation. J Physiol (Lond) 447:83–102

24. January CT, Fozzard HA (1988) Delayed afterdepolarization in heart muscle: Mechanisms and relevance. Pharmacol Rev 40:219–227

25. Capogrossi MC, Kort AA, Spurgeon HA, Lakatta EG (1986) Single adult rabbit and rat cardiac myocytes retain the Ca^{2+}- and species-dependent systolic and diastolic contractile properties of the intact muscle. J Gen Physiol 88:589–613

26. Parrat JR, Wainright CL, Fagbemi O (1988) Effect of dopexamine hydrochloride in the early stage of experimental myocardial infarction and comparison with dopamine and dobutamine. Am J Cardiol 62:18C–23C

27. Aass H, Skomedal T, Osnes J-B (1988) Increase of cyclic AMP in subcellular fractions of rat heart muscle after β-adrenergic stimulation: prenalterol and isoprenaline caused different distribution of bound cyclic AMP. J Mol Cell Cardiol 20:847–860

28. Hohl CM, Li Q (1991) Compartmentation of cAMP in adult canine ventricular myocytes: relation to single-cell free Ca^{2+} transient. Circ Res 69:1369–1379

29. Wegener AD, Simmerman HKB, Lindemann JP, Jones LR (1989) Phospholamban phosphorylation in intact ventricles: phosphorylation of serine 16 and threonine 17 in response to β-adrenergic stimulation. J Biol Chem 264:11468–11474

30. Wegener AD, Jones LR (1984) Phosphorylation-induced mobility shift in phospholamban in sodium dodecyl sulfate-polyacrylamide gel. J Biol Chem 259:1834–1841

31. Lindemann JP, Jones LR, Hathaway DR, Henry BG, Watanabe AM (1983) β-adrenergic stimulation of phospholamban phosphorylation and Ca^{2+}-ATPase activity in guinea pig ventricles. J Biol Chem 258:464–471

32. Sham JSK, Jones LR, Morad M (1991) Phospholamban mediates the β-adrenergic-enhanced Ca^{2+} uptake in mammalian ventricular myocytes. Am J Physiol 261:H1344–H1349

33. Lemoine H, Kaumann AJ (1991) Regional differences of β₁- and β₂-adrenoceptor-

mediated functions in feline heart: a β_2-adrenoceptor-mediated positive inotropic effect possibly unrelated to cyclic AMP. Naunyn Schmiedebergs Arch Pharmacol 344:56–69

34. Borea PA, Amerini S, Masini I, Cerbai E, Ledda F, Mantelli L, Varani K, Mugelli A (1992) β_1- and β_2-adrenoceptors in sheep cardiac ventricular muscle. J Mol Cell Cardiol 24:753–764

35. Altschuld RA, McCune SA, Hamlin RL, Phillips RM, Hensley J, Castillo LC, Starling RC, Hohl CM (1994) Cardiac myocytes and heart failure. J Mol Cell Cardiol 26:CXLV

36. Altschuld RA, Starling RC, Hamlin RL, Billman GE, Hensley J, Castillo L, Fertel RH, Hohl CM, Robitaille P-ML, Jones LR, Xiao R-P, Lakatta EG (1995) Response of failing canine and human heart cells to β_2-adrenergic stimulation. Circulation 92:1612–1618

37. Bassani JWM, Bassani RA, Bers DM (1994) Relaxation in rabbit and rat cardiac cells: species-dependent differences in cellular mechanisms. J Physiol 476(2):279–293

38. Bassani RA, Bassani JWM, Bers DM (1994) Relaxation in ferret ventricular myocytes: unusual interplay among calcium transport systems. J Physiol 476(2):295–308

39. Xiao R-P, Hohl CM, Ji X, Ziman BD, Altschuld RA, Lakatta EG (1994) Adenosine antagonizes β_2-adrenoceptor stimulated increases in the Ca_i transient and contraction in canine heart cells via a cAMP-independent mechanisms. Circulation 90:I-414

40. Ventura C, Spurgeon H, Lakatta EG, Guarnieri C, Capogrossi MC (1992) κ and δ opioid receptor stimulation affects cardiac myocyte function and Ca^{2+} release from an intracellular pool in myocytes and neurons. Circ Res 70:66–81

41. Sakai M, Danziger RS, Xiao R-P, Spurgeon H, Lakatta EG (1992) Contractile response of individual ventricular cardiac myocytes to norepinephrine declined with senescence. Am J Physiol 262:H184–H189

42. Negishi M, Namba T, Sugimoto Y, Irie A, Katada T, Narumiya S, Ichikawa A (1993) Opposite coupling of prostaglanding E receptor EP_{3C} with G_s and G_o. J Biol Chem 268:26067–26070

43. Brechler V, Pavoine C, Hanf R, Garbarz E, Fischmeister R, Pecker F (1992) Inhibition by glucagon of the cGMP-inhibited low-K_m cAMP phosphodiesterase in heart is mediated by a pertussis toxin-sensitive G-protein. J Biol Chem 267:15496–15501

44. Milligan G (1993) Mechanisms of multifunctional signalling by G protein-linked receptors. Trends Pharmacol Sci 14:239–244

45. Xiao R-P, Ji X, Lakatta EG (1995) Functional coupling of β_2-adrenoceptor to a pertussis toxin-sensitive G protein in cardiac myocytes. Mol Pharmacol 47:322–329

46. Bean BP, Nowycky MC, Tsein RW (1984) β-Adrenergic modulation of calcium channels in frog ventricular heart cells. Nature 307:371–375

47. Spurgeon HA, Stern MD, Baartz G, Raffaeli S, Hansford RG, Talo A, Lakatta EG, Capogrossi MC (1990) Simultaneous measurements of Ca^{2+}, contraction, and potential in cardiac myocytes. Am J Physiol 258:H574–H586

48. Laemmli UK (1970) Cleavage of structural proteins during the assembly of the head of bacteriophage T_4. Nature 227:680–685

Receptor-Mediated Regulation of Cardiac Contractility: Inotropic Effects of Alpha-Adrenoceptor Stimulation with Phenylephrine and Noradrenaline in Failing Human Hearts

Hasso Scholz, Thomas Eschenhagen, Joachim Neumann,
and Birgitt Stein

Summary. In the failing human heart, the beta-adrenergic positive inotropic effect (PIE) is attenuated. It is conceivable that in compensation alpha-adrenoceptor-mediated inotropism may gain importance under these conditions. The number of alpha-adrenoceptors has been shown to be enhanced in hearts explanted from patients with endstage myocardial failure. However, previous studies with phenylephrine (Ph) revealed only small PIEs. Therefore, the effect of noradrenaline (NA) as an agonist was compared to that of Ph. Trabeculae were obtained from the hearts of patients undergoing cardiac transplantation because of idiopathic dilated cardiomyopathy. NA ($100\,\mu M$ in the presence of $10\,\mu M$ propranolol) increased force of contraction by about 90% of the predrug value. Subsequently applied carbachol ($10\,\mu M$) had no negative inotropic effect, indicating both complete blockade of beta-adrenoceptors and the absence of a cAMP-dependent effect. Prazosin ($1\,\mu M$) and the alpha$_{1A}$-antagonist WB 4101 blocked the PIE of NA but the alpha$_{1B}$-antagonist chloroethylclonidine was nearly ineffective. The PIE of Ph ($100\,\mu M$) was much smaller than that of NA. Thus, in the failing human heart the magnitude of the alpha$_1$-receptor-mediated PIE apparently is agonist-dependent, and alpha-adrenergic effects of the physiological agonist NA might be important to sustain contractility under conditions of impaired beta-adrenergic stimulation.

Key words: Alpha-adrenoceptor—Failing human heart—Noradrenaline—Phenylephrine—WB 4101—Chloroethylclonidine

Introduction

In the mammalian heart, the endogenous sympathomimetic agents adrenaline and noradrenaline induce positive inotropic and positive chronotropic effects. These effects are mainly mediated by beta-adrenoceptors, but there are alpha-adrenoceptors in the heart that also mediate an increase in contractility.

This chapter describes characteristics, possible mechanisms, and the potential biological significance of the alpha-adrenoceptor-mediated positive inotropic response in the mammalian heart including experiments with noradrenaline in human

Pharmakologisches Institut, Universitäts-Krankenhaus Eppendorf, Universität Hamburg, D-20246 Hamburg, Germany

failing myocardium. For further references, more detailed reviews may be consulted [1–6].

Characteristics of the Alpha-Adrenergic Positive Inotropic effect

The alpha-adrenoceptors mediating positive inotropic effects are of the alpha$_1$ type. The synthetic agonists mainly used are phenylephrine or methoxamine, although these agents are far from being selective. The experiments with these drugs are therefore usually performed in the presence of beta-adrenoceptor blockers to avoid beta-sympathomimetic effects.

The alpha-sympathomimetic positive inotropic effect develops relatively slowly within several minutes and is accompanied by a lengthening of the contraction. In hypothermia and hypothyroidism, the alpha-sympathomimetic positive inotropic effect is more pronounced than under normal conditions, and an enhanced sensitivity of diabetic hearts to alpha-adrenoceptor stimulation was also reported [7]. This might be linked to an increased alpha-adrenergic phosphoinositide breakdown [8]. Moreover, the alpha-adrenergic positive inotropic effect is not inhibited by parasympathomimetic agents or by adenosine. Carbachol and adenosine, for example, antagonize the positive inotropic effect of isoprenaline while they do not affect the positive inotropic effects of phenylephrine or methoxamine [9,10].

Species Dependence of the Alpha-Adrenergic Positive Inotropic Effect

The alpha-adrenergic positive inotropic effect is not equally well pronounced in all species. It is only poorly developed or lacking in dog and guinea pig heart [11–13]. However, in the human myocardium distinct alpha-adrenergic positive inotropic effects have been described, both in the atrium [14] and in the ventricle [15–18]. Direct intracoronary infusion of phenylephrine also led to an alpha-adrenoceptor-mediated increase in contractility in patients [19].

The number of myocardial alpha-adrenoceptors is also species dependent. It is relatively small in the human heart [17,20–23] and in the heart of guinea pigs and rabbits, while a relatively high density of alpha-adrenoceptors is observed in rat heart (for review, see [13,23]).

Possible Mechanisms of the Alpha-Adrenergic Positive Inotropic Effect

It is generally agreed that an increase in cardiac contractility may be caused by two basic mechanisms: (1) an increase in the amount of Ca available for interaction with the contractile proteins or (2) a change in the sensitivity of the contractile proteins for Ca. Some years ago, we studied the effect of phenylephrine on Ca inward current with Ca-dependent slow action potentials and with the voltage-clamp method [24]. Phenylephrine induced an increase in the maximum rate of depolarization of slow action potentials, and mechanical and electrophysiological effects showed similar time patterns. In the voltage-clamp experiments, phenylephrine also increased the magnitude of slow Ca inward current and the decay of the slow Ca inward current was delayed, which thus was increased not only in terms of its magnitude but also of its duration.

These studies showed also that the effect of phenylephrine on slow Ca inward current was only about half as strong as that of isoprenaline in equi-effective inotropic concentrations.

These findings are in agreement with those of Miura et al. [25], who observed that phenylephrine triggers slow, phentolamine-sensitive action potentials in rabbit papillary muscle. However, in more recent studies with adult mammalian single cardiomyocytes, alpha-adrenoceptor agonists failed to produce changes in slow Ca inward current [26–30]. On the other hand, an alpha-adrenergic increase in L-type calcium channel current was recently found in neonatal rat ventricular cells [31,32]. These discrepancies are not fully explained at present, although the use of different preparations (different species, multicellular preparations versus cardiomyocytes, adult versus neonatal cells) may be of importance. The effects of phenylephrine or noradrenaline in neonatal rat cells were blocked by WB 4101 and were thus of the alpha$_{1A}$-adrenoceptor type.

It thus seems conceivable that an increase in slow Ca inward current contributes to alpha-sympathomimetic positive inotropy. However, because the alpha-sympathomimetic increase in Ca inward current is relatively small in comparison with the effect of beta-sympathomimetic agents, there are probably additional mechanisms involved. Endoh and Blinks [33] demonstrated, in experiments with the photoprotein aequorin, that phenylephrine increases the sensitivity of the contractile proteins to Ca. Terzic et al. [34] have provided evidence that alpha-adrenoceptor stimulation activates the Na/H-antiporter, leading to intracellular alkalinization and, via an increased myofibrillar Ca sensitivity, to positive inotropy. This view is in accord with the findings of Endoh and Blinks [33] and with the alpha-adrenergic effects on phosphoinositide metabolism discussed next.

Alpha-Adrenergic Positive Inotropic Effects and Phosphoinositide Metabolism

Another question arising is whether the alpha-adrenergic positive inotropic effect is mediated by one or more second messengers. A possible effect on phosphoinositide metabolism is of particular interest. Experiments performed with phenylephrine in the presence of propranolol in rat isolated left auricles have shown that the positive inotropic effect of alpha-adrenoceptor agonists is accompanied by an increase in inositol 1,4,5-trisphosphate (IP$_3$) and in inositol 1,3,4,5-tetrakisphosphate (IP$_4$) [35]. Both positive inotropic effect and increase in inositol phosphates were similarly time- and concentration dependent. An alpha-adrenergic increase in IP$_3$ was also observed in human cardiac muscle [36].

It is, however, still unclear how inositol phosphates may lead to an increase in force of contraction. In many tissues, IP$_3$ has been shown to release calcium from intracellular stores. However, in cardiac sarcoplasmic reticulum some authors found an IP$_3$-induced calcium release [37] although others did not [38,39]. The function of IP$_4$ in the heart is also unknown, but in sea urchin eggs, IP$_4$ has been shown to initiate calcium entry from the extracellular space [40] (see also [41]). Moreover, in skinned cardiac muscle fibers, IP_3 and IP_4 induced an increase in calcium sensitivity of the contractile proteins [42]. This might at least in part contribute to the positive inotropic effect of phenylephrine as discussed previously.

One should also keep in mind that activation of phospholipase C and the resulting increase in diacylglycerol and IP_3 may lead to intracellular alkalinization. Thus, it is also conceivable that stimulation of phosphoinositide metabolism and positive inotropy are interrelated by changes in pH and that primary changes in Ca concentration are only of minor importance [6,34,43].

Alpha-Adrenergic Positive Inotropic Effect in Myocardial Failure

Experiments performed with phenylephrine in ventricular preparations isolated from human nonfailing or failing hearts have shown that the maximal alpha-adrenergic positive inotropic effect is greatly reduced in failing preparations [22]. However, alpha-adrenoceptor density was increased or unchanged in failing hearts [17,20–22]. Thus, changes in the number of alpha-adrenoceptors cannot account for the decreased alpha-adrenergic effect. More recent experiments have provided evidence that the alpha-adrenergic agonist used is of importance. Noradrenaline in the presence of propranolol produced pronounced positive inotropic effects in ventricular trabeculae isolated from failing, explanted human hearts. These effects developed relatively slowly (Fig. 1), were not antagonized by carbachol (Figs. 1, 3, 4, and 5), and the duration of the contraction was prolonged rather than shortened (Fig. 2).

The effects of noradrenaline were much more pronounced than those of phenylephrine (Fig. 3) and were antagonized by the alpha$_{1A}$-antagonist WB 4101 [44] (Fig. 4) but not by the alpha$_{1B}$-antagonist chloroethylclonidine (CEC) [44] (Fig. 5). They are thus similar to the alpha$_{1A}$-adrenergic effects seen in neonatal rat ventricular

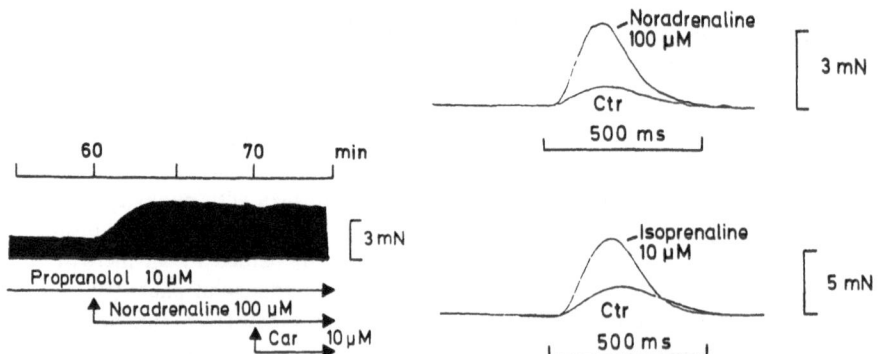

FIG. 1. Effect of 100 μM noradrenaline on force of contraction in an electrically driven (frequency, 0.5 Hz) ventricular trabecula isolated from a failing human heart. The muscle was first exposed to 10 μM propranolol for 60 min. Thereafter, noradrenaline and later 10 μM carbachol were added at the indicated times. Note the slow development of the inotropic effect and the absence of a negative inotropic effect of carbachol (*Car*) (experiment 15039210)

FIG. 2. Effect of noradrenaline in the presence of 10 μM propranol or isoprenaline (alone) on force of contraction in ventricular trabeculae from failing human hearts (experiment 16049307)

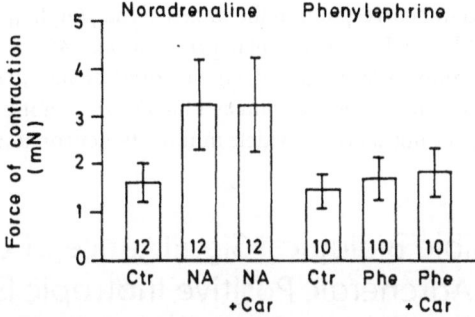

FIG. 3. Effect of noradrenaline (*NA*, 100 μM) and *phenylephrine* (*Phe*, 100 μM) on force of contraction in isolated electrically driven (0.5 Hz) ventricular trabeculae isolated from failing human hearts. All preparations were first treated with 10 μM propranolol for 60 min. Incubation periods were 10 and 15 min for NA and Phe, respectively. Note the absence of a negative inotropic effect of carbachol (*Car*, 10 μM). Numbers in brackets are number of preparations isolated from four hearts

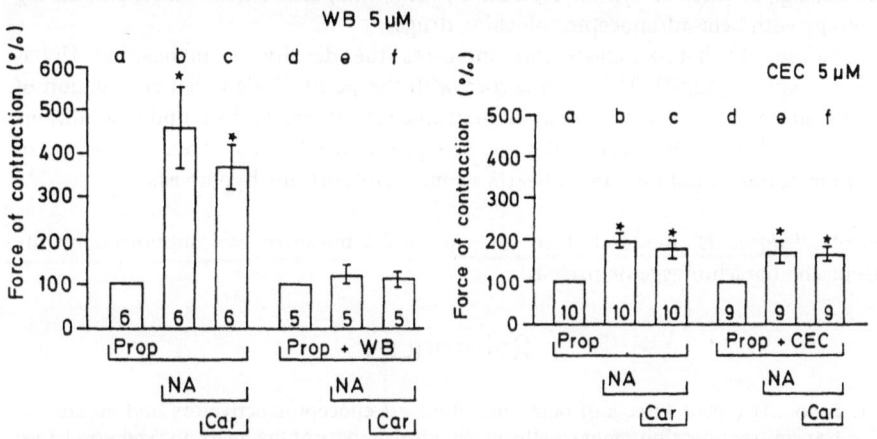

FIG. 4. Effect of noradrenaline on force of contraction in electrically driven (0.5 Hz) ventricualr trabeculae isolated from failing human hearts. All preparations were first treated with 10 μM propranolol for 60 min (*a*). Thereafter, muscles were stimulated with 100 μM noradrenaline for 10 min (NA, *b*) and subsequently carbachol was added for 10 min (Car, *c*). Thereafter, the compounds were washed out and muscles were again treated, first with propranolol and the alpha$_{1A}$-antagonist WB 4101 (*WB*, 5 μM) (*d*); then noradrenaline (*e*) and carbachol (*f*) were added. Ordinate, increase in force of contraction in percent of control (*upper panel*). Numbers in brackets, number of trabeculae isolated from three hearts; *, significant differences vs control conditions ($P < 0.05$ vs a,d)

FIG. 5. Effect of noradrenaline on force of contraction in electrically driven (0.5 Hz) ventricular trabeculae isolated from failing human hearts. All preparations were first treated with 10 μM propranolol for 60 min (*a*). Thereafter, muscles were stimulated with 100 μM noradrenaline for 10 min (NA, *b*) and subsequently carbachol was added for 10 min (Car, *c*). Thereafter, the compounds were washed out and muscles were again treated, first with propranolol and the alpha$_{1B}$-antagonist chloroethylclonidine (*CEC*, 5 μM) (*d*); then noradrenaline (*e*) and carbachol (*f*) were added. Ordinate, increase in force of contraction in percent of control (*upper panel*). Numbers in brackets, number of trabeculae isolated from three hearts; *, significant differences vs control conditions ($P < 0.05$ vs a,d)

cells [31,32,45] but do not correspond to the mixed alpha$_{1A}$/alpha$_{1B}$-adrenergic effects observed in adult rabbit and rat ventricular preparations [46,47]. It should also be emphasized that the alpha-adrenergic effects of noradrenaline, whose existence in human hearts have been described previously [48–50], were not blocked by cocaine or hydrocortisone (data not shown), which inhibit its neuronal and extraneuronal uptake, respectively [51].

Possible Biological Significance of the Alpha-Adrenergic Positive Inotropic Effect

The biological significance of the alpha-adrenergic positive inotropic effect is not entirely clear. Not all alpha-sympathomimetic agents (e.g., oxymetazoline) exert a positive inotropic effect, which suggests that cardiac and vascular alpha-adrenergic receptors differ from each other. The physiological singnificance of myocardial alpha-receptors it is probably not great under normal conditions. However, if stimulation of normally prevailing beta-adrenergic receptors is relatively low, they may in fact play a role, e.g., in cases of hypothyroidism, hypothermia, at low heart rates, and during therapy with beta-adrenoceptor blocking drugs.

Blockade of beta-adrenoceptors increases the density of myocardial alpha-adrenoceptors [52,53]. This is in accord with the point of view that stimulation of alpha-adrenoceptors may serve as an inotropic reserve mechanism under conditions of impaired beta-adrenergic influence. The pronounced alpha-adrenergic effects of noradrenaline in failing human hearts strongly support this hypothesis.

Acknowledgments. Research from the authors' laboratory was supported by the Deutsche Forschungsgemeinschaft.

References

1. Scholz H (1980) Effects of beta- and alpha-adrenoceptor activators and adrenergic transmitter releasing agents on the mechanical activity of the heart. In: Szekeres L (ed) Handbook of experimental pharmacology, 54/I. Springer, Berlin Heidelberg New York, pp 651–733
2. Endoh M (1982) Adrenoceptors and the myocardial inotropic response: do alpha and beta receptor sites functionally coexist? In: Kalsner S (ed) Trends in autonomic pharmacology, vol 2. Urban and Schwarzenberg, Baltimore, pp 303–322
3. Brückner R, Mügge A, Scholz H (1985) Existence and functional role of alpha$_1$-adrenoceptors in the mammalian heart. J Mol Cell Cardiol 17:639–645
4. Benfey BG (1990) Function of myocardial α-adrenoceptors. Life Sci 46:743–757
5. Endoh M (1991) Myocardial α-adrenoceptors: multiplicity of subcellular coupling processes. Asia Pac J Pharmacol 6:171–186
6. Terzic A, Pucéat M, Vassort G, Vogel SM (1993) Cardiac α$_1$-adrenoceptors: an overview. Pharmacol Rev 45:147–175
7. Downing SE, Lee JC, Fripp RR (1983) Enhanced sensitivity of diabetic hearts to alpha-adrenoceptor stimulation. Am J Physiol 245:H808–H813
8. Xiang H, McNeill J (1991) α$_1$-Adrenoceptor-mediated phosphoinositide breakdown and inotropic response in diabetic hearts. Am J Physiol 260:H557–H562
9. Endoh M, Motomura S (1979) Differentiation by cholinergic stimulation of positive inotropic actions mediated via α-adrenoceptors and β-adrenoceptors in the rabbit heart. Life Sci 25:759–768

10. Endoh M, Yamashita S (1980) Adenosine antagonizes the positive inotropic action mediated via β-, but not α-adrenoceptors in the rabbit papillary muscle. Eur J Pharmacol 65:445–448

11. Endoh M, Shimizu T, Yanagisawa T (1978) Characterization of adrenoceptors mediating positive intropic responses in the ventricular myocardium of the dog. Br J Pharmacol 64:53–61

12. Shibata S, Seriguchi DG, Iwadare S, Ishida Y, Shibata T (1980) The regional and species differences on the activation of myocardial alpha-adrenoceptors by phenylephrine and methoxamine. Gen Pharmacol 11:173–180

13. Shen YT, Gagnon HE, Vatner DE, Vatner SF (1989) Species differences in regulation of α-adrenergic receptor function. Am J Physiol 257:R1110–R1116

14. Schümann HJ, Wagner J, Knorr A, Reidemeister JC, Sadony V, Schramm G (1978) Demonstration in human atrial preparations of α-adrenoceptors mediating positive inotropic effects. Naunyn-Schmiedeberg's Arch Pharmacol 302:333–336

15. Brückner R, Meyer W, Mügge A, Schmitz W, Scholz H (1984) α-Adrenoceptor-mediated positive inotropic effect of phenylephrine in isolated human ventricular myocardium. Eur J Pharmacol 99:345–347

16. Schmitz W, Scholz H, Erdmann E (1987) Effects of α- and β-adrenergic agonists, phosphodiesterase inhibitors and adenosine on isolated human heart muscle preparations. Trends Pharmacol Sci 8:447–450

17. Böhm M, Diet F, Feiler G, Kemkes B, Erdmann E (1988) Alpha-adrenoceptors and alpha-adrenoceptor-mediated positive inotropic effects in failing human myocardium. J Cardiovasc Pharmacol 12:357–361

18. Jakob H, Nawrath H, Rupp J (1988) Adrenoceptor-mediated changes of action potential and force of contraction in human isolated ventricular heart muscle. Br J Pharmacol 94:584–590

19. Landzberg JS, Parker JD, Gauthier DF, Colucci WS (1991) Effects of myocardial α_1-adrenergic receptor stimulation and blockade on contractility in humans. Circulation 84:1608–1614

20. Bristow MR, Minobe W, Rasmussen R, Hershberger RE, Hoffman BB (1988) α_1-Adrenergic receptors in nonfailing and failing human heart. J Pharmacol Exp Ther 247:1039–1045

21. Vago T, Bevilacqua M, Norbiato G, Baldi G, Chebat E, Bertora P, Baroldi G, Accinni R (1989) Identification of $alpha_1$-adrenergic receptors on sarcolemma from normal subjects and patients with idiopathic dilated cardiomyopathy: characteristics and linkage to GTP-binding protein. Circ Res 64:474–481

22. Steinfath M, Danielsen W, von der Leyen H, Mende U, Meyer W, Neumann J, Nose M, Reich T, Schmitz W, Scholz H, Starbatty J, Stein B, Döring V, Kalmar P, Haverich A (1992) Reduced α_1- and β_2-adrenoceptor-mediated positive inotropic effects in human end-stage heart failure. Br J Pharmacol 105:463–469

23. Steinfath M, Chen YY, Lavicky J, Magnussen O, Nose M, Rosswag S, Schmitz W, Scholz H (1992) Cardiac α_1-adrenoceptor densities in different mammalian species. Br J Pharmacol 107:185–188

24. Brückner R, Scholz H (1984) Effects of alpha-adrenoceptor stimulation with phenylephrine in the presence of propranolol on force of contraction, slow inward current and cyclic AMP content in the bovine heart. Br J Pharmacol 82:223–232

25. Miura Y, Inui J, Imamura I (1978) Alpha-adrenoceptor-mediated restoration of calcium-dependent potential in the partially depolarized rabbit papillary muscle. Naunyn-Schmiedeberg's Arch Pharmacol 301:201–205

26. Apkon M, Nerbonne JM (1988) $Alpha_1$-adrenergic agonists selectively suppress voltage-dependent K^+ currents in rat ventricular myocytes. Proc Natl Acad Sci USA 85:8756–8760

27. Hescheler J, Nawrath H, Tang M, Trautwein W (1988) Adrenoceptor-mediated changes of excitation and contraction in ventricular heart muscle from guinea-pigs and rabbits. J Physiol (Camb) 397:657–670

28. Hartmann HA, Mazzocca NJ, Kleimann RB, Houser SR (1988) Effects of phenylephrine on calcium current and contractility of feline ventricular myocytes. Am J Physiol 255:H1173–H1180

29. Ravens U, Wang XL, Wettwer E (1989) Alpha adrenoceptor stimulation reduces outward currents in rat ventricular myocytes. J Pharmacol Exp Ther 250:364–370

30. Wang XL, Wettwer E, Gross G, Ravens U (1991) Reduction of cardiac outward currents by alpha-1 adrenoceptor stimulation: a subtype-specific effect? J Pharmacol Exp Ther 259:783–788

31. Liu QY, Karpinski E, Pang PKT (1994) The L-type calcium channel current is increased by alpha-1 adrenoceptor activation in neonatal rat ventricular cells. J Pharmacol Exp Ther 271:935–943

32. Liu QY, Karpinski E, Pang PKT (1994) L-Channel modulation by alpha-1 adrenoceptor activation in neonatal rat ventricular cells: intracellular mechanisms. J Pharmacol Exp Ther 271:944–951

33. Endoh M, Blinks JR (1988) Actions of sympathomimetic amines on the Ca transients and contractions of rabbit myocardium: reciprocal changes in myofibrillar responsiveness to Ca mediated through α- and β-adrenoceptors. Circ Res 62:247–265

34. Terzic A, Pucéat M, Clément O, Scamps F, Vassort G (1992) α_1-Adrenergic effects on intracellular pH and calcium and on myofilaments in single rat cardiac cells. J Physiol (Camb) 447:275–292

35. Kohl C, Schmitz W, Scholz H, Scholz J (1990) Evidence for the existence of inositol tetrakisphosphate in mammalian heart. Effect of α_1-adrenoceptor stimulation. Circ Res 66:580–583

36. Kohl C, Schmitz W, Scholz H, Scholz J, Toth M, Döring V, Kalmar P (1989) Evidence for α_1-adrenoceptor mediated increase in inositol phosphate in the human heart. J Cardiovasc Pharmacol 13:324–327

37. Nosek TM, Williams TF, Zeigler ST, Godt RE (1986) Inositol trisphosphate enhances calcium release in skinned cardiac and skeletal muscle. Am J Physiol 250:C807–C811

38. Movsesian MA, Thomas AP, Selak M, Williamson JR (1985) Inositol trisphosphate does not release Ca from permeabilized cardiac myocytes and sarcoplasmic reticulum. FEBS Lett 185:328–332

39. Zhu Y, Nosek TM (1991) Inositol trisphosphate enhances Ca^{2+} oscillations but not Ca^{2+}-induced Ca^{2+} release from cardiac sarcoplasmic reticulum. Pflügers Arch 418:1–6

40. Irvine RF, Moor RM (1986) Micro-injection of inositol 1,3,4,5-tetrakisphosphate activates sea urchin eggs by a mechanism dependent on external Ca. Biochem J 240:917–920

41. Taylor CW (1987) Receptor regulation of calcium entry. Trends Pharmacol Sci 8:79–80

42. Brückner R, Armah B, Traupe B, Schmitz W, Scholz H (1988) Effects of inositol phosphates on Ca-sensitivity in skinned porcine cardiac muscle fibers. Naunyn-Schmiedeberg's Arch Pharmacol 338[Suppl 1]:R44

43. Iwakura K, Hori M, Watanabe Y, Kitabatake A, Cragoe EJ Jr, Yoshida H, Kamada T (1990) α_1-Adrenoceptor stimulation increases intracellular pH and Ca^{2+} in cardiomyocytes through Na^+/H^+ and Na^+/Ca^{2+} exchange. Eur J Pharmacol 186:29–40

44. Bylund DB, Eikenberg DC, Hieble JP, Langer SZ, Lefkowitz RJ, Minneman KP, Molinoff PB, Ruffolo RR Jr (1994) International Union of Pharmacology nomenclature of adrenoceptors. Pharmacol Rev 46:121–136

45. Balzo U, Rosen MR, Malfatto G, Kaplan LM, Steinberg SF (1990) Specific α_1-adrenergic receptor subtypes modulate catecholamine-induced increases and decreases in ventricular automaticity. Circ Res 67:1535–1551

46. Takanashi M, Norota I, Endoh M (1991) Potent inhibitory action of chlorethylclonidine on the positive inotropic effect and phosphoinositide hydrolysis mediated via myocardial alpha$_1$-adrenoceptors in the rabbit ventricular myocardium. Naunyn-Schmiedeberg's Arch Pharmacol 343:669–673

47. Williamson AP, Seifen E, Lindemann JP, Kennedy RH (1994) Effects of WB4101 and chloroethylclonidine on the positive and negative inotropic actions of phenylephrine in rat cardiac muscle. J Pharmacol Exp Ther 268:1174–1182

48. Skomedal T, Aass H, Osnes JB, Fjeld NB, Klingen G, Langslet A, Semb G (1985) Demonstration of an alpha adrenoceptor-mediated inotropic effect of norepinephrine in human atria. J Pharmacol Exp Ther 233:441–446
49. Aass H, Skomedal T, Osnes JB, Fjeld NB, Klingen G, Langslet A, Svennevig J, Semb G (1986) Noradrenaline evokes an alpha-adrenoceptor-mediated inotropic effect in human ventricular myocardium. Acta Pharmacol Toxicol 58:88–90
50. Borthne K, Haga P, Langslet A, Lindberg H, Skomedal T, Osnes JB (1995) Endogenous norepinephrine stimulates both α_1- and β-adrenoceptors in myocardium from children with congenital heart defects. J Mol Cell Cardiol 27:693–699
51. Graefe KH (1981) The disposition of ^{3}H-(-)-noradrenaline in the perfused cat and rabbit heart. Naunyn-Schmiedeberg's Arch Pharmacol 318:71–82
52. Mügge A, Reupcke C, Scholz H (1985) Increased myocardial alpha$_1$ adrenoceptor density in rats chronically treated with propranolol. Eur J Pharmacol 112:249–252
53. Steinkraus V, Nose M, Scholz H, Thormählen K (1989) Time course and extent of α_1-adrenoceptor density changes in rat heart after β-adrenoceptor blockade. Br J Pharmacol 96:441–449

The Role of Phosphoinositide Hydrolysis in the Regulation of Cardiac Function via α-Adrenergic, Endothelin, and Angiotensin Receptors

Masao Endoh[1], Hideyuki Morita[1], and Junko Kimura[2]

Summary. Activation of myocardial α_1-adrenergic, endothelin, and angiotensin receptors leads to acceleration of the hydrolysis of phosphoinositide, with resultant production of inositol 1,4,5-trisphosphate (IP_3) and diacylglycerol. In spite of the wide range of species-dependent variation in the induction of the positive inotropic effect among mammalian species, there is an excellent correlation between the extent of acceleration of the hydrolysis of phosphoinositide and the positive inotropic effect under most experimental conditions after the administration of the respective agonists in the rabbit ventricular muscle. Moreover, the positive inotropic effect of the agonists of these receptors is consistently associated with a negative lusitropic effect and an increase in the sensitivity of myofilaments to Ca^{2+} ions. Furthermore, the positive inotropic effect can be selectively inhibited by inhibitors of protein kinase C such as staurosporine, NA 0345, and H-7, with little associated effect on the hydrolysis of phosphoinositide and the positive inotropic effect of isoproterenol and Bay K 8644 in the rabbit ventricular muscle. An activator of protein kinase C, phorbol 12,13-dibutyrate (PDBu), likewise selectively inhibited the positive inotropic effect and acceleration of phosphoinositide hydrolysis induced by these receptor agonists in the rabbit. By contrast, the regulation of action potentials and membrane ionic currents induced by these receptor agonists shows quite a wide range of variation in rabbit ventricular cardiomyocytes. α-Adrenoceptor agonists cause monophasic prolongation of the action potential, while endothelin-1 and angiotensin II elicit a biphasic change in the duration of action potential, namely a transient abbreviation that is followed by a long-lasting prolongation. Endothelin-1 also modifies the calcium current (I_{Ca}) in a biphasic manner, while α-agonists scarcely affected I_{Ca} and angiotensin II has a weak and variable effect on I_{Ca}. The potassium current, I_{K1}, is suppressed by α-agonists, whereas it is transiently activated by angiotensin II. Angiotensin II activates a slowly developing Cl^- current, while endothelin-1 does not induce such a current. These results suggest that the products of hydrolysis of phosphoinositide might play a crucial role as intracellular messengers in the regulation of cardiac function that is induced upon activation of angiotensin, endothelin, and α-adrenergic receptors in the rabbit ventricular myocardium. The signal-transduction process subsequent to

[1] Department of Pharmacology, Yamagata University School of Medicine, Yamagata 990-23, Japan
[2] Department of Pharmacology, Fukushima Medical College, Fukushima 960-12, Japan

acceleration of the hydrolysis of phosphoinositide might, however, show a wide range of variable types of coupling to regulatory proteins in the heart. Alternatively, additional regulatory processes that are specifically triggered by activation of the respective receptors might operate in parallel with the acceleration of phosphoinositide hydrolysis. Thus, the activation of receptors that belong to this class could be involved in diverse types of physiological as well as pathophysiological regulation of myocardial cell function in the mammalian heart.

Key words. Angiotensin—Endothelin—Phenylephrine—Methoxamine—Phosphoinositide hydrolysis—Positive inotropic effect

Introduction

Various types of receptor are densely distributed on the membranes of myocardial cells. These receptors are activated by neurotransmitters, neuropeptides, autacoids, and cytokines for the subsequent rapid functional and metabolic adaptation that must occur in response to physiological and pathophysiological stimuli. It has been established that cyclic adenosine $3',5'$-monophosphate (cAMP) plays an important role in the regulation of cardiac function. However, increasing interest has been focused on the pathway that involves the receptor-mediated acceleration of the hydrolysis of phosphoinositide and on the resultant production of inositol 1,4,5-trisphosphate (IP_3) and diacylglycerol that activates protein kinase C. Although various endogenous transmitters and hormones, including catecholamines, muscarinic receptor agonists, endothelin, angiotensin II, ATP, vasopressin, and histamine, stimulate this hydrolytic process, the role of this process in the regulation of the function of myocardial cells is poorly understood. This process is coupled to multiple regulatory processes, which include the operation of various types of ion channel, such as the Ca^{2+}, K^+ and Cl^- channels, ion-transport systems that include Na^+-H^+ exchange, and the responsiveness to Ca^{2+} ions of contractile proteins (for reviews, see [1–5]). This transduction process varies widely among different mammalian species. A comparison of the effects mediated by the various types of receptor that result in acceleration of the hydrolysis of phosphoinositide might help us to understand the role of this signal-transduction process in greater detail. Therefore, this chapter focuses on similarities and dissimilarities of the regulation of contractile function and ion-channel activity induced by angiotensin II and endothelin, in a comparison with the regulation induced by α-adrenoceptor agonists, such as phenylephrine and methoxamine. The results discussed were obtained from studies of the ventricular myocardium of the rabbit and other mammals and are mainly based on observations from our own laboratory.

While the present chapter is confined to a summary of the effect of these agonists on cardiac contractile function, these agonists do also have a pronounced vasoconstrictor effect on the coronary artery and cause the release of endogenous substances. For example, when endothelin is administered directly into the perfused rabbit heart, it induces vasoconstriction, facilitates the outflow of prostacyclin, and prevents diastolic relaxation [6]. Thus, the modulation induced by further divergent regulatory factors must be taken into consideration if we are to understand the pathophysiological relevance of these agonists in situ.

Regulation of Contractile Function

The regulation of cardiac contractility, induced by receptor agonists that stimulate the hydrolysis of phosphoinositide in cardiac myocytes, has definite characteristics that are clearly distinct from cAMP-mediated regulation. We shall first discuss the relationship between the positive inotropic effect and the acceleration of phosphoinositide hydrolysis in the rabbit ventricular myocardium. Then we shall focus on the negative lusitropic effect and the increase in myofibrillar Ca^{2+} sensitivity that is induced by the various receptor agonists. Finally, species-dependent differences in regulation and the inhibitory regulation of cardiac function mediated by endothelin and α_1-adrenergic receptors will be described in this section.

Cardiac Contractility and the Hydrolysis of Phosphoinositide

In rabbit ventricular slices that have been prelabeled with myo-[^{3}H]inositol, α-adrenoceptor agonists (methoxamine and phenylephrine) [7,8], endothelin isopeptides (endothelin-1 and endothelin-3) [9–11], and angiotensin II [12] produce a concentration-dependent accumulation of [^{3}H]IP$_1$, [^{3}H]IP$_2$ and [^{3}H]IP$_3$.

Figure 1 shows the time courses of the accumulation of inositol phosphates and the development of the positive inotropic effect that are induced by methoxamine in the presence of bupranolol, a β-adrenoceptor blocking agent [8]. Accumulation of [^{3}H]IP$_1$ increased continuously during the period of investigation, while that of [^{3}H]IP$_3$ and [^{3}H]IP$_2$ was transient and levels of these latter compounds returned to basal values at 30 min after the administration of methoxamine, when the positive inotropic effect had reached a steady level. The accumulation of [^{3}H]IP$_3$ induced by endothelin-1 was also transient [10].

An excellent correlation between the positive inotropic effect and the extent of acceleration of the hydrolysis of phosphoinositide was found during activation of α_{1B}-adrenoceptors in the rabbit ventricular myocardium [13]. By contrast, activation of α_{1A}-adrenoceptors elicited a positive inotropic effect without or with only a small alteration in the levels of inositol phosphates [8]. It is postulated therefore that activation of α_{1B}-adrenoceptors is predominantly coupled to acceleration of phosphoinositide hydrolysis and positive inotropic effect, whereas activation of α_{1A}-adrenoceptors mediates the positive inotropic effect via a process independent of the hydrolysis. The various pieces of evidence supporting the above postulate were obtained by using subtype-selective adrenoceptor antagonists. Chlorethylclonidine was used as an α_{1B} antagonist [13], while (+)-niguldipine [14], HV723 [15], and WB 4101 [8] were used as α_{1A}-receptor antagonists in these studies.

An excellent correlation between the positive inotropic effect and hydrolysis of phosphoinositide was also found during determinations of the dependence on time and concentration of the increases in both parameters induced by endothelin-1, as shown in Fig. 2 [10], and by angiotensin II [12] in rabbit ventricular muscle.

Dissociation to a certain extent of contractile force from changes in the rate of phosphoinositide hydrolysis was also evident after administration of endothelin isopeptides and endothelin receptor antagonists. First, while the ability of endothelin-3 to elicit the acceleration of phosphoinositide hydrolysis was lower than that of endothelin-1 [11], the maximal inotropic response to endothelin-3 was slightly larger than that to endothelin-1. This difference might be partly due to the fact that

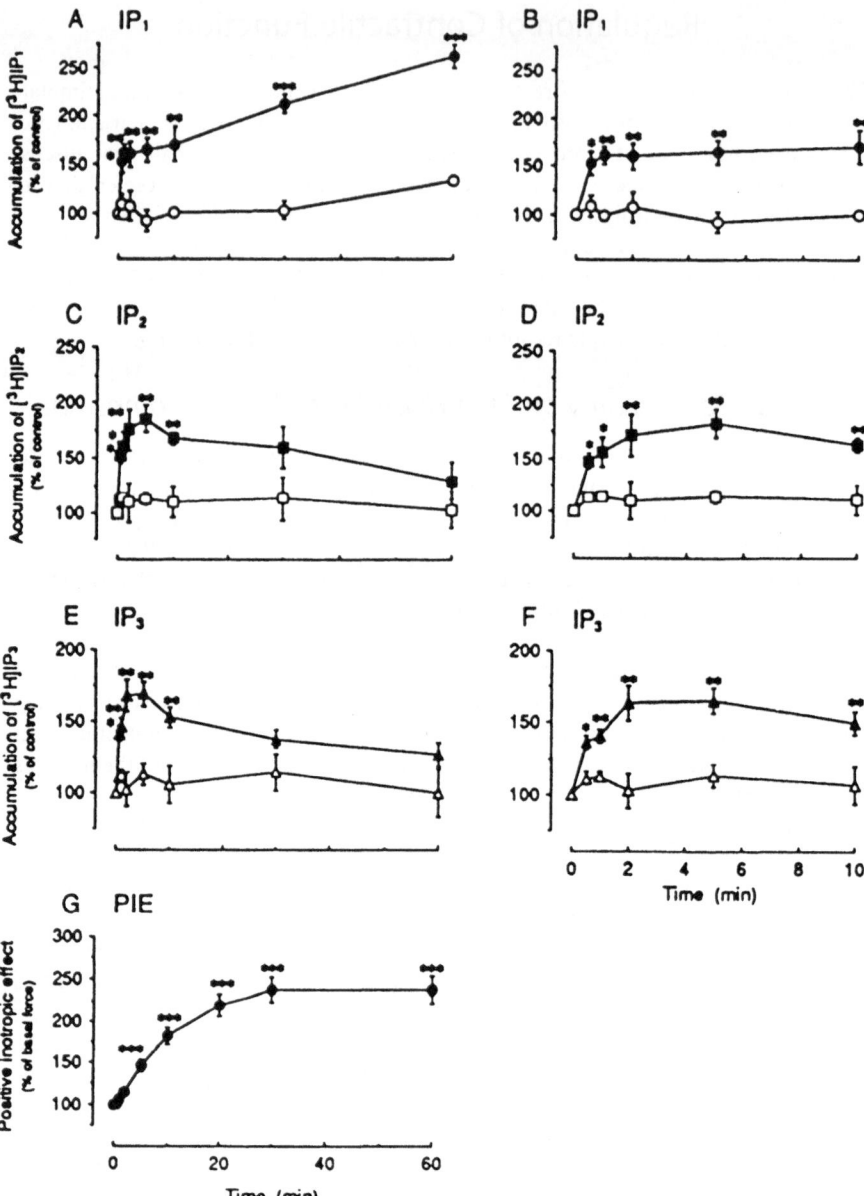

FIG. 1. Time course of accumulation of [³H]IP₁ (A, B), [³H]IP₂ (C, D), and [³H]IP₃ (E, F), and of the positive inotropic effect (*PIE*, G) induced by 10^{-4} M methoxamine in rabbit ventricular muscle in the presence of 3×10^{-7} M bupranolol. *Closed symbols*, values in the presence of 10^{-4} M methoxamine (*n* = 5 each); *open symbols*, controls in the absence of methoxamine (*n* = 3 each). *$P < 0.05$; **$P < 0.01$ and ***$P < 0.001$ *vs* the control values. In B, D, and F the time scale is amplified. (From [8] with permission)

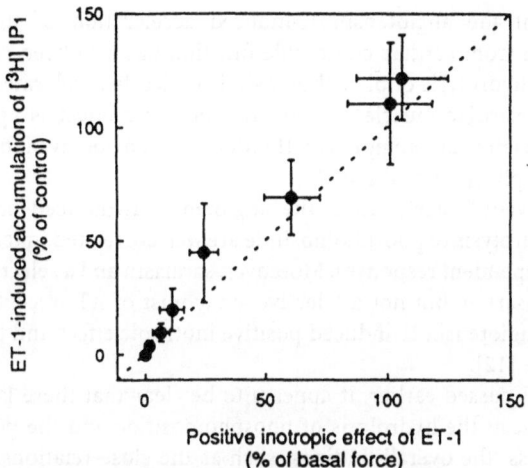

FIG. 2. Correlation between the positive inotropic effect of endothelin-1 (*ET-1*) and endothelin-1-induced accumulation of [³H]IP₁, both expressed as the percentage of control values in the absence of endothelin-1 in the rabbit ventricular muscle. Values were obtained during determination of the concentration-response relationship for endothelin-1, 30 min after its administration. *Dotted line*, a line with a slope of unity. (From [10] with permission)

endothelin-1 activates a subtype of endothelin receptor that is coupled to inhibitory regulation of contractile function: in the presence of the selective ET_A-receptor antagonist FR139317, the concentration-response curve for the positive inotropic effect of endothelin-1 becomes steeper. By contrast, the rate of phosphoinositide hydrolysis induced by endothelin-1 decreased by 20% in the presence of FR139317, with the relationship between the two parameters in the presence of endothelin-1 and FR139317 being similar to that in the presence of endothelin-3 alone. Consistent with the findings with FR139317, another ET_A-receptor antagonist, namely BQ-123, also slightly enhanced the positive inotropic effect of endothelin-1 over a high concentration range in the rabbit papillary muscle [11]. It has been reported that endothelin receptors are coupled to various processes [16–18] that include an inhibitory response in rat and guinea pig cardiac myocytes [16,19,20]. The predominant mechanism of inhibitory regulation in the studies discussed herein involves the coupling of endothelin receptors to suppression of the activity of adenylate cyclase via the pertussis toxin-sensitive G protein.

While FR139317 abolished the positive inotropic effect of endothelin-3, approximately 40% of the endothelin-3-induced stimulation of phosphoinositide hydrolysis remained uninhibited in the presence of FR139317 at a concentration at which it completely inhibited the positive inotropic effect of endothelin-3. This result indicates that a definite fraction of phosphoinositide hydrolysis is not coupled to the positive inotropic effect. Dissociation of both parameters was also observed with vasopressin and α_1-adrenoceptor agonists in rabbit ventricular muscle. Vasopressin elicited the concentration-dependent accumulation of IP₁ with little change in the contractile force [21], while methoxamine accelerated phosphoinositide hydrolysis but inhibited the positive inotropic effect that was mediated by the activation of α_1-adrenoceptors [8].

Dissociation of the angiotensin II-induced acceleration of the hydrolysis of phosphoinositide from cardiac contractile function has also been reported. For example, while the hydrolysis of phosphoinositide is clearly accelerated by angiotensin II in guinea pig cardiac muscle, no positive inotropic effect is apparent [22]. By contrast, in the avian heart, angiotensin II induces both a positive inotropic effect and the hydrolysis of phosphoinositide [23].

In the rabbit ventricular muscle, the angiotensin II-induced positive inotropic effect and the hydrolysis of phosphoinositide are well correlated in terms of time- and concentration-dependent responses. Moreover, saralasin and a selective antagonist of AT_1-receptors, losartan, but not a selective antagonist of AT_2-receptors, PD 123319, antagonize the angiotensin II-induced positive inotropic effect and the hydrolysis of phosphoinositide [12].

As has been discussed earlier, it appears to be clear that there is some extent of discrepancy between the hydrolysis of phosphoinositide and the positive inotropic effect. Nonetheless, the overall findings, such as the close relationship between the positive inotropic effect and phosphoinositide hydrolysis under various experimental conditions, as well as the similarity of the contractile regulation that is associated with a negative lusitropic effect and the increase in Ca^{2+} sensitivity, imply that the hydrolysis of phosphoinositide may play an important role in the positive inotropic effect induced by these receptor agonists.

The accumulation of IP_3 is transient and the level of IP_3 returns to the basal value during induction of the positive inotropic effect as shown, for example, in Fig. 1. Moreover, there is evidence that the activation of protein kinase C is involved in long-term regulation, in the case of hypertrophy of myocardial cells. Thus, the receptor-mediated activation of protein kinase C might play a more important role than IP_3 in cardiac regulation. To examine this hypothesis, we studied the effects of inhibitors and activators of protein kinase C in rabbit ventricular muscle. Although over a certain range of concentrations, staurosporine, NA 0345, and H-7 had selective inhibitory actions on the α_1-adrenoceptor-mediated positive inotropic effect, as compared to their actions on the β-mediated effect, the extent of the selective inhibition was only 20%–30% of the total response [24]. When these inhibitors were used at higher concentrations, the β-mediated inotropic effect was also suppressed. Therefore, while it is difficult to delineate the extent of the contribution of protein kinase C to the inotropic effect, the experimental evidence implies that activation of protein kinase C might require additional process(es) for full functional regulation.

Whereas we expected that phorbol 12,13-dibutyrate (PDBu), which activates protein kinase C in vitro, might mimic the effect of receptor activation, it had more pronounced inhibitory actions than inhibitors of protein kinase C on the positive inotropic effects of α-adrenoceptor agonists, endothelin, and angiotensin II in rabbit ventricular myocardium. PDBu at 3×10^{-8} M and at 10^{-7} M did not affect the positive inotropic effects of isoproterenol or Bay K 8644, but it markedly decreased the positive inotropic effect of phenylephrine [25,26] and of endothelin-1 [9,27], and it abolished the positive inotropic effect of angiotensin II [12]. Since it was found that the acceleration of phosphoinositide hydrolysis induced by the agonists is similarly inhibited by PDBu, it is postulated that, in the rabbit ventricular muscle, PDBu administered externally might have a site of action that differs from the site of action of an endogenous activator of protein kinase C, namely diacylglycerol. Supporting this postulate, we note that α-adrenoceptor agonists and endothelin isopeptides do not cause tachyphylaxis when they induce a positive inotropic effect. Angiotensin II causes limited tachyphylaxis upon its repeated administration to rabbit papillary muscle (our unpublished observations). Since the binding characteristics of α_1-adrenoceptors are unaffected by PDBu when the rate of acceleration of the hydrolysis of phosphoinositide induced by α_1-stimulation is decreased, PDBu might cause uncoupling of the activation of the receptor and phospholipase C, probably via an effect on the GTP-binding protein, G_q, or by a direct effect on phospholipase C [24,26].

The effect of PDBu is dependent on the species of animal examined. While PDBu has an inhibitory effect on the receptor-mediated process in the rabbit ventricular muscle, it has been reported that PDBu enhances the positive inotropic effect of α-adrenoceptor agonists in the left ventricular muscle of the rat [28].

Although these pieces of evidence imply a close relationship between the hydrolysis of phosphoinositide and the positive inotropic effect induced by these receptor agonists, the role of IP_3 and activation of protein kinase C in the regulation of cardiac contractility has not yet been unequivocally established.

It has been shown that in ventricular myocytes of the adult rat, the endothelin-induced stimulation of the hydrolysis of phosphoinositide is insensitive to treatment with pertussis toxin [16,17,29]. In ventricular cardiomyocytes of the adult cat, endothelin stimulates the hydrolysis of phosphoinositide and elicits a positive inotropic effect; the former effect is insensitive, while the latter is sensitive, to inhibition by pertussis toxin [29].

The regulation of cardiac function mediated by endothelin receptors is also dependent on the age of animals. The density of endothelin receptors decreases as rats age [30]. In addition, endothelin-1 (10 nM) elicits a negative inotropic effect, acidification of cytoplasm, and a decrease in Ca^{2+} transients in chick embryonic and rat neonatal cardiomyocytes—effects that contrast strongly with those on the corresponding adult cardiomyocytes [18].

In cultures of neonatal rat cardiomyocytes, endothelin-1 induces hypertrophy of the cardiomyocytes that is associated with the induction of transcription of muscle-specific genes, perhaps via the acceleration of phosphoinositide hydrolysis and activation of the protein kinase C or via mobilization of intracellular Ca^{2+} ions [31,32]. Similar results have been obtained with α-adrenoceptor agonists and angiotensin II (for reviews, see [1–5]).

Negative Lusitropic Effects of Receptor Agonists that Stimulate the Hydrolysis of Phosphoinositide

The positive inotropic effects of α_1-adrenoceptor agonists [33,34], endothelin isopeptides [9,11], and angiotensin II [12] in the isolated rabbit papillary muscle are consistently associated with a concentration-dependent negative lusitropic effect. Figure 3 shows that the total duration of contraction time, time to peak force, and half relaxation time were all prolonged by endothelin-1 in a concentration-dependent manner. These phenomena are indicative of a negative lusitropic effect [9]. The changes associated with isometric contractions are in strong contrast to those produced by stimulation of β-adrenoceptors, and they are very similar to those induced by newly developed cardiotonic agents that act essentially by an increase in sensitivity to Ca^{2+} ions and are termed "Ca^{2+} sensitizers" (for review, see [3]).

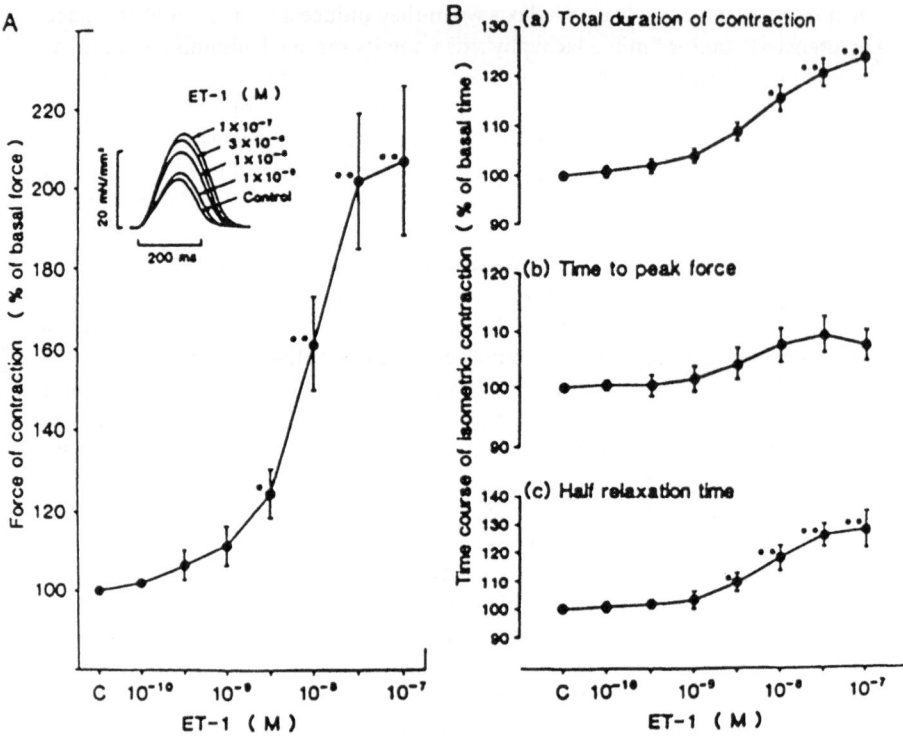

FIG. 3. A Positive inotropic effect of endothelin-1 (*ET-1*). B Changes in the time course of isometric contractions induced by endothelin-1 in isolated rabbit papillary muscle in the presence of 3×10^{-7} M ($\pm$)-bupranolol. *$P < 0.05$; **$P < 0.01$ *vs* corresponding control values. (From [9] with permission)

Increases in the Sensitivity of Myofilaments to Ca^{2+} Ions

Most sympathomimetic amines, including norepinephrine, epinephrine, dopamine, denopamine, and phenylephrine, modulate intracellular Ca^{2+} transients during induction of a positive inotropic effect via activation of α_1-adrenoceptors. While stimulation of α-adrenoceptors increases both the amplitude of Ca^{2+} transients and the force of contraction in aequorin-injected papillary muscles of the rabbit, the increase in Ca^{2+} transients is much smaller than that induced by elevation of the extracellular concentration of Ca^{2+} ions ($[Ca^{2+}]_o$) or stimulation of β-adrenoceptors. The maximum increase in Ca^{2+} transients is less than 10% of the maximum response to isoproterenol [3,34]. The maximal increase in the contractile force induced by stimulation of α-adrenoceptors is about 50%–60% of that induced by isoproterenol. Hence, for a given increase in the contractile force, stimulation of α-adrenoceptors produces a much smaller change in the amplitude of Ca^{2+} transients than does elevation of $[Ca^{2+}]_o$ or β-stimulation, an indication that the positive inotropic effect of α-stimulation might be due, in large part, to an increase in myofibrillar responsiveness to Ca^{2+} ions. In support of this postulate, we noted that stimulation of α-adrenoceptors elicits contrary changes in the duration of contraction and in Ca^{2+} transients. Thus, for example, dopamine reduces the duration of Ca^{2+} transients in association with a prolongation of isometric contractions (Fig. 4). The activation of myocardial α_1-adrenoceptors might therefore produce a positive inotropic effect through both an increase in mobilization of intracellular Ca^{2+} ions and an increase in the myofibrillar responsiveness to Ca^{2+} ions.

An increase in sensitivity to Ca^{2+} ions upon stimulation of α-adrenoceptors has been demonstrated in various mammalian species (for reviews, see [1–5]). A similar finding has been reported for activation of endothelin and angiotensin receptors in mammalian cardiac muscle. Endothelin has also been shown to increase Ca^{2+} sensitivity in the ferret papillary muscle [35] and in rat ventricular myocytes [36,37]. Angiotensin II had a positive inotropic effect, the predominant mechanism of which did not involve an increase in $[Ca^{2+}]_i$ but rather involved, in part, an increase in the Ca^{2+} sensitivity of myofilaments that was associated with intracellular alkalinization [38]. Thus, an increase in Ca^{2+} sensitivity of myofilaments appears to be a common regulatory process that is generally induced by receptor agonists that stimulate the hydrolysis of phosphoinositide in cardiac muscle [3].

The mechanism responsible for the increase in myofibrillar responsiveness to Ca^{2+} ions that is caused by the receptor agonists that stimulate phosphoinositide hydrolysis remains unknown. The possible involvement of two processes has been postulated: (1) an intracellular alkalinization induced by activation of the Na^+-H^+ exchanger, and (2) the phosphorylation of contractile proteins. It has been suggested that the contribution of the former mechanism might be of lesser significance in the rat because an α_1-mediated increase in myofibrillar responsiveness to Ca^{2+} ions was elicited even in the presence of an inhibitor of the Na^+-H^+ exchange, namely ethylisopropylamiloride (EIPA) at $0.1\,\mu M$ [39]. However, Gambassi and co-workers [40] demonstrated that EIPA at $10\,\mu M$ abolished the alkalinization and the increase in myofibrillar responsiveness to Ca^{2+} ions that was induced by stimulation of α-adrenoceptors in rat ventricular myocytes. Since the selectivity of EIPA for the Na^+-H^+ exchange system is not especially high, further studies with more selective agents

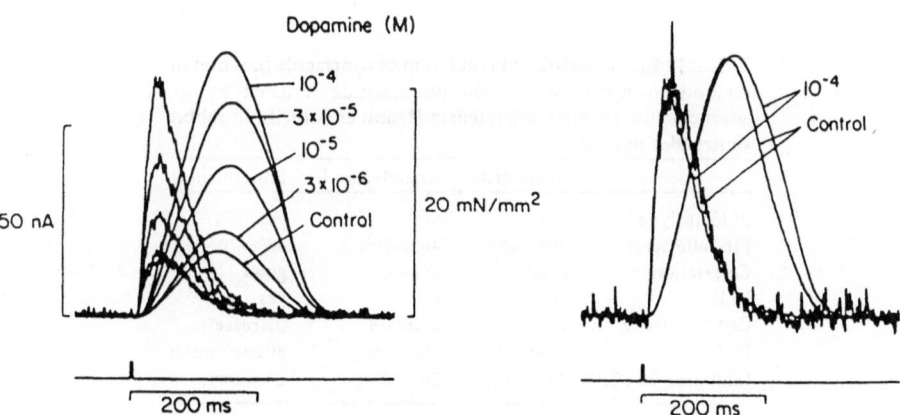

FIG. 4. Effects of dopamine on aequorin light signals and isometric contractions of an isolated rabbit papillary muscle injected with aequorin. ($\pm$)-Bupranolol ($3 \times 10^{-7}\,M$) was present throughout the experiment. **Left** Aequorin signals and contractions. **Right** Signals recorded in the presence of $10^{-4}\,M$ dopamine are superimposed on the control signals with adjustment of the amplitude. Muscle length, 7.0 mm; cross-sectional area, $0.46\,mm^2$; stimulus interval, 1 s; temperature, 37.5°C; 128 signals were averaged. (From [34] with permission)

are necessary before we can draw any firm conclusions about the significance of alkalinization.

Considering a rather different system, we note that it has long been known that protein kinase C phosphorylates both troponin I and troponin T in vitro [41,42]. However, Edes and Kranias [43] failed to detect the phosphorylation of troponin in the perfused guinea pig heart in vivo. Although it has been proposed that such phosphorylation might be related to the negative inotropic effect induced by externally applied phorbol esters in cardiac muscles from various experimental animals, including chicks and mammals [44–48], a low concentration of phorbol esters in the cardiac muscles of certain species has been found to have a positive inotropic effect [24,26,49,50]. Clearly, the physiological significance of the protein kinase C-induced phosphorylation of contractile proteins requires further study.

Features of the regulation of contractile function, as it relates to the hydrolysis of phosphoinositide in response to stimulation by α-adrenoceptor agonists, endothelin, and angiotensin II, are summarized in Table 1. The characteristics of cardiac regulation induced by the various agonists appear to be quite similar.

Species-Dependent Differences in Regulation

One characteristic feature of the regulation that is induced by receptor agonists which stimulate the hydrolysis of phosphoinositide is the wide range of species-dependent variations even among mammals. For example, α-agonists [50], endothelin [9], and angiotensin II [52] all fail to elicit a definite positive inotropic effect in the dog heart. In addition, the nature of the regulation also differs between the atrial and ventricular myocardium. This observation contrasts strongly with the β-adrenoceptor-mediated regulation of contraction that can be observed in all parts of the hearts of experimental animals.

Figure 5 shows the inotropic effects of endothelin-1 in ventricular muscle from various mammals [9]. Endothelin-1 elicited the most pronounced positive inotropic

TABLE 1. Characteristics of regulation of contractile function in relation to hydrolysis of phosphoinositide induced by α-adrenoceptor agonists, angiotensin II, and endothelin in rabbit ventricular muscle.

	α-Agonists	Angiotensin II	Endothelin
PI hydrolysis	yes	yes	yes
PIE (efficacy)[a]	50%–60%	40%–50%	60%–70%
Correlation	good	good	good
NLE	yes	yes	yes
Ca^{2+} sensitivity	increase[b]	increase[c]	increase[d]
PDBu	attenuation	abolition	attenuatation
Inhibition by STP	20%–30%	20%–30%	20%–30%

PI, phosphoinositide; PIE, positive inotropic effect; NLE, negative lusitropic effect; PDBu, phorbol 12,13-dibutyrate; STP, staurosporine.
[a] Percentage of maximum response to isoproterenol.
[b] [34].
[c] [38].
[d] In the ferret [35].

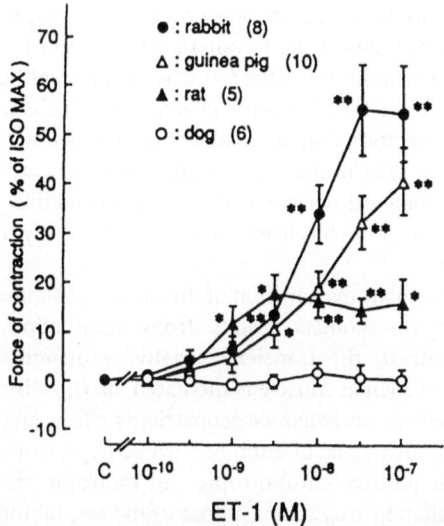

FIG. 5. Concentration-response curves for the positive inotropic effect of endothelin-1 (*ET-1*) in isolated rabbit, guinea pig, and rat papillary muscles and in right ventricular trabeculae of the dog. All muscle preparations were driven electrically at 1 Hz except for the ventricular trabeculae (0.5 Hz) at 37°C in the presence of 3×10^{-7} M ($\pm$)-bupranolol. *$P < 0.05$; **$P < 0.01$ *vs* the respective control. *Numbers in parentheses* are numbers of experiments. (From [9] with permission)

effect in the rabbit. In the rat, the potency of endothelin-1 was high but its efficacy was lower than in the rabbit. The inotropic effect of endothelin was intermediate in the guinea pig. Although endothelin-1 had no inotropic effect in the dog, quite a high density of specific binding sites for [^{125}I]endothelin-1 was found in a membrane fraction derived from the dog ventricle [9]. Moreover, it has recently been shown that subtypes of endothelin receptor differ markedly among cardiac muscles of different animals. For example, in the rat, the ET_A subtype appears to mediate the positive inotropic effect of endothelin-1 because BQ-123, a selective ET_A receptor antagonist, antagonizes the inotropic effect of endothelin-1 [17]. By contrast in the rabbit, the inotropic effect of endothelin-1 is resistant to BQ-123 [11].

The species-dependence of the positive inotropic effect of α-agonists resembles that of endothelin, with the exception that α-agonists are less effective in the guinea pig and α-agonists induce a triphasic inotropic response in the rat [28,53].

The distribution of subtypes of α_1-adrenoceptors also differs between rat and rabbit myocardial membranes. The ratio of the number of α_{1A}-receptors to that of α_{1B}-receptors is approximately 1 to 4 in the rat [54,55] and 2 to 3 in the rabbit [13]. In rabbit ventricular muscle, α_{1B}-adrenoceptors play a crucial role in mediating the positive inotropic effect and in the acceleration of the hydrolysis of phosphoinositide, each of which is inhibited by chlorethylclonidine with a similar dependence on concentration. Selective α_{1A}-antagonists, namely WB 4101 and 5-methylurapidil, each produce a parallel shift to the right in the concentration-response curve for phenylephrine (α_1-mediated effect) and partially inhibit the hydrolysis of phosphoinositide [8,56]. By contrast, another selective α_{1A}-antagonist, namely, (+)-

niguldipine, does not produce such a parallel shift but suppresses the maximum response by approximately 20% [14]. Denopamine [57] and low concentrations of HV723 [15] have a similar inhibitory effect to that of (+)-niguldipine. The inhibitory effects of (+)-niguldipine and HV723 are not associated with changes in the hydrolysis of phosphoinositide. Therefore, it appears likely that further subtypes of myocardial α_{1A}-adrenoceptors might exist in the rabbit ventricular myocardium [8]. The physiological and pathophysiological relevance of signal-transduction processes mediated by myocardial α_1-adrenoceptors has been discussed extensively in recent reviews [1–5].

In the atrial and ventricular myocardium of the rat, the sustained positive inotropic effect of α_1-adrenoceptor agonists results from stimulation of α_{1A}- and α_{1B}-adrenoceptors. By contrast, the transient negative inotropic component of the triphasic response in ventricular muscle is mediated via α_{1B}-adrenoceptors [58].

In addition to its well-documented vasoconstrictor effect, angiotensin II also has specific cardiac effects, such as facilitation of cardiac hypertrophy and induction of fibrosis [59], as well as positive chronotropic and inotropic effects in avian hearts [23,60] and in mammalian hearts, such as those of the cat, rabbit, calf [61], neonatal rat [62,63], and human [64,65]. The inotropic effects of angiotensin II resemble those of α-agonists and endothelin insofar as the induction of a positive inotropic effect by angiotensin II is markedly dependent on a variety of modulatory factors, which include location (atrial or ventricular), species, and the presence or absence of endothelium [66]. For example, in preparations of isolated heart from the dog and the adult rat, angiotensin II does not have a positive inotropic effect [52], whereas it does have positive inotropic and chronotropic effects, mediated by the direct activation of cardiac receptors for angiotensin II, in the isolated blood-perfused dog heart [67] and in the pithed rat heart [68]. It has been reported that angiotensin II does not have any positive inotropic effects in guinea pig atrial and ventricular muscles [22,60]. However, angiotensin II was shown recently to have a positive inotropic effect in guinea pig atria [69]. Rabbit cardiac muscle contains receptors with a high affinity for angiotensin II [70,71], and it responds consistently to angiotensin II with a pronounced positive inotropic effect [12,52,60,72].

Although angiotensin II does not produce a positive inotropic effect in the ventricular muscle of the rat, ferret, or dog, the specific binding sites for [^{125}I]angiotensin II are found in membrane fractions derived from these animals, and angiotensin II accelerates the hydrolysis of phosphoinositide [52], an indication that an important mechanism that contributes to the species-dependence of the inotropic effect of angiotensin II operates at a site distal to the acceleration of phosphoinositide hydrolysis (Table 2).

TABLE 2. Species-dependent regulation of myocardial contractility induced by receptor agonists that accelerate the hydrolysis of phosphoinositide in mammalian ventricular muscle

	α-Agonists	Angiotensin II	Endothelin
Receptor density	Rat > others	identical	Rab > Gp = F = Rat >> Dog
PI hydrolysis	yes	yes	yes
PIE	Rab > Rat > F > Gp > Dog	Rabbit >> others	Rab > Gp = F = Rat >> Dog

PI, phosphoinositide; PIE, positive inotropic effect; Rab, rabbit; Gp, guinea pig; F, ferret.

The Subtype of Receptors Involved in Inhibitory Regulation

Activation of myocardial α_1-adrenoceptors in certain cardiac tissues is coupled to cellular processes that can induce a decrease in $[Ca^{2+}]_i$ or that can counteract an increase in $[Ca^{2+}]_i$. For example, in canine Purkinje fibers, α_1-stimulation activates an Na^+,K^+ ATPase via the pertussis toxin-sensitive G protein. This activation can reduce $[Na^+]_i$ and thereby cause a decrease in $[Ca^{2+}]_i$ [73,74]. In guinea pig ventricular myocytes, the activation of protein kinase C by phorbol esters and/or stimulation by α_1-adrenoceptors activates the delayed rectifier K^+ current, I_K [75], and the K^+ current that is activated via muscarinic ACh receptors, $I_{K,ACh}$ [76], which also leads to a decrease in $[Ca^{2+}]_i$. These divergent signal-transduction processes, triggered by activation of myocardial α_1-adrenoceptors, contribute to the wide range of species-dependent variations in the α_1-mediated positive inotropic effect [3,53]. Species-dependent variations in the distribution of α_1-adrenoceptors might also contribute to the species-dependent variations in functional regulation [7].

In the rabbit ventricular myocardium, methoxamine is approximately ten times less potent than phenylephrine in terms of its ability to stimulate phosphoinositide hydrolysis. However the concentration-response curves for methoxamine and phenylephrine are parallel and the efficacy of both agonists is equivalent [8]. By contrast, the positive inotropic effect of methoxamine is much smaller than that of phenylephrine and, furthermore, methoxamine antagonizes the positive inotropic effect of phenylephrine in the rabbit ventricular muscle. Methoxamine also inhibits the positive inotropic effect of endothelin isopeptides, and the α_1-adrenoceptor antagonists, such as prazosin, WB 4101, and ($\pm$)-tamsulosin, antagonize the inhibitory action of methoxamine. By contrast, methoxamine does not affect the positive inotropic effects of $[Ca^{2+}]_o$, Bay K 8644, dihydroouabain, and forskolin [77]. These observations indicate that there exists a subtype of α_1-adrenoceptors responsible for selective inhibition of the positive inotropic effect that is elicited in association with the acceleration of the hydrolysis of phosphoinositide.

Endothelin inhibits adenylate cyclase in cardiomyocytes from the adult rat, and this effect is inhibited by pretreatment of animals with pertussis toxin [16,17]. The rank order of potency of endothelin isopeptides and sarafotoxin 6c, the inhibition of the effect by BQ-123, and the competition with [^{125}I]endothelin-1 for specific binding together imply that these effects of endothelin are mediated by ET_A receptors [16,17].

In guinea-pig ventricular cardiomyocytes, endothelin-1 also decreases the β-adrenoceptor-mediated accumulation of cAMP that is mediated by the pertussis toxin-sensitive, G protein-coupled ET_A receptor and, in this way, it antagonizes the β-adrenoceptor-mediated activation of the Cl^- current [19].

Regulation of Ion Channels and Ion-Transport System

Various modes of regulation of ion channels and ion-transport systems, triggered by activation of α_1-adrenergic, endothelin, and angiotensin receptors, have been demonstrated in the cardiac myocytes of several animal species. These modes of regulation include an increase in the influx of Ca^{2+} ions through L-type Ca^{2+} channels, the activation of Na^+-H^+ exchange with the resultant modulation of Na^+-Ca^{2+} exchange [39,78–80], and various types of K^+ channel, which might be responsible for the agonist-induced changes in action potential and the mobilization of Ca^{2+} ions by direct and indirect mechanisms, as discussed next.

Regulation of the Action Potential

In single ventricular myocytes from the rabbit, phenylephrine prolongs the action potential in a monophasic manner (Fig. 6A). This effect is consistent with the effect in a multicellular preparation that is induced in parallel to the development of the positive inotropic effect [7]. By contrast, the effects of endothelin-1 (Fig. 6B) and

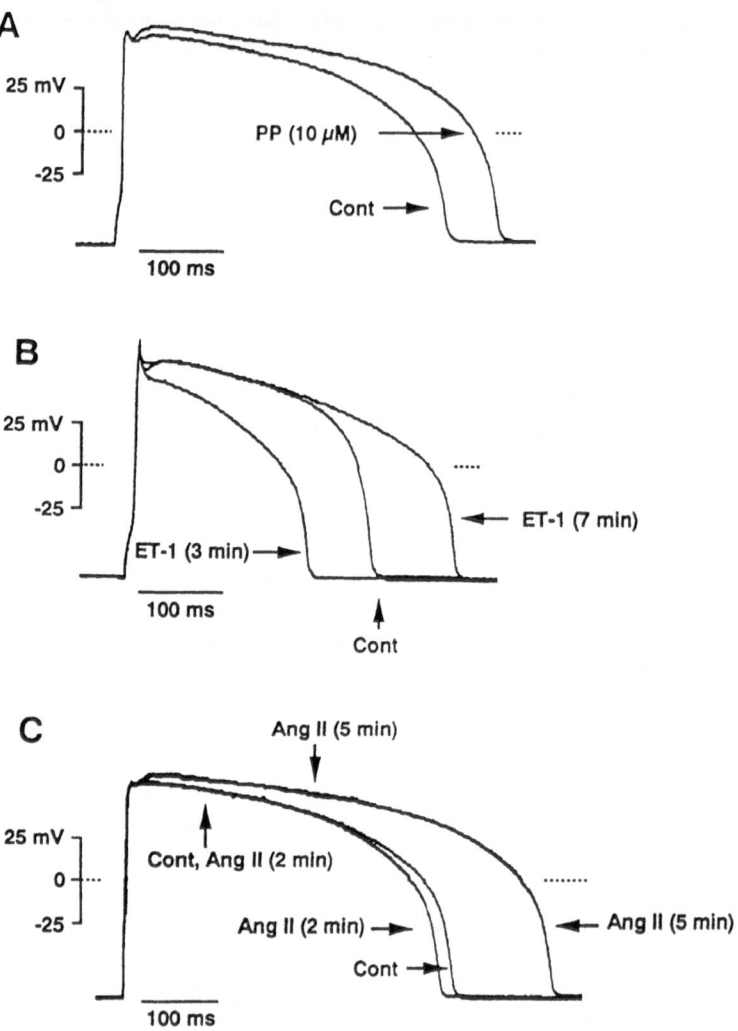

FIG. 6. Effects of phenylephrine (*PP*, A), endothelin-1 (*ET-1*, B), and angiotensin II (*Ang II*, C) on the action potential in rabbit ventricular cardiomyocytes. Action potentials were elicited by suprathreshold current pulses of 2 ms at 1 Hz. Superimposed action potentials recorded from the control (*Cont*) and from treated samples at various times after application of the receptor agonists. Experiments were carried out at 36°C (unpublished data)

angiotensin II (Fig. 6C) on the duration of action potential are biphasic, namely, a long-lasting prolongation is preceded by a transient abbreviation. The change in duration of the action potential induced by endothelin-1 in rabbit cardiomyocytes is consistent with that in the development of the positive inotropic effect in rabbit papillary muscle [10].

Regulation of L-type Ca^{2+} Channels

The activation of L-type Ca^{2+} channels is not directly facilitated by activation of α_1-adrenoceptors in whole-cell voltage-clamped ventricular cardiomyocytes of various mammalian species [81–83]. Hence, the activity of L-type Ca^{2+} channels might be increased indirectly for the most part via inhibition of K^+ channels and the resultant prolongation of the duration of action potentials induced by stimulation of α_1-adrenoceptors (Fig. 6A).

The positive inotropic effect of α_1-adrenoceptor stimulation is more sensitive to the inhibitory action of organic Ca^{2+} antagonists (nifedipine, verapamil, and diltiazem) than is the β-mediated inotropic effect [84], an indication of a significant contribution of L-type Ca^{2+} channels to the α_1-mediated positive inotropic effect.

Tohse and co-workers [85] reported that, in guinea pig ventricular myocytes, endothelin-1 decreases the amplitude of I_{Ca}, as measured under whole-cell voltage-clamp conditions. By contrast, in rabbit cardiomyocytes, when GTP ($100\,\mu M$) is added to the pipette solution that is used to dialyze the inside of the cell, endothelin-1 causes a large, reproducible increase in the peak I_{Ca} via a process that is insensitive to pertussis toxin [86]. As shown in Fig. 7, we found that endothelin-1 had a biphasic effect on I_{Ca} in whole-cell patch-clamped rabbit ventricular myocytes.

It has been postulated that the cellular mechanism of the angiotensin II-induced positive inotropic effect involves facilitation of the opening of L-type Ca^{2+} channels because the slow inward current (I_{si}) is increased by angiotensin II [60,61].

Regulation of K^+ Channels

Currents through cardiac K^+ channels, including the transient outward current (I_{to}), have been shown to be suppressed by stimulation of α-adrenoceptors in rabbit atrial myocytes [87] and in rat ventricular myocytes [85,88,89]. By contrast, in rabbit ventricular myocytes, the inwardly rectifying K^+ current (I_{K1}) is suppressed by stimulation of α_1-adrenoceptors (Fig. 8 and [90]). The change in the current induced by angiotensin II is quite different from that induced by α_1-stimulation (Fig. 9). Therefore, it appears that angiotensin II activates a current that is different from the I_{K1} that is suppressed by methoxamine (Fig. 10). The current that is activated by angiotensin II has been shown to be a Cl^- current [91,92], as will be discussed in detail later.

Habuchi and co-workers [93] showed that, in guinea pig ventricular myocytes, endothelin-1 enhances the delayed rectifier K^+ current (I_K), without affecting the L-type Ca^{2+} current, via phospholipase C-mediated activation of protein kinase C and intracellular mobilization of Ca^{2+} ions, as do α_1-adrenoceptor agonists. By contrast, the activity of rat cardiac K^+ channels (carrying I_K) expressed in *Xenopus* oocytes is suppressed by endothelin-1. This suppression occurs via coexpressed receptors for endothelin in a process that probably involves the hydrolysis of phosphoinositide [94]. In spontaneously contracting atrial cells of the rat, all three isopeptides of endothelin decrease the rate of beating and cause an increase in the I_{K1}, with endothelin-3 being the most potent of the three isopeptides in this regard [95].

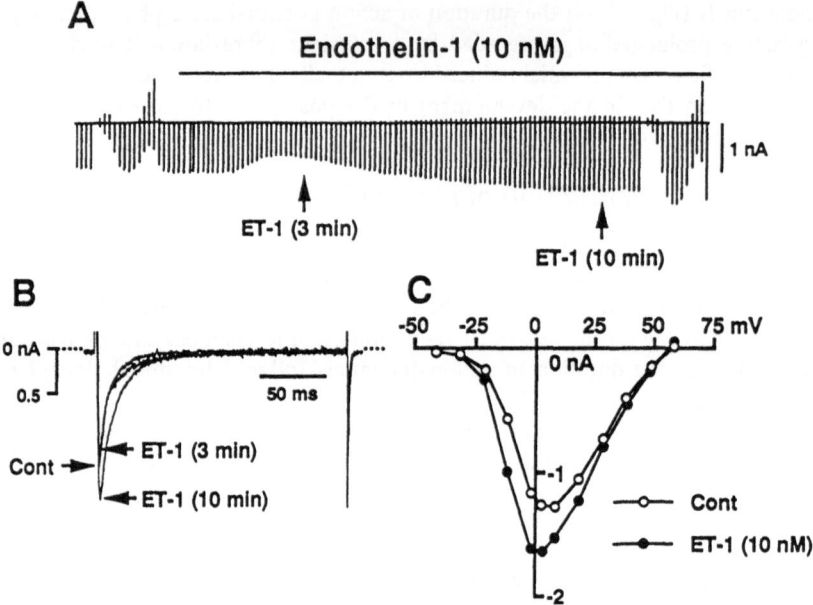

FIG. 7A–C. Effects of endothelin-1 on I_{Ca} in rabbit ventricular cardiomyocytes. **A** Currents obtained with 200-ms pulses with steps of 50 mV from a holding potential of –50 mV, applied at intervals of 8.5 s. **B** Superimposed I_{Ca} currents before (*Cont*) and 3 and 10 min after superfusion with 10 nM endothelin-1. **C** Isochronal I-V curves determined at the peak current. Experiments were carried out at 36°C (unpublished data)

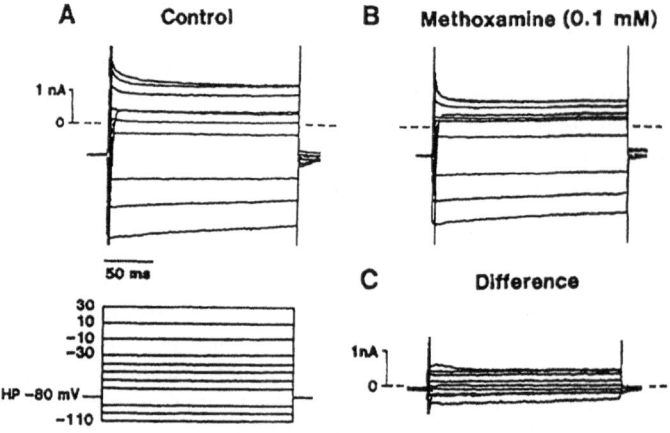

FIG. 8A–C. Effects of methoxamine on the inwardly rectifying K^+ current (I_{K1}) in a rabbit ventricular cardiomyocyte. **A** Control current in the voltage range between –110 and +30 mV with a holding potential (*HP*) of –80 mV. **B** Currents recorded by the same pulse protocol as in A in the presence of methoxamine (10^{-4} M). Methoxamine suppressed the current in both the hyperpolarization and the depolarization range of voltage. **C** The difference in current induced by methoxamine, obtained by subtracting B from A, which represents the extent of suppression. Experiments were carried out at 36°C (unpublished data)

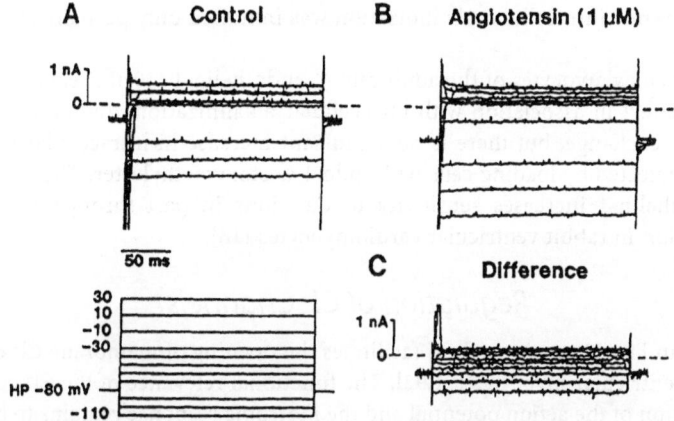

FIG. 9A–C. Effects of angiotensin on the current detected under the same condition as used to detect I_{K1} in rabbit ventricular cardiomyocytes. A Control current in the voltage range between −110 and +30 mV with a holding potential (*HP*) of −80 mV. B Currents recorded by the same pulse protocol as in A in the presence of angiotensin II (10^{-6} M). Angiotensin II increased the current more prominently in the hyperpolarization range. C The difference in current induced by angiotensin II, obtained by subtracting A from B, which represents the extent of facilitation. Experiments were carried out at 36°C (unpublished data)

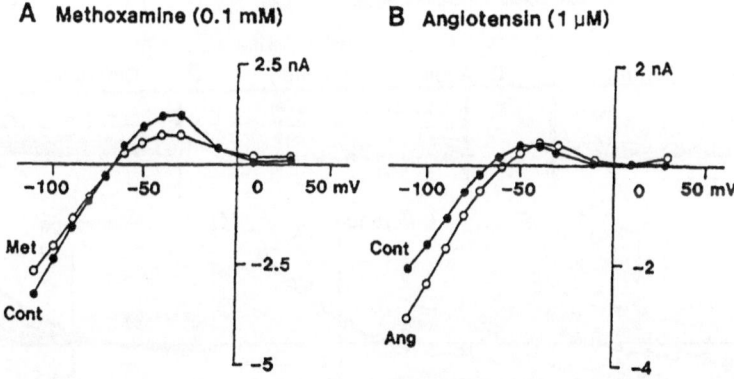

FIG. 10. Comparison of the effects on the I-V curves induced by 10^{-4} M methoxamine (A) and 10^{-6} M angiotensin II (B) in rabbit ventricular myocytes. Data were obtained from the experiments for which results are shown in Figs. 8 and 9. A Two I-V curves cross at about −70 mV, that is, near E_K. B I-V curves cross at about −40 mV, an indication that angiotensin II affects a current that is different from the current affected by methoxamine (unpublished data)

Regulation of the Na⁺-H⁺ Exchanger

The positive inotropic effect of endothelin in the ventricular myocytes of the adult rat is due in part to stimulation of the sarcolemmal Na⁺-H⁺ exchanger by a protein kinase C-mediated pathway, with resultant intracellular alkalinization and sensitization of cardiac myofilaments to Ca^{2+} ions [36,37]. The positive inotropic effect of endothelin in these ventricular myocytes has been reported to be inhibited by pertussis toxin

[28,36,37], while intracellular alkalinization was inhibited only partially by pertussis toxin [37].

In ventricular myocytes of the adult rabbit, endothelin-1 (10 nM) elicits a positive inotropic effect in association with intracellular alkalinization, due to activation of the Na^+-H^+ exchange, but there is no significant increase in intracellular Ca^{2+} transients, as detected by loading cells with indo-1-acetoxymethylester. Thus, it appears that endothelin-1 increases sensitivity to Ca^{2+} ions in part through intracellular alkalinization in rabbit ventricular cardiomyocytes [18].

Regulation of Cl⁻ Channels

As shown in Fig. 11, angiotensin II facilitates the opening of membrane Cl⁻ channels in rabbit ventricular myocytes [91,92]. The functional relevance of the Cl⁻ current to the regulation of the action potential and the inotropic response remains to be established. Since this current is not facilitated by endothelin-1, the relationship of the regulation of this current to the hydrolysis of phosphoinositide also remains to be clarified.

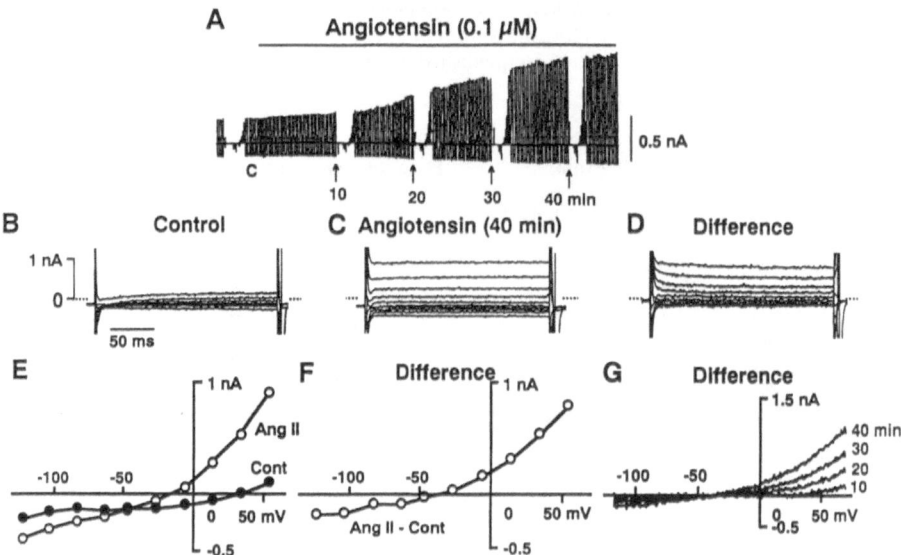

FIG. 11A–G. Effects of angiotensin II on the Cl⁻ current in the absence of K⁺ ions in rabbit ventricular cardiomyocytes. No external K⁺ ions were applied, and internal K⁺ ions were replaced by Cs⁺ ions. A The time course of the change in current during superfusion with angiotensin II at 0.1 μM. C, Control. Ramp pulses were applied every 15 s and a series of square pulses was applied at 10-min intervals. The holding potential was −50 mV. Approximately 40 min were required for the current to reach a maximum steady state. B Control currents obtained with 200-ms pulses with steps of 20 mV from a holding potential of −50 mV. C Currents recorded with the same protocol but after 40 min of superfusion with angiotensin II at 0.1 μM. D The angiotensin II-induced current, obtained by subtracting the current shown in B from that shown in C. E Isochronal I-V curves generated from results obtained 100 ms after the onset of the square pulses for the currents shown in B (*closed circles*) and C (*open circles*). F I-V relationship for the angiotensin II-induced current shown in D. G I-V curves for the net angiotensin II-induced current, recorded at 10-min intervals, as indicated by *arrows* in A. The control current at time 0 was subtracted from each current. (From [92] with permission)

Regulation of Atrial Function

The regulation of atrial function induced by endothelin and angiotensin II is quite different from that of ventricular function. For example, in spontaneously contracting rat atrial cells, endothelin isopeptides have a potent negative chronotropic effect. They activate $I_{K(ACh)}$ via a pertussis toxin-sensitive G protein and, again, endothelin-3 is the most potent isoform [95]. By contrast, in guinea pig atria, endothelin-1, and not endothelin-3, elicits hyperpolarization and shortens the duration of action potential by activation of $I_{K(ACh)}$. It also inhibits I_{Ca} in association with a decrease in the accumulation of cAMP. Endothelin-1 induces these effects by activation of ET_A receptors that are coupled to a pertussis toxin-sensitive G protein [20].

Conclusion

Activation of receptors for α_1-agonists, endothelin, and angiotensin II, which is coupled in each case to acceleration of the hydrolysis of phosphoinositide in cardiac muscle, produces an inotropic response, and the response is very similar for all members of these classes of receptor. By contrast, the regulation of action potentials, and membrane ionic currents induced by activation of these receptors, show a certain extent of variation among individual receptors (Table 3). The physiological and pathophysiological relevance of the acceleration of the hydrolysis of phosphoinositide that is triggered by the activation of these receptors remains to be clarified. The wide

TABLE 3. Characteristics of the regulation of action potentials, ionic currents, and intracellular pH in relation to the hydrolysis of phosphoinositide induced by α-adrenoceptor agonists, angiotensin II, and endothelin in mammalian ventricular muscle.

	α-Agonists	Angiotensin II	Endothelin
DAP	prolongation	biphasic	biphasic
I_{Ca}	no	no[a]	biphasic
I_{K1}	decrease[b]	transient increase	—
I_{to}	decrease[c]	decrease	decrease[d]
I_K	increase[e]	—	increase[f]
I_{Cl}	slight increase	increase (mimicked by PDBu)	no
pH_i	alkalinization[g]	alkalinization[h]	alkalinization[i]

DAP, Duration of the action potential; —, not yet determined; I_{Ca}, calcium current; I_{K1}, inwardly rectifying K+ current; I_{to}, transient outward current; I_K, delayed rectifier K+ current; I_{Cl}, Cl- current; pH_i intracellular pH.

[a] [38].
[b] [90].
[c] [96].
[d] 4-Aminopyridine inhibits the prolongation of action potential duration (APD) in rabbit (unpublished data).
[e] In the guinea pig [97].
[f] In the guinea pig [93].
[g] In the rat [78].
[h] [38].
[i] [18].

range of variation in regulatory processes, probably due both to species-dependent differences and to as yet undefined differences in experimental conditions, hampers our efforts to delineate the general features of regulation.

Acknowledgments. This work was supported in part by Grants-in-Aid (nos. 06274202 and 06274201) for Scientific Research on Priority Areas and by a Grant-in-Aid for Scientific Research (B)(no. 06454155) from the Ministry of Education, Science and Culture, Japan, and by the Mitsubishi Foundation (1994–1995).

References

1. Endoh M (1991) Myocardial α-adrenoceptors: multiplicity of subcellular coupling processes. Asia Pac J Pharmacol 6:171–186
2. Endoh M (1991) Signal transduction of myocardial α_1-adrenoceptors: regulation of ion channels, intracellular calcium, and force of contraction—a review. J Appl Cardiol 6:379–399
3. Endoh M (1995) The effects of various drugs on the myocardial inotropic responses. Gen Pharmacol 26:1–31
4. Fedida D, Braun AP, Giles WR (1993) α_1-Adrenoceptors in myocardium: functional aspects and transmembrane signaling mechanisms. Physiol Rev 73:469–487
5. Terzic A, Pucéat M, Vassort G, Vogel SM (1993) Cardiac α_1-adrenoceptors: an overview. Pharmacol Rev 45:147–175
6. Karwatowska-Prokopczuk E, Wennmalm A (1990) Effects of endothelin on coronary flow, mechanical performance, oxygen uptake, and formation of purines and on outflow of prostacyclin in the isolated rabbit heart. Circ Res 66:46–54
7. Endoh M, Hiramoto T, Ishihata A, Takanashi M, Inui J (1991) Myocardial α_1-adrenoceptors mediate positive inotropic effect and changes in phosphatidylinositol metabolism. Species differences in receptor distribution and the intracellular coupling process in mammalian ventricular myocardium. Circ Res 68:1179–1190
8. Yang H-T, Endoh M (1994) Dissociation of the positive inotropic effect of methoxamine from the hydrolysis of phosphoinositide in rabbit ventricular myocardium: a comparison with the effects of phenylephrine and the subtype of the *alpha*-1 adrenoceptor involved. J Pharmacol Exp Ther 269:732–742
9. Takanashi M, Endoh M (1991) Characterization of positive inotropic effect of endothelin on mammalian ventricular myocardium. Am J Physiol 261:H611–H619
10. Takanashi M, Endoh M (1992) Concentration- and time-dependence of phosphoinositide hydrolysis induced by endothelin-1 in relation to the positive inotropic effect in the rabbit ventricular myocardium. J Pharmacol Exp Ther 262:1189–1194
11. Kasai H, Takanashi M, Takasaki C, Endoh M (1994) Pharmacological properties of endothelin receptor subtypes mediating positive inotropic effects in rabbit heart. Am J Physiol 266:H2220–H2228
12. Ishihata A, Endoh M (1993) Pharmacological characteristics of the positive inotropic effect of angiotensin II in the rabbit ventricular myocardium. Br J Pharmacol 108:999–1005
13. Takanashi M, Norota I, Endoh M (1991) Potent inhibitory action of chlorethylclonidine on the positive inotropic effect and phosphoinositide hydrolysis mediated via myocardial alpha$_1$-adrenoceptors in the rabbit ventricular myocardium. Naunyn Schmiedebergs Arch Pharmacol 343:669–673
14. Endoh M, Takanashi M, Norota I (1992) Effect of (+)-niguldipine on myocardial α_1-adrenoceptors in the rabbit. Eur J Pharmacol 223:143–151
15. Kohi M, Yang H-T, Endoh M (1993) Myocardial α_1-adrenoceptor subtypes in rabbit: differentiation by a selective antagonist, HV723. Eur J Pharmacol 250:95–101

16. Hilal-Dandan R, Urasawa K, Brunton LL (1992) Endothelin inhibits adenylate cyclase and stimulates phosphoinositide hydrolysis in adult cardiac myocytes. J Biol Chem 267:10620–10624

17. Hilal-Dandan R, Merck DT, Lujan JP, Brunton LL (1994) Coupling of the type A endothelin receptor to multiple responses in adult rat cardiac myocytes. Mol Pharmacol 45:1183–1190

18. Kohomoto O, Ikenouchi H, Hirata Y, Momomura S, Serizawa T, Barry WH (1993) Variable effects of endothelin-1 on $[Ca^{2+}]_i$ transients, pH_i, and contraction in ventricular myocytes. Am J Physiol 265:H793–H800

19. James AF, Xie L-H, Fujitani Y, Hayashi S, Horie M (1994) Inhibition of the cardiac protein kinase A-dependent chloride conductance by endothelin-1. Nature 370:297–300

20. Ono K, Tsujimoto G, Sakamoto A, Eto K, Masaki T, Ozaki Y, Satake M (1994) Endothelin-A receptor mediates cardiac inhibition by regulating calcium and potassium currents. Nature 370:301–304

21. Endoh M, Takanashi M, Norota I (1992) Effects of vasopressin on phosphoinositide hydrolysis and myocardial contractility. Eur J Pharmacol 218:355–358

22. Baker KM, Singer HA (1988) Identification and characterization of guinea pig angiotensin II ventricular and atrial receptors: coupling to inositol phosphate production. Circ Res 62:896–904

23. Baker KM, Aceto JA (1989) Characterization of avian angiotensin II cardiac receptors: coupling to mechanical activity and phosphoinositide metabolism. J Mol Cell Cardiol 21:375–382

24. Endoh M, Norota I, Takanashi M, Kasai H (1993) Inotropic effects of staurosporine, NA 0345 and H-7, protein kinase C inhibitors, on rabbit ventricular myocardium: selective inhibition of the positive inotropic effect mediated by α_1-adrenoceptors. Jpn J Pharmacol 63:17–26

25. Endoh M, Otomo J, Norota I (1990) Phorbol-12,13-dibutyrate antagonizes the α_1-adrenoceptor-mediated positive inotropic effect in the rabbit ventricular myocardium. Br J Clin Pharmacol 30:115S–117S

26. Endoh M, Otomo J, Norota I, Takanashi M (1993) Selective inhibition by phorbol 12,13-dibutyrate of the α_1-receptor-mediated positive inotropic effect. Int J Cardiol 40:191–201

27. Endoh M, Takanashi M (1991) Differential inhibitory action of phorbol-12,13-dibutyrate on the positive inotropic effect of endothelin-1 and Bay K 8644 in the isolated rabbit papillary muscle. J Cardiovasc Pharmacol 17 [Suppl VII]:S165–S168

28. Otani H, Otani H, Das DK (1988) α_1-Adrenoceptor-mediated phosphoinositide breakdown and inotropic response in rat left ventricular papillary muscles. Circ Res 62:8–17

29. Jones LG, Rozich JD, Tsutsui H, Cooper G IV (1992) Endothelin stimulates multiple responses in isolated adult ventricular cardiac myocytes. Am J Physiol 263:H1447–H1454

30. Gu XH, Ou RC, Casley DJ, Daly MJ, Nayler WG (1992) Effect of age on endothelin-1 binding sites in rat cardiac ventricular membranes. J Cardiovasc Pharmacol 19:764–769

31. Shubeita HE, McDonough PM, Harris AN, Knowlton KU, Glembotski CC, Brown JH, Chien KR (1990) Endothelin induction of inositol phospholipid hydrolysis, sarcomere assembly, and cardiac gene expression in ventricular myocytes. A paracrine mechanism for myocardial cell hypertrophy. J Biol Chem 265:20555–20562

32. Ito H, Hirata Y, Hiroe M, Tsujino M, Adachi S, Takamoto T, Nitta M, Taniguchi K, Marumo F (1991) Endothelin-1 induces hypertrophy with enhanced expression of muscle-specific genes in cultured neonatal rat cardiomyocytes. Circ Res 69:209–215

33. Endoh M (1986) Regulation of myocardial contractility via adrenoceptors: differential mechanisms of α- and β-adrenoceptor-mediated actions. In: Grobecker H, Philippu A, Starke K (eds) New aspects of the role of adrenoceptors in the cardiovascular system. Springer, Berlin Heidelberg, pp 78–105

34. Endoh M, Blinks JR (1988) Actions of sympathomimetic amines on the Ca^{2+} transients and contractions of rabbit myocardium: reciprocal changes in myofibrillar responsiveness to Ca^{2+} mediated through α- and β-adrenoceptors. Circ Res 62:247–265

35. Wang JX, Paik G, Morgan JP (1991) Endothelin-1 enhances myofilament Ca^{2+}-responsiveness in aequorin-loaded ferret myocardium. Circ Res 69:582–589

36. Keely RA, Eid H, Krämer BK, O'Neil M, Liang BT, Reers M, Smith TW (1990) Endothelin enhances the contractile responsiveness of adult rat ventricular myocytes to calcium by a pertussis toxin-sensitive pathway. J Clin Invest 86:1164–1171

37. Krämer BK, Smith TW, Keely RA (1991) Endothelin and increased contractility in adult rat ventricular myocytes: role of intracellular alkalosis induced by activation of the protein kinase C-dependent N^+-H^+ exchanger. Circ Res 68:269–279

38. Ikenouchi H, Barry WH, Bridge JHB, Weinberg EO, Apstein CS, Lorell BH (1994) Effects of angiotensin II on intracellular Ca^{2+} and pH in isolated beating rabbit hearts and myocytes loaded with the indicator indo-1. J Physiol (Lond) 480:203–215

39. Terzic A, Pucéat M, Clément O, Scamps F, Vassort G (1992) $α_1$-Adrenergic effects on intracellular pH and calcium and on myofilaments in single rat cardiac cells. J Physiol (Lond) 447:275–292

40. Gambassi G, Spurgeon HA, Lakatta EG, Blank PS, Capogrossi MC (1992) Different effects of α- and β-adrenergic stimulation on cytosolic pH and myofilament responsiveness to Ca^{2+} in cardiac myocytes. Circ Res 71:870–882

41. Katoh N, Wise BC, Kuo JF (1983) Phosphorylation of cardiac troponin inhibitory subunit (troponin I) and tropomyosin-binding subunit (troponin T) by cardiac phospholipid-sensitive Ca^{2+}-dependent protein kinase. Biochem J 209:189–195

42. Noland TA Jr, Raynor RL, Kuo JF (1989) Identification of sites phosphorylated in bovine cardiac troponin I and troponin T by protein kinase C and comparative substrate activity of synthetic peptides containing the phosphorylation sites. J Biol Chem 264:20778–20785

43. Edes I, Kranias EG (1990) Phospholamban and troponin I are substrates for protein kinase C in vitro but not in intact beating guinea pig hearts. Circ Res 67:394–400

44. Leatherman GF, Kim D, Smith TW (1987) Effect of phorbol esters on contractile state and calcium flux in cultured chick heart cells. Am J Physiol 253:H205–H209

45. Yuan S, Sunahara FA, Sen AK (1987) Tumor-promoting phorbol esters inhibit cardiac functions and induce redistribution of protein kinase C in perfused beating rat heart. Circ Res 61:372–378

46. Dösemeci A, Dhallan RS, Cohen NM, Lederer WJ, Rogers TB (1988) Phorbol ester increases calcium current and simulates the effects of angiotensin II on cultured neonatal rat heart myocytes. Circ Res 62:347–357

47. Capogrossi MC, Kaku T, Filburn CR, Pelto DJ, Hansford RG, Spurgeon HA, Lakatta EG (1990) Phorbol ester and dioctanoylglycerol stimulate membrane association of protein kinase C and have a negative inotropic effect mediated by changes in cytosolic Ca^{2+} in adult rat cardiac myocytes. Circ Res 66:1143–1155

48. Gwathmay JK, Hajjar RJ (1990) Effect of protein kinase C activation on sarcoplasmic reticulum function and apparent myofibrillar Ca^{2+} sensitivity in intact and skinned muscles from normal and diseased human myocardium. Circ Res 67:744–752

49. Teutsch I, Weible A, Siess M (1987) Differential inotropic and chronotropic effects of various protein kinase C activators on isolated guinea pig atria. Eur J Pharmacol 144:363–367

50. MacLeod KT, Harding SE (1991) Effects of phorbol ester on contraction, intracellular pH and intracellular Ca^{2+} in isolated mammalian ventricular myocytes. J Physiol (Lond) 444:481–498

51. Endoh M, Shimizu T, Yanagisawa T (1978) Characterization of adrenoceptors mediating positive inotropic responses in the ventricular myocarium of the dog. Br J Pharmacol 64:53–61

52. Ishihata A, Endoh M (1995) Species-related differences in inotropic effects of angiotensin II in mammalian ventricular muscle: receptors, subtypes and phosphoinositide hyrolysis. Br J Pharmacol 114:447–453

53. Endoh M (1982) Adrenoceptors and the myocardial inotropic response: do alpha and beta receptor sites functionally coexist? In: Kalsner S (ed) Trends in autonomic pharmacology, vol 2. Urban and Schwarzenberg, Baltimore, pp 303–322

54. Gross G, Hanft G, Rugevics C (1988) 5-Methyl-urapidil discriminates between subtypes of the α_1-adrenoceptor. Eur J Pharmacol 151:333–335

55. Sallès J, Gascón S, Ivorra D, Badia A (1994) In vivo recovery of α_1-adrenoceptors in rat myocardial tissue after alkylation with phenoxybenzamine. Eur J Pharmacol 266:35–42

56. Endoh M, Takanashi M, Norota I (1992) Role of alpha$_{1A}$ adrenoceptor subtype in production of the positive inotropic effect mediated via myocardial alpha$_1$ adrenoceptors in the rabbit papillary muscle: influence of selective alpha$_{1A}$ subtype antagonists WB 4101 and 5-methylurapidil. Naunyn Schiedebergs Arch Pharmacol 345:578–585

57. Kohi M, Norota I, Takanashi M, Endoh M (1993) On the mechanism of action of the *beta*-1 partial agonist denopamine in regulation of myocardial contractility: effects on myocardial *alpha* adrenoceptors and intracellular Ca^{++} transients. J Pharmacol Exp Ther 265:1292–1300

58. Williamson AP, Seifen E, Lindemann JP, Kennedy RH (1994) Effects of WB4101 and chloroethylclonidine on the positive and negative inotropic actions of phenylephrine in rat cardiac muscle. J Pharmacol Exp Ther 268:1174–1182

59. Timmermans PBMWM, Wong PC, Chiu AT, Herblin WF, Benfield P, Carini DJ, Lee RJ, Wexler RR, Saye JAM, Smith RD (1993) Angiotensin II receptors and angiotensin II receptor antagonists. Pharmacol Rev 45:205–251

60. Freer RJ, Pappano AJ, Peach MJ, Bing KT, McLean MJ, Vogel S, Sperelakis N (1976) Mechanism for the positive inotropic effect of angiotensin II on isolated cardiac muscle. Circ Res 39:178–182

61. Kass RS, Blair ML (1981) Effects of angiotensin II on membrane current in cardiac Purkinje fibers. J Mol Cell Cardiol 13:797–809

62. Rogers TB, Gaa ST, Allen IS (1986) Identification and characterization of functional angiotensin II receptors on cultured heart myocytes. J Pharmacol Exp Ther 236:438–444

63. Kem DC, Johnson EIM, Capponi AM, Chardonnens D, Lang U, Blondel B, Koshida H, Vallotton MB (1991) Effect of angiotensin II on cytosolic free calcium in neonatal rat cardiomyocytes. Am J Physiol 261:C77–C85

64. Moravec CS, Reynolds EE, Stewart RW, Bond M (1989) Endothelin is a positive inotropic agent in human and rat heart in vitro. Biochem Biophys Res Commun 159:14–18

65. Chen S-A, Chang M-S, Chiang BN, Cheng K-K, Lin C-I (1991) Electromechanical effects of angiotensin in human atrial tissues. J Mol Cell Cardiol 23:483–493

66. Meulemans AL, Andries LJ, Brutsaert DL (1990) Does endocardial endothelium mediate positive inotropic response to angiotensin I and angiotensin II? Circ Res 66:1591–1601

67. Kobayashi M, Furukawa Y, Chiba S (1978) Positive chronotropic and inotropic effects of angiotensin II in the dog heart. Eur J Pharmacol 50:17–25

68. Zhang J, Pfaffendorf M, van Zwieten PA (1993) Positive inotropic action of angiotensin II in the pithed rat. Naunyn Schmiedebergs Arch Pharmacol 347:658–663

69. Feolde E, Vigne P, Frelin C (1993) Angiotensin AT$_1$ receptors mediate a positive inotropic effect of angiotensin II in guinea pig atria. Eur J Pharmacol 245:63–66

70. Wright GB, Alexander RW, Ekstein LS, Gimborne MA Jr (1983) Characterization of the rabbit ventricular myocardial receptor for angiotensin II. Mol Pharmacol 24:213–221

71. Baker KM, Campanile CP, Trachte GJ, Peach MJ (1984) Identification and characterization of the rabbit angiotensin II myocardial receptor. Circ Res 54:286–293

72. Bonnardeaux JL, Park WK, Regoli D (1977) Effects of angiotensins and catecholamines on the transmembrane potential and isometric force of rabbit isolated atria. Arch Int Pharmacodyn 229:83–94

73. Shah A, Cohen IS, Rosen MR (1988) Stimulation of cardiac alpha receptors increases Na/K pump current and decreases g_K via a pertussis toxin-sensitive pathway. Biophys J 54:219–225

74. Zaza A, Kline RP, Rosen MR (1990) Effects of α-adrenergic stimulation on intracellular sodium activity and automaticity in canine Purkinje fibers. Circ Res 66:416–426

75. Tohse N, Kameyama M, Irisawa H (1987) Intracellular Ca^{2+} and protein kinase C modulate K^+ current in guinea pig heart cells. Am J Physiol 253:H1321–H1324

76. Kurachi Y, Ito H, Sugimoto T, Miki I, Ui M (1989) α-Adrenergic activation of the muscarinic K^+ channel is mediated by arachidonic acid metabolites. Pflugers Arch 414:102–104

77. Yang H-T, Norota I, Zhu Y, Endoh M (1996) Methoxamine-induced inhibition of the positive inotropic effect of endothelin via α_1-adrenoceptors in the rabbit heart. Eur J Pharmacol (in press)

78. Iwakura K, Hori M, Watanabe Y, Kitabatake A, Cragoe EJ Jr, Yoshida H, Kamada T (1990) α_1-Adrenoceptor stimulation increases intracellular pH and Ca^{2+} in cardiomyocytes through Na^+/H^+ and Na^+/Ca^{2+} exchange. Eur J Pharmacol 186:29–40

79. Otani H, Otani H, Uriu T, Hara M, Inoue M, Omori K, Cragoe EJ Jr, Inagaki C (1990) Effects of inhibitors of protein kinase C and Na^+/K^+ exchange on α_1-adrenoceptor-mediated inotropic responses in the rat left ventricular papillary muscle. Br J Pharmacol 100:207–210

80. Pucéat M, Clément O, Lechene P, Pelosin JM, Ventura-Clapier R, Vassort G (1990) Neurohormonal control of calcium sensitivity of myofilaments in rat single cells. Circ Res 67:517–524

81. Hartmann HA, Mazzocca NJ, Kleiman RB, Houser SR (1988) Effects of phenylephrine on calcium current and contractility of feline ventricular myocytes. Am J Physiol 255:H1173–H1180

82. Hescheler J, Nawrath H, Tang M, Trautwein W (1988) Adrenoceptor-mediated changes of excitation and contraction in ventricular heart muscle from guinea pigs and rabbits. J Physiol (Lond) 397:657–670

83. Fedida D, Bouchard RA (1992) Mechanisms for the positive inotropic effect of α_1-adrenoceptor stimulation in rat cardiac myocytes. Circ Res 71:673–688

84. Kushida H, Hiramoto T, Endoh M (1990) The preferential inhibition of α_1- over β-adrenoceptor-mediated positive inotropic effect by organic calcium antagonists in the rabbit papillary muscle. Naunyn Schmiedebergs Arch Pharmacol 341:206–214

85. Tohse N, Hattori Y, Nakaya H, Endou M, Kanno M (1990) Inability of endothelin to increase Ca^{2+} current in guinea pig heart cells. Br J Pharmacol 99:437–438

86. Lauer MR, Gunn MD, Clusin WT (1992) Endothelin activates voltage-dependent Ca^{2+} current by a G protein-dependent mechanism in rabbit cardiac myocytes. J Physiol (Lond) 448:729–747

87. Fedida D, Shimoni Y, Giles WR (1990) α-Adrenergic modulation of the transient outward current in rabbit atrial myocytes. J Physiol (Lond) 423:257–277

88. Apkon M, Nerbonne JM (1988) α_1-Adrenergic agonists selectively suppress voltage-dependent K^+ currents in rat ventricular myocytes. Proc Natl Acad Sci USA 85:8756–8760

89. Ravens U, Wang X-L, Wettwer E (1989) *Alpha* adrenoceptor stimulation reduces outward currents in rat ventricular myocytes. J Pharmacol Exp Ther 250:364–370

90. Fedida D, Braun AP, Giles WR (1991) α_1-Adrenoceptors reduce background K^+ current in rabbit ventricular myocytes. J Physiol (Lond) 441:673–684

91. Endoh M, Morita H, Kimura J (1993) Activation of chloride channel via AT_1 angiotensin receptors in rabbit ventricular myocytes. Circulation 88[Suppl II] I-31

92. Morita H, Kimura J, Endoh M (1995) Angiotensin II activation of a chloride current in rabbit cardiac myocytes. J Physiol (Lond) 483:119–130

93. Habuchi Y, Tanaka H, Furukawa T, Tsujimura Y, Takahashi H, Yoshimura M (1992) Endothelin enhances delayed potassium current via phospholipase C in guinea pig ventricular myocytes. Am J Physiol 262:H345–H354

94. Ishii K, Numoki K, Murakoshi H, Taira N (1992) Cloning and modulation by endothelin-1 of rat cardiac K channel. Biochem Biophys Res Commun 184:1484–1489

95. Kim D (1991) Endothelin activation of an inwardly rectifying K^+ current in atrial cells. Circ Res 69:250–255

96. Shimoni Y, Banno H (1993) α-Adrenergic modulation of transient outward current in hyperthyroid rabbit myocytes. Am J Physiol 264:H74–H77
97. Dirsken RT, Sheu SS (1990) Modulation of ventricular action potential by α_1-adrenoceptors and protein kinase C. Am J Physiol 258:H907–H911

The NO Pathway in Cardiovascular Regulation: Constitutive and Inducible Nitric Oxide Synthase in Cardiac Myocytes and Microvascular Endothelial Cells

Jean-Luc Balligand[1], Xinqiang Han[1], William W. Simmons[1],
David M. Kaye[1], Wendy L. Gross[2], Ralph A. Kelly[1],
and Thomas W. Smith[1]

Summary. Nitric oxide (NO) is a ubiquitous autocrine- and paracrine-acting signalling autacoid that, among other functions, has been shown to regulate cardiac contractile responsiveness to β-adrenergic and muscarinic cholinergic agonists. Cellular constituents of cardiac muscle, including ventricular myocytes as well as microvascular endothelial cells, have been shown to express the "endothelial constitutive" isoform of NO synthase (ecNOS or NOS III) in vivo, and both cell types also express the NO synthase isoform induced by specific inflammatory cytokines (iNOS or NOS II) in vivo and in vitro. While NO-dependent intracellular signalling in cardiac myocytes clearly involves the activation of guanylate cyclase and downstream signalling by cyclic guanosine monophosphate (cGMP), there is accumulating evidence that non-cGMP-dependent regulatory signalling events are also initiated by NO. In addition, decreased contractile responsiveness of cardiac myocytes to β-adrenergic agonists, following induction of NOS II by inflammatory cytokines, requires the presence of insulin and the coinduction of enzymes responsible for production of tetrahydrobiopterin, a NOS cofactor. Inappropriate or excessive production of NO by cardiac myocytes and by microvascular endothelial cells probably contributes to the cardiac contractile dysfunction characteristic of the systemic inflammatory response syndrome and cardiac allograft rejection.

Key words. Guanylate cyclase—β-Adrenergic agonist—Muscarinic cholinergic agonist—Tetrahydrobiopterin—Insulin

Introduction

Evidence has been reported recently from several laboratories documenting that exogenous nitric oxide (NO) donors such as nitroprusside can alter the inotropic and lusitropic contractile function of isolated hearts and of cardiac myocytes in vitro as well as in the intact heart in situ in a number of species, including humans [1–3]. Similarly, endogenous NO generated by the "high-output" inflammatory cytokine-inducible NO synthase in cellular constituents of cardiac muscle, including

---

[1]Cardiovascular Division, Department of Medicine and [2]Department of Anesthesiology, Brigham and Women's Hospital and Harvard Medical School, Boston, MA 02115, USA

microvascular endothelial cells anc cardiac myocytes, causes a reduction in the contractile responsiveness of myocytes to some positive inotropic stimuli, including β-
adrenergic agonists [4–9]. In this review, we examine the evidence for NO generation
within cellular constituents of cardiac muscle and the physiologic roles of endogenous
NO signalling pathways in the heart.

NO Synthase Isoforms

NO is a highly reactive form of nitrogen monoxide with an oxidation state of +2 and
a neutral charge. It reacts readily in biological systems with molecular oxygen as well
as transition metal ions, resulting in a short biological half-time. NO is formed by the
oxidation of one of two equivalent guanidino nitrogens in L-arginine by O_2 to form
NO and L-citrulline. This reaction is catalyzed by a family of enzymes termed NO
synthases. The reaction requires several redox cofactors, including reduced nicotinamide adenine dinucleotide phosphate (NADPH) and the flavin nucleotides flavin
adenine dinucleotide (FAD) and flavin mononucleotide (FMN).

To date, three distinct isoforms of NO have been identified. Each represents the
product of a separate gene, and each has been cloned, sequenced, and identified in a
number of diverse cell types [10–12]. The constitutive isoform first identified in the
brain (i.e., ncNOS) has recently been found to be expressed in skeletal muscle cells
[13]. The cytokine-inducible isoform was first characterized in a macrophage cell line,
and is now known to be expressed in a wide variety of cells after stimulation with
inflammatory mediators [10], including adult cardiac myocytes [5]. A second constitutively expressed isoform was originally characterized in large vessel endothelial
cells (i.e., ecNOS) [14]. A numerical nomenclature recently proposed by Nathan
and Xie [10] identifies ncNOS, iNOS, and ecNOS as NOS I, NOS II, and NOS III,
respectively, and will be used here.

The activity of the constitutively active NOS isoenzymes (i.e., NOS I and NOS III)
identified to date is believed to be regulated by Ca^{2+} and calmodulin, and control
occurs within the physiologically relevant range of intracellular Ca^{2+} activity. These
isoenzymes can also be phosphorylated by cyclic adenosine monophosphate (cAMP)-
dependent protein kinase, protein kinase C, and the Ca^{2+}/calmodulin-dependent protein kinase with consequent regulation of activity [15]. Endothelial constitutive NOS
activity may also be regulated under physiologic circumstances by shear stress related
to blood flow and by hypoxia. Several neurotransmitters and autacoids appear to
activate NOS III in endothelial cells, including muscarinic cholinergic agonists, substance P, bradykinin, and thrombin [16,17]. NO synthase activity in microvascular
beds of specific tissues has been less well studied than NOS III activity in large vessel
endothelium. Among other factors thought to regulate NOS III in endothelial cells,
tumor necrosis factor-α (TNF-α) appears to limit NOS III mRNA stability, and inflammatory cytokines may also downregulate the generation of cofactors such as
tetrahydrobiopterin necessary for generation of NO from L-arginine by NOS [18]. In
cardiac myocytes, in which a constitutively active NO synthase activity has also been
detected, NOS activity increases in response to β-adrenergic agonists. NO has been
shown to diminish the influx of Ca^{2+} into myocytes through L-type voltage-sensitive
ion channels (i.e., I_{Ca-L}) and to blunt their inotropic response to β-adrenergic agonists
[5,19,20]. Even in the absence of adrenergic agonists, constitutive NOS activity is

increased by uniform electric field pacing in isolated adult rat ventricular myocytes in a frequency-dependent manner [21].

In contrast to the properties of the constitutive NOS isoenzymes, the cytokine-inducible NOS isoenzyme (NOS II) does not appear to be regulated by Ca^{2+} within the physiologic range. Calmodulin also appears to be necessary for its activation, although it is unlikely to play an important role in the physiologic regulation of NOS II in most cells. Control of the activity of the NOS II in the presence of excess cofactors and substrate (i.e., L-arginine) appears to be largely pretranslational. Induction of NOS II transcription and synthesis in macrophages, hepatocytes, and vascular smooth muscle cells is induced by inflammatory cytokines, including interleukin-1 (IL-1) and interferon-γ (IFN-γ). It may also be induced by lipopolysaccharide (LPS; endotoxin), either alone when given in vivo, or in the presence of serum in vitro, as necessary sources of LPS-binding protein and, in the case of nonimmunocytes, soluble CD14 [22].

NO-Dependent Signalling Pathways

Although the half-life of NO in aqueous media is very short, it is sufficient to permit diffusion of several hundred microns before redox reactions, principally with O_2, result in largely inert products such as nitrite (NO_2^-) and nitrate (NO_3^-). NO, however, readily diffuses through lipid bilayers, providing a potential means for transmission to adjacent cells. In addition, NO forms relatively stable adducts which can subsequently donate bioactive NO. These include S-nitrosocysteine and S-nitrosothiols present on proteins in plasma [23]. These relatively stable physiologic NO donors may, together with NO, comprise the biologic activities originally attributed to endothelium-derived relaxing factor (EDRF).

A principal molecular target of NO as a signalling molecule is the hemeprosthetic group of soluble guanylyl cyclase [16,24]. By mechanisms not yet well understood, this results in a substantially higher rate of cGMP synthesis by this enzyme. Our own studies [4,5] and those from other laboratories [25,26] suggest that the cardiac myocyte contractile dysfunction observed following exposure to inflammatory cytokines is due in large part to an interruption in cAMP-mediated signal transduction pathways. Our experiments indicate that the increase in cAMP levels following isoproterenol exposure in cytokine-treated myocytes was significantly lower in cells that had been exposed to inflammatory mediators [27]. Our findings confirmed prior observations on the relationship between cytosolic levels of cAMP and cytokine-induced contractile abnormalities in isolated cultured myocytes [25,26]. It is possible that increased levels of cGMP following activation of soluble guanylyl cyclase would activate protein kinase G, and could also lower cAMP levels by activation of cGMP-dependent cAMP phosphodiesterase. This would be expected to diminish cardiac myocyte Ca^{2+} influx via L-type Ca^{2+} channels, exerting downstream effects on Ca^{2+} release from the sarcoplasmic reticulum that would tend to diminish their inotropic responsiveness to β-adrenergic agonists [28].

A growing number of non-cGMP-mediated actions of NO have now been described. These include not only formation of potentially toxic intermediates, such as peroxynitrite ($OONO^-$), that could serve a role in host defense, but also, depending on the redox status of the cell, regulation of the activity of ion channels, enzymes, and nuclear regulatory factors, among other proteins, by binding to transition metals or sulfhydryl groups at or near regulatory or catalytic sites [10–12]. In skeletal muscle, Kobzik et al. [13] have recently shown that activation of cGMP signalling pathways could account for only a modest portion of the suppressive effect of increased endogenous NO production on the force-frequency relationship of electrically stimulated muscle fibers. These authors speculated that either S-nitrosylation of Ca^{2+} regulatory proteins in the sarcoplasmic reticulum, or a direct suppression of mitochondrial respiration by NO, could have accounted for some of the actions of NO in this model [13]. Indeed, NO is known to rapidly and reversibly decrease mitochondrial membrane potential ($\Delta\psi$) in isolated brain and liver mitochondria when exposed to respiratory substrates such as pyruvate, but not by ATP [29,30]. Shen et al. [31] have also shown that whole-animal oxygen consumption could be increased in experimental animals with systemic infusion of an L-arginine analog NO synthase antagonist, but did not change in animals treated with a drug that mimicked the cardiovascular effects of L-noradrenaline (L-NA), but which did not affect endogenous NO signalling pathways directly.

These data suggest that endogenous NO, among other functions, regulates the energy metabolism of both resting and contracting muscle [13,31]. Preliminary evidence from this laboratory indicates that exogenous NO donors can decrease the "contractile reserve" of the heart by, among other mechanisms, altering high-energy phosphate metabolism [32]. In isolated adult rat hearts exposed to a concentration of the NO donor S-nitrosoacetylcysteine (SNAC, 5 mM) that resulted only in a moderate increase in coronary blood flow in a retrogradely perfused Langendorff perfusion model, SNAC abolished the contractile responsiveness of these hearts to a high Ca^{2+} buffer. Interestingly, although ATP levels fell in these hearts with SNAC, as determined by [^{31}P]NMR spectroscopy, phosphocreatinine levels were preserved, suggesting that NO generated by SNAC could have been acting at sites within the cell in addition to, or other than, the mitochondrial respiratory chain [32].

NOS II in Cardiac Myocytes and Cardiac Microvascular Endothelial Cells

We have recently reported that the cytokine-inducible isoform of NO synthase (NOS II) is expressed by both cardiac myocytes and by microvascular endothelial cells in the heart [5–7]. Studies in vitro indicate that the extent of NOS II induction is strongly dependent on the specific cytokines present. Interferon-γ (IFN-γ) has been reported in several experimental models to potentiate both the effect of endotoxin [33] and of other cytokines [5,7]. The NOS II promoter in macrophages has recently been characterized, and contains several IFN-γ response elements [33]. However, when the NOS II promoter was linked to the chloramphenicol aminotransferase (CAT) gene in appropriate expression systems, the presence of IFN-γ response elements alone did not suffice to induce CAT activity in the presence of IFN-γ. If such a differential responsiveness to IFN-γ occurred in vivo in cellular constituents of cardiac muscle, it could mean that NOS II induction would be dependent, at least in part, on the recruitment of specific inflammatory cell subtypes to potentiate NO production in response to myocardial inflammation, and that specific inflammatory cell subtypes might be required to produce myocardial dysfunction in the presence of high levels of circulating cytokines.

Other cytokines, including transforming growth factor-β (TGF-β), attenuate NOS II induction triggered by inflammatory cytokines in vivo [34–36] and in isolated cardiac myocytes and microvascular endothelial cells in vitro [5]. This observation supports the view that the level of NOS II induction in the heart in response to local or systemic inflammatory mediators is complex and finely tuned in the intact organism.

The specific mechanism or mechanisms by which induction of the "high-output" NOS II isoform produces contractile dysfunction in cardiac myocytes are under continuing study. The contractile dysfunction observed in vitro in response to TNF-α has been reported to be reversible [37] and irreversible [38] by inhibitors of NOS. Studies from our own laboratory have demonstrated the induction of NOS activity following 24 h of exposure of primary isolates of adult rat ventricular myocytes to TNF-α, IL-1β and IFN-γ [5]. Specific culture conditions were required, however, to elicit a decline in myocardial contractile responses to β-adrenergic agonists, despite the induction of NOS II by cytokines. Several essential cofactors are required for NOS activity, in addition to the availability of substrate. These cofactors include tetrahydrobiopterin (THB4), which is synthesized de novo by GTP cyclohydrolase I and dihydrofolate reductase. These enzymes are also induced by cytokines [39]. GTP cyclohydrolase I inhibitors have been shown to reduce NOS activity in smooth muscle cells incubated in the presence of cytokines [40]. In addition, we have demonstrated in a preliminary report that inflammatory cytokines induce GTP cyclohydrolase I and THB4 synthesis in cardiac myocytes [41]. Thus, it would appear that cytokines can alter the NOS II activity through the increasing expression of the protein and also by influencing substrate or cofactor availability.

Insulin is also required in the culture medium in order for the decreased contractile responsiveness of cardiac myocytes to β-adrenergic agonists to become apparent following NOS II induction [42]. The mechanism(s) by which this effect of insulin is manifested is the subject of ongoing investigation by this laboratory.

Importantly, induction of NOS II in cardiac microvascular endothelial cells in vitro and in vivo contribute to the decreased contractile responsiveness of cardiac myocytes to inotropic stimuli [5,7]. Unlike most large conduit vessel endothelial cells, microvascular endothelium does express NOS II as well as the "constitutive endothelial" NOS III isoform. In vitro coincubation of freshly isolated cardiac myocytes from adult rat ventricular muscle with cardiac microvascular endothelial cells that had been preincubated with inflammatory cytokines resulted in an immediate decline in their inotropic responsiveness to isoproterenol that could be reversed with NO synthase antagonists [42]. The microvascular endothelium within cardiac muscle may therefore play an important role in the genesis of certain forms of pathophysiologic cardiac contractile dysfunction, such as in the systemic inflammatory response syndrome [43].

NOS III Activity in Cardiac Myocytes and Microvascular Endothelial Cells

Despite the recognition of multiple roles of NO in the nervous system and the vasculature, among other tissues, the potential role of NO in the regulation of cardiac muscle function has emerged only recently. The role of the autonomic nervous system as a regulator of cardiac function, particularly the β-adrenergic and muscarinic cholinergic-mediated signal transduction pathways, mediated in part by cAMP and cGMP, respectively, forms the basis for recent observations from this and other laboratories, indicating that a constitutive from of NOS present in cardiac myocytes generates NO that appears to modulate both of these autonomic nervous system signalling pathways [19,20]. Under culture conditions in which NOS II induction, either within cardiac myocytes themselves or by nonmyocyte cellular contaminants of primary myocyte isolates, could be excluded, NO synthase antagonists were found to augment the contractile response of isolated, electrically paced adult rat ventricular myocytes to β-adrenergic agonists [20]. Similarly, these NO antagonists could diminish the negative inotropic action of muscarinic cholinergic agonists and the spontaneous beating rate of neonatal rat ventricular myocytes in primary culture [20]. Han and colleagues have also demonstrated that sinoatrial nodal cells obtained from adult guinea pig hearts contained an endogenous NO signalling pathway that appeared to couple muscarinic cholinergic signalling to L-type calcium channel conductance (I_{Ca-L}) [19].

In isolated adult rat ventricular myocytes, we have recently confirmed that suppression of β-adrenergic agonist-induced increases in I_{Ca-L} by the muscarinic cholinergic agonist carbamylcholine was also mediated by the activation of an endogenous NO synthase isoform in these cells [44] (Fig. 1). This endogenous NO synthase activity could be detected constitutively in the absence of inflammatory cytokines and, unlike NOS II, did not appear to be located in the cytosol, but rather was consistently partitioned with the "particulate" fraction on subcellular localization. This NOS was definitively identified as the constitutive endothelial NOS III isoform by independent and complementary techniques, including reverse-transcriptase polymerase chain reaction (RT-PCR) amplification of NOS II mRNA—but not NOS I or NOS II mRNA—from total RNA isolated from highly purified adult rat ventricular myocyte primary isolates [44]. This NOS III PCR product coded for a portion of the NOS III protein in rat that was 91% identical to the originally identified bovine endothelial NOS III [14]. Using this PCR product as a probe for the Northern blot analysis, NOS III mRNA was detectable in primary isolates of ventricular myocytes. Antibodies to NOS III also identified the protein in cardiac myocyte isolates by Western blot, and in cardiac myocytes in vivo and in vitro by immunohistochemistry. Interestingly, microvascular endothelial cells abundantly express NOS III in intact cardiac muscle as well as in situ, but rapidly decrease NOS III expression following isolation and primary culture [7,44]. Indeed, we have to date not been able to establish culture conditions in which cardiac microvascular endothelial cells will reexpress NOS III in vitro although, as noted earlier, they readily express NOS II in response to inflammatory cytokines.

Conclusion

In conclusion, cardiac myocytes and microvascular endothelial cells both express NOS III constitutively in vivo and can be induced to express NOS II in response to inflammatory cytokines in vivo and in vitro. The constitutively expressed NOS isoform appears to act to regulate the contractile responsiveness of cardiac myocytes to autonomic nervous system agonists, in part by activating guanylate cyclase, although additional mechanisms are likely and are the subject of intense investigations in many laboratories. In addition, increased NO production following induction of NOS II in one or both cell types, as well as other cellular constituents of cardiac

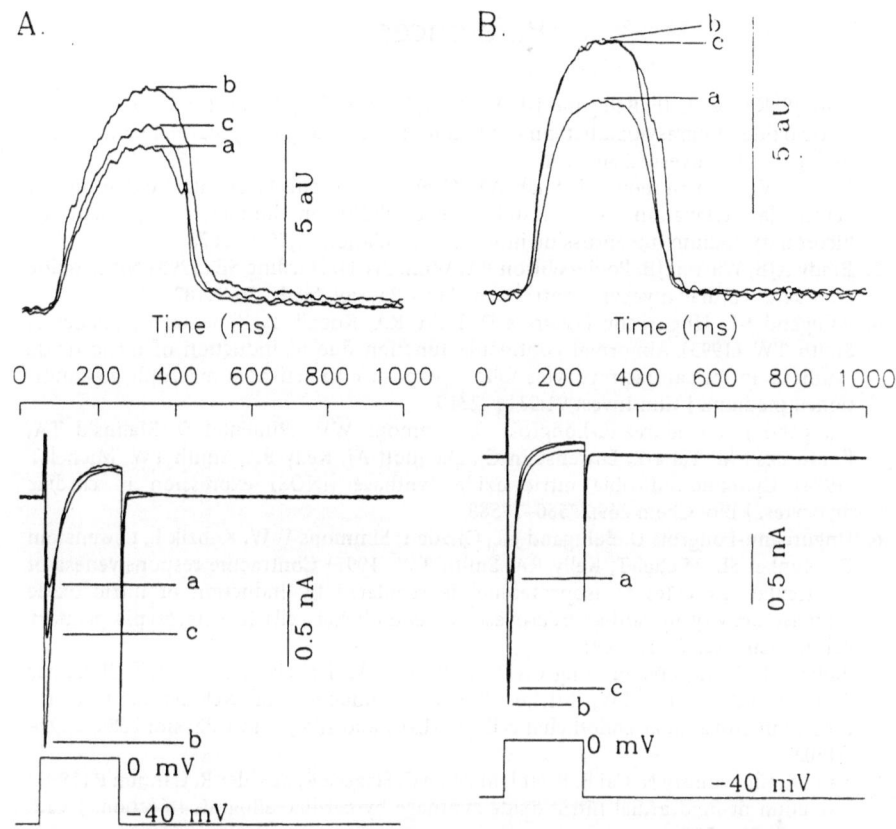

FIG. 1A,B. NO antagonists block muscarinic cholinergic-induced attenuation of L-type Ca^{2+} current (I_{Ca-L}) induced by β-adrenergic agonists in adult rat ventricular myocytes. Simultaneous recordings of I_{Ca-L} and cell shortening were obtained in single freshly isolated adult rat ventricular myocytes as described elsewhere [44]. A Representative superimposed tracings showing cell shortening amplitude (*upper panel*) and I_{Ca-L} (*lower panel*) in response to a cellular depolarization in the absence (a) and presence (b) of 1 μM isoproterenol, and (c) in the presence of isoproterenol and 1 μM carbamylcholine. B The same experiment as in A, except that cells were internally dialyzed with 20 μM methylene blue during each experimental intervention. Similar results were obtained with myocytes internally dialyzed with 1 mM L-N-monomethyl-arginine [44]

muscle, including infiltrating inflammatory cells, probably contribute to the decreased cardiac function seen in advanced systemic sepsis, some inflammatory cardiomyopathies, and perhaps in cardiac allograft rejection [45]. The ultimate biological and clinical significance of this cytokine-mediated contractile dysfunction, however, remains unclear [43]. Efforts to modify the NO signalling pathway in vivo have met with both beneficial [46,47] and deleterious [48–50] outcomes. Thus, while it is likely that induction of NOS in the myocardium does contribute to cardiac dysfunction in some patients, much further work is needed to reach an understanding of the pathophysiologic role of the NO pathway, and to exploit the possible therapeutic benefits that might accrue from pharmacologic manipulation of the NO pathway.

References

1. Hare JS, Keaney Jr JF, Balligand J-L, Loscalzo J, Smith TW, Colucci WS (1995) Role of nitric oxide in parasympathetic modulation of β-adrenergic myocardial contractility in dogs. J Clin Invest 95:360–366
2. Paulus WJ, Vantrimpont PJ, Shah AM (1994) Acute effects of nitric oxide on left ventricular relaxation and diastolic distensibility in humans: assessment by bicoronary sodium nitroprusside infusion. Circulation 89:2070–2078
3. Brady AJB, Warren JB, Poole-Wilson PA, Williams TJ, Harding SE (1993) Nitric oxide attenuates cardiac myocyte contraction. Am J Physiol 265:H176–H182
4. Balligand J-L, Ungureanu-Longrois D, Kelly RA, Kobzik L, Pimental D, Michel T, Smith TW (1993) Abnormal contractile function due to induction of nitric oxide synthesis in rat cardiac myocytes follows exposure to activated macrophage-conditioned medium. J Clin Invest 91:2314–2319
5. Balligand J-L, Ungureanu-Longrois D, Simmons WW, Pimental D, Malinski TA, Kapturczak M, Taha Z, Lowenstein CJ, Davidoff AJ, Kelly RA, Smith TW, Michel T (1994) Cytokine-inducible nitric oxide synthase (iNOS) expression in cardiac myocytes. J Biol Chem 269:27580–27588
6. Ungureanu-Longrois D, Balligand J-L, Okada I, Simmons WW, Kobzik L, Lowenstein CJ, Kunkel SL, Michel T, Kelly RA, Smith TW (1995) Contractile responsiveness of ventricular myocytes to isoproterenol is regulated by induction of nitric oxide synthase activity in cardiac microvascular endothelial cells in heterotypic primary culture. Circ Res 77:486–493
7. Balligand J-L, Ungureanu-Longrois D, Simmons WW, Kobzik L, Lowenstein CJ, Lamas S, Kelly RA, Smith TW, Michel T (1995) Induction of NO synthase in rat cardiac microvascular endothelial cells by IL-1β and IFNγ. Am J Physiol 268:H1293–H1303
8. Yang X, Chowdhury N, Cai B, Brett J, Marboe C, Sciacca R, Michler R, Cannon P (1994) Induction of myocardial nitric oxide synthase by cardiac allograft rejection. J Clin Invest 94:714–721
9. Brady A, Poole-Wilson P, Harding S, Warren J (1992) Nitric oxide production within cardiac myocytes reduces their contractility in endotoxemia. Am J Physiol 263:H1963–H1966
10. Nathan C, Xie Q-W (1994) Nitric oxide synthases: roles, tolls, and controls. Cell 78:915–918
11. Schmidt HHH, Walter U (1994) NO at work. Cell 78:919–925
12. Stamler JS (1994) Redox signaling: nitrosylation and related target interactions of nitric oxide. Cell 78:931–936
13. Kobzik L, Reid MB, Bredt DS, Stamler JS (1994) Nitric oxide in skeletal muscle. Nature 372:546–548
14. Lamas S, Marsden PA, Li GK, Tempst P, Michel T (1992) Endothelial nitric oxide synthase: molecular cloning and characterization of a distinct constitutive enzyme isoform. Proc Natl Acad Sci USA 88:6348–6352
15. Marletta MA (1993) Nitric oxide synthase structure and mechanism. J Biol Chem 268:12231–12234
16. Moncada S, Palmer RMJ, Higgs EA (1991) Nitric oxide: physiology, pathophysiology, and pharmacology. Pharmacol Rev 43:109–142
17. Moncada S, Higgs A (1993) The L-arginine-nitric oxide pathway. N Engl J Med 329:2002–2010
18. Yoshizumi M, Perrella MA, Burnett JC, Jr Lee M-E (1993) Tumor necrosis factor downregulates an endothelial nitric oxide synthase mRNA by shortening its half-life. Circ Res 73:205–209
19. Han X, Shimoni Y, Giles WR (1994) An obligatory role for nitric oxide in autonomic control of mammalian heart rate. J Physiol (Lond) 476:309–314

20. Balligand J-L, Kelly RA, Marsden PA, Smith TW, Michel T (1993) Control of cardiac muscle cell function by an endogenous nitric oxide signalling system. Proc Natl Acad Sci USA 90:347–351

21. Kaye DM, Simmons WW, Balligand J-L, Kelly RA, Smith TW (1994) Contractile activity activates a constitutive nitric oxide synthase in adult rat ventricular myocytes. Circulation 90:I-33

22. Pugin J, Schurer-Maly C-C, Leturco D, Moriarty A, Ulevitch RJ, Tobias PS (1993) Lipopolysaccharide activation of human endothelial and epithelial cells is mediated by lipopolysaccharide-binding proteins and soluble CD14. Proc Natl Acad Sci USA 90:2744–2748

23. Stamler JS, Simon DI, Osborne JA, Mullins ME, Jaraki O, Michel T, Singel DJ, Loscalzo J (1992) S-nitrosylation of proteins with nitric oxide: Synthesis and characterization of biologically active compounds. Proc Natl Acad Sci USA 89:444–448

24. Garbers DL (1992) Guanylyl cyclase receptors and their endocrine, paracrine, and autocrine ligands. Cell 71:1–14

25. Lange LG, Schreiner GF (1992) Immune cytokines and cardiac disease. Trends Cardiovasc Med 2:145–151

26. Gulick TS, Chung MK, Pieper SJ, Lange LG, Schreiner GF (1989) Interleukin-1 and tumor necrosis factor inhibit cardiac myocyte β-adrenergic responsiveness. Proc Natl Acad Sci USA 86:6753–6757

27. Balligand J-L, Ungureanu-Longrois D, Schussheim A, Mäki T, Kelly RA, Smith TW (1993) Induction of nitric synthase activity in ventricular myocytes reduces cAMP response to β-adrenergic agonists. Circulation 88:I-384

28. Mery P-F, Lohmann SM, Walter U, Fischmeister R (1991) Ca²⁺ current is regulated by cyclic GMP-dependent protein kinase in mammalian cardiac myocytes. Proc Natl Acad Sci USA 88:1197–1201

29. Schweizer M, Richter C (1994) Nitric oxide potently and reversibly deenergizes mitochondria at low oxygen tension. Biochem Biophys Res commun 204:169–175

30. Brown GC, Cooper CE (1994) Nanomolar concentrations of nitric oxide reversibly inhibit synaptosomal respiration by competing with oxygen at cytochrome oxidase. FEBS Lett 356:295–298

31. Shen W, Xu X, Ochoa M, Zhao G, Wolin MS, Hintze TH (1994) Role of nitric oxide in the regulation of oxygen consumption in conscious dogs. Circ Res 75:1086–1095

32. Gross WL, Balligand J-L, Kelly RA, Smith TW, Ingwall JS (1994) Nitric oxide and the heart: Infusion of an exogenous niric oxide donor alters cardiac high-energy phosphate metabolism and contractile reserve. Circulation 90:I-193

33. Lowenstein CJ, Alley EW, Raval P, Snowman AM, Snyder SH, Russell SW, Murphy WJ (1993) Macrophage nitric oxide synthase gene—Two upstream regions mediate induction by interferon-γ and lipopolysaccharide. Proc Natl Acad Sci USA 90:9730–9734

34. Roberts AB, Vodovotz Y, Roche NS, Sporn MB, Nathan CF (1992) Role of nitric oxide in antagonistic effects of transforming growth factor-β and interleukin-1β on the beating rate of cultured cardiac myocytes. Mol Endocrinol 6:1921–1930

35. Pfeilschifter J, Vosbeck K (1991) Transforming growth factor beta 2 inhibits interleukin 1 beta- and tumor necrosis factor alpha-induction of nitric oxide synthase in rat renal mesangial cells. Biochem Biophys Res Commun 175:372–379

36. Vodovotz Y, Bogdan C, Paik J, Xie QW, Nathan C (1993) Mechanisms of suppression of macrophage nitric oxide release by transforming growth factor-β. J Exp Med 178:605–613

37. Finkel MS, Oddis CV, Jacob TD, Watkins SC, Hattler BG, Simmons RL (1992) Negative inotropic effects of cytokines on the heart mediated by nitric oxide. Science 257:387–389

38. Yokoyama T, Vaca L, Rossen RD, Durante W, Hazarika P, Mann DL (1993) Cellular basis for the negative inotropic effects of tumor necrosis factor-α in the adult mammalian heart. J Clin Invest 92:2303–2312

39. Werner ER, Werner-Felmayer G, Wachter H (1993) Tetrahydrobiopterin and cytokines. Proc Soc Exp Biol Med 203:1–12
40. Gross SS, Levi R (1992) Tetrahydrobiopterin synthesis. An absolute requirement for cytokine-induced nitric oxide generation by vascular smooth muscle. J Biol Chem 267:25722–25729
41. Simmons WW, Balligand J-L, Ungureanu-Longrois D, Michel T, Kelly RA, Smith TW (1994) Dexamethasone regulates inducible nitric oxide synthase activity in cardiac microvascular endothelial cells by suppressing tetrahydrobiopterin synthesis. Circulation 90:I-627
42. Ungureanu-Longrois D, Balligand J-L, Okada I, Simmons WW, Kobzik L, Lowenstein CJ, Kunkel S, Michel T, Kelly RA, Smith TW (1995) Induction of nitric oxide synthase activity by cytokines in ventricular myocytes is necessary but not sufficient to decrease contractile responsiveness to β-adrenergic agonists. Circ Res 77:494–502
43. Ungureanu-Longrois D, Balligand J-L, Kelly RA, Smith TW (1995) Myocardial contractile dysfunction in the systemic inflammatory response syndrome: Role of a cytokine-inducible nitric oxide synthase in cardiac myocytes. J Mol Cell Cardiol 27:155–167
44. Balligand J-L, Kobzik L, Han X, Kaye DM, Belhassen L, O'Hara DS, Kelly RA, Smith TW, Michel T (1995) Nitric oxide-dependent parasympathetic signalling is due to activation of constitutive endothelial (Type III) NO synthase in cardiac myocytes. J Biol Chem 270:14582–14586
45. Yang X, Chowdhury N, Cai B, Brett J, Marboe C, Sciacca R, Michler R, Cannon P (1994) Induction of myocardial nitric oxide synthase by cardiac allograft rejection. J Clin Invest 94:714–721
46. Kilbourn RG, Gross SS, Jubran A, Adams J, Griffith OW, Levi R, Lodato RJ (1990) NG-methyl-arginine inhibits tumor necrosis factor-induced hypotension: Implications for the involvement of nitric oxide. Proc Natl Acad Sci USA 87:3629–3632
47. Kilbourn RG, Jubran A, Gross SS, Griffith OW, Levi R, Adams J, Lodato RJ (1990) Reversal of endotoxin-mediated shock by NG-methyl-L-arginine, an inhibitor of nitric oxide synthesis. Biochem Biophys Res Commun 172:1132–1138
48. Petros A, Lamb G, Leone A, Moncada S, Bennett D, Vallance P (1994) Effects of a nitric oxide synthase inhibitor in humans with septic shock. Cardiovasc Res 28:34–39
49. Wright CE, Rees DD, Moncada S (1992) Protective and pathological roles of nitric oxide in endotoxin shock. Cardiovasc Res 26:48–57
50. Billiar TR, Curran RD, Harbrecht BG, Stuehr DJ, Demetris AJ, Simmons RL (1990) Modulation of nitrogen oxide synthesis in vivo: NG-monomethyl-L-arginine inhibits endotoxin-induced nitrate/nitrate biosynthesis while promoting hepatic damage. J Leukoc Biol 48:565–569

Calcium Sensitizers and Molecular Mechanisms of Altered Response of Cardiac Myofilaments to Calcium

R. John Solaro

Summary. In this chapter I consider a current perception of the molecular interactions by which Ca-binding to the myofilaments regulates the activity of heart cells, and the response to Ca^{2+} is modulated. Control of the actin-myosin reaction is not only through Ca^{2+}-binding to troponin C (TnC), but also through steric, cooperative and allosteric processes involving all of the main myofilament proteins—actin, myosin, tropomyosin (Tm), TnC, troponin T (TnT), and troponin I (TnI). The process is modulated by covalent and noncovalent mechanisms. Apart from the importance of these mechanisms in the basic physiological control of heart function, an understanding of control of myofilament activation has taken on new importance for the following reasons: First, it is now clear that altered response of the myofilaments to Ca^{2+} is a cause of heart failure associated with familial hypertrophic cardiac myopathies as well as in diverse pathologies such as acidosis, ischemia, and stunning. Second, the response of cardiac myofilaments to Ca^{2+} can be manipulated pharmacologically. Pharmacological agents from a variety of chemical classes increase responsiveness of the myofilaments to Ca^{2+} by promoting Ca^{2+} binding to TnC, by altering the transduction of the Ca^{2+}-binding signal, and by promoting the actin-myosin reaction.

Key words. Actin—Myosin—Troponin—Tropomyosin—Inotropic agents—Phosphorylation

Physiological Changes in the Response of Cardiac Myofilaments to Ca^{2+}

There are compelling reasons to think that there is physiological control of the myofilament response to Ca^{2+}. Altered response of myofilaments to Ca^{2+} is important in the most prominent cardiac control devices, which exert intrinsic control and extrinsic control by neural and neurohumoral mechanisms. The sensitivity of the myofilaments to Ca^{2+} depends on the sarcomere length [1–3]. This length-dependence of myofilament activation is likely to be an important determinant of the relation between end-systolic volume and end-systolic pressure and thus the basis of Starling's Law. Neural and neurohumoral regulation of cardiac muscle cell activity also involves an altered

Department of Physiology and Biophysics, College of Medicine (M/C 901), University of Illinois-Chicago, Chicago, IL 60612-7342, USA

myofilament response to Ca^{2+}. There is substantial evidence that adrenergic stimulation of the heart is associated with phosphorylation of the myofilaments by activation of signaling pathways involving cyclic adenosine monophosphate (cAMP) and cyclic guanosine monophosphate (cGMP) and protein kinases A and G, phospholipase C, diacylglycerol, and protein kinase C as well as Ca-calmodulin dependent protein kinase (myosin light chain kinase) [4,5]. More recent evidence indicates that the control of working cardiac myocytes by vascular endothelium or by endocardial endothelium may also involve a change in myofilament response to Ca^{2+} [6]. The mediators of this potentially important mechanism are not clear but may involve NO or peptides released from the endothelial cells. Long-term alterations in myofilament response to Ca^{2+} also occur with isoform switching of myofilament proteins during development and possibly with physiological changes in cardiac loading with exercise and aging [7,8].

Mechanisms of Physiological Alterations in the Myofilament Response to Ca^{2+}

Before discussing these mechanisms, it is important to consider what we think happens in the transition from the diastolic (relaxed) to the systolic (active) state. Ca^{2+} ions released into the myofilament space bind to a single regulatory site on troponin C (TnC) [9,10]. and activate force and shortening. The amounts of Ca^{2+} bound to myofilament TnC in basal physiological states are considerably smaller than the number of TnC sites; the proportion is likely to be some 20% of the sites [9]. Ca-TnC triggers contraction through a series of protein-protein interactions involving troponin I (TnI), troponin T (TnT), and tropomyosin (Tm) (Fig. 1). The triggering of contraction by Ca-TnC thus involves an allosteric process acting at some distance from the cross-bridge binding site on actin. This allosteric mechanism may involve the following types of processes: a release of the actin-cross-bridge reaction from a blocked state and/or an increase in the rate constants for transition from a weak actin-cross-bridge state to a strong binding (force-generating) state [11,12]. It is apparent that the allosteric mechanism induces a movement of tropomyosin or TnI (and potentially TnT) from a blocking position in a few functional units. Close neighbor cross-bridges promote further activation of the thin filament; thus activation spreads and more functional units are engaged in the contraction [2,11,13]. In this way, a particular contractile state may be perceived as a balance between the allosteric activation of the myofilaments by Ca^{2+} and the cooperative activation of the myofilaments by cross-bridges. The force that is generated is a function of the distribution of cross-bridge states and force generated by each state.

Ca-TnC Induced Activation of Cardiac Myofilaments and Its Modulation in Physiological and Pathophysiological States

The reaction of Ca^{2+} with TnC undoubtedly triggers the transition of cross-bridges from weak-binding or blocked states to force-generating states [1,2,11]. Yet there is no clear resolution between different hypotheses on how Ca-TnC acts. One hypothesis is that Ca^{2+} acts as a switch and promotes the transition from the weak/blocked to the

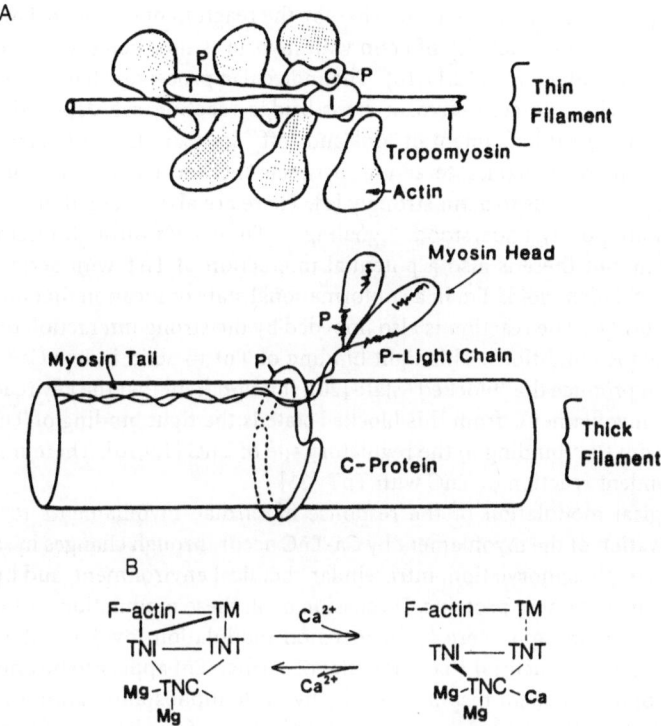

FIG. 1A,B. Schematic representation of protein-protein interactions involved in activation of cardiac myofilaments. A Proteins of the myofilaments. *T, TnT; I, TnI; C, TnC; P,* site of covalent phosphorylation. B Model of interactions among thin filament proteins in diastole (*left*) and in systole (*right*)

strong state in an "all-or-none" fashion [13,14]. According to this idea, Tm acts to enhance the affinity of cross-bridges for actin, and relative activation of the myofilaments by Ca²⁺, for example at the 50% level, would involve 50% of the cross-bridges "recruited" to the strong state. A second hypothesis is that Ca²⁺ increases the rate of transition from the weak to the strong state in a "graded" fashion [15,16]. Here, a 50% relative activation of the myofilaments could involve all of the cross-bridges in an activated state, but with the forward rate of transition between weak and strong states at some submaximal level. The distinction between these hypotheses has been difficult in that the conclusions from particular experiments appear to depend on the methods used and may also be model-dependent [13,14]. However, the actions of Tm are difficult to explain by a pure steric effect and in some cases are more readily explained by allosteric effects on actin structure. A model restricted to the idea that simple movement of Tm or Tn permits binding of myosin heads is probably too simple, and some allosteric effects on actin structure seem likely. Another aspect of the mode of regulation has to do with the kinetics of the processes. It appears possible that both ideas may be accommodated by a difference in the timing of the switch and the graded activation. For example, switching on the functional unit might be a rapid, non-rate-limiting process, whereas graded activation follows with a slower, more rate-limiting process.

Whatever the case, the mechanism whereby the reaction of Ca^{2+} with TnC is transduced to promote the reactivity of actin with myosin is now being sorted out in the case of heart myofilaments [12,17,18]. The molecular processes that are believed to occur in triggering the actin-myosin cross-bridge reaction are depicted in Fig. 1, which illustrates the thin filament in "on" and "off" states. In the "off" state with low cytosolic Ca^{2+}, there are weak interactions between TnC and TnI and possibly between TnC and TnT; TnI binds to actin strongly [1]. There are also interactions of TnI with TnT, which are poorly understood. Signaling to Tm occurs through interactions of TnT with Tm, but there is also a potential interaction of TnT with actin [19]. The signaling mechanism holds Tm in a conformational state or location that impedes the actin-cross-bridge. The reaction is also impeded by the strong interaction of TnI with actin in relaxing conditions. This tight binding of TnI to actin in low Ca^{2+} has been speculated to produce the "blocked" state [20]. It is apparent that the key reaction that releases the myofilaments from this blocked state is the tight binding of TnC to TnI, associated with Ca^{2+} binding to the regulatory site of TnC [1,9,10]. There may also be a Ca^{2+}-dependent reaction of TnC with TnT [21].

Physiological modulation of the response of cardiac myofilaments to Ca^{2+} that modify activation of the myofilament by Ca-TnC occur through changes in sarcomere length, protein phosphorylation, intracellular chemical environment, and by isoform switching of myofilament proteins. Discussion of all these modulations is beyond the scope of this monograph. Here I will focus on modulation involving the TnC-TnI interaction. Special structural characteristics of cardiac TnI appear to be important in the control of myofilament response to Ca^{2+} by protein phosphorylation [4,5] and in the relatively big effect of acidic pH on Ca-activation of cardiac myofilaments [22] compared to skeletal myofilaments [23]. The cardiac variant of TnI (cTnI) contains an amino-terminal extension of 32 amino acids that is not present in the fast or slow skeletal variants. This stretch of amino acids contains two serines that are substrates for protein kinase A (PKA) [4,5]. Phosphorylation of cTnI either in vitro or in vivo by the PKA pathway results in a decreased responsiveness of the myofilaments to Ca^{2+}. Studies on the topology of the interactions between TnC and TnI indicate that the proteins are arranged antiparallel, that is, the N domain of cTnC is opposite the C domain of cTnI [17]. Moreover, we [18] have also shown that myofilaments reconstituted with deletion mutants containing no amino-terminal extension demonstrate Ca^{2+} activation of ATPase activity that is the same as that of native myofilaments. Our hypothesis is that the unique N domain of cardiac TnI is important only when it is phosphorylated. Alterations in the response of the myofilaments to Ca^{2+} also occur during conditions associated with depressed cardiac function. One example is during acidosis, in which it has been shown that force-generating capabilities of heart muscle are considerably depressed under conditions in which the amplitude of the Ca^{2+}-transient during the twitch is, in fact, increased [22]. Moreover, when compared to slow skeletal muscle myofilaments, the effect of acidic pH on the pCa-force relation is greater than with cardiac myofilaments [24]. The major effector of this difference appears to be the difference in TnI isoforms [25]. Slow skeletal TnI is the embryonic and neonatal isoform of TnI in the heart, which is important with regard to development of functional properties of the heart. There are also potential long-term changes in structure/function relations of the myofilaments associated with breakdown of TnI and TnT [26] or altered gene expression [27–29] that may affect the myofilament response to Ca^{2+}. A strong tie between altered gene expression and heart failure is the identification of mutations in the myosin heavy chain gene that form the molecular basis of familial hypertrophic cardiomyopathy [28]. More recent evidence also ties missense mutations in TnT and in Tm to this same syndrome, which is emerging as a "sarcomeric" disease [29]. Reexpression of a fetal isoform of TnT has also been correlated with the well-known depression in maximum myofibrillar ATPase activity in various forms of heart failure [27].

Switching the Thin Filament "On" Through Strong Cross-Bridges

It is now clear that in striated muscle, myosin is not only a molecular motor but is also involved in activation of the thin filament [1,2,11]. This action of myosin heads was first clearly demonstrated in vitro in the studies of Bremel et al. [30], who showed that rigor (nucleotide-free) cross-bridges bound to actin could, in the presence of Tm or Tn-Tm, cooperatively turn on the thin filament even in the absence of Ca^{2+}. That binding of S-1 affects further binding of S-1 was also shown by the experiments of Lehrer and Ishii [31], who probed the number of active Tm units using a fluorescent tag reporting the "on" configuration. These experiments showed that turning on of the thin filament is largely dependent on myosin head (S-1) binding and relatively weakly affected by Ca^{2+} binding to Tn. The cooperative turning on of the thin filament lies in two mechanisms. One is through Tm, which covers 7 actins; therefore, with binding of S-1, 7 actins are activated. The other is through end-to-end interactions between adjacent Tm molecules. Thus, a functional unit consisting of actin : Tm : Tn in a 7 : 1 : 1 ratio influences its close neighbors upon binding of S-1 [1,2,11].

Pharmacologically Induced Alterations in the Response of Myofilaments to Ca²⁺

The complexity of myofilament regulation suggests a rich array of possible mechanisms by which myofilament response to Ca^{2+} might be manipulated pharmacologically. The following three general types of agents are discussed here: (1) agents (MCI 154 and UDCG 115BS, also known as pimobendan or acardi) acting at the level of TnC; (2) agents (levosimendan) acting on transduction of the Ca-binding signal; and (3) agents (EMD 57033) acting at the actin-cross-bridge interface.

Agents that increase Ca-binding to TnC

There are two prominent examples of agents that increase the response of cardiac myofilaments to Ca^{2+} by increases in Ca-binding to myofilament TnC. One is pimobendan, which we [32] showed had stereoselective effects on myofilament Ca-sensitivity that fit with its effects on amounts of Ca bound to the regulatory site of cardiac myofilament TnC. This inotropic agent now known as acardi is also an inhibitor of cAMP phosphodiesterase (type III) [33]. Acardi is the first Ca-sensitizer to be introduced into wide clinical use, and it is apparent that its use in the treatment of heart failure in Japan shows early promise. However, evaluation of the use of such agents must await more extensive clinical experience and trials. A second agent that increases the myofilament response by a mechanism involving enhanced affinity of myofilament TnC for Ca^{2+} is MCI-154. MCI-154 increases the response of guinea pig heart myofilaments to Ca^{2+}. It has been reported that MCI-154 enhances the responses to Ca^{2+} in saponin-treated skinned fiber bundles of guinea pig ventricles [34], canine ventricles [35], and human failing hearts [36]. MCI-154 has also been shown to increase the affinity of TnC for Ca^{2+} in canine heart myofilaments [36]. MCI-154 has no effect on the activity of actin-activated myosin and myosin ATPase in preparations for dog hearts [36]. Yet there is the possibility that the effect of MCI-154 is not exclusively on TnC; rather, it may involve other regulatory proteins such as TnI, TnT, or tropomyosin. For example, we have found that there was a diminished effect of MCI-154 on myofilament force in preparations from transgenic mouse hearts, which overexpressed skeletal β-tropomyosin isoform when compared with that in nontransgenic mouse hearts, which overexpressed only α-type tropomyosin isoform [37].

The action of MCI-154 on myofilament force is opposite that which occurs with acidosis on the cardiac myofilament, in which case the affinity of TnC for TnI is reduced [22]. It has been shown that MCI-154 restored the decrease in active force induced by acidic pH in skinned fiber bundles of the guinea pig ventricles [34]. More recent studies indicate that the Ca-sensitizing action of MCI-154 may alter the energy requirements for pumping function of the failing heart. Evidence that MCI-154 affects cardiac energetics in humans comes from studies [38] showing that the compound reduced the oxygen cost of nonmechanical work [39]. This is what one would expect from a compound that increases myofilament mechanical activity by increased responsiveness to Ca^{2+}.

Agents that Alter Transduction of the Ca-Binding Signal

A unique and exciting example of this class of Ca-sensitizing agent is levosimendan ((R)-[[4-(1,4,5,6-tetrahydro-4-methyl-6-oxo-3-pyridazinyl)-phenyl] hydrazono] propanedinitrile). This compound, which was synthesized by Orion-Farmos, is the first cardiotonic agent specifically screened for its ability to bind to cardiac TnC [40,41]. Levosimendan docks at the amino-terminal region of TnC near the regulatory Ca^{2+}-binding domain and in the region of TnC that is believed to react with TnI in a Ca-dependent manner. It has been hypothesized that occupancy of this site with levosimendan is associated with stabilization of the Ca^{2+} bound conformation [41]. This stabilization is thought to increase the level of thin-filament activation. Interestingly, as is the case with Ca-sensitizers MCI-154 and pimobendan, levosimendan is also a phosphodiesterase inhibitor. We [42] have shown that levosimendan is without effect on Ca-binding to myofilament TnC. Thus, levosimendan appears to act in the cascade of protein-protein reactions triggered by Ca-TnC rather than by increasing the affinity of TnC for Ca^{2+}. We [42] have shown that levosimendan (0.03 −10 μM) reversibly increases force generated by detergent-extracted fiber bundles over a range of submaximally activating free Ca^{2+} concentrations with no significant effect on maximum force. In isolated perfused hearts, relatively low concentrations of levosimendan increased +dP/dt, but had no effect on the speed of relaxation or tissue cAMP levels. Higher levosimendan concentrations significantly increased cAMP levels in the heart, and there was an increase in the phosphorylation of phospholamban, TnI, and C protein. These results suggested to us that at low concentrations (<0.1 μM), the action of levosimendan as a Ca^{2+}-sensitizer predominates. At higher concentrations, though, its action as a phosphodiesterase inhibitor appears to contribute to the positive inotropic effect.

Agents Acting at the Actin-Myosin Interface

A new direction in the search for inotropic agents occurred with the introduction of a novel class of inotropic agent, the diazinones, which promote the reaction of myosin with actin. Studies on the racemic mixtures of the thiadiazinone (EMD 53998;(5-[1-(3,4-dimethoxybenzoyl)-1,2,3,4-tetrahydro-6-quinolyl]-6-methyl-3,6-dihydro-2H-1,3,4-thiadiazin-2-one)) indicated that it might work by direct actions on the myofilaments [43–45]. In skinned fiber bundles, the pCa-force relation was shifted to the left in the presence of EMD 53998 [43,46]. In intact muscle preparations and myocytes, force and shortening were increased with no increase in the peak amplitude of the Ca-transient [44–46]. Yet the racemic mixture is a potent inhibitor of phosphodiesterase (PDE)III, and it was not clear to what extent Ca-sensitization formed the basis of the effect on cardiac muscle. Studies on enantiomers of EMD 53998 showed that one enantiomer had the potent PDE inhibitory activity, whereas the other enantiomer had the potent Ca-sensitizer activity [45,46]. To investigate the mechanism of action of these compounds, we [46] studied the effects of racemic thiadiazinone (EMD 53998) and its enantiomers on Ca²⁺-signaling in dog heart myocytes, myofilaments, and myofilament proteins. When treated with the (+) enantiomer EMD 57033, intact ventricular myocytes responded with an increase in the extent of shortening during twitch contractions with no increase in the peak amplitude of the Ca²⁺-transient. On the other hand, as expected from its activity as a PDE inhibitor, EMD 57439, the (−)enantiomer, increased both the extent of shortening and the peak amplitude of the Ca²⁺-transient in a concentration-dependent manner. EMD 57439 had no effect on the pCa-actomyosin MgATPase activity relation of heart myofibrils. However, treatment of myofibrils with EMD 57033 induced a left shift in the pCa-MgATPase activity relation. This stereoselective stimulation of MgATPase activity occurred even in preparations from which Tn-Tm had been extracted. We also determined the effect of the enantiomers on the actin-myosin interaction in experiments in which we measured actin filament sliding on myosin heads adhered to nitrocellulose-coated cover slips. EMD 57033 stimulated the velocity of actin filament sliding, whereas EMD 57439 did not. These results strongly indicated that the mechanism of action of EMD 57033 on myocyte contractility is a direct promotion of the actin-myosin reaction. We further proposed that the increased myofilament sensitivity to Ca²⁺ induced by EMD 57033 is due to cross-bridge-dependent activation of thin filaments.

Conclusion

Modulation of the response of cardiac myofilaments to Ca²⁺ occurs in intrinsic and extrinsic regulation of cardiac contraction. This modulation appears to be causal in some forms of acute and long-term pathologies of the heart. Manipulation of the response of myofilaments to Ca²⁺ occurs with diverse pharmacological agents acting at various steps in the activation pathways. These agents may prove useful in heart failure and may also be important tools in understanding the mechanisms by which Ca²⁺ and cross-bridges regulate the level of thin-filament activation.

Acknowledgments. I dedicate this article to Professor Norio Taira on the occasion of his retirement. Work described here is supported by research grants NIH RO1-

HL22231 and R01 HL49934. I am grateful to the many colleagues who collaborated on the studies referred to in this manuscript.

References

1. Solaro RJ (1995) Control mechanisms regulating contractile activity of cardiac myofilaments. In: Sperelakis N (ed) Physiology and pathophysiology of the heart, 3rd edn. Kluwer Academic, Boston, pp 355–366
2. Moss RL (1992) Ca^{2+} regulation of mechanical properties of striated muscle: mechanistic studies using extraction and replacement of regulatory proteins. Circ Res 70:865–884
3. Allen DG, Kentish JC (1985) The cellular basis of the length–tension relation in cardiac muscle. J Mol Cell Cardiol 17:821–840
4. Solaro RJ (1986) Protein phosphorylation and the cardiac myofilaments. In: Solaro RJ (ed) Protein phosphorylation in heart. CRC, Boca Raton, pp 129–156
5. Solaro RJ (1993) Modulation of activation of cardiac myofilaments by beta-adrenergic agonists. In: Lee JA, Allen DG (eds) Modulation of cardiac calcium sensitivity. Oxford University Press, Oxford, pp 161–177
6. Brutsaert DL, Andries LJ (1992) The endocardial endothelium. Am J Physiol 263 (Heart Circ Physiol 32):H985–H1002
7. Pagani ED, Solaro RJ (1983) Thyroid state, cardiac myosin isoenzymes and swimming exercise in rat. Am J Physiol 245:H713–H720
8. Ball KL, Solaro RJ (1994) Discoordinate regulation of contractile protein gene expression in the senescent rat myocardium. J Mol Cell Cardiol 26:519–525
9. Pan B-S, Solaro RJ (1987) Calcium binding properties of troponin C in detergent skinned heart muscle fibers. J Biol Chem 262:7339–7349
10. Holroyde MJ, Robertson SP, Johnson JD, Solaro RJ, Potter JD (1980) The Ca^{2+} and Mg^{2+} binding sites on cardiac troponin and their role in the regulation of adenosine triphosphatase. J Biol Chem 255:11688–11693
11. Lehrer S (1994) The regulatory switch of the muscle thin filament: Ca^{2+} or myosin heads? J Muscle Res Cell Motility 15:232–236
12. Zot AS, Potter JD (1987) Structural aspects of troponin-tropomyosin regulation of skeletal muscle contraction. Ann Rev Biophys Biophys Chem 16:535–559
13. Millar N, Homsher E (1990) The effect of phosphate and Ca on force generation in glycerinated rabbit skeletal muscle fibers. J Biol Chem 265:20234–20240
14. Kress M, Huxley HE, Faruqi AR, Hendrix J (1986) Structural changes during activation of frog muscle studied by time-resolved X-ray diffraction. J Mol Biol 188:325–342
15. Brenner B (1993) Changes in calcium sensitivity at the cross-bridge level. In: Lee JA, Allen DG (eds) Modulation of cardiac calcium sensitivity. Oxford University Press, Oxford, pp 197–214
16. Walker JW, Lu Z, Moss RL (1992) Effects of Ca^{2+} on the kinetics of phosphate release in skeletal muscle. J Biol Chem 267:2459–2466
17. Krudy G, Kleerkoper Q, Guo X, Howarth JW, Solaro RJ, Rosevear PR (1994) NMR studies delineating spatial relationships within the cardiac troponin I-troponin C complex. J Biol Chem 269:23731–23735
18. Guo X, Wattanapermpool J, Palmiter KA, Murphy AM, Solaro RJ (1994) Mutagenesis of cardiac troponin I: Role of the unique NH_2-terminal peptide in myofilament activation. J Biol Chem 269:15210–15216
19. Heeley DH, Smillie LB (1988) Interaction of rabbit skeletal muscle troponin T and F-actin at physiological ionic strength. Biochemistry 27:8227–8231
20. Geeves MA, Lehrer SS (1994) Dynamics of the muscle thin filament regulatory switch: the size of the cooperative unit. Biophys J 67:273–282
21. Potter JD, Sheng Z, Pan B-S, Zhao J (1995) A direct regulatory role for troponin T and a dual role for troponin C in the regulation of muscle contraction. J Biol Chem 270:2557–2562

22. Solaro RJ, Lee J, Kentish J, Allen DA (1988) Differences in the response of adult and neonatal heart muscle to acidosis. Circ Res 63:779–787

23. Ball KA, Johnson MA, Solaro RJ (1994) Isoform specific interactions of troponin I and troponin C determine pH sensitivity of myofibrillar Ca^{2+}-activation. Biochemistry 33:8464–8471

24. Wattanapermpool J, Reiser PJ, Solaro RJ (1995) Troponin I isoforms as determinants of differential effects of acidic pH on Ca^{2+}-activation of soleus and cardiac myofilaments. Am J Physiol:Cell 268:C323–C330

25. Martin AM, Ball K, Gao L, Kumar PK, Solaro RJ (1991) Identification and functional significance of troponin I isoforms in neonatal rat heart myofibrils. Circ Res 69:1244–1252

26. Westfall MV, Solaro RJ (1992) Alterations in myofibrillar function and protein profiles following global ischemia in rat hearts. Circ Res 70:302–313

27. Anderson PAW, Malouf NN, Oakeley A, Pagani ED, Allen PD (1991) Troponin T isoform expression in humans: A comparison among normal and failing adult heart, fetal heart, and adult and fetal skeletal muscle. Circ Res 60:1226–1233

28. Tanigawa G, Jarcho JA, Kass S, Solomon SD, Vosberg JG, Seidman JG, Seidman CE (1990) A molecular basis for familial hypertrophic cardiomyopathy: an α/β cardiac myosin heavy chain hybrid gene. Cell 622:991–998

29. Thierfelder L, Watkins H, MacRae C, et al (1994) Alpha-tropomyosin and cardiac troponin T mutations cause familial hypertrophic cardiomyopathy: a disease of the sarcomere. Cell 77:701–712

30. Bremel R, Murray J, Weber A (1973) Manifestations of cooperative behavior in the regulated actin filament during actin-activated ATP hydrolysis in the presence of calcium. Cold Spring Harbor Symp Quant Biol 37:267–275

31. Lehrer S, Ishii Y (1988) Fluorescence properties of acrylodan-labeled tropomyosin and tropomyosin-actin: Evidence for myosin subfragment 1-induced changes in geometry between tropomyosin and actin. Biochemistry 27:5899–5906

32. Fujino K, Sperelakis N, Solaro RJ (1988) Sensitization of dog and guinea pig cardiac myofilaments to Ca^{2+}-activation and inotropic effect of pimobendan: Comparison with milrinone. Circ Res 63:911–922

33. Rüegg JC, Solaro RJ (1993) Calcium-sensitizing positive inotropic drugs. In: Gwathmey JK, Briggs GM, Allen PD (eds) Heart failure: Basic science and clinical aspects. Dekker, New York, pp 457–477

34. Kitada Y, Narimatsu A, Matsumura N, Endo M (1987) Increase in Ca^{2+} sensitivity of the contractile system by MCI-154, a novel cardiotonic agent, in chemically skinned fibers from guinea pig papillary muscles. J Pharmacol Exp Ther 243:633–638

35. Kitada Y, Kobayashi M, Narimatsu A, Ohizumi Y (1989) Potent stimulation of myofilament force and adenosine triphosphatase activity of canine cardiac muscle through a direct enhancement of troponin C Ca^{++} binding by MCI-154, a novel cardiotonic agent. J Pharmacol 250:272–277

36. Perrault CL, Brozovich FV, Ransil BJ, Morgan JP (1989) Effects of MCI-154 on Ca^{2+} activation of skinned human myocardium. Eur J Pharmacol 165:305–308

37. Kitada Y, Solaro RJ (1995) The myofilament Ca^{2+}-sensitizing effect of levosimendan, which binds to the NH$_2$-terminus of cardiac troponin C (TNC), is blocked by phosphorylation of the NH$_2$-terminus of troponin I (TNI) (abstract). Biophysical J 68:258

38. Kitada Y, Abe Y, Narimatsu A, Tobe A (1991) MCI-154, a novel cardiotonic agent, reverses the acid pH-induced decrease in responses of cardiac myofilament to Ca^{++}: Comparison with sulmazole and pimobendan. J Pharmacol Exp Ther 257:812–819

39. Mori M, Takeuchi M, Takaoka H, et al (1994) New Ca^{2+} sensitizer, MCI-154, reduces myocardial oxygen consumption for non-mechanical work in diseased human hearts. Circulation I:217

40. Pollesello P, Ovaska M, Kaivola J, Tilgmann C, Lundstrom K, Kalkkinen N, Ulmanen I, Nissinen E, Takinen J (1994) Binding of a new Ca^{2+} sensitizer, levosimendan, to recombinant human cardiac troponin C. J Biol Chem 269:28584–28590

41. Haikala H, Nissinen E, Etemadzadeh E, Linden I-B, Pohto P (1992) Levosimendan increases calcium sensitivity without enhancing myosin ATPase activity and impairing relaxation. J Mol Cell Cardiol 24[Suppl V]:S97
42. Edes I, Kiss E, Kitada Y, Papp JG, Kranias EG, Solaro RJ (1995) Effects of levosimendan, a cardiotonic agent targeted to troponin C, on cardiac function and on phosphorylation and Ca^{2+}-sensitivity of cardiac myofibrils and sarcoplasmic reticulum in guinea pig heart. Circ Res 77:107–113
43. Beier N, Jonas R, Klockow M, Lues I, Wolf G (1991) The two mechanisms of action of the racemic cardiotonic EMD 53998, Ca-sensitization and PDE-inhibition, reside in different enantiomers. J Mol Cell Cardiol 23[Suppl V]:P37
44. Lee JA, Allen DG (1991) EMD 53998 sensitizes the contractile proteins to calcium in intact ferret ventricular muscle. Circ Res 77:107–113
45. Gambassi G, Capogrossi MC, Klockow M, Lakatta EG (1993) Enantiomeric dissection of the effects of the inotropic agent, EMD 53998, in single cardiac myocytes. Am J Physiol 264:H728–H738
46. Solaro RJ, Gambassi G, Warshaw DM, Keller MR, Spurgeon HA, Beier N, Lakatta EG (1993) Stereoselective actions of thiadiazinones on dog cardiac myocytes and myofilaments. Circ Res 73:981–990

Cardiac Mechanics and Energetics

Hiroyuki Suga, Miyako Takaki, Hiromi Matsubara,
and Junichi Araki

Summary. This review summarizes the first author's almost 30-year research carried
out with his co-workers for a better understanding of the mechanics and energetics of
the canine heart beating under various normal and abnormal conditions of preload,
afterload, heart rate, and contractility. This research began with Suga's proposal of
E_{max} (end-systolic maximum elastance) as an index of ventricular contractility on the
basis of the left ventricular (LV) pressure-volume (P-V) relationship and its time-
varying elastance model. This model demonstrates a temporal and spatial integration
of crossbridge activities within the ventricular wall. On the basis of this model, Suga
further established PVA (systolic P-V area) as a measure of the total mechanical
energy generated by ventricular contraction. We then experimentally found that PVA
closely correlates with myocardial oxygen consumption (Vo_2) at a given E_{max} and that
the Vo_2-PVA relation shifts up and down with increases and decreases, respectively,
in E_{max}. The Vo_2-PVA relation indicates the oxygen cost of PVA and separates Vo_2 into
PVA-independent and PVA-dependent components. The PVA-independent Vo_2-E_{max}
relation indicates the oxygen cost of E_{max}. Our two-decade research has indicated
that this Vo_2-PVA-E_{max} framework is a new paradigm to characterize the
mechanoenergetics of normal and pathological hearts.

Key words. Heart—Ventricle—Contractility—Pressure-volume relation—Myocardial oxygen consumption

Introduction

Characterization of the mechanics and energetics of the heart has long been among
the central themes in cardiac physiology and cardiology. This problem remains to be
more thoroughly elucidated not only for a better understanding of normal hearts but
also for better diagnosis, treatment, and prevention of cardiac diseases [1-3].

According to current knowledge, myocardial contraction is a process of converting
free energy of ATP into mechanical energy by crossbridge (CB) cycling for force
development and shortening against load. Myocardial relaxation is a process in which
the ATP-consuming and force-generating CB cycling in the contractile machinery
ceases and ATP is replenished in the aerobic metabolism in the mitochondria. For the

Department of Physiology II, Okayama University Medical School, Okayama 700, Japan

373

switch between contraction and relaxation, the sarcoplasmic calcium ion (Ca^{2+}) plays a key role in excitation-contraction (E-C) coupling. Sarcoplasmic free Ca^{2+} comes mainly from the sarcoplasmic reticulum (SR) and partly from outside the cell. It binds with troponin C (TnC) and triggers CB cycling. Ca^{2+} then dissociates itself from the Ca^{2+}-bound TnC and is removed mainly by the SR Ca^{2+} pump and partly by the sarcolemmal Na^+/Ca^{2+} exchanger for relaxation. Membrane excitation preceding E-C coupling involves Na^+ influx and K^+ efflux followed by the restoration of transsarcolemmal gradients of Na^+ and K^+ concentrations by the Na^+-K^+ pump. This pump also corrects the Na^+ imbalance produced by the Na^+/Ca^{2+} exchanger.

Thus, excitation, E-C coupling, and CB cycling are essential steps in cardiac contraction and performance in the circulatory system. These processes require considerable ATP consumption. Figure 1 shows the known stoichiometries of these ATP-consuming processes. Besides, a small amount of ATP is consumed for producing cyclic adenosine monophosphate (cAMP), phosphorylation of the Ca^{2+} channel, troponin I and phospholamban, and ATP futile cycling.

Although these subcellular mechanisms have increasingly been elucidated, the mechanical determinants of myocardial energetics have not yet been constitutively and quantitatively accounted for by those microscopic terms. Since we have been interested in a better understanding of cardiac contraction in the circulatory system,

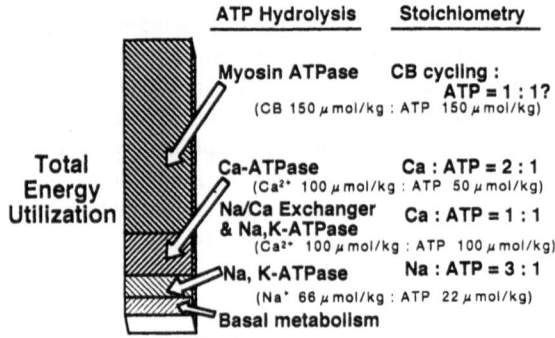

FIG. 1. Stoichiometries of ATP hydrolysis in myocardial excitation, excitation-contraction (E-C) coupling, and contraction. Total energy consumption consists of basal metabolism, excitation energy (Na^+-K^+ handling energy mainly by Na^+-K^+ ATPase), E-C coupling energy (Ca^{2+} handling energy mainly by Ca^{2+} ATPase and secondarily by a combination of Na^+/Ca^{2+} exchanger and Na^+-K^+ ATPase), and mechanical contraction energy (crossbridge cycling energy by myosin ATPase). When the total amount of crossbridges (*CB*) is 150 μmol/kg, and if every CB cycles once (or twice) per twitch, ATP consumption would be 150 (or 300) μmol/kg at a CB : ATP stoichiometry of 1 : 1. However, recently, this stoichiometry has seemed to increase a few times with loading conditions, as indicated by the question mark. If all Ca^{2+} ions, e.g., a maximum level of 100 μmol/kg, are removed by the sarcoplasmic reticulum (SR) Ca^{2+} pump, ATP consumption would be 50 μmol/kg at a Ca^{2+} : ATP stoichiometry of 2 : 1. However, if the same amount of Ca^{2+} is removed entirely by the sarcolemmal Na^+/Ca^{2+} exchanger, the Na^+ influx has to be removed by the Na^+-K^+ pump and the net Ca^{2+} : ATP stoichiometry decreases to 1 : 1. This doubles the ATP consumption for Ca^{2+} handling by the SR Ca^{2+} pump. If part of the sequestered Ca^{2+} leaks from the SR as in the ryanodine-treated heart, the net Ca^{2+} : ATP stoichiometry decreases. Therefore, even when the same amount of Cad^{2+} is involved in the E-C coupling, the E-C coupling energy will change. If the Na^+ influx, e.g., a maximum level of 66 μmol/kg, during the action potential is removed by the Na^--K^- pump, ATP consumption would be 22 μmol/kg at the 3 : 1 Na^- : ATP stoichiometry

we have continued to investigate cardiac mechanics and energetics in a macroscopic or systems-physiological manner [1–3].

History

Cardiac contraction has been viewed scientifically on different levels over a century. In 1895, Frank characterized the (frog's) ventricular function in the pressure-volume (P-V) diagram and viewed the heart as a compression chamber [4]. In 1918, Starling viewed the heart as a pump to generate flow against afterload as a function of preload, and proposed that cardiac tone (contractility) could be assessed by the height of the cardiac output versus preload curve. The cardiac output curve is the basis of the Starling law of the heart [5]. Its mechanisms have been examined up to and including molecular levels such as CB, Ca^{2+} channels, receptors, and intracellular signal transduction—topics which are still attracting cardiac scientists to this day [5]. In 1955, Sarnoff applied the Starling law to the stroke work–preload relation and proposed that ventricular contractility could be assessed by the height of the ventricular function curve. Although this relation cannot be a unique function of preload because of the afterload-dependence of external work, Sarnoff's idea still survives in the preload-recruitable stroke work in in situ hearts [6]. In 1962, Sonnenblick characterized the papillary muscle's isotonic contractions by applying Hill's force–velocity relation, and assessed contractility by the maximum unloaded shortening velocity V_{max} [7]. This index was applied to in situ beating hearts, and their contractility assessed by circumferential fiber shortening velocity (V_{cf}). However, the complex morphological and functional relations between a papillary muscle and the ventricle seem to limit the utility of the force–velocity relation in evaluating ventricular contractility.

In the late 1960s, Suga scrutinized left ventricular (LV) P-V relations at end-systole, end-diastole, and other intermediate time points under various loading conditions in canine hearts. Figure 2 shows a representative example of such tracings, superimposed on each other. Suga's first important observation was that the left upper shoulders of the P-V loops could be connected by a line called the end-systolic P-V relation (ESPVR), as shown in panel a. His second important observation was that the P-V relation increased its slope during contraction (isovolumic contraction phase and ejection phase) and decreased the slope during relaxation (isovolumic relaxation phase and filling phase), as shown in panel a. He first considered that the ESPVR passed through the origin of the P-V diagram. When he plotted these changes in the slope [i.e., $E(t) = P(t)/V(t)$] as a function of time, he obtained the mutually superimposable curves as seen in panel b. The peaks (E_{max}) of these curves correspond to the end-systolic points of the P-V loops. These innovative observations led Suga to hypothesize a time-varying elastance model of a contracting cardiac chamber by the analogy of a variable elasticity [8–10]. Although several circulatory system modellers had already adopted a time-varying capacitance or elastance model of the heart, none had validated the model in physiological experiments [8–10]. Suga's model was reconfirmed after he joined Sagawa at the Johns Hopkins University [2,11–14]. Although almost 30 years have passed since Suga's proposal of the time-varying elastance model, no better model of ventricular global performance has yet been proposed. The reason for this situation seems to be due to the following advantages of the P-V diagram in which the $E(t)$ model and E_{max} are defined.

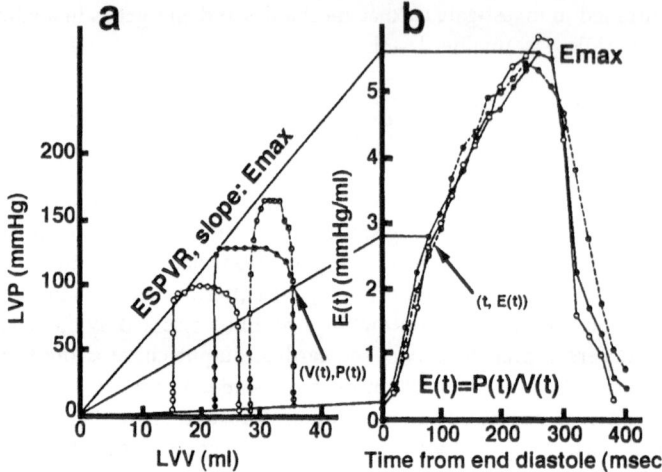

FIG. 2. Left ventricular (*LV*) pressure (*P*)-volume (*V*) diagram with P-V loops and two P-V relations (ESPVR and one at an intermediate time) under three different loading conditions in a stable contractile state (**a**) and their time-varying elastance curves (**b**) in an in situ canine heart. Left ventricular volume (*LVV*) was measured by a combination of an electromagnetic flow meter on the aorta and an indicator (hypertonic saline) dilution method. *ESPVR*, end-systolic P-V relation; E_{max}, slope of the ESPVR; *E(t)*, time-varying elastance obtained by dividing P(t) by V(t). In this study, the volume intercept of the ESPVR was assumed to be zero. E_{max}, maximum E(t) value at end-systole

Advantages of P-V Diagram

The P-V diagram has several advantages in providing a grasp of cardiac mechanoenergetics, as shown in Fig. 3 [1–3,12]. First, as this diagram used to be called the "work diagram", the area within a loop drawn in the diagram quantifies mechanical work that the ventricle (or any chamber) has performed. A working point moves counterclockwise on the loop when the work is performed by the ventricle to the load. This is the basis of the determination of stroke (or external, or mechanical) work in this diagram. When the loop moves clockwise, work is done to the heart. Second, a P-V relation curve in a certain state of the ventricle shows a stress–strain relation, and its slope, whether linear or nonlinear, shows the elastance, or more specifically volume elastance, of the chamber. This is the basis of the end-systolic maximum volume elastance (E_{max}) of the cardiac chamber Suga first proposed; he and his co-workers then further developed this concept as an index of contractility of the ventricle [8–15]. Third, the area under the P-V relation curve above the volume axis at zero pressure quantifies the mechanical (or elastic) potential energy that the chamber wall has generated and stores. This is the basis of the systolic P-V area (PVA) that Suga proposed as a measure of the total mechanical energy that a ventricular contraction generates [1–3,12,15,16].

One more advantage is that the P-V diagram temporally and spatially integrates mechanoenergetics (i.e., force, length, work, and energy) of all the CBs within the chamber wall, as shown in Fig. 4. This advantage is the basis of the successful applications of the E_{max} and PVA concepts not only to the LV but also to the right ventricle, right and left atria, ventricular wall regions, and papillary muscles in different animal

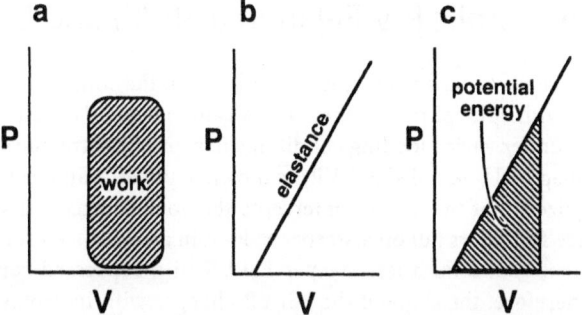

FIG. 3a–c. Physical and physiological significance of the P-V diagram. The area of a working P-V loop quantitates mechanical (or external) work of the chamber (a). When the loop rotates counterclockwise, the work is positive, or the work is done by the chamber. When the loop rotates clockwise, the work is negative, or the work is given to the chamber. A P-V relation line (or curve) in a certain state represents elastance of the chamber (b). A steeper line means greater elastance or smaller compliance. When the line changes its slope with time, the chamber wall has a time-varying elastance. The area under the elastance line (or curve) on the origin side of a working volume quantitates the potential energy that is contained in the elastic chamber. P, pressure; V, volume

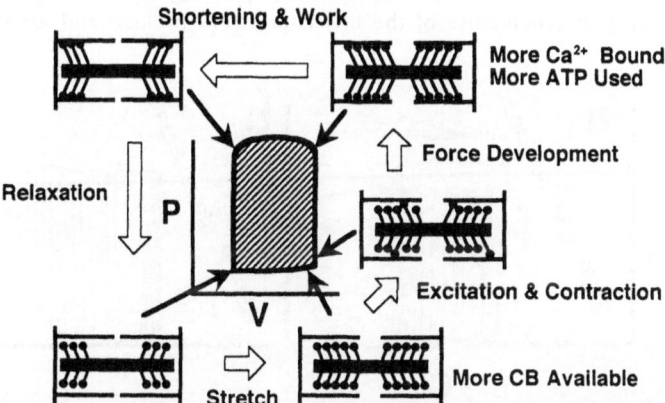

FIG. 4. Macromicro correspondence of cardiac mechanoenergetics. Different working points of a P-V loop correspond to different stretches of the sarcomere and numbers of attached crossbridges in one cardiac cycle (stretch → excitation-contraction coupling → force development → shortening and work → relaxation)

species including humans [17–23]. In these respects, the P-V diagram we favor is advantageous over many other diagrams such as Starling's cardiac output-preload, Sarnoff's stroke work-preload, and Sonnenblick's force-velocity diagrams of the cardiac chamber.

Thanks to these advantages, E_{max} and PVA in the P-V diagram have been a powerful tool in understanding the cardiac mechanics and energetics [1,2,12] as reviewed below. This situation will probably hold until a better or ideal methodology is devised that enables us to know directly the detailed mechanoenergetics of all the individual contractile elements and then integrate them to derive P-V information in a constitutive manner.

End-Systolic P-V Relation (ESPVR) and E_{max}

Figure 5 shows a representative example of P-V loops in the control and an enhanced contractile state with epinephrine in the LV of a canine heart. The left upper corners of the P-V loops under varied loading conditions in a given contractile state fall on or near a straight diagonal line called ESPVR, as shown in panels a and b of Fig. 5 [13,14]. We have recognized that the ESPVR intercepts the volume axis at a small positive volume V_0. These shoulders fall on a steeper ESPVR in an enhanced contractile state, as shown in panel c, and on a less steeper ESPVR in a depressed contractile state (not shown). Therefore, the slope of the ESPVR changes with inotropism. The slope quantitates the end-systolic elastance (or more correctly, volume elastance) of the ventricular chamber. This finding is the basis of E_{max} as an index of ventricular contractility [8–15]. The "E" in "E_{max}" is the first letter of "elastance". The "max" in "E_{max}" means the maximum elastance reached at end-systole. [Strictly, the slope of the ESPVR is called Ees (end-systolic elastance) and is slightly different from E_{max}, which is defined in each contraction. However, this difference can be ignored for the purposes of explaining the E_{max} and PVA concepts.]

Moreover, the time-varying elastance E(t) model can reasonably account for the instantaneous P-V relation during systole. Figure 6 shows representative examples of the time curves of LVP(t), V(t), and $E(t) = P(t)/[V(t) - V_0]$ obtained with an analog computer [9,19]. Independence of the E(t) curve from preload and afterload and

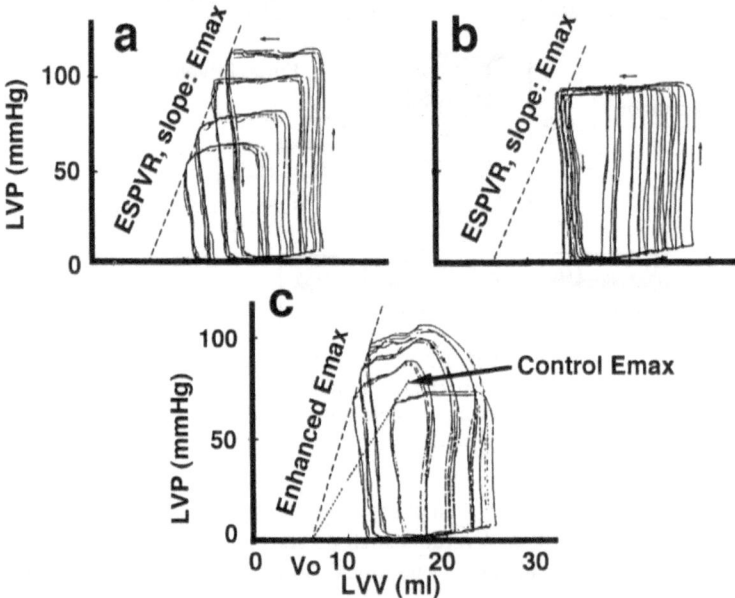

FIG. 5. Left ventricular (*LV*) pressure (*P*)-volume (*V*) loops of contractions under different loading conditions in a stable control contractile state (**a,b**) and in an enhanced contractile state (**c**) in a canine heart. The *left upper* (end-systolic) *corners* of the P-V loops obtained under different afterloads fall on a line called ESPVR (end-systolic pressure-volume relation) in **a**. On the same ESPVR fall the *left upper corners* of the P-V loops with different stroke volumes under a constant afterload in **b**. Epinephrine was given to double E_{max} in **c**. A steeper E_{max} line connects the end-systolic corners of these P-V loops

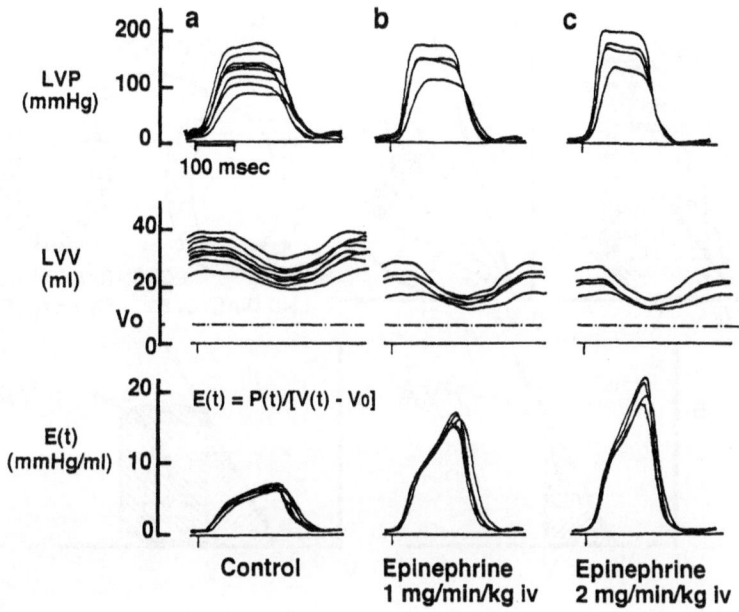

FIG. 6. Left ventricular (LV) pressure (P), LV volume (V), and time-varying elastance ($E(t)$) of variously loaded contractions in a control contractile state (a) and two enhanced contractile states with epinephrine (b,c) in a canine heart. P, V, and E(t) curves of variously loaded contractions are superimposed. V_0, dead volume at which peak systolic pressure is zero

dependence of E(t) on contractility (or inotropism) are explicit. The peak value of E(t) corresponds to E_{max}.

Soon after the publication of E_{max} in *Circulation Research* [13,14], cardiologists started the clinical application of E_{max} [20–22]. Thereafter, many investigators tested E_{max}, coming up with various results. The majority supported the utility, feasibility, and advantages of E_{max}, but some encountered difficulties and limitations in E_{max} application. These limitations include difficulty of accurate ventricular volumetry, nonlinearity of ESPVR, negative V_0, load-dependence of ESPVR, difficulty of E_{max} normalization for heart size, etc. [2,15].

Despite these problems, the E_{max} concept has gradually spread globally and is still favored by many groups as an index of the contractile state of a cardiac chamber, not only of the LV but also of the right ventricle and the right or left atrium [2,15].

The E_{max} concept has also been applied to ventricular wall regions and shown to be useful to compare end-systolic elastances between different regions with different contractilities [17,23]. Sugawara et al. devised a method to obtain myocardial end-systolic elastance normalized for unit muscle mass which is hence clinically applicable to different-sized hearts [23].

Systolic P-V Area (PVA) and Myocardial Energetics

On the basis of the time-varying elastance model of the ventricle, Suga proposed an innovative idea in 1976 that the total mechanical energy of ventricular contraction could be quantitated in the P-V diagram [16]. Figure 7 is a schematic illustration of the

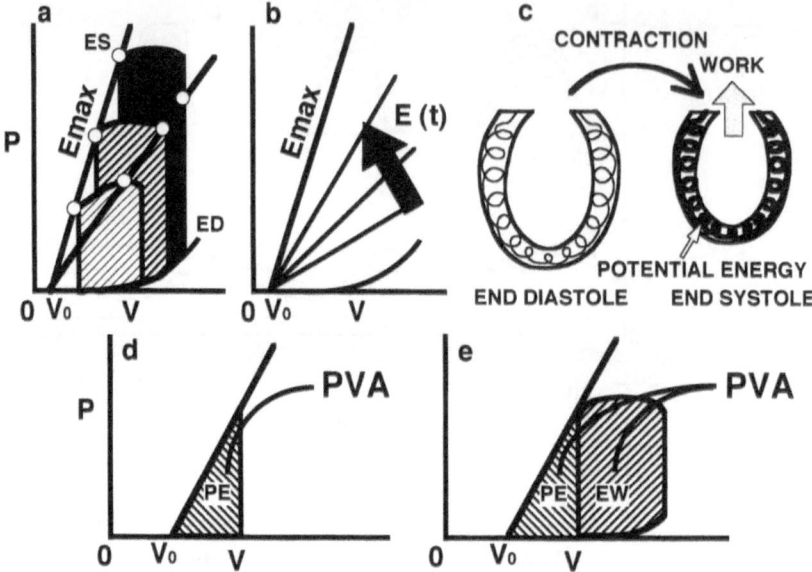

FIG. 7. Schematic illustration of three ventricular pressure (*P*)-volume (*V*) loops and their E_{max} line in a stable contractile state (a), time-varying elastance (*E(t)*) to simulate a "family" of instantaneous P-V relations (b), and the time-varying elastance model at end-diastole and end-systole (c). The pressure-volume area (*PVA*) represents the total mechanical energy of an isovolumic contraction (d) and an ejecting contraction (e). PVA consists of the sum of potential energy (*PE*) and external work (*EW*) if any. V_0, dead volume at which end-systolic pressure is zero; *ES*, end-systole; *ED*, end-diastole

time-varying P-V relation (panels a and b), which is the basis of the time-varying elastance model of the ventricle (panel c). Panels d and e illustrate the specific areas in the P-V diagram, "systolic P-V area," or PVA, representing the total mechanical energy that the ventricle generated in an isovolumic contraction (D) and an ejecting contraction (E). PVA is the sum of potential energy (PE) and external mechanical work (EW) if any. The derivation of the PVA concept is physically sound [16], but its physiological validity had to be examined experimentally. Suga then hypothesized that PVA in the real ventricle would somehow correlate with myocardial oxygen consumption (Vo_2), which represents the total energy utilization of the heart under aerobic conditions [16].

Suga and his co-workers then tested this hypothesis in the excised, cross-circulated canine heart preparation [1–3,24–27]. Its LV was connected to a custom-made volume servo pump, and its coronary flow and arteriovenous oxygen content difference were accurately and continuously measured with a flow meter and an oxygen content difference analyzer (our custom-made PWA-200S, Shoe Technica, Chiba, Japan) placed in the coronary arterial and venous cross-circulation tubing. Vo_2 was obtained as the product of the mean coronary flow and arteriovenous oxygen content difference. It was divided by heart rate to obtain Vo_2 per beat in steady state.

Figure 8 is a representative example of the experimentally obtained relation between LV Vo_2 and PVA on a per-beat basis. Panel a shows data plots in isovolumic contractions at different preloads. Panel b shows data plots in variously preloaded and afterloaded ejecting contractions in the same canine LV in the same stable con-

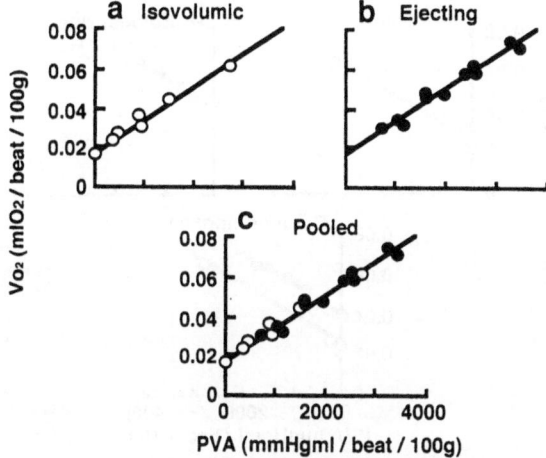

FIG. 8. Relationship between left ventricular oxygen consumption (Vo_2) and pressure-volume area (PVA) of isovolumic contractions at different preloads (a) and ejecting contractions at different preloads and afterloads (b) in a stable contractile state in a canine heart. c pools all the data in a and b

tractile state (a constant E_{max}). Panel c superimposes these two data sets. We found that LV Vo_2 linearly correlated with PVA in a given heart over a wide range of preload and afterload in a stable contractile state [25]. This contention was corroborated by a series of successive studies using various types of contractions [1–3,12,26]. The empirical equation we obtained was $Vo_2 = a \cdot PVA + b$, where both Vo_2 (ml O_2, 1 ml O_2 = 20 J) and PVA (mmHg $\cdot$ ml, 1 mmHg $\cdot$ ml = 1.33×10^{-4} J) are per-beat values normalized for 100 g LV. The $a \cdot PVA$ is the PVA-dependent fraction of Vo_2 and coefficient a is the slope of the relation. Constant b is the PVA-independent fraction of Vo_2 and corresponds to the Vo_2 of unloaded contraction [1–3].

Figure 9 is a representative set of experimentally obtained Vo_2-PVA relations in a control (panel a) and in an enhanced contractile state (enhanced E_{max}) with epinephrine (panel b) at the same atrial pacing rate in the same canine LV [1–3]. Panel c superimposes the data plots in panels a and b. Epinephrine-enhanced E_{max} elevated the Vo_2-PVA relation in a parallel manner. Various positive inotropic interventions enhanced E_{max} and simultaneously elicited similar parallel elevations of the Vo_2-PVA relation [1–3]. They included isoproterenol, norepinephrine, dobutamine, denopamine, calcium, digitalis, paired pulse stimulation, and some new cardiotonic agents such as milrinone, amrinone, sulmazole, vesnarinone, DPI 201-106, pimobendan, and EMD-53998 [1–3]. Various negative inotropic interventions such as Ca^{2+} antagonists, β-blockers, pentobarbital, nipradilol, and low coronary perfusion depressed E_{max} and lowered the Vo_2-PVA relation in a parallel manner [1–3,27]. From these results, we expanded the empirical equation to $Vo_2 = a \cdot PVA + c \cdot E_{max} + d$, where $c \cdot E_{max} + d$ has replaced b. The $c \cdot E_{max}$ term is the E_{max}-dependent fraction of the PVA-independent Vo_2 and d is basal metabolic Vo_2 at zero PVA and zero E_{max} [1–3].

We interpreted the terms of the empirical equation as follows: $a \cdot PVA$ represents energy utilization primarily by CB cycling [1–3] and $c \cdot E_{max}$ represents energy utilization primarily by the active transport of ions (mostly Ca^{2+} and secondarily Na^+ as seen in Fig. 1) in excitation and E-C coupling. Although Ca^{2+} and H^+ removal by the Na^+/

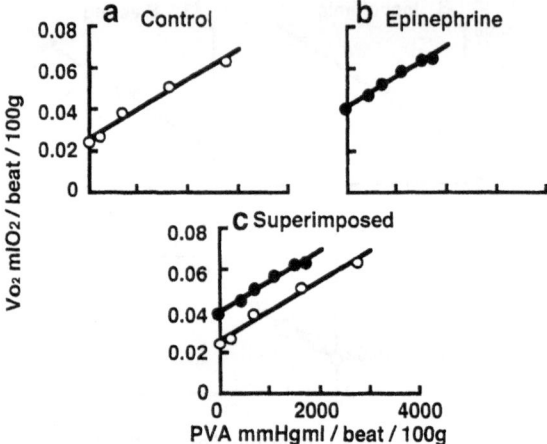

Fig. 9. Relationship between left ventricular oxygen consumption (Vo_2) and pressure-volume area (PVA) of variously loaded contractions in control (a) and an enhanced contractile state (b) in a canine heart. c superimposes all the data in a and b

Ca^{2+} and Na^+/H^+ exchangers do not consume ATP, ATP is eventually consumed when the exchanged Na^+ is removed by the Na^+-K^+ pump.

We also confirmed that basal metabolic Vo_2 under KCl arrest was virtually un-changed by positive and negative inotropic agents and by increased preload [28]. Therefore, the increases in PVA-independent Vo_2 with E_{max} could primarily be attri-buted to increases in the Vo_2 component for Ca^{2+} handling in E-C coupling. This Ca^{2+} handling seems to involve primarily the SR Ca^{2+} pump, secondarily the combination of the Na^+/Ca^{2+} exchanger and the Na^+-K^+ pump, and negligibly the sarcolemmal Ca^{2+} pump.

Figure 10 schematically shows the Vo_2-PVA relationship of variously loaded con-tractions in a stable control contractile state (panel a) and in three different contrac-tile states (or E_{max} levels) (panel b). Note that the Vo_2-PVA relation ascends with an increase in E_{max} and descends with a decrease in E_{max} in a parallel manner. Panel c relates PVA-independent Vo_2 (b) with E_{max}. Coefficients a and c indicate the slopes of the Vo_2-PVA relation and the PVA-independent Vo_2-E_{max} relation, respectively. These slopes a and c signify the O_2 cost of PVA (ventricular total mechanical energy) and the O_2 cost of E_{max} (ventricular contractility), respectively. These costs mean O_2 costs for unit increments in PVA and E_{max}, respectively. The parallelism of the Vo_2-PVA rela-tions for different E_{max} levels means no change in O_2 cost of PVA.

Oxygen Cost of PVA and Oxygen Cost of E_{max}

Figure 11 compares the O_2 cost of PVA (panel a) and O_2 cost of E_{max} (panel b) for various positive and negative inotropic interventions. We have found that most ino-tropic agents shift the Vo_2-PVA relation without affecting the O_2 cost of PVA (a) in panel a [1–3]. In panel a, we eliminated any parallel shift of the Vo_2-PVA relation because we only need to compare changes in a. The upward or downward shift of the Vo_2-PVA relation with E_{max} by these inotropic interventions mean a positive O_2 cost of E_{max} in panel b. Moreover, the O_2 cost of E_{max} was comparable among the most positive

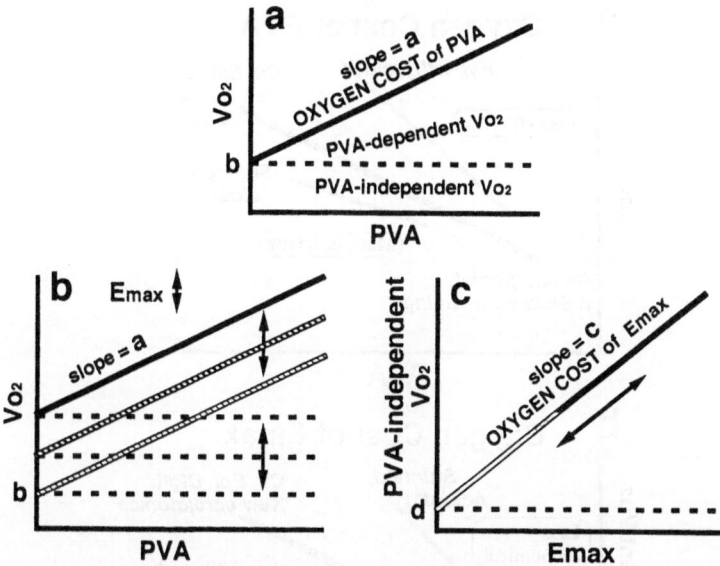

FIG. 10. Relationship between left ventricular oxygen consumption (Vo_2) and pressure-volume area (PVA) of variously loaded contractions in a stable contractile state (a) and in three different contractile states (E_{max}) (b). c relates the changes in PVA-independent Vo_2 (b) to E_{max}. The slope (a) of the Vo_2-PVA relation at a given E_{max} represents the oxygen cost of PVA. The Vo_2-PVA relation divides Vo_2 at b into PVA-independent and PVA-dependent components of Vo_2. The slope (c) of the PVA-independent Vo_2-E_{max} relation represents the oxygen cost of E_{max}. Its intercept (d) indicates basal metabolism. The *arrows* correspond to E_{max} changes

and negative inotropic interventions [1–3]. These results are intriguing to us because we had expected that different mechanisms of inotropism would have resulted in different responses of the O_2 costs of PVA and E_{max}. However, no difference in O_2 cost of PVA may reflect no effect of these inotropic interventions on crossbridge cycling kinetics, although they affect E-C coupling in different ways. No difference in the O_2 cost of E_{max} for different inotropic interventions seems to reflect no difference in the relation between contractility and Ca^{2+} handling energy.

For example, an increased intracoronary Ca^{2+} concentration first increases transsarcolemmal Ca^{2+} influx via the sarcolemmal Ca^{2+} channel, next the amount of Ca^{2+} within the sarcoplasmic reticulum (SR), then the Ca^{2+} transient, and finally the amount of Ca^{2+} bound to troponin C. Catecholamines bind with the β-receptor and increase cAMP, which augments Ca^{2+} influx, Ca^{2+} uptake by the SR, the Ca^{2+} transient, and Ca^{2+} bound troponin C, although cAMP decreases the Ca^{2+} sensitivity of troponin C. The primary determinant of the PVA-independent Vo_2 is the total amount of Ca^{2+} to be handled in E-C coupling. No difference in the O_2 cost of E_{max} between Ca^{2+} and catecholamines despite the difference of the pharmacological mechanisms therefore suggests that the amount of Ca^{2+} involved in the E-C coupling is comparable unless the SR Ca^{2+} pump is dysfunctional [1–3]. Similar situations probably hold true for digitalis, various new cardiotonic agents, paired pulse stimulation, etc., which show a comparable O_2 cost of E_{max}.

There are a few exceptional inotropic interventions that showed an abnormal O_2 cost of E_{max} [1–3]. Cardiac cooling enhanced E_{max} but did not elevate the Vo_2-PVA relation or change its slope [29]. On the contrary, cardiac warming depressed E_{max} but

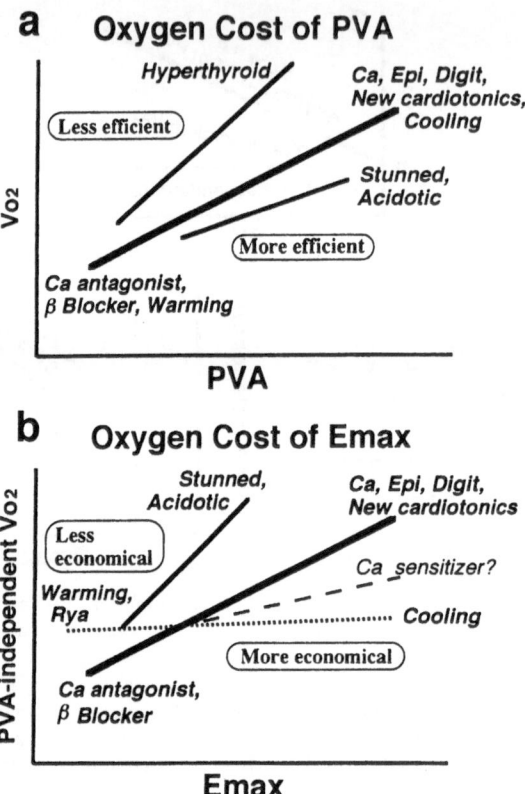

FIG. 11. Oxygen cost of PVA (a) and of E_{max} (b) under various inotropic interventions and pathophysiological conditions. The *thick solid lines* represent normal oxygen costs of PVA and E_{max} determined using various inotropic agents and interventions. *Ca*, Ca^{2+}; *Epi*, epinephrine and other catecholamines; *Digit*, ouabain; *New cardiotonics*, various new cardiotonic agents (see text); *Cooling*, hypothermia; *Hyperthyroid*, hyperthyroidism in the rabbit; *Stunned*, postischemic stunning and postacidotic stunning; *Ca antagonist*, Ca^{2+} antagonists verapamil and nifedipine; β-*Blocker*, β-blocker propranolol; *Warming*, hyperthermia; *Acidotic*, hypercapnic acidosis; *Rya*, ryanodine (40 nM). Oxygen cost of PVA is the slope of the Vo_2-PVA relation. A steeper slope means a greater oxygen cost of PVA which implies a smaller efficiency of energy conversion from Vo_2 to PVA. Oxygen cost of E_{max} is the slope of the PVA-independent Vo_2-E_{max} relation. A steeper slope represents a greater oxygen cost of E_{max}, which means smaller economy of contractility. The reason to use economy rather than efficiency is that E_{max}, with dimensions of mmHg/ml, is not an energy parameter, unlike PVA with dimensions of mmHg·ml. For efficiency, input and output must have the same dimensions of energy or power, like Vo_2 (1 ml $O_2 = 20$ J) and PVA (1 mmHg·ml $= 1.33 \times 10^{-4}$ J). As for the *dotted line* for cooling, warming, and ryanodine, the oxygen cost of E_{max} appears to be almost zero. However, this is not the true oxygen cost of E_{max} because this line is a composite line for different oxygen costs of E_{max}

did not lower the Vo_2-PVA relation or change its slope [30]. In both cases, the O_2 cost of E_{max} for graded cooling or warming was almost zero. These results mean that changing E_{max} by temperature accompanies no change in PVA-independent Vo_2. This suggests no change in the amount of Ca^{2+} to be handled in the E-C coupling despite the positive and negative inotropism of temperature [29,30]. Another case is myocardial vibration which depressed E_{max} without decreasing PVA-independent Vo_2 and showed a nearly zero O_2 cost of E_{max} [31]. Considering the low sensitivity of basal metabolism to these physical inotropic interventions, we speculate that Ca^{2+} handling energy does not change with temperature or with vibration.

Some more exceptions are myocardial postischemic stunning, postacidotic stunning and hypercapnic acidosis [32–34]. Although a very low coronary perfusion pressure (33 mmHg) lowered the Vo_2-PVA relation and slightly decreased its slope, this decreased slope was the result of decreased E_{max} with increases in PVA because of a severely insulted coronary reserve [35]. However, stunned hearts 1–2 h under 15-min-postischemic reperfusion had a decreased E_{max} as well as a decreased slope of the Vo_2-PVA relation with almost no change in its elevation. Although we do not know the mechanism underlying the decreased O_2 cost of PVA, this suggests the existence of an as yet unknown mechanism to increase the efficiency of CB cycling. The unchanged elevation of the Vo_2-PVA relation despite the decreased E_{max} indicates an increased O_2 cost of E_{max}, which means an uneconomical O_2 waste for contractility. We speculated this waste to reflect a decreased Ca^{2+} responsiveness of the contractile machinery, increased Ca^{2+} futile cycling in the SR, and increased Na^+/Ca^{2+} exchange accompanied by augmented Na^+-K^+ pumping [32]. Similar simulations seem to hold true in acidotic hearts and postacidotic stunned hearts [33,34]. The increased O_2 cost of E_{max} indicates that O_2 waste has occurred in the Ca^{2+} handling in these pathological hearts.

Ryanodine produced a considerable O_2 waste in the Ca^{2+} handling [36]. This agent infused into the coronary artery (40 nM) leaves the Ca^{2+} release channel of the SR open and elicits futile cycling of Ca^{2+} between the SR and sarcoplasm, increasing PVA-independent Vo_2 despite decreases in E_{max}.

Another exception is an increased O_2 cost of PVA in thyrotoxic rabbit hearts [37]. This change probably reflects the massive isomyosin shift from the economical β-type to the less economical α-type. The underlying mechanism of the increased PVA cost seems to involve a higher myosin ATPase activity and a faster CB cycling rate of the α-type myosin. However, thyrotoxic canine hearts did not have an increased PVA cost despite a 20% increased CB cycling rate [38]. This may partly be due to a minor shift of the myosin isozyme from β- to α-type.

Our recent study showed intriguingly that a short-term Ca^{2+} overloading protocol produced a failing heart without an increased O_2 cost of E_{max} [39] despite a comparable decrease in E_{max} to the stunned heart [32]. This failing heart rather looks similar in mechanoenergetic terms to the heart depressed by a Ca^{2+} antagonist or a β-blocker [1–3]. This finding indicates that all types of Ca^{2+}-overloaded myocardium should not be characterized equally by an increased O_2 cost of E_{max} despite their similar contractile failure.

Ca^{2+} sensitizers are expected to decrease the amount of Ca^{2+} involved in E-C coupling for the same contractility. We therefore expected a decrease in Vo_2 for the same E_{max} and hence a decreased O_2 cost of E_{max} compared to the control. However, there is so far no supportive evidence for this expectation [40]. Our unpublished data on EMD53998 (T. Nishioka et al.) supported de Tombe et al.'s [40] observation. For this reason, we put a question mark after Ca^{2+} sensitizer in panel b of Fig. 11.

Figure 12 shows our hypothesis on the O_2 cost of E_{max}. This illustrates a "family" of lines for different O_2 costs of E_{max} when E_{max} is changed by Ca^{2+} and its antagonist. A steeper line means a greater O_2 cost of E_{max}, which means that the heart manifests contractility less economically. A less steep line means a smaller O_2 cost of E_{max}, which means that the heart manifests contractility more economically. The control line of the O_2 cost of E_{max} has been observed with Ca^{2+} or catecholamines in normal hearts [1–

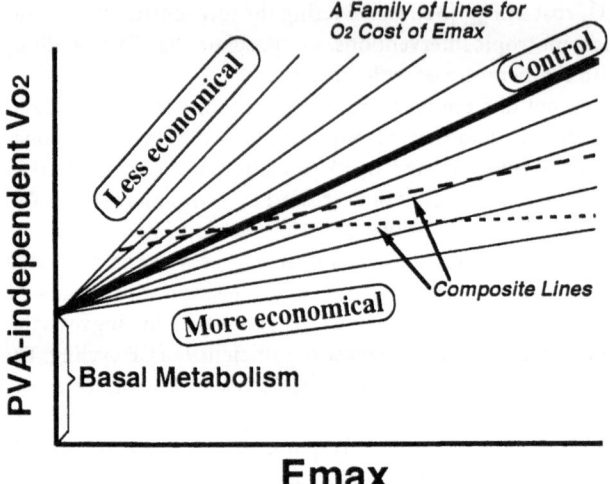

FIG. 12. Hypothesized schema of a "family" of lines (*solid*) for the oxygen cost of E_{max} and two composite lines (*dashed*) crossing the family of lines. The family of O_2-cost-of-E_{max} lines can be obtained by changing the intracoronary Ca^{2+} concentration under various fixed pathophysiological conditions that have different values for the O_2 cost of E_{max}. The composite O_2 cost lines can be obtained by gradually changing the pathophysiological conditions without changing the intracoronary Ca^{2+} level. Changing E_{max} in various ways in isovolumic contractions at a fixed end-diastolic volume could yield all these lines. A steeper O_2-cost-of-E_{max} line (*thin solid lines*) than the control line (*thick solid line*) means smaller economy (or greater energy) in manifesting contractility. This condition has been identified in postischemic stunning, postacidotic stunning, hypercapnic acidosis, and hyperthermia in canine left ventricles. A less steep O_2-cost-of-E_{max} line (*thin solid lines*) than the control line (*thick solid line*) means a greater economy (or smaller energy) in manifesting contractility. This condition has not yet been directly recognized, but is expected to exist in hypothermia and with Ca^{2+} sensitizers. The flat composite lines have been observed when cardiac temperature was changed gradually, the ventricular wall was vibrated, ventricular pacing was applied, and intraventricular block occurred

3,39]. A steeper line of the O_2 cost of E_{max} has been observed with Ca^{2+} in stunned and acidotic hearts [32–34]. Although we have described cardiac cooling and warming as having a near-zero O_2 cost of E_{max} in Fig. 11, this is a confusing expression because this O_2 cost of E_{max} was obtained as the slope of a composite line as shown by the dashed line in Fig. 12. A true O_2 cost of E_{max} at a low or high temperature should be obtained with Ca^{2+} at a fixed temperature. In fact, the O_2 cost of E_{max} for Ca^{2+} at 41°C was significantly greater than that at 36°C [30]. Thus, much more work remains to be done to obtain the O_2 cost of E_{max} with Ca^{2+} in a fixed pathophysiological state than to obtain an apparent O_2 cost of E_{max} as the slope of a composite line.

Conclusion

The O_2 costs of PVA and E_{max} based on the Vo_2-PVA-E_{max} framework have thus provided an entirely new physically and physiologically sound paradigm to characterize normality and abnormality of mechanoenergetics of hearts under various physiological and pathological conditions. This framework established in canine hearts has been basically confirmed in human hearts [41–43]. We hope that the present framework will greatly facilitate the conquest of heart diseases in a scientific manner.

Acknowledgments. This study was partly supported by Grants-in-Aid for Scientific Research (04237219, 04557041, 05221224, 05305007, 06213226, 06770494) from the Ministry of Education, Science and Culture; a Research Grant for Cardiovascular Diseases (4C-4) and a Research Grant on Aging and Health from the Ministry of Health and Welfare; a Joint Research Grant Utilizing Regional Scientific and Technological Potential from the Science and Technology Agency; and a research grant from the Terumo Life Science Foundation, all of Japan.

References

1. Suga H (1990) Ventricular energetics. Physiol Rev 70:247–277
2. Sagawa K, Maughan WL, Suga H, Sunagawa K (1988) Cardiac contraction and the pressure-volume relationship. Oxford University Press, New York
3. Suga H, Goto Y (1991) Cardiac oxygen costs of contractility (Emax) and mechanical energy (PVA): New key concepts in cardiac energetics. In: Sasayama S, Suga H (eds) Recent progress in failing heart syndrome. Springer, Berlin Heidelberg New York Tokyo, pp 61–115
4. Frank O (1899) Die Grundform des arteriellen Pulses. Z Biol 37:483–526. [Translated into English by Sagawa K et al (1990) J Mol Cell Cardiol 22:253–277]
5. Ter Keurs HEDL, Noble MIM (eds) (1988) Starling's law of the heart revisited. Kluwer Academic, Dordrecht
6. Takaoka H, Suga H, Goto Y, Hata K, Takeuchi M (1995) Cardiodynamic conditions for the linearity of preload recruitable stroke work. Heart Vessels 10:57–68
7. Sonnenblick EH (1962) Force–velocity relations in mammalian heart muscle. Am J Physiol 202:931–939
8. Suga H (1969) Analysis of left ventricular pumping by its pressure-volume coefficient (in Japanese with English abstract). Jpn J Med Electr Biol Eng 7:406–415
9. Suga H (1971) Theoretical analysis of a left-ventricular pumping model based on the systolic time-varying pressure/volume ratio. IEEE Trans Bio-Med Eng 18:47–55
10. Suga H (1971) Left ventricular time-varying pressure/volume ratio in systole as an index of myocardial inotropism. Jpn Heart J 12:153–160
11. Sagawa K (1978) Pressure-volume diagram revisited. Circ Res 43:677–687
12. Suga H (1994) Paul Dudley White international lecture: Cardiac performance as viewed through the pressure-volume window. Jpn Heart J 35:263–280 [or its abstract (1993) Circulation 88 [Suppl part 2]:I-C]
13. Suga H, Sagawa K, Shoukas AA (1973) Load independence of the instantaneous pressure-volume ratio of the canine left ventricle and effects of epinephrine and heart rate on the ratio. Circ Res 32:314–322
14. Suga H, Sagawa K (1974) Instantaneous pressure-volume relationships and their ratio in the excised, supported canine left ventricle. Circ Res 35:117–126
15. Suga H (1990) Cardiac mechanics and energetics—from Emax to PVA—Front Med Biol Eng 2:3–22, 1990
16. Suga H (1979) Total mechanical energy of a ventricle model and cardiac oxygen consumption. Am J Physiol 236:H498–H505
17. Goto Y, Suga H, Yamada O, Igarashi Y, Saito M, Hiramori K (1986) Left ventricular regional work from wall tension-area loop in the canine left ventricle. Am J Physiol 250:H151–H158
18. Hisano R, Cooper G (1987) Correlation of force-length area with oxygen consumption in ferret papillary muscle. Circ Res 61:318–328

19. Suga H, Sagawa K (1972) Mathematical interrelationship between instantaneous ventricular pressure-volume ratio and myocardial force-velocity relations. Ann Biomed Eng 1:160–181

20. Weisfeldt ML, Shoukas AA, Weiss JL, Dashkoff N, Conic P, Griffith LSC, Achuff SC, Ducci H, Sagawa K (1976) Emax as a new contractility index in man (abstract). Circulation 54 [Suppl II]:II-31

21. Sasayama S, Takahashi M, Osakada G, Hamashima H, Nishimura T, Sakurai T, Hirose K, Kawai C, Kotura H (1977) Evaluation to left ventricular function in clinical patients. Analysis of end-systolic length-tension relation and force-velocity relation (abstract). Jpn Circ J 41:778

22. Grossman W, Braunwald E, Mann T, McLaurin LP, Green LH (1977) Contractile state of the left ventricle in man as evaluated from end-systolic pressure-volume relations. Circulation 56:845–852

23. Sugawara M, Tamiya K, Nakano K (1985) Regional work of the ventricle. Wall tension-area relation. Heart Vessels 1:133–144

24. Khalafbeigui F, Suga H, Sagawa K (1979) Left ventricular systolic pressure-volume area correlates with oxygen consumption. Am J Physiol 237:H566–H789

25. Suga H, Hayashi T, Shirahata M (1981) Ventricular systolic pressure-volume area as predictor of cardiac oxygen consumption. Am J Physiol 240:H39–H44

26. Suga H, Hayashi T, Suehiro S, Hisano R, Shirahata M, Ninomiya I (1981) Equal oxygen consumption rates of isovolumic and ejecting contractions with equal systolic pressure-volume areas in canine left ventricle. Circ Res 49:1082–1091

27. Namba T, Takaki M, Araki J, Ishioka K, Suga H (1994) Energetics of the negative and positive inotropism of pentobarbitone sodium in the cane left ventricle. Cardiovasc Res 28:557–565

28. Nozawa T, Yasumura Y, Futaki S, Tanaka N, Suga H (1988) No significant increase in O_2 consumption of KCl-arrested dog heart with filling and dobutamine. Am J Physiol 255:H807–H812

29. Suga H, Goto Y, Igarashi Y, Yasumura Y, Nozawa T, Futaki S, Tanaka N (1988) Cardiac cooling increases Emax without affecting relation between O_2 consumption and systolic pressure-volume area in dog left ventricle. Circ Res 63:61–71

30. Saeki A, Goto Y, Hata K, Takasago T, Nishioka T, Suga H (1992) Hyperthermia increases oxygen cost of contractility in dog left ventricle. Circulation 86 [Suppl I]:I-428

31. Nishoka T, Goto Y, Hata K, Takasago T, Saeki A, Taylor TW, Suga H (1996) Mechanoenergetics of negative inotropism of ventricular wall vibration in dog heart. Am J Physiol 270 (in press)

32. Ohgoshi Y, Goto Y, Futaki S, Yaku H, Kawaguchi O, Suga H (1991) Increased oxygen cost of contractility in stunned myocardium of dog. Circ Res 69:975–988

33. Hata K, Goto Y, Kawaguchi O, Takasago T, Saeki A, Nishioka T, Suga H (1994) Hypercapnic acidosis increases oxygen cost of contractility in the dog left ventricle. Am J Physiol 266:H730–H740

34. Hata K, Takasago T, Saeki A, Nishioka T, Goto Y (1994) Stunned myocardium after rapid correction of acidosis. Increased oxygen cost of contractility and the role of the Na^+-H^+ exchange system. Circ Res 74:795–805

35. Suga H, Goto Y, Yasumura Y, Nozawa T, Futaki S, Tanaka N, Uenishi M (1988) O_2 consumption of dog heart under decreased coronary perfusion and propranolol. Am J Physiol 254:H292–H303

36. Takasago T, Goto Y, Kawaguchi O, Hata K, Saeki A, Nishioka T, Suga H (1993) Ryanodine wastes oxygen consumption for Ca^{2+} handling in the dog heart. A new pathological heart model. J Clin Invest 92:823–830

37. Goto Y, Slinkier BK, LeWinter MM (1990) Decreased contractile efficiency and increased nonmechanical energy cost in hyperthyroid rabbit heart. Circ Res 66:999–1011

38. Suga H, Tanaka N, Ohgoshi Y, Saeki Y, Nakanishi T, Futaki S, Yaku H, Goto Y (1991) Hyperthyroid dog left ventricle has the same oxygen consumption versus pressure-volume area (PVA) relation as euthyroid dog. Heart Vessels 6:71–83

39. Araki J, Takaki M, Namba T, Mori M, Suga H (1995) Ca^{2+}-free, high-Ca^{2+} coronary perfusion suppresses contractility and excitation-contraction coupling energy. Am J Physiol 268:H1061–H1070

40. de Tombe PP, Burkhoff D, Hunter WC (1992) Effects of calcium and EMD53998 on oxygen consumption in isolated canine hearts. Circulation 86:1945–1954

41. Kameyama T, Asanoi H, Ishizaka S, Yamanishi K, Fujita M, Sasayama S (1992) Energy conversion efficiency in human left ventricle. Circulation 85:988–996

42. Takaoka H, Takeuchi M, Yokoyama M (1992) Assessment of myocardial oxygen consumption (Vo_2) and systolic pressure-volume area (PVA) in human hearts. Eur Heart J 13 [Suppl E]:85–90

43. Takaoka H, Takeuchi M, Odake M, Hayashi Y, Hata K, Mori M, Yokoyama M (1993) Comparison of hemodynamic determinants for myocardial oxygen consumption under different contractile states in human ventricle. Circulation 87:59–69

Part 4

Pathophysiological Modulation of Regulatory Mechanisms

Human Myocardial β-Adrenergic Receptors: Properties, Function, and Changes in Chronic Heart Failure

Otto-Erich Brodde

Summary. In the human heart there exist many receptor systems that regulate heart rate and contractility. Among these the β-adrenergic receptor–G protein(s)–adenylyl cyclase–cyclic AMP pathway is the most powerful mechanism to acutely increase contractility and heart rate. Compared with the heart of commonly used laboratory animals, the human heart shows quite an unusual feature: it contains β_1- *and* β_2-adrenergic receptors that can mediate both positive chronotropic *and* inotropic effects in vitro and in vivo: the β_2-adrenergic receptors are much more efficiently coupled to adenylyl cyclase than are the β_1-adrenergic receptors. In chronic heart failure human, the cardiac β_1-adrenergic receptor number and inotropic responsiveness are decreased presumably due to down-regulation by the released endogenous noradrenaline which is enhanced locally in the heart and is a rather selective β_1-adrenergic receptor agonist. The cardiac β_2-adrenergic receptor number may or may not be reduced; however, its functional responsiveness is impaired, possibly due to the increased levels of the inhibitory G protein G_i and corresponding mRNA or due to enhanced phosphorylation by β-adrenergic receptor kinase and subsequent uncoupling from the adenylyl cyclase.

Key words. Human cardiac β_1-adrenergic receptors—Human cardiac β_2-adrenergic receptor—G proteins—Adenylyl cyclase—Heart failure

Introduction

It is now generally accepted that in the heart of various species, including man, catecholamines exert their effects through activation of β- and α-adrenergic receptors. In this chapter, we discuss properties and functional importance of β- and α-adrenergic receptors in the nonfailing human heart and give some insights into their alterations in chronic heart failure.

Institute of Pharmacology and Toxicology, Martin-Luther-University of Halle-Wittenberg, D-06097 Halle (Saale), Germany

Adrenergic Receptors in the Nonfailing Human Heart

β-Adrenergic Receptors

In the human heart both β_1- and β_2-adrenergic receptors coexist; this was first demonstrated by radioligand binding studies, and has been subsequently confirmed in functional experiments (for reviews, see [1–3]). The number of β-adrenergic receptors is quite evenly distributed in right- and left-atrial and ventricular tissue; however, the proportion of β_2-adrenergic receptors is somewhat higher in the atria (approximately one-third of the total β-adrenergic receptor population) than in ventricular myocardium (about 20% of the total β-adrenergic receptor population [3,4]), and may be even higher (to 50%) in the atrioventricular conducting system [5]. On the other hand, β_3-adrenergic receptors have not been found in the human heart, either in functional studies [6] or in studies on the tissue distribution of mRNA for β_1-, β_2- and β_3-adrenergic receptors in humans [7].

Both β_1- and β_2-adrenergic receptors couple to adenylyl cyclase and cause increases in the intracellular amount of cyclic AMP [8–11]. Interestingly, in the human heart adenylyl cyclase is preferentially activated by β_2-adrenergic receptor stimulation although β_1-adrenergic receptors predominate: in human right-atrial membranes, β_2-adrenergic receptor-selective agonists such as fenoterol, procaterol, and terbutaline caused activation of adenylyl cyclase activity that amounted to about 50%–70% of that of isoprenaline (for references, see [3]), although only 30% of the total β-adrenergic receptor population is of the β_2-subtype. Similarly, in ventricular membranes of the human heart, the β_2-adrenergic receptor agonists terbutaline and zinterol caused 50% of maximal isoprenaline activation [9,12] and isoprenaline, adrenaline, and noradrenaline evoked their stimulatory effects on adenylyl cyclase activity, predominantly via β_2-adrenergic receptor stimulation [9,10], although only 20% of the whole β-adrenergic receptor population is of the β_2-subtype (see earlier).

The mechanism underlying the different coupling efficiencies of human cardiac β_1- and β_2-adrenergic receptors to adenylyl cyclase is not known at present. However, Green et al. [13] recently showed that in the mammalian fibroblast cell line CHW-1102 transfected with β_1- or β_2-adrenergic receptor cDNAs, the β_2-adrenergic receptor exhibited a much greater functional coupling to the adenylyl cyclase than the β_1-adrenergic receptor. Similarly, Levy et al. [14] have expressed human β_1- and β_2-adrenergic receptors in permanent cell lines and found that activation of β_2-adrenergic receptors caused much greater activation of adenylyl cyclase than did β_1-adrenergic receptors. Thus, it might be a general phenomenon that β_2-adrenergic receptors couple more efficiently to adenylyl cyclase than β_1-adrenergic receptors.

In vitro experiments have convincingly shown that both β_1- and β_2-adrenergic receptors mediate the positive inotropic effects of β-adrenergic receptor agonists in isolated electrically driven atrial and ventricular preparations (for references, see [1–3,10,15]); this has also been demonstrated in single myocytes from human ventricle [16]. Among the classical catecholamines, isoprenaline and adrenaline cause their positive inotropic effects via stimulation of β_1- and β_2-adrenergic receptors, while noradrenaline, the endogenous transmitter of the sympathetic nervous system, evokes its positive inotropic effect almost exclusively via β_1-adrenergic receptor stimulation [10,17]. In right and left atria, β_1- and β_2-adrenergic receptor stimulation can evoke maximum positive inotropic effects, while on right and left ventricles only β_1-adrenergic receptor stimulation can evoke maximum positive inotropic effects and

β_2-adrenergic receptor stimulation only submaximal positive inotropic effects (Fig. 1) [10,17,18].

In vivo experiments in humans have confirmed that β_2-adrenergic receptors can mediate positive chronotropic and inotropic effects of β-adrenergic receptor agonists. Several studies have shown that isoprenaline-induced tachycardia in humans is mediated by both β_1-and β_2-adrenergic receptors to about the same degree, while exercise-induced tachycardia (which is mainly caused by neuronally released noradrenaline) is mediated solely by β_1-adrenergic receptor stimulation (for references, see [3,19]), in close agreement with the in vitro data on isolated human right atria [10,17].

Moreover, in healthy volunteers the positive chronotropic effect caused by intravenous infusions of terbutaline was only marginally affected by the β_1-adrenergic receptor-selective antagonists atenolol and bisoprolol (Fig. 2) given in doses that markedly inhibited β_1-adrenergic receptor-mediated effects [12,20,21]. Finally, Hall et al. [22] have demonstrated that the positive chronotropic effect of salbutamol induced by injections into the right coronary artery of patients with chronic stable angina (thereby avoiding any systemic effects) was not affected by the β_1-adrenergic receptor-selective antagonist practolol, but was significantly antagonized by propranolol indicating that it is mediated exclusively by (cardiac) β_2-adrenergic receptor stimulation. It is interesting to note, however, that in contrast to the in vitro data (see forgoing) adrenaline appears to cause its positive chronotropic effect in vivo solely via (cardiac) β_2-adrenergic receptor stimulation. Thus, several authors have shown that adrenaline-induced tachycardia is not affected by β_1-selective antagonists such as metoprolol [23], atenolol [24], or bisoprolol (Fig. 2) [25], but is completely abolished by the β_2-selective antagonist ICI 118, 551 [26] or by the nonselective β-adrenergic receptor antagonist propranolol (Fig. 2) [25].

Using the β_2-adrenergic receptor agonist terbutaline, at least two groups have convincingly shown that cardiac β_2-adrenergic receptors can in vivo also mediate

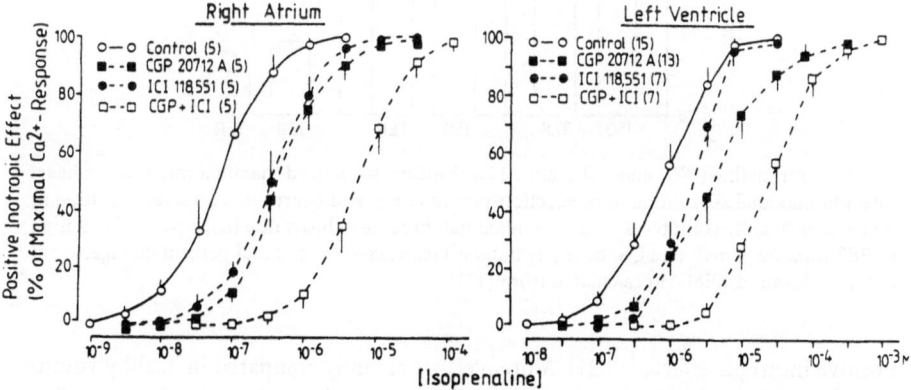

FIG. 1. Effects of the β_1-adrenergic receptor antagonist CGP 20712 A ($3 \times 10^{-7} M$) and of the β_2-adrenergic receptor antagonist ICI 118,551 ($3 \times 10^{-8} M$) on the positive inotropic effect of isoprenaline in isolated electrically driven right atria and left ventricles of the nonfailing human heart. *Ordinate,* positive inotropic effect in percent of maximal Ca^{2+} response; *abscissa,* molar concentrations of isoprenaline. Note that in right atria both β-adrenergic receptor antagonists shifted the isoprenaline curve to the right to about the same extent, while in left ventricles ICI 118,551 shifted only the lower part and CGP 20712 A mainly the upper part of the curve to the right. (From [17] with modifications)

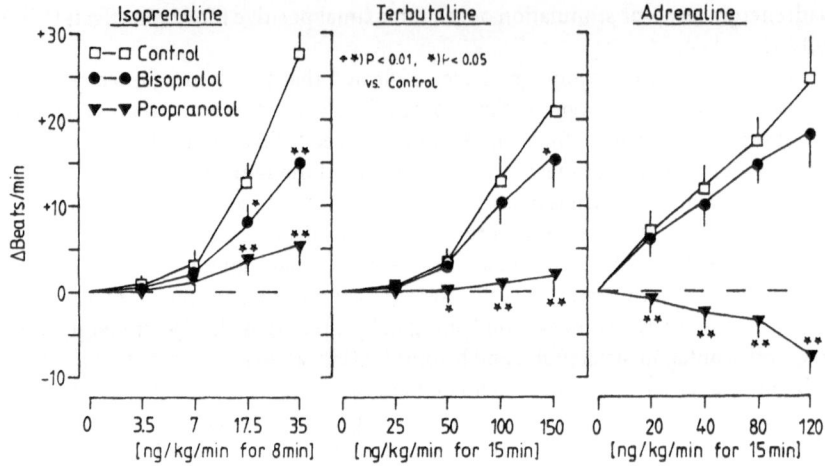

FIG. 2. Effect of bisoprolol (15 mg orally 2 h before infusion) or propranolol (5 mg i.v. 45 min before infusion) on isoprenaline (*left panel*), terbutaline (*middle panel*), or adrenaline (*right panel*) infusion-induced increase in heart rate in eight healthy male volunteers. *Ordinate*, increase in heart rate in Δ beats/min; *abscissae*, dose of the agonists in ng kg^{-1} min^{-1}. Means ± SEM. (Modified from [25])

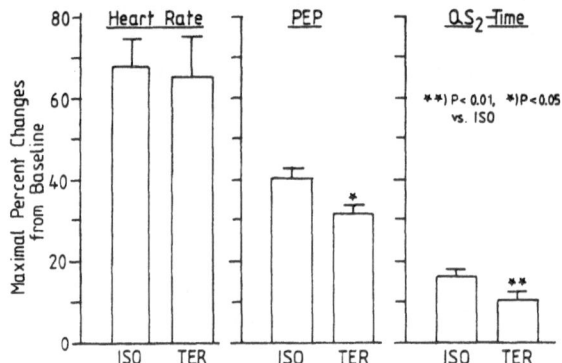

FIG. 3. Isoprenaline (*ISO*) and terbutaline (*TER*) infusion-induced maximal increases in heart rate and maximal shortening of preejection-period (*PEP*) and heart rate corrected QS$_2$ time in seven male healthy volunteers. Ordinate, maximal increase in heart rate (*left panel*), shortening of PEP (*middle panel*), and QS$_2$ time (*right panel*) expressed as maximal percent changes from baseline. Means ± SEM. (Recalculated from [12])

positive inotropic effects [12,21]. Moreover, we recently compared in healthy volunteers the positive chrono- and inotropic effects induced by infusions of isoprenaline and terbutaline, and found that at doses which caused the same increase in heart rate isoprenaline caused larger positive inotropic effects than did terbutaline (Fig. 3) [12], in close agreement with the in vitro observation (see earlier) that in the human right atrium both β_1- and β_2-adrenergic receptors cause maximal positive inotropic effects, while in the ventricular myocardium only β_1-adrenergic receptor stimulation caused maximal positive inotropic effects and β_2-adrenergic receptor stimulation evoked only submaximal positive inotropic effects.

α-Adrenergic Receptors

There can be no doubt that, in the heart of various species including man, in addition to β-adrenergic receptors α_1-adrenergic receptors exist that can bring about positive inotropic effects without changes in the intracellular levels of cyclic AMP in vitro [27–30] and in vivo [31,32]. The number of α_1-adrenergic receptors varies among species, being quite high in the rat heart and very low in the human heart [33–35]. In the human heart α_1-adrenergic receptor-mediated positive inotropic effects have been demonstrated in atrial [36–38] and ventricular preparations [35,39–41].

The mechanism of α_1-adrenergic receptor-mediated inotropic effects is still a matter of debate: α_1-adrenergic receptors couple via a pertussis toxin- (PTX-) insensitive G protein (possibly $G_{q/11}$) [42,43] to phospholipase C that causes formation of two second messengers, 1,4,5-inositoltrisphosphate (IP_3, mediating the release of Ca^{2+} from intracellular stores) and diacylglycerol (DAG); whether these are also responsible for the increases in the Ca^{2+}-sensitivity of myofilaments or transsarcolemmal Ca^{2+} influx and intracellular alkalinization via activation of the Na^+/H^+-antiporter that have been observed after α_1-adrenergic receptor activation (for recent review, see [44]) is not completely understood at present. Among the three known α_1-adrenergic receptor subtypes (α_{1A}, α_{1B}, or α_{1D}, [45]), the α_{1A}-subtype seems to be the predominant subtype at the mRNA level in the human heart [46,47], but it is not known at present whether this holds true also at the protein level.

Adrenergic Receptor Changes in the Failing Human Heart

β-Adrenergic Receptors

Heart failure is a disease that is primarily attributed to an inadequate perfusion of peripheral organs and to pulmonary and venous congestion. Reflectively, various neurohumoral systems are activated including the renin-angiotensin system and the sympathetic nervous system [48]. Chronic activation of the sympathetic nervous system is accompanied by changes in adrenergic receptors and their signaling pathways. Thus, a general feature of chronic heart failure is that cardiac β-adrenergic receptor number *and* function decrease. Numerous studies have confirmed the original observation of Bristow et al. [49] that the β_1-adrenergic receptor number is decreased in patients with chronic failure from dilated cardiomyopathy. This appears to be true for heart failure of all causes, and the extent of reduction in β-adrenergic receptor number is directly related to the severity of the disease (often judged by *New York Heart Association* [NYHA] classification; for recent reviews, see [1–3,50–52]). On the other hand, it is still controversial whether the β_2-adrenergic receptor number decreases or not; some authors described unchanged numbers, and others found a simultaneous decrease of β_2- together with β_1-adrenergic receptors, possibly dependent on the etiology of the disease (Fig. 4). However, independent of whether the β_2-adrenergic receptor number is decreased or not, there appears to be general agreement that β_2-adrenergic receptor function (i.e., induction of positive inotropic effects) is also decreased in patients with chronic heart failure (Fig. 5) [3,50].

Recent studies have given some insights into the mechanisms underlying β-adrenergic receptor desensitization in chronic heart failure. In general, β-adrenergic receptor desensitization (for recent review, see [53]) can be caused (1) by phosphorylation

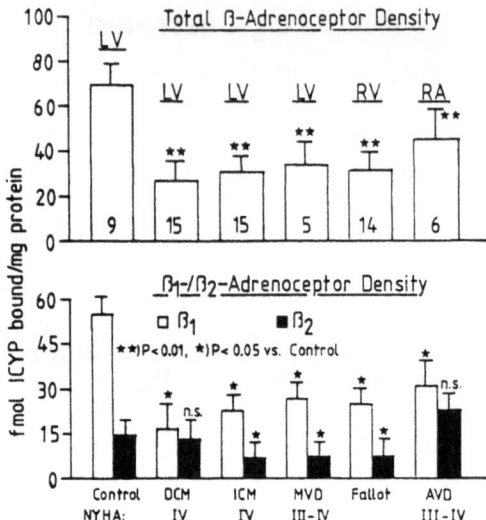

FIG. 4. Total β-, β₁-, and β₂-adrenergic receptor changes in different forms of heart failure. *Upper panel*, total β-adrenergic receptor density, determined from Scatchard analysis of (−)-[¹²⁵I]iodocyanopindolol (ICYP) binding, in femtomoles ICYP specifically bound per milligram protein. *Lower panel*, β₁- and β₂-adrenergic receptor densities in femtomoles ICYP specifically bound per milligram protein. *DCM*, idiopathic dilated cardiomyopathy; *ICM*, ischemic cardiomyopathy; *MVD*, mitral valve disease; *Fallot*, tetralogy of Fallot; *AVD*, aortic valve disease; *RA*, right atrium; *RV* and *LV*, right and left ventricle. Means ± SEM; number of experiments at the bottom of the columns. (From [90], with permission, and unpublished data)

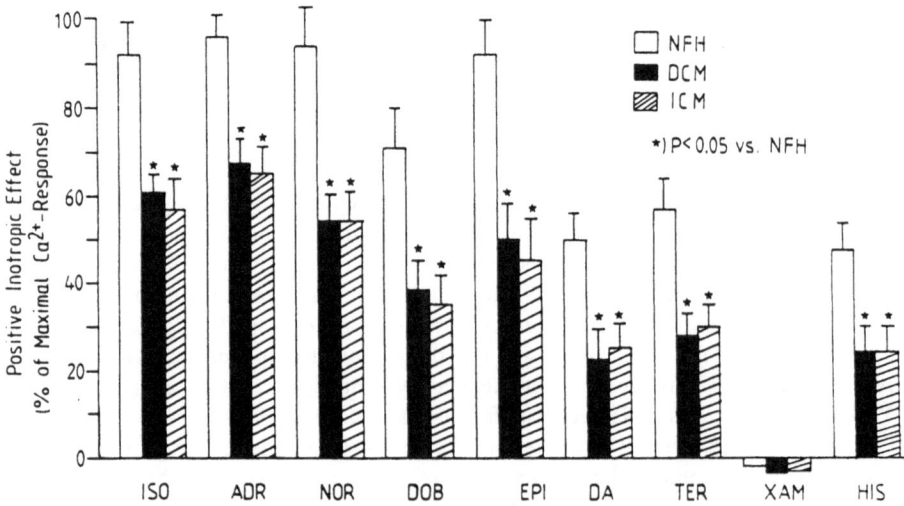

FIG. 5. Maximal positive inotropic effects of various β-adrenergic receptor agonists and histamine on isolated electrically driven left-ventricular trabeculae from nonfailing hearts (*NFH*, unshaded bars, n = 6), patients with end-stage idiopathic dilated cardiomyopathy (*DCM*, solid bars, n = 9) and patients with end-stage ischemic cardiomyopathy (*ICM*, shaded bars, n = 11). *Ordinate*, positive inotropic effect in percent of maximal Ca²⁺ response (that is not changed in heart failure; see [3,50]). *ISO*, isoprenaline; *ADR*, adrenaline; *NOR*, noradrenaline; *DOB*, dobutamine; *EPI*, epinine; *DA*, dopamine; *TER*, terbutaline; *XAM*, xamoterol; *HIS*, histamine. Means ± SEM. (Brodde OE, unpublished observations)

of the receptor through the enzyme β-adrenergic receptor kinase (βARK), which acts only if receptors are occupied by agonists (homologous desensitization) and enhances the binding of the inhibitor protein β-arrestin; binding of β-arrestin to the phosphorylated receptor inhibits interaction of the receptor with the G_s protein, or (2) by phosphorylation through the cyclic AMP-dependent protein kinase A (PKA) (and possibly through protein kinase C, PKC), which obviously does not involve the action of β-arrestin. While βARK-induced desensitization is primarily homologous (i.e., agonist-specific), PKA-induced desensitization can be heterologous (i.e., various G_s-coupled receptors can be desensitized). There are two major differences between βARK- and PKA-induced desensitization: (a) βARK-induced phosphorylation is considerably faster than PKA-induced effects and (b) PKA-induced phosphorylation occurs at much lower agonist concentrations than does βARK phosphorylation. β-Adrenergic receptor desensitization can also be caused by (3) transient internalization of the receptors into a still unknown intracellular compartment where they are not accessible to hydrophilic ligands; these internalized receptors are functionally intact and can be recycled; or by (4) downregulation, i.e., a decrease in the available number of receptors which can be caused either by enhanced degradation of the receptors or by diminished synthesis.

In chronic heart failure, internalization seems not to play an important role as several groups have shown no differences in the amount of β-adrenergic receptors in a light vesicular fraction of nonfailing and failing human hearts [54–56]. PKA seems not to be changed, as a recent study by Böhm et al. [57] found that the potency and efficacy of cyclic AMP in activating PKA in the failing human heart is not changed. Nevertheless, PKA-induced phosphorylation could contribute to β-adrenergic receptor desensitization in chronic heart failure, because in this setting PKA will be chronically activated by enhanced endogenous noradrenaline. Although it has been shown in the human neuroblastoma cell line SK-N-MC that PKA can phosphorylate and desensitize $β_1$-adrenergic receptors [58], $β_2$-adrenergic receptors are much more susceptible to PKA phosphorylation than are $β_1$-adrenergic receptors, possibly because $β_2$-adrenergic receptors contain two potential PKA phosphorylation sites and $β_1$-adrenergic receptors only one [59].

On the other hand, βARK mRNA levels and βARK activity [60], but not β-arrestin mRNA and β-arrestin levels [61], have been found to be increased in hearts of patients with end-stage dilated and ischemic cardiomyopathy. This might contribute to the desensitization process, possibly more for the $β_2$- than the $β_1$-adrenergic receptor, because in various cell line experiments it has been shown that the $β_2$-adrenergic receptor is much more phosphorylated by βARK than is the $β_1$-adrenergic receptor, possibly because the $β_2$-adrenergic receptor contains more potential βARK phosphorylation sites than the $β_1$-adrenergic receptor [59]. Thus, the downregulation of $β_1$-adrenergic receptors could be caused by the decrease in mRNA levels that have been recently demonstrated in the hearts of patients with dilated and ischemic cardiomyopathy [60,62], while mRNA levels for $β_2$-adrenergic receptors were not altered in the failing human heart.

In addition to downregulation of $β_1$-adrenergic receptors and desensitization ("uncoupling") of $β_2$-adrenergic receptors, the amount and function of G proteins appear to be altered in chronic heart failure. There is general agreement that $G_{sα}$ is not changed in chronic heart failure, neither when determined on the protein level by cholera toxin-catalyzed adenosine diphosphate (ADP) ribosylation or quantitative Western blotting nor on mRNA levels (for reviews, see [3,63,64]) or functionally in a reconstitution assay using cyc^- cells [65]. On the other hand, $G_{i\alpha}$ was found to be increased in the majority of studies [3,63,64]. This has been initially demonstrated by pertussis toxin- (PTX-) catalyzed ADP ribosylation [65–69]; the use of quantitative Western and Northern blotting to differentially determine expression of G_i isoforms at the protein or mRNA levels, however, has led to controversies as to which of the three $G_{i\alpha}$s is increased in end-stage dilated and ischemic cardiomyopathy. Thus, one group [68] found $G_{i\alpha-3}$ to be the predominant form in human heart; the amount of this isoform was unchanged in heart failure assessed on the protein level (by quantitative Western blotting) but functionally increased (assessed by decreased Gpp(NH)p- but not NaF-induced adenylyl cyclase activation). Subsequently, this group [70] also described mRNA levels of $G_{i\alpha-3}$ to be unchanged in chronic heart failure. On the other hand, two other groups showed $G_{i\alpha-2}$ to be the predominant form in human heart, and this was found to be increased both on protein and mRNA levels [71,72].

Thus, it appears at present that PTX substrates in human heart failure are increased and that this could be restricted to $G_{i\alpha-2}$. Such an increase in G_i that leads to inhibition of cyclic AMP formation could contribute to the diminished response of β_2- or β_1-adrenergic receptors in chronic heart failure. Three lines of evidence favor this hypothesis. First, in ventricular membranes obtained from end-stage heart failure activation of adenylyl cyclase by guanosine triphosphate (GTP) or its nonhydrolyzable analogue Gpp(NH)p (involving G_s and G_i) and forskolin is diminished, while that induced by NaF (involving only G_s) and Mn^{2+} (activating directly the catalytic unit of the adenylyl cyclase) are unchanged (for references, see [3]). Second, Feldman et al. [65] showed that pretreatment of cardiac membranes from severely failing hearts with PTX restores the previously decreased adenylyl cyclase response to isoprenaline, and third, Brown and Harding [73] have shown, in isolated human cardiomyocytes, that pretreatment with PTX restored the previously reduced maximal inotropic response to isoprenaline. In addition, the increase in G_i might also explain why in the failing human heart activation of adenylyl cyclase by β_2-adrenergic receptor stimulation (even in those settings where β_2-adrenergic receptor number is not changed, cf. Fig. 4), but also by histamine through H_2-receptor stimulation and serotonin through $5-HT_4$-receptor stimulation, is diminished (Fig. 6).

The mechanisms underlying the increase in G_i are not completely understood. It has been speculated that it is caused by the increased activity of the sympathetic nervous system and hence increased noradrenaline levels. This hypothesis is based on findings that (a) chronic exposure to noradrenaline increased G_i in rat neonatal cardiomyocytes [74], and (b) chronic treatment of rats with isoprenaline caused an increase in myocardial G_i [75] that was accompanied by increases in the mRNA levels of $G_{i\alpha-2}$ and $G_{i\alpha-3}$ [76,77]. Thus it could be that noradrenaline via increasing cyclic AMP and activating a cyclic AMP response element in the G_i gene might lead to increased expression in chronic heart failure. Because the gene for $G_{i\alpha-2}$ contains a possible consensus sequence of cyclic AMP response element [78,79] while the $G_{s\alpha}$ gene does not [80], this would also explain why in chronic heart failure G_i but not G_s increases.

In this context it is interesting to note that the aging human heart shows some similarities with the failing human heart; it is well known that the aging human heart exerts reduced responses to β-adrenergic stimulation (for references see [81,82]). We have recently studied the mechanism underlying this effect in more detail [83]. For this purpose we determined, in right atria from 52 patients of different ages (7 days– 83 years) undergoing open heart surgery without apparent heart failure, β-adrenergic receptor number and subtype distribution, G_s and G_i proteins, and adenylyl cyclase

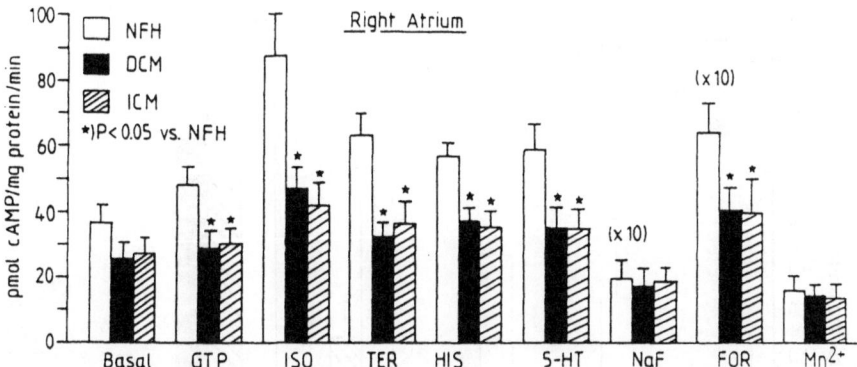

FIG. 6 Adenylyl cyclase activity in right-atrial membranes from nonfailing hearts (*NFH, un-shaded bars, n* = 6), patients with end-stage idiopathic dilated cardiomyopathy (*DCM, solid bars, n* = 9) and patients with end-stage ischemic cardiomyopathy (*ICM, shaded bars, n* = 11). *Ordinate*, net increase in right-atrial adenylyl cyclase activity on stimulation in picomoles cAMP formed per milligram protein per minute. Means ± SEM. *Basal*, basal adenylyl cyclase activity; *GTP*, 10 μM guanosine triphosphate-stimulated adenylyl cyclase activity; *ISO*, 100 μM isoprenaline-stimulated adenylyl cyclase activity; *TER*, 100 μM terbutaline-stimulated adenylyl cyclase activity; *HIS*, 100 μM histamine-stimulated adenylyl cyclase activity; *5-HT*, 100 μM sero-tonin-stimulated adenylyl cyclase activity; *NaF*, 10 mM NaF-stimulated adenylyl cyclase activity; *FOR*, 100 μM forskolin-stimulated adenylyl cyclase activity; *Mn²⁺*, 10 mM Mn²⁺-stimulated adenylyl cyclase activity. (Brodde EO, unpublished observations)

activity. We found that GTP-, isoprenaline-, histamine-, serotonin- (5-HT-), forskolin-, NaF-, and Mn^{2+}-activated adenylyl cyclase significantly decreased with increasing age of the patients (Fig. 7); moreover, all these adenylyl cyclase parameters were significantly negatively correlated with the age of the patients [83]. In addition, $G_{i\alpha}$ increased with age; β-adrenergic receptor number and subtype distribution, how-ever, were unchanged.

These results indicate that the reduction in β-adrenergic responsiveness with age might be caused by a reduction in the activity of the catalytic unit of the adenylyl cyclase, which leads to impairment of cyclic AMP formation. An increase in G_i might enhance that effect. Thus, with both chronic heart failure and age, β-adrenergic receptor-mediated effects and all other cyclic AMP-dependent effects are depressed and G_i protein is increased. However, the basic mechanisms underlying these pro-cesses must be different: in chronic heart failure β-adrenergic receptor number is markedly reduced while it is not changed in the aging human heart. On the other hand, an impairment of the activity of the catalytic unit of adenylyl cyclase appears to be the prominent change in the aging human heart while in chronic heart failure adenylyl cyclase activity is unaltered, with the exception of a decreased activity of the catalytic unit in right-ventricular preparations from hearts subjected to pressure overload [84].

α-Adrenergic Receptors

There appears to be general agreement that the number of α_1-adrenergic receptors (although very low in the human heart) is increased in patients with chronic heart failure [41,50,85]; the mechanism underlying this phenomenon is not completely understood but may be due to the fact that in a cell line it has been shown that chronic

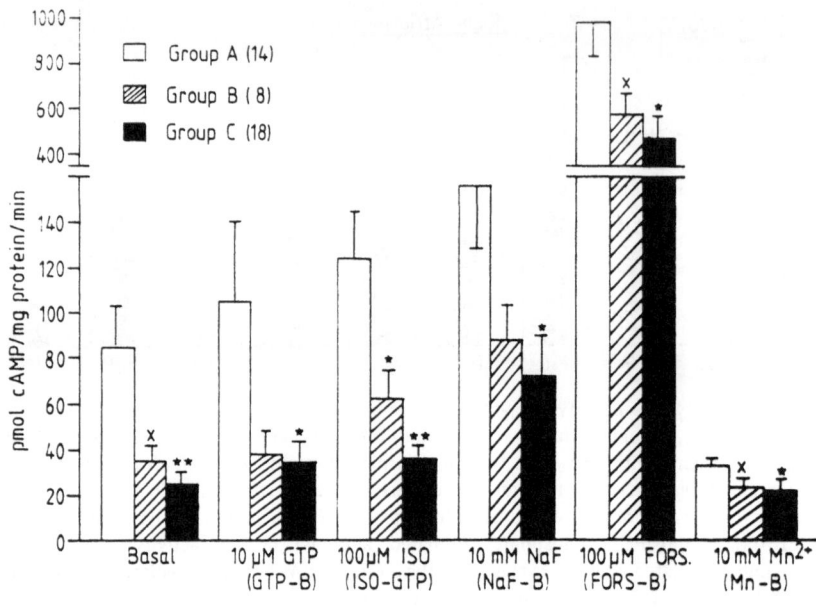

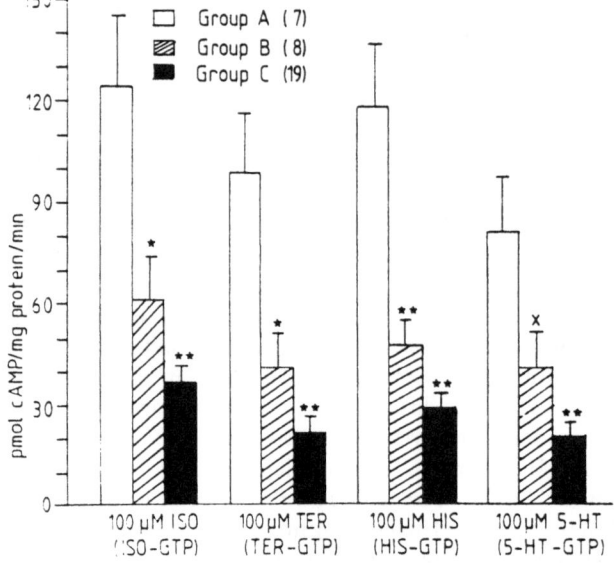

FIG. 7. Age dependency of adenylyl cyclase activity in right-atrial membranes from three groups of patients of different ages without apparent heart failure undergoing open heart surgery; group A (*unshaded bars*, 0–19 years), group B (*shaded bars*, 20–50 years), and group C (*solid bars*, 51–83 years). *Ordinate*, net increase in right-atrial adenylyl cyclase activity on stimulation in picomoles cAMP formed per milligram protein per minute. Means ± SEM; number of experiments in parentheses. B, Basal adenylyl cyclase activity; *ISO*, isoprenaline; *FORS*, forskolin; *TER*, terbutaline; *HIS*, histamine; *5-HT*, serotonin. **, $P < 0.01$ *vs* 0–19 years; *, $P < 0.05$ *vs* 0–19 years; x, $0.1 > P > 0.05$ *vs* 0–19 years. (From [83], with permission)

β-adrenergic stimulation increases the amount of α_1-adrenergic receptor mRNA [86]. On the other hand, in rats chronically treated with the β-adrenergic receptor antagonist propranolol, α_1-adrenergic receptors also increase [87,88], which might argue against the cross-regulation hypothesis. Despite increased number, α_1-adrenergic receptor-mediated inositol phosphate accumulation is unchanged in the failing human heart [50], as is the inositol phosphate response to stimulation of two other PLC/ IP_3 DAG-coupled receptors unchanged in chronic heart failure: the endothelin ET_A receptor [89] and the muscarinic M_2 receptor [50].

Controversies exist whether the positive inotropic effect induced by α_1-adrenergic receptor activation is altered in chronic heart failure. Although Böhm et al. [35] found it be unchanged in left-ventricular preparations from patients with severe chronic heart failure, Steinfath et al. [41] demonstrated in this preparation a marked decreased response to phenylephrine and noradrenaline; these in vitro data have been recently confirmed in an in vivo study by Landzberg et al. [32], who demonstrated that after intracoronary injections of phenylephrine its positive inotropic effect was markedly reduced in patients with severe heart failure when compared with healthy controls. Thus, taken together the increased number, the unchanged inositol phosphate response and the (presumably) decreased inotropic response indicate that in chronic heart failure cardiac α_1-adrenergic receptors are uncoupled from the response.

Acknowledgment. Part of the author's work cited in this article was supported by the Deutsche Forschungsgemeinschaft (DFG Br 526/3-1; Br 526/3-2).

References

1. Jones CR, Molenaar P, Summers RJ (1989) New views of human cardiac β-adrenoceptors. J Mol Cell Cardiol 21:519–535
2. Bristow MR, Hershberger RE, Port JD, Gilbert EM, Sandoval A, Rasmussen R, Cates AE, Feldman AM (1990) β-Adrenergic pathways in nonfailing and failing human ventricular myocardium. Circulation 82[Suppl I]:I-12-I-25
3. Brodde O-E (1991) β_1- and β_2-Adrenoceptors in the human heart: properties, function, and alterations in chronic heart failure. Pharmacol Rev 43:203–242
4. Steinfath M, Lavicky J, Schmitz W, Scholz H, Döring V, Kalmar P (1992) Regional distribution of β_1- and β_2-adrenoceptors in the failing and nonfailing human hearts. Eur J Clin Pharmacol 42:607–612
5. Elnatan J, Molenaar P, Summers RJ (1991) Density and distribution of β-adrenoceptor subtypes in human atrioventricular conducting system (abstract). Clin Exp Pharmacol Physiol 18 [Suppl]:16
6. Kaumann AJ (1989) Is there a third heart β-adrenoceptor? Trends Pharmacol Sci 10:316–320
7. Krief S, Lönnqvist F, Raimbault S, Baude B, Van Spronsen A, Arner P, Strosberg D, Ricquier D, Emorine LJ (1993) Tissue distribution of β_3-adrenoceptor mRNA in man. J Clin Invest 91:344–349
8. Brodde O-E, O'Hara N, Zerkowski H-R, Rohm N (1984) Human cardiac β-adrenoceptors: both β_1- and β_2-adrenoceptors are functionally coupled to the adenylate cyclase in right atrium. J Cardiovasc Pharmacol 6:1184–1191
9. Bristow MR, Hershberger RE, Port JD, Minobe W, Rasmussen R (1989) β_1- And β_2-adrenoceptor-mediated adenylate cyclase stimulation in nonfailing and failing human ventricular myocardium. Mol Pharmacol 35:295–303
10. Kaumann AJ, Hall JA, Murray KJ, Wells FC, Brown MJ (1989) A comparison of the effects of adrenaline and noradrenaline on human heart: the role of β_1- and β_2-

adrenoceptors in the stimulation of adenylate cyclase and contractile force. Eur Heart J 10[Suppl B]:29–37

11. Ikezono K, Michel MC, Zerkowski H-R, Beckeringh JJ, Brodde O-E (1987) The role of cyclic AMP in the positive inotropic effect mediated by β_1- and β_2-adrenoceptors in isolated human right atrium. Naunyn-Schmiedeberg's Arch Pharmacol 335:561–566

12. Schäfers RF, Adler S, Daul A, Zeitler G, Vogelsang M, Zerkowski H-R, Brodde O-E (1994) Positive inotropic effect of the beta$_2$-adrenoceptor agonist terbutaline in the human heart: effects of long-term beta$_1$-adrenoceptor antagonist treatment. J Am Coll Cardiol 23:1224–1233

13. Green SA, Holt BD, Liggett SB (1992) β_1- And β_2-adrenoceptors display subtype-selective coupling to G_s. Mol Pharmacol 41:889–893

14. Levy FO, Zhu X, Kaumann AJ, Birnbaumer L (1993) Efficacy of β_1-adrenoceptors is lower than that of β_2-adrenoceptors. Proc Natl Acad Sci USA 90:10798–10802

15. Feldman AM, Bristow MR (1990) The β-adrenergic pathway in the failing human heart: implications for inotropic therapy. Cardiology 77[Suppl 1]:1–32

16. Del Monte F, Kaumann AJ, Poole-Wilson PA, Wynne DG, Pepper J, Harding SE (1993) Coexistence of functioning β_1- and β_2-adrenoceptors in single myocytes from human ventricle. Circulation 88:854–863

17. Motomura S, Zerkowski H-R, Daul A, Brodde O-E (1990) On the physiologic role of beta-2 adrenoceptors in the human heart: in vitro and in vivo studies. Am Heart J 119:608–619

18. Bristow MR (1989) Myocardial cell surface membrane receptors in heart failure. Heart Failure 5:47–50

19. McDevitt DG (1989) In vivo studies on the function of cardiac β-adrenoceptors in man. Eur Heart J 10(suppl B):22–28

20. Strauss MH, Reeves RA, Smith DL, Leenen FHH (1986) The role of cardiac beta-1 receptors in the hemodynamic response to a beta-2 agonist. Clin Pharmacol Ther 40:108–115

21. Levine MAH, Leenen FHH (1989) Role of β_1-receptors and vagal tone in cardiac inotropic and chronotropic responses to a β_2-agonist in humans. Circulation 79:107–115

22. Hall JA, Petch MC, Brown MJ (1989) Intracoronary injections of salbutamol demonstrate the presence of functional β_2-adrenoceptors in the human heart. Circ Res 65:546–553

23. Johnsson G (1975) Influence of metoprolol and propranolol on hemodynamic effects induced by adrenaline and physical work. Acta Toxicol 36[Suppl]:59–68

24. Leenen FHH, Chan YK, Smith DL, Reeves RA (1988) Epinephrine and left ventricular function in humans: effects of beta-1 vs nonselective beta-blockade. Clin Pharmacol Ther 43:519–528

25. Daul A, Hermes U, Schäfers RF, Wenzel R, Von Birgelen C, Brodde O-E (1995) The β-adrenoceptor subtype(s) mediating adrenaline- and dobutamine-induced blood pressure and heart rate changes in healthy volunteers. Int J Clin Pharmacol Ther 33:140–148

26. Brown MJ, Brown DC, Murphy MB (1983) Hypokalemia from beta$_2$-receptor stimulation by circulating epinephrine. N Engl J Med 309:1414–1419

27. Wagner J, Brodde O-E (1979) On the presence and distribution of α-adrenoceptors in the heart of various mammalian species. Naunyn-Schmiedeberg's Arch Pharmacol 302:239–254

28. Scholz H (1980) Effects of beta- and alpha-adrenoceptor activators and adrenergic transmitter releasing agents on the mechanical activity in the heart. In: Szekeres L (ed) Handbook of experimental pharmacology, vol 54/I. Adrenergic activators and inhibitors Springer, Verlag, Berlin Heidelberg New York, pp 651–733

29. Benfey BG (1982) Function of myocardial α-adrenoceptors. Life Sci 31:101–112

30. Endoh M (1982) Adrenoceptors and the myocardial inotropic response: do alpha and beta receptor sites functionally coexist? In: Kalsner S (ed) Trends in autonomic pharmacology, vol 2. Urban & Schwarzenberg, Baltimore, pp 304–322

31. Curiel R, Perez-Gonzalez J, Brito N, Zerpa R, Tellez D, Cabrera J, Curiel C, Cubeddu L (1989) Positive inotropic effects mediated by α_1-adrenoceptors in intact human subjects. J Cardiovasc Pharmacol 14:603-615
32. Landzberg JS, Parker JD, Gauthier DF, Colucci WS (1991) Effects of myocardial α_1-adrenoceptor stimulation and blockade on contractility in humans. Circulation 84:1608-1614
33. Steinfath M, Chen Y-L, Lavicky J, Magnussen O, Nose M, Rosswag S, Schmitz W, Scholz H (1992) Cardiac α_1-adrenoceptor densities in different mammalian species. Br J Pharmacol 107:185-188
34. Bristow MR, Minobe W, Rasmussen R, Hershberger RE, Hoffman BB (1988) Alpha-1 adrenoceptors in the nonfailing and failing human heart. J Pharmacol Exp Ther 247:1039-1045
35. Böhm M, Diet F, Feiler G, Kemkes B, Erdmann E (1988) α-Adrenoceptors and α-adrenoceptor-mediated positive inotropic effects in failing human myocardium. J Cardiovasc Pharmacol 12:357-364
36. Schümann HJ, Wagner J, Knorr A, Reidemeister JC, Sadony V, Schramm G (1978) Demonstration in human atrial preparations of alpha-adrenoceptors mediating positive inotropic effects. Naunyn-Schmiedeberg's Arch Pharmacol 302:333-336
37. Skomedal T, Aass H, Osnes J-B, Fjeld NB, Klingen G, Langslet A, Semb G (1985) Demonstration of an alpha adrenoceptor-mediated inotropic effect of norepinephrine in human atria. J Pharmacol Exp Ther 233:441-446
38. Jahnel U, Jakob H, Nawrath H (1992) Electrophysiologic and inotropic effects of α-adrenoceptor stimulation in human isolated atrial heart muscle. Naunyn-Schmiedeberg's Arch Pharmacol 346:82-87
39. Brückner R, Meyer W, Mügge A, Schmitz W, Scholz H (1984) Alpha-adrenoceptor-mediated positive inotropic effect of phenylephrine in isolated human ventricular myocardium. Eur J Pharmacol 99:345-347
40. Aass H, Skomedal T, Osnes J-B, Fjeld NB, Klingen G, Langslet A, Svennevig J, Semb G (1986) Noradrenaline evokes an α-adrenoceptor-mediated inotropic effect in human ventricular myocardium. Acta Pharmacol Toxicol 58:88-90
41. Steinfath M, Danielsen W, Von der Leyen H, Mende U, Meyer W, Neumann J, Nose M, Reich T, Schmitz W, Scholz H, Starbatty J, Stein B, Döring V, Kolmer P, Haverich A (1992) Reduced α_1- and β_2-adrenoceptor-mediated positive inotropic effects in human end-stage heart failure. Br J Pharmacol 105:463-469
42. Kohl C, Schmitz W, Scholz H, Scholz J, Toth M, Döring V, Kalimar P (1989) Evidence for alpha$_1$-adrenoceptor-mediated increase of inositol trisphosphate in the human heart. J Cardiovasc Pharmacol 13:324-327
43. Schmitz W, Scholz H, Scholz J, Steinfath M, Lohse M, Puurunen J, Schwabe U (1987) Pertussis toxin does not inhibit the alpha$_1$-adrenoceptor-mediated effect on inositol phosphate production in the heart. Eur J Pharmacol 134:377-378
44. Terzic A, Puceat M, Vassort G, Vogel SM (1993) Cardiac α_1-adrenoceptors: an overview. Pharmacol Rev 45:147-175
45. Bylund DB, Eikenberg DC, Hieble PJ, Langer SZ, Lefkowitz RJ, Minneman KP, Molinoff PB, Ruffolo RR, Trendelenburg U (1994) International Union of Pharmacology: Nomenclature of adrenoceptors. Pharmacol Rev 46:121-136
46. Hirasawa A, Horie K, Tanaka T, Takagaki K, Murai M, Yano J, Tsujimoto G (1993) Cloning, functional expression and tissue distribution of human cDNA for the α_{1c}-adrenergic receptor. Biochem Biophys Res Commun 195:902-909
47. Price DT, Lefkowitz RJ, Caron MG, Berkowitz D, Schwinn DA (1994) Localization of mRNA for three distinct α_1-adrenergic receptor subtypes in human tissues: implications for human α-adrenergic physiology. Mol Pharmacol 45:171-175
48. Packer M (1992) Pathophysiology of chronic heart failure. Lancet 340:88-92
49. Bristow MR, Ginsburg R, Minobe W, Cubicciotti RS, Sageman WS, Lurie K, Billingham ME, Harrison DC, Stinson EB (1982) Decreased catecholamine sensitivity and β-adrenergic-receptor density in failing human hearts. N Engl J Med 307:205-211

50. Bristow MR (1993) Changes in myocardial and vascular receptors in heart failure. J Am Coll Cardiol 22[Suppl 4]:61A–71A
51. Brodde O-E (1994) Beta-adrenoceptors in cardiac disease. Pharmacol Ther 60:405–430
52. Harding SE, Brown LA, Wynne DG, Davies CH, Poole-Wilson PA (1994) Mechanisms of β-adrenoceptor desensitization in the failing human heart. Cardiovasc Res 28:1451–1460
53. Lohse MJ (1993) Molecular mechanisms of membrane receptor desensitization. Biochim Biophys Acta 1179:171–188
54. Denniss AR, Colucci WS, Allen PD, Marsh JD (1989) Distribution and function of human ventricular beta adrenoceptors in congestive heart failure. J Mol Cell Cardiol 21:651–660
55. Murphree SS, Saffitz JE (1989) Distribution of β-adrenoceptors in failing human myocardium. Implications for mechanisms of down-regulation. Circulation 79:1214–1225
56. Pitschner HF, Droege A, Mitze M, Schlepper M, Brodde O-E (1993) Down-regulated β-adrenoceptors in severely failing human ventricles: uniform regional distribution, but no increased internalization! Basic Res Cardiol 88:179–191
57. Böhm M, Reiger B, Schwinger RHG, Erdmann E (1994) cAMP concentrations, cAMP-dependent protein kinase activity, and phosphoplamban in non-failing and failing myocardium. Cardiovasc Res 28:1713–1719
58. Zhou X-M, Fishman PH (1991) Desensitization of the human β₁-adrenoceptor. Involvement of the cyclic AMP-dependent but not a receptor-specific protein kinase. J Biol Chem 266:7462–7468
59. Hausdorff WP, Caron MG, Lefkowitz RJ (1990) Turning off the signal: desensitization of β-adrenoceptor function. FASEB J 4:2881–2889
60. Ungerer M, Böhm M, Elce JS, Erdmann E, Lohse MJ (1993) Altered expression of β-adrenoceptor kinase and β₁-adrenergic receptors in the failing human heart. Circulation 87:454–463
61. Ungerer M, Parruti G, Böhm M, Puzicha M, DeBlasi A, Erdmann E, Lohse MJ (1994) Expression of β-arrestin and β-adrenoceptor kinases in the failing human heart. Circ Res 74:206–213
62. Bristow MR, Minobe WA, Raynolds MV, Port JD, Rasmussen R, Ray PE, Feldman AM (1993) Reduced β₁ receptor messenger RNA abundance in the failing human heart. J Clin Invest 92:2737–2745
63. Feldman AM (1991) Experimental issues in assessment of G protein function in cardiac disease. Circulation 84:1852–1861
64. Eschenhagen T (1993) G Proteins and the heart. Cell Biol Int 17:723–749
65. Feldman AM, Cates AE, Veazey WB, Hershberger RE, Bristow MR, Baughman KL, Baumgartner WA, van Dop C (1988) Increase in the 40,000 mol wt pertussis toxin substrate (G-protein) in the failing human heart. J Clin Invest 82:189–197
66. Neumann J, Schmitz W, Scholz H, von Meyerinck L, Döring V, Kalmar P (1988) Increase of myocardial Gᵢ-proteins in human heart failure. Lancet II:936–937
67. Böhm M, Gierschik P, Jakobs K-H, Pieske B, Schnabel P, Ungerer M, Erdmann E (1990) Increase of Gᵢₐ in human hearts with dilated but not ischemic cardiomyopathy. Circulation 82:1249–1265
68. Feldman AM, Jackson DG, Bristow MR, Cates AE, van Dop C (1991) Immunodetectable levels of the inhibitory guanine nucleotide binding regulatory proteins in failing human heart: discordance with measurements of adenylate cyclase activity and levels of pertussis toxin substrate. J Mol Cell Cardiol 23:439–452
69. Bristow MR, Anderson FL, Port JD, Skerl L, Hershberger RE, Larrabee P, O'Connell JB, Renlund DG, Volkman K, Murray J, Feldman AM (1991) Differences in β-adrenergic neuroeffector mechanisms in ischemic versus idiopathic dilated cardiomyopathy. Circulation 84:1024–1039
70. Feldman AM, Ray PE, Bristow MR (1991) Expression of α-subunits of G proteins in failing human heart: a reappraisal utilizing polymerase chain reaction. J Mol Cell Cardiol 23:1355–1358

71. Eschenhagen T, Mende U, Nose M, Schmitz W, Scholz H, Haverich A, Hirt S, Döring V, Kalmar P, Höppner W, Seitz HJ (1992) Increased messenger RNA level of the inhibitory G-protein α-subunit $G_{i\alpha-2}$ in human end-stage heart failure. Circ Res 70:688–696

72. Böhm M, Eschenhagen T, Gierschik P, Larisch K, Lensche H, Mende U, Schmitz W, Schnabel P, Scholz H, Steinfath M, Erdmann E (1994) Radioimmunochemical quantification of $G_{i\alpha}$ in right and left ventricles from patients with ischaemic and dilated cardiomyopathy and predominant left ventricular failure. J Mol Cell Cardiol 26:133–149

73. Brown LA, Harding SE (1992) The effect of pertussis toxin on β-adrenoceptor responses in isolated cardiac myocytes from noradrenaline-treated guinea-pigs and patients with cardiac failure. Br J Pharmacol 106:115–122

74. Reithmann C, Gierschik P, Sidiropoulos D, Werdan K, Jakobs KH (1989) Mechanism of noradrenaline-induced heterologous desensitization of adenylate cyclase stimulation in rat heart muscle cells: increase in the level of inhibitory G-protein α-subunits. Eur J Pharmacol 172:211–221

75. Mende U, Eschenhagen T, Geertz B, Schmitz W, Scholz H, Schulte am Esch J, Sempell R, Steinfath M (1992) Isoprenaline-induced increase in the 40/41 kDa pertussis toxin substrates and functional consequences on contractile response in rat heart. Naunyn-Schmiedeberg's Arch Pharmacol 345:44–50

76. Eschenhagen T, Mende U, Nose M, Schmitz W, Scholz H, Warnholtz A, Wüstel JM (1991) Isoprenaline-induced increase in mRNA levels of inhibitory G-protein α-subunits in rat heart. Naunyn-Schmiedeberg's Arch Pharmacol 343:609–615

77. Eschenhagen T, Mende U, Nose M, Schmitz W, Scholz H, Schulte am Esch J, Warnholtz A (1992) Long-term β-adrenoceptor-mediated upregulation of $G_{i\alpha}$- $G_{o\alpha}$-mRNA levels and pertussis toxin sensitive G-proteins in rat heart. Mol Pharmacol 42:773–783

78. Weinstein JS, Spiegel AM, Carter AD (1988) Cloning and characterization of the human gene for the α-subunit of G_{i2}, a GTP-binding signal transduction protein. FEBS Lett 232:333–340

79. Hadcock JR, Ros M, Watkins DC, Malbon CC (1990) Cross-regulation between G-protein mediated pathways. J Biol Chem 265:14784–14790

80. Kozasa T, Itoh H, Tsukamoto T, Kaziro Y (1988) Isolation and characterization of the human $G_{s\alpha}$ gene. Proc Natl Acad Sci USA 85:2081–2085

81. Docherty JR (1990) Cardiovascular responses in ageing: a review. Pharmacol Rev 42:103–125

82. Lakatta EG (1993) Deficient neuroendocrine regulation of the cardiovascular system with advancing age in healthy humans. Circulation 87:631–636

83. Brodde O-E, Zerkowski H-R, Schranz D, Broede-Sitz A, Michel-Reher M, Schäfer-Beisenbusch E, Piotrowski JA, Oelert H (1995) Age-dependent changes of the β-adrenoceptor-G-protein(s)-adenylyl cyclase system in human right atrium. J Cardiovasc Pharmacol 26:20–26

84. Bristow MR, Minobe W, Rasmussen R, Larrabee P, Skerl L, Klein JW, Anderson FL, Murray J, Mestroni L, Karwande SV, Fowler M, Ginsburg R (1992) β-Adrenergic neuroeffector abnormalities in the failing human heart are produced by local rather than systemic mechanisms. J Clin Invest 89:803–815

85. Vago T, Bevilacqua M, Norbiato G, Baldi G, Chebat E, Bertora P, Baroldi G, Accinni R (1989) Identification of α_1-adrenergic receptors on sarcolemma from normal subjects and patients with idiopathic dilated cardiomyopathy: characteristics and linkage to GTP-binding protein. Circ Res 64:474–481

86. Morris GM, Hadcock JR, Malbon CC (1991) Cross-regulation between G-protein-coupled receptors: activation of β_2-adrenergic receptors increases α_1-adrenoceptor mRNA levels. J Biol Chem 266:2233–2238

87. Mügge A, Reupcke CH, Scholz H (1985) Increased myocardial $alpha_1$-adrenoceptor density in rats chronically treated with propranolol. Eur J Pharmacol 112:249–252

88. Steinkraus V, Nose M, Scholz H, Thormählen K (1989) Time course and extent of alpha$_1$-adrenoceptor density changes in rat heart after beta-adrenoceptor blockade. Br J Pharmacol 96:441–449

89. Broede-Sitz A, Zerkowski H-R, Brodde O-E (1995) Einfluss von Endothelin auf Inositol Phosphat Bildung und Adenylat Zyklase Aktivität im menschlichen Herzen (abstract). Z Kardiol 84[Suppl I]:219

90. Brodde O-E (1992) Pathphysiology of the β-adrenoceptor system in chronic heart failure: consequences for treatment with agonists, partial agonists or antagonists? Eur Heart J 12[Suppl F]:54–62

Role of the Renin-Angiotensin System in the Development of Hypertensive Left Ventricular Hypertrophy

ICHIRO SHIOJIMA, TSUTOMU YAMAZAKI, ISSEI KOMURO, RYOZO NAGAI, and YOSHIO YAZAKI

Summary. Previous studies have demonstrated that angiotensin II (AII) acts as a growth-promoting factor on cardiac myocytes and that treatment with angiotensin-converting enzyme (ACE) inhibitors induces reduction of left ventricular mass and suppression of ventricular remodeling. These results suggest that the renin-angiotensin system (RAS) may play an important role in the development of hypertensive left ventricular hypertrophy (LVH). Moreover, it has recently been demonstrated that gene expression of angiotensinogen and ACE is augmented in pressure-overloaded left ventricles, suggesting that endogenous AII produced by the activated cardiac RAS may contribute to the formation of LVH. To elucidate the role of the RAS in the progression of cardiac hypertrophy, we evaluated the effect of the type 1 AII receptor (AT_1 receptor) antagonist on LVH in spontaneously hypertensive rats (SHR) and investigated the molecular mechanisms by which antagonism of AII receptors reduces cell hypertrophy of myocytes using the in vitro model of mechanical stretching. In the in vivo study, we treated SHR with a nonpeptide AT_1 receptor antagonist, TCV-116. Treatment with TCV-116 reduced anatomical left ventricular (LV) weight, echocardiographic LV wall thickness, transverse diameter of myocytes, and the relative amount of V_3 myosin heavy-chain and interstitial collagen volume fraction. In the in vitro study, neonatal rat cardiomyocytes were cultured on deformable silicone dishes and mechanically stretched with or without pretreatment of CV-11974, an active metabolite of TCV-116. Pretreatment of cultured cardiomyocytes with CV-11974 partially inhibited an increase in MAP kinase activity, *c-fos* gene expression and [^{3}H] phenylalanine incorporation induced by stretching of cardiomyocytes. These results indicate that (1) the RAS plays a critical role not only in the development of hypertensive LVH but also in the ventricular remodeling associated with LVH, which subsequently leads to the impairment of cardiac function and (2) endogenous AII produced by the cardiac RAS contributes to the pathogenesis of LVH.

Keywords. Angiotensin II—Pressure overload—Ventricular remodeling—AT_1 receptor antagonist

Third Department of Medicine, University of Tokyo School of Medicine, Bunkyo-ku, Tokyo 113, Japan

Introduction

Cardiac hypertrophy has been regarded as a secondary adaptation to an increase in hemodynamic workload [1]. Recent studies, however, have demonstrated that left ventricular hypertrophy (LVH) has both physiological and pathological aspects at the same time and that LVH is clinically one of the most important risk factors for congestive heart failure, ischemic heart disease, and sudden cardiac death in hypertensive patients [2,3]. Furthermore, a sustained increase in hemodynamic load, even though it may be temporarily compensated by the development of LVH, finally leads to the impairment of cardiac function. Therefore, it is imperative in cardiovascular research to understand the mechanisms of the development of cardiac hypertrophy and to establish effective measures to prevent it.

Humoral factors such as angiotensin II (AII), as well as the increased hemodynamic load, have been implicated in the pathogenesis of hypertensive LVH. In many clinical and experimental studies, angiotensin-converting enzyme (ACE) inhibitors reduced left ventricular (LV) mass significantly in hypertensive subjects, while other vasodilators, such as hydralazine, did not cause regression of LVH in spite of a significant decrease in blood pressure [4–9]. In addition, AII has been demonstrated in in vitro studies to act as a growth factor on cardiomyocytes [10,11]. These results suggest the putative role of the renin-angiotensin system (RAS) in the formation of LVH. Of course, the effect of ACE inhibitors antagonizing the growth-promoting influence of AII can never be dissociated from the concomitant systemic hemodynamic effect of these agents. However, a previous study indicating that even a nonantihypertensive dose of ACE inhibitor reversed LVH in thoracic aorta-constricted rats [12] strongly suggests the direct involvement of the RAS in the pathogenesis of LVH.

Moreover, previous studies in animal models also indicated that ACE inhibitors suppressed hypertrophy-associated ventricular remodeling such as the shift of myosin heavy chain (MHC) isoforms from V_1 to V_3 or the interstitial fibrosis of myocardium [13,14], suggesting that the RAS may contribute not only to the development of LVH but also to the progression of ventricular remodeling associated with LVH.

In addition to the growing body of evidence which supports the existence of tissue RAS in individual organs including the heart [15–17], recent studies have shown that (a) the cardiac RAS is activated in hypertrophied left ventricles: the mRNA level of angiotensinogen and ACE is upregulated by pressure overload [18,19] and (b) the AII content in the left ventricles correlates with LV weight in spontaneously hypertensive rats (SHR) [20]. These results suggest that endogenous AII produced by the cardiac tissue RAS plays a more important role than circulating AII in the development of LVH.

Recently a novel nonpeptide antagonist to the AT_1 receptor, TCV-116, was developed. It has selectively high affinity for the AT_1 site and noncompetitively inhibits the binding between AII and the AT_1 receptor [21]. Therefore, TCV-116 and CV-11974, an active metabolite of TCV-116, are thought to be useful tools in studying the functional significance of the RAS. Furthermore, we have previously established an in vitro system of stretching cultured cardiomyocytes, by which we can impose a mechanical stress on cultured cells without incurring any effect of circulating humoral factors, and have demonstrated that mechanical loading applied to cultured myocytes activates phosphorylation cascades including mitogen-activated protein (MAP) kinase, induces protooncogene expression, and increases protein synthesis [22–24]. This system, when combined with the use of AII receptor antagonist, is considered to be a beneficial apparatus for analyzing the effect of endogenous AII on stretch-induced hypertrophy of cardiomyocytes.

To explore the precise role of the RAS in the pathogenesis of LVH, we examined (1) the effect of TCV-116 on the development of LVH and on the progression of ventricular remodeling in vivo using SHR and (2) the effect of CV-11974 on stretch-mediated cardiomyocyte hypertrophy in vitro using cultured cardiac myocytes.

Regression of LVH and Suppression of Ventricular Remodeling by an AT$_1$ Receptor Antagonist: An In Vivo Study

As mentioned above, ACE inhibitors have been demonstrated to induce regression of LVH in hypertensive subjects. However, the effect of ACE-independently formed AII is not blocked by ACE inhibitors [25] and there remains a possibility that the antihypertrophic effect of ACE inhibitors may be due to the effect of increased kinins [26]. We therefore treated SHR with the AT$_1$ receptor antagonist TCV-116 and examined its effect on the development of LVH.

In SHR, treatment with TCV-116 significantly decreased anatomical LV weight, echocardiographic LV wall thickness, and transverse diameter of cardiac myocytes compared with vehicle-treated SHR. Treatment with hydralazine, however, did not exhibit significant antihypertrophic effect in spite of the almost identical antihypertensive effect of this agent [27]. These results suggest that AII contributes to the development of hypertensive LVH not only with its systemic hemodynamic effect but also with its growth-promoting effect via the AT$_1$ receptor subtype.

Previous studies demonstrating that ACE inhibitors suppressed the remodeling of pressure-overloaded myocardium [13,14] indicate that ACE inhibitors are cardioprotective. To investigate the role of the RAS in progression of LVH-associated ventricular remodeling, we examined the effect of TCV-116 on MHC isoforms, myocardial fibrosis, and hyperplasia of vascular smooth muscle cells. Treatment of SHR with TCV-116 significantly reduced the relative amount of V$_3$ MHC, interstitial collagen volume fraction, and medial thickening of coronary arteries compared with vehicle-treated controls [27], which demonstrates the beneficial effect of AT$_1$ receptor antagonist on cardiac hypertrophy not only with regard to quantitative parameters of LV mass but also in terms of qualitative features of the myocardium. Our preliminary results using cultured cardiac fibroblasts, which demonstrated that AII stimulates collagen synthesis possibly via autocrine release of transforming growth factor (TGF)-β1, also support the hypothesis that RAS contributes to the formation of cardiac remodeling. These results suggest that (1) the RAS plays an important role both in the development of LVH and in the progression of ventricular remodeling and (2) the AT$_1$ receptor antagonist as well as the ACE inhibitor are cardioprotective.

Inhibition of Stretch-Induced Cardiomyocyte Hypertrophy by an AT₁ Receptor Antagonist: An In Vitro Study

To elucidate the molecular mechanisms by which mechanical stress is transduced into intracellular signals that regulate gene expression and protein synthesis in cardiac myocytes, we previously constructed an in vitro cultured cardiac myocyte stretching model and demonstrated that mechanical load applied to myocytes induces phosphatidyl inositol turnover, activation of MAP kinase subsequent to protein kinase C activation, expression of protooncogenes, and increase in protein synthesis [22–24]. On the other hand, AII has been demonstrated in in vitro studies to activate MAP kinase, stimulate protooncogene expression, and increase protein synthesis in cultured cardiac myocytes [10,11]. Therefore, stretch-induced signaling pathways have a strong analogy with those induced by AII, suggesting that stretch-induced cardiomyocyte hypertrophy is mediated, at least in part, by endogenous AII. To test this hypothesis, we treated cultured cardiac myocytes with CV-11974, an active metabolite of TCV-116, and imposed a passive stretch.

Pretreatment of cultured cardiac myocytes with CV-11974 partially inhibited the activation of MAP kinase, expression of *c-fos* mRNA, and increase in protein synthesis provoked by mechanical stretching [27]. These results indicate that endogenous AII produced by the cardiac tissue RAS plays an important role in the development of stretch-induced cardiomyocyte hypertrophy and, at the same time, that AII is not the only constituent promoting the growth of cardiomyocytes in response to mechanical stimuli.

Many questions, however, remain to be elucidated as for the functional significance of the cardiac RAS. For example, the precise localization of AII production or distribution of AT₁ receptors in cardiac tissue is still unknown. Further investigations are needed regarding the contribution of the cardiac tissue RAS to the pathogenesis of hypertensive LVH.

Possible Mechanisms Leading to the Dysfunction of Pressure-Overloaded Hearts

The increase in LV mass and ventricular remodeling induced by pressure overload are thought to be adaptational responses to an increased external load: hypertrophy of cardiac myocytes with isoform transition of MHC increases contractile force, while collagen accumulation in the interstitium provides a framework for supporting the hypertrophied myofibrils. At the same time, however, these adaptational phenomena may lead to the impairment of cardiac function mainly by imposing relative ischemia on the myocardium: inadequate proliferation of capillaries and decreased myocardial/arteriolar compliance due to interstitial fibrosis and coronary medial thickening induce reduction of myocardial blood flow. Accordingly, our study, indicating that the RAS is involved both in cellular hypertrophy of cardiomyocytes and in the progression of ventricular remodeling, further implies that the RAS contributes not only to the development of cardiac hypertrophy but also to the progression of cardiac failure in hypertrophied left ventricle induced by pressure overload (Fig. 1).

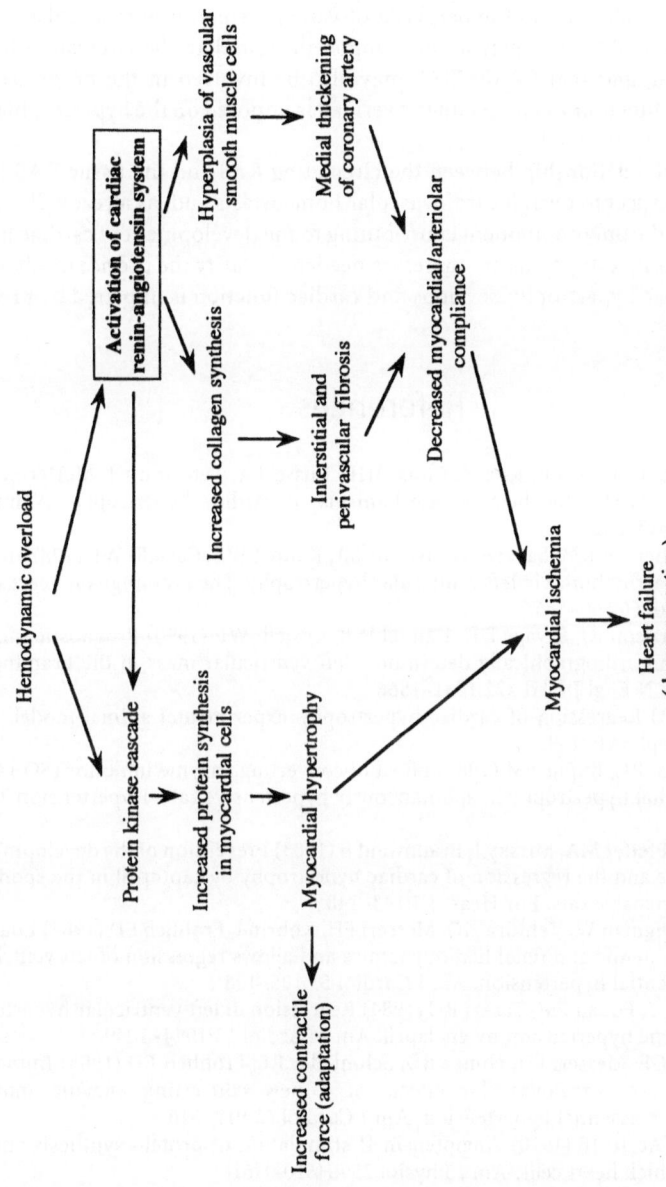

FIG. 1. Involvement of the renin-angiotensin system in the development of cardiac hypertrophy and failure

Conclusions and Future Directions

In our study using the AT_1 receptor antagonist, we have found that (1) the RAS is involved in the development of individual myocyte hypertrophy and in the progression of ventricular remodeling such as the shift of MHC isoforms, interstitial and perivascular fibrosis, and hyperplasia of vascular smooth muscle cells; that (2) the cardiac tissue RAS may play a more important role than the circulating RAS in LVH formation; and that (3) the RAS may also be involved in the progression of ventricular dysfunction when sustained overload is imposed on the hypertrophied left ventricle.

However, the relationship between the circulating RAS and the tissue RAS is still unclear with respect to overall cardiovascular homeostasis and, as already discussed, the RAS is not the only component contributing to the development of cardiac hypertrophy. Further investigations are therefore needed to clarify the precise mechanisms by which cardiac hypertrophy develops and cardiac function is impaired by pressure overload.

References

1. Morgan HE, Gordon EE, Kita Y, Chua BHL, Russo LA, Peterson CJ, McDermott PJ, Watson PA (1987) Biochemical mechanisms of cardiac hypertrophy. Annu Rev Physiol 49:533–543
2. Levy D, Anderson KM, Savage DD, Balkus SA, Kannel WB, Castelli WP (1987) Risk of ventricular arrhythmias in left ventricular hypertrophy: The Framingham heart study. Am J Cardiol 60:560–565
3. Levy D, Garrison RJ, Savage DD, Kannel WB, Castelli WP (1990) Prognostic implications of echocardiographically determined left ventricular mass in the Framingham heart study. N Engl J Med 322:1561–1566
4. Sen S (1983) Regression of cardiac hypertrophy: experimental animal model. Am J Med 75[Suppl 6A]:87–93
5. Sen S, Tarazi RC, Bupus FM (1983) Effect of converting enzyme inhibitor (SQ 14,225) on myocardial hypertrophy in spontaneously hypertensive rats. Hypertension 2:169–176
6. Pfeffer JM, Pfeffer MA, Mirsky I, Braunwald E (1983) Prevention of the development of heart failure and the regression of cardiac hypertrophy by captopril in the spontaneously hypertensive rats. Eur Heart J 4:143–148
7. Dunn FG, Oigman W, Ventura HO, Messeri FH, Kobrin I, Frohlich ED (1984) Enaiapril improves systemic and renal hemodynamics and allows regression of left ventricular mass in essential hypertension. Am J Cardiol 53:105–108
8. Nakashima Y, Fouad FM, Tarazi RC (1984) Regression of left ventricular hypertrophy from systemic hypertension by enalapril. Am J Cardiol 53:1044–1049
9. Garavaglia GE, Messeri FH, Nunez BD, Schmieder RE, Frohlich ED (1988) Immediate and short-term cardiovascular effects of a new converting enzyme inhibitor (lisinopril) in essential hypertension. Am J Cardiol 62:912–916
10. Baker KM, Aceto JF (1990) Angiotensin II stimulation of protein synthesis and cell growth in chick heart cells. Am J Physiol 259:H610–H618
11. Katoh Y, Komuro I, Shibasaki Y, Yamaguchi H, Yazaki Y (1989) Angiotensin II induces hypertrophy and oncogene expression in cultured cardiac myocytes. Circulation 80:[Suppl II]:II-450
12. Scholkens BA, Linz W, Martorana PA (1991) Experimental cardiovascular benefits of angiotensin-converting enzyme inhibitors: beyond the blood pressure. J Cardiovasc Pharmacol 18[Suppl II]:S26–S30

13. Childs TJ, Adams MA, Mak AS (1990) Regression of cardiac hypertrophy in spontane-ously hypertensive rats by enalapril and the expression of contractile proteins. Hyper-tension 16:662–668
14. Brilla CG, Janicki JS, Weber KT (1991) Cardioprotective effects of lisinopril in rats with genetic hypertension and left ventricular hypertrophy. Circulation 83:1771–1779
15. Dzau VJ (1988) Cardiac renin-angiotensin system: Molecular and functional aspects. Am J Med 84[Suppl 3A]:22–27
16. Lindpaintner K, Ganten D (1991) The cardiac renin-angiotensin system: An appraisal of present experimental and clinical evidence. Circ Res 68:905–921
17. Griendling KK, Murphy TJ, Alexander RW (1993) Molecular biology of the renin-angiotensin system. Circulation 87:1816–1828
18. Baker KM, Chernin MI, Wixson SK, Aceto JF (1990) Renin-angiotensin system in-volvement in pressure-overload cardiac hypertrophy in rats. Am J Physiol 259:H324–H332
19. Schunkert H, Dzau VJ, Tang SS, Hirsch AT, Apstein CS, Lorell BH (1990) Increased rat cardiac angiotensin converting enzyme activity and mRNA expression in pressure overload left ventricular hypertrophy: Effect on coronary resistance, contractility, and relaxation. J Clin Invest 86:1913–1920
20. Mizuno K, Tani M, Hashimoto S, Niimura S, Sanada H, Watanabe H, Ohtsuki M, Fukuchi S (1992) Effects of losartan, a nonpeptide angiotensin II receptor antagonist, on cardiac hypertrophy and tissue angiotensin II content in spontaneously hypertensive rats. Life Sci 51:367–374
21. Noda M, Shibouta Y, Inada Y, Ojima M, Wada T, Sanada T, Kubo K, Kohara Y, Naka T, Nishimawa K (1993) Inhibition of rabbit aortic angiotensin II (AII) receptor by CV-11974, a new nonpeptide AII antagonist. Biochem Pharmacol 46:311–318
22. Komuro I, Kaida T, Shibazaki Y, Kurabayashi F, Takaku F, Yazaki Y (1990) Stretching cardiac myocytes stimulates proto oncogene expression. J Biol Chem 265:3595–3598
23. Komuro I, Katoh Y, Kaida T, Shibazaki Y, Kawaguchi M, Hoh E, Takaku F, Yazaki Y (1991) Mechanical loading stimulates cell hypertrophy specific gene expression in cultured rat cardiac myocytes. J Biol Chem 266:1265–1268
24. Yamazaki T, Tobe K, Hoh E, Maemura K, Kaida T, Komuro I, Tamemoto H, Kadowaki T, Nagai R, Yazaki Y (1993) Mechanical loading activates mitogen-activated protein kinase and S6 peptide kinase in cultured rat cardiac myocytes. J Biol Chem 268:12069–12076
25. Urata H, Healy B, Stewart RW, Bumpus FM, Husain A (1990) Angiotensin II-forming pathways in normal and failing human hearts. Circ Res 66:883–890
26. Linz W, Schölkens BA (1992) A specific B_2-bradykinin receptor antagonist HOE 140 abolishes the antihypertrophic effect of ramipril. Br J Pharmacol 105:771–772
27. Kojima M, Shiojima I, Yamazaki T, Komuro I, Yunzeng Z, Ying W, Mizuno T, Ueki K, Tobe K, Kadowaki T, Nagai R and Yazaki Y (1994) Angiotensin II receptor antagonist TCV-116 induces regression of hypertensive left ventricular hypertrophy in vivo and inhibits intracellular signaling pathway of stretch-mediated cardiomyocyte hypertro-phy in vitro. Circulation 89:2204–2211

The Role of Alpha-Adrenergic Activity in Cardioprotection Against Ischemic Injury

Masatsugu Hori, Masafumi Kitakaze, and Takenobu Kamada

Summary. It is well recognized that sympathetic stimulation increases heart rate and enhances the contractile function through beta-adrenoceptors. Less attention, however, has been paid to alpha-adrenergic activation in the heart, probably because direct effects of alpha-adrenoceptor stimulation on the functional properties of the heart are much less than beta-adrenoceptor stimulation. Alpha-adrenoceptor activation may exert various metabolic effects through phosphatidyl inositol hydrolysis and activation of protein kinase C. We reported that alpha-adrenoceptor stimulation activates 5′-nucleotidase activity, which synthesizes adenosine from 5′-AMP. In isolated rat cardiomyocytes subjected to hypoxia, norepinephrine increased adenosine release, which was inhibited by prazosin. Activation of protein kinase C by phorbol ester (PMA) also increased the release of adenosine and inhibited GF109203X, an inhibitor of protein kinase C. In dogs, also, adenosine release from the heart was markedly inhibited by treatments of the alpha-adrenoceptor antagonists phentolamine and prazosin, but not by propranolol and yohimbine. Thus, alpha$_1$-adrenoceptor stimulation during ischemia may augment adenosine release from the ischemic heart. Adenosine is cardioprotective against ischemic injury through multifactorial effects: (1) attenuation of cardiac oxygen demand in the beta-adrenoceptor-stimulated hearts, (2) inhibition of Ca influx, (3) augmentation of coronary blood flow, and (4) inhibition of platelet activation and neutrophil activation. Augmented release of adenosine by alpha-adrenoceptor activation during myocardial ischemia may exert beneficial effects on ischemic hearts. Intracoronary administration of methoxamine attenuates myocardial stunning (sustained dysfunction after brief ischemia) but prazosin augments stunning. Infarct size-limiting effects of ischemic preconditioning are mediated by adenosine, and we demonstrated that alpha-adrenoceptor activation during ischemic preconditioning augments adenosine release, which limits infarct size in dogs. Augmentation of adenosine release by ischemic preconditioning is caused by activation of ecto-5′-nucleotidase through alpha$_1$-adrenoceptor activation. Abolishments of infarct size-limiting effects by prazosin, AOPCP (an inhibitor of ecto-5′-nucleotidase), and GF 109203X support this hypothesis. Thus, our results strongly suggest that alpha$_1$-adrenoceptor activation during cardiac ischemia plays a pivotal role in cardioprotection aganst ischemic injury of the heart.

First Department of Medicine, Osaka University, School of Medicine, Suita, Osaka 565, Japan

Key words. Alpha-adrenoceptor activity—Adenosine—Cardioprotection—Myocardial stunning—Ischemic preconditioning—Adenosine receptors—Ischemic injury

Role of Sympathetic Activity in Normal and Ischemic Hearts

In the basal condition, the heart is rhythmically beating, pumping the blood to the peripheral blood vessels even without autonomic nerve control. Sympathetic nerves play a central role when the demand for systemic blood supply is increased. During exercise, heart rate is increased and blood pressure is elevated by activated sympathetic activity; norepinephrine is released from the sympathetic nerve terminals and binds to adrenoceptors on the myocardial cells and vascular smooth muscles, triggering intracellular signal transduction. Beta$_1$-adrenoceptors, predominantly distributed on the myocardial cells, are coupled with G$_s$ proteins and enhance cyclic AMP synthesis, exerting a positive inotrophic action [1]. Alpha-adrenoceptors, predominantly distributed on vascular smooth muscles, are coupled with phosphatidyl inositol turnover, and increase intracellular Ca concentration and Ca sensitivity to contractile proteins, exerting vasoconstriction [2].

Alpha-adrenoceptors are classified into alpha$_1$- and alpha$_2$-receptors. Alpha$_1$-adrenoceptors, abundantly located on the vascular walls, play a pivotal role in regulation of vascular tone. The proximal portions of the coronary arteries have plenty of alpha$_1$-adrenoceptors, and thus alpha-adrenergic control of vascular tone is predominant at the epicardial coronary arteries [3]. In contrast to epicardial large arteries, in the visceral organs and skin small resistance vessels are sensitive to alpha-adrenergic activity. The difference of sensitivity to alpha-adrenergic activity among organs may cause redistribution of the blood under various conditions.

Another important factor in neural regulation of vascular tone is the interaction between alpha-adrenoceptor activity and vasoactive substances. Several substances are modulated by alpha-adrenoceptor stimulation. Alpha$_2$-adrenoceptor stimulation enhances the release of endothelium-derived relaxing factor (EDRF) from endothelial cells [4]; norepinephrine-induced vasoconstriction is affected by the presence or absence of endothelium. Although the mechanism by which alpha$_2$-adrenoceptor stimulation increases nitric oxide (NO) production is yet to be elucidated, NO is a potent vasodilator and inhibits platelet aggregation. Recent reports suggest that NO attenuates the contractile function through accumulation of cyclic guanosine monophosphate (cGMP) [5]. Furthermore, alpha$_2$-adrenoceptor stimulation inhibits norepinephrine release from sympathetic nerve endings [6] and thus decreases in coronary arterial vascular tone. Alpha$_2$-adrenoceptor stimulation also increases the release of histamine in skeletal muscles [7]. On the other hand, alpha$_1$-adrenoceptor stimulation increases adenosine release in ischemic conditions [8]. This mechanism is critically important in the role of alpha-adrenoceptor activity in cardioprotection against ischemic injury of the heart.

It should be noticed that sympathetic activity is activated during myocardial ischemia because myocardial ischemia is a potent trigger of norepinephrine release from local sympathetic nerve terminals [9]. During myocardial ischemia, however, activation of the nerve terminals is not influenced by central sympathetic nerve activity. Release of norepinephrine is observed in the Langendorff rat heart preparation, and the amount of norepinephrine release is dependent on the ischemic period

[10]. Schomig et al. [9] reported that norepinephrine is released from the ischemic heart within 10 min after the onset of ischemia. Wollenberger et al. [10] also observed that a large amount of norepinephrine overflowed during 3–4 min of ischemia in an isolated rat heart. In canine hearts in vivo, coronary occlusion for 2.5 min caused a release of norepinephrine [11]. Thus, during brief myocardial ischemia local sympathetic nerves are activated, stimulating alpha- and beta-adrenoceptors in the ischemic myocardium.

Adenosine as a Cardioprotective Mediator for the Ischemic Heart

Adenosine is a degradative product of ATP, exerting a potent biological action in the ischemic heart although it is rapidly metabolized. The effects of adenosine are mediated by two types of adenosine receptors, A_1- and A_2-receptors. A_1-receptors are predominantly distributed on the myocardial cells and A_2-receptors are distributed on the coronary vascular walls [12]. The coronary vasodilatory effect of adenosine is mediated by A_2-receptors. Although it is controversial whether the autoregulation of coronary blood flow is mediated by adenosine [12], adenosine is released to maintain coronary blood flow when the coronary perfusion pressure falls below 80 mmHg because of coronary arterial narrowings. A significant contribution of endogenous adenosine to the maintenance of coronary circulation is clearly shown by the fact that blockade of adenosine receptors with 8-phenyltheophylline during hypoperfusion decreases blood flow and increases lactate production, causing worsening myocardial ischemia.

In canine hearts subjected to coronary microembolization, we also observed the continuous release of adenosine, which could ameliorate the ischemic changes [13,14]. These results indicate that adenosine release in the ischemic heart may serve to attenuate the ischemic insults, either in coronary narrowings or in coronary microcirculatory disturbances. Thromboembolism in the small coronary arteries is often observed in ischemic heart disease, and this may cause the non-reflow after reperfusion in acute myocardial infarction. Endogenous adenosine could prevent thromboembolism with platelet aggregations through A_2-receptors [15]. In dogs, we observed the progressive decrease of coronary blood flow because of platelet aggregations when 8-phenytheophylline was administered in the narrowed coronary artery. Adenosine also inhibits the free radical formation in leukocytes through A_2-receptors [16,17] and thus could attenuate myocardial injury from neutrophil filtration. As is discussed later, ischemic preconditioning augments adenosine release from the ischemic heart, which attenutes activation of neutrophils after reperfusion and allows salvage of the ischemic myocardium [18].

Adenosine also attenuates the contractility enhanced by beta-adrenoceptor stimulation through A_1-receptors [19]. Beta-adrenoceptor stimulation activates G_s proteins that are antagonized by activation of G_i proteins from A_1-receptor stimulation. It should be noted, however, that stimulation of A_1-receptors does not exert a negative inotropic effect in basal conditions, and attenuation of contractile function is only observed when the beta-adrenoceptors are activated, such as during exercise and myocardial ischemia. Therefore, in the ischemic heart, this mechanism is substantially realized. We observed that blockade of adenosine receptors by 8-phenyltheophylline substantially augmented contractile function in the ischemic canine hearts when beta-adrenoceptors were stimulated by isoproterenol (see Fig. 1) [20]. This negative effect of adenosine in the ischemic heart, however, plays a beneficial role in cardioprotection because attenuation of inotropic effects by endogenous adenosine could improve metabolic dysfuntion in the ischemic heart, i.e., by decreasing lactate production and attenuating tissue acidosis.

It is well known that contractile dysfunction is not recovered quickly after reperfusion following brief ischemia, and this sustained contractile abnormality is called "myocardial stunning," as is often observed in the clinical setting after coronary recanalization in patients with acute myocardial infarction [21]. Adenosine could also attenuate myocardial stunning. Several lines of evidence suggest that myocardial stunning is caused by intracellular Ca overload during an early period of reperfusion, mainly through Na/Ca exchange [22]. It has been reported that adenosine inhibits this iron exchange and may attenuate the Ca influx on reperfusion [23]. Indeed, administration of adenosine markedly improved the cardiac function after 15 min occlusion of the coronary artery in the dog (Fig. 2). Beneficial effects of adenosine were confirmed by the deterioration of contractile function when adenosine receptors were blocked by 8-phenyltheophylline. The subtypes of adenosine receptors involved in this improvement of myocardial stunning could be clarified by administration of selective adenosine receptor agonists, N-6-cyclohexyladenosine (CHA) for A_1-receptors and 5'-N-ethylcarboxyamidoadenosine (NECA) for A_2 receptors. We observed that both adenosine receptor agonists improved myocardial stunning in the canine heart to a similar extent, indicating that both A_1- and A_2-receptors are responsible for attenuating myocardial stunning [24].

Because propranolol does not affect the stunning of the heart, a mechanism whereby adenosine attenuates beta-stimulated inotropic action may not be involved, but A_1-receptor-mediated effects may be attributable to attenuation of Ca influx. On

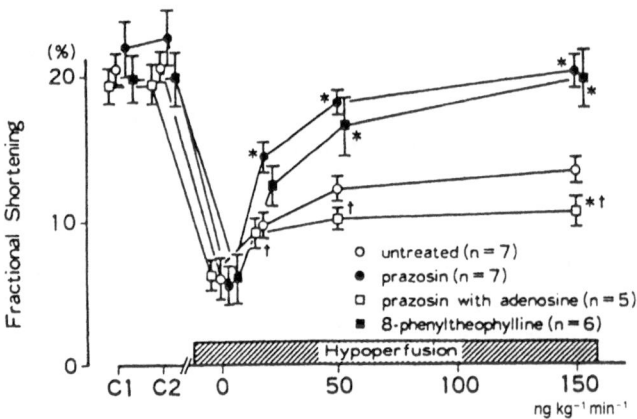

FIG. 1. Dose–response relations of isoproterenol to fractional shortening in hypoperfused canine hearts. Fractional shortening was increased by intravenous infusion of isoproterenol in a dose-dependent manner, but the increments of fractional shortening were significantly augmented in the 8-phenyltheophylline- and prazosin-treated hearts. The effect of prazosin was abolished by intracoronary infusion of adenosine, indicating that the beta-adrenoceptor-mediated inotropic response is attenuated by endogenous adenosine in the ischemic heart. Bars, mean + SEM; *, $P < 0.05$ vs untreated group; †, $P < 0.01$ vs prazosin-treated group. (From [20] with permission)

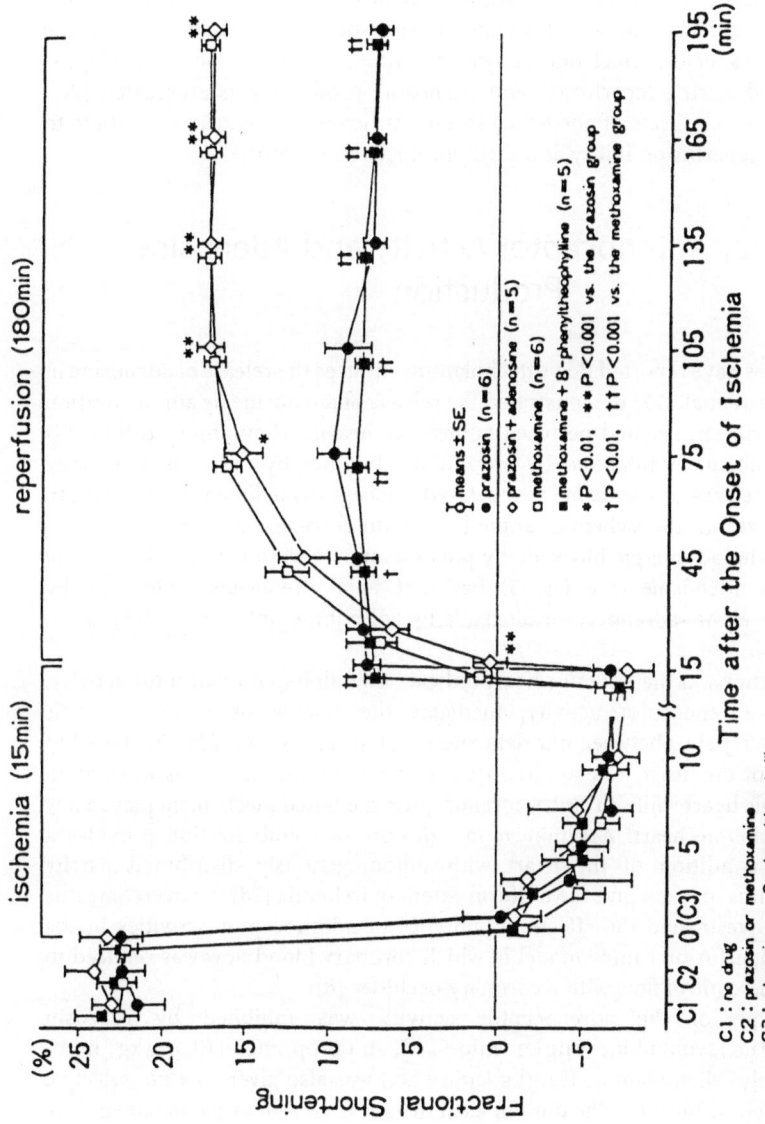

FIG. 2. Effect of exogenous adenosine in the prazosin-treated (4.0μg·kg⁻¹·min⁻¹ i.c.) group and 8-phenyltheophylline in the methoxamine-treated (1.0μg·kg⁻¹·min⁻¹ i.c.) group on fractional shortening after 15-min occlusion of the coronary artery in the dog. In the prazosin-treated group, administration of adenosine significantly increased the fractional shortening, indicating that adenosine could improve the myocardial stunning, while inhibition of adenosine receptors with 8-phenyltheophylline decreased fractional shortening in the methoxamine-treated group in which adenosine release was augmented. (From [36], with permission)

the other hand, stimulation of A_2-receptors increases hyperemic flow and inhibits activation of neutrophils and platelets. However, papaverine does not improve stunning, suggesting that increases in coronary blood flow per se may not contribute to improvement of stunning. Alternatively, it is suggested that microcirculatory abnormalities are involved in part as a cause of myocardial stunning. Indeed, oxygen-derived free radicals are generated in stunned myocardium, and radical scavengers attenuate myocardial stunning [25]. Because oxygen-derived free radicals inactivate enzyme activities, ecto-5'-nucleotidase, which synthetizes adenosine from AMP, is also inactivated during reperfusion and adenosine production is attenuated [26]. Thus, multifactorial effects of adenosine in the cardiovascular system contribute to attenuation of reperfusion injury as a cardioprotective mediator.

Alpha$_1$-Adrenoceptor Activity and Adenosine Production

Previous studies have reported that catecholamine induces the release of adenosine in the heart. DeWitt et al. [27] demonstrated the release of adenosine by administration of norepinephrine in isolated perfused guinea pig hearts. They observed that this release of adenosine is inhibited by propranolol but not by prazosin; thus, they attributed the release of adenosine to a beta-adrenoceptor-mediated mechanism. In contrast, however, in the ischemic canine heart with coronary embolization we reported that alpha-adrenergic blockade by phentolamine and prazosin did attenuate the release of adenosine (see Fig. 3) but that beta-adrenoceptor blockade by propranolol or alpha$_2$-adrenoceptor blockade by yohimbine only minimally attenuated release [8].

Our observations in the ischemic heart indicate that alpha$_1$-adrenoceptor activity, but not beta-adrenoceptor activity, mediates the release of adenosine. This appararent discrepancy between our data and previous reports may be attributed to the condition of the heart; a beta-adrenoceptor-mediated mechanism is working in the nonischemic heart while an alpha-adrenoceptor-mediated mechanism plays a key role in the ischemic heart. A canine model of coronary embolization provides a characteristic condition of the heart with inhomogenously distributed patchy ischemia and thus may not give the uniform extent of ischemia [28]. To overcome this problem, we investigated the effects of subtypes of adrenoceptor activities in the coronary hypoperfusion canine model in which coronary blood flow was reduced to one-third of the control flow with a coronary occluder [8].

Each subtype of the adrenoceptor activity was inhibited by prazosin ($4\mu g kg^{-1} min^{-1}$ i.c.), yohimbine ($9\mu g kg^{-1} min^{-1}$ i.c.), and propranolol ($0.3\mu g kg^{-1} min^{-1}$ i.c.), respectively. Phentolamine ($9\mu g kg^{-1} min^{-1}$ i.c.) was also given as a nonselective alpha-adrenoceptor blocker. The dose of each drug was chosen at the maximal dose that affects neither baseline coronary blood flow nor hemodynamic parameters. In treatment by yohimbine or phentolamine, the metabolic effects of norepinephrine release caused by presynaptic alpha antagonism were prevented by propranolol. In the untreated condition, adenosine release was progressively increased after the onset of hypoperfusion and reached a peak at 5 min, gradually decreased to a steady state thereafter (Fig. 4). The steady-state release of adenosine was still higher than the control level. Treatments of propranolol and yohimbine did not attenuate adenosine

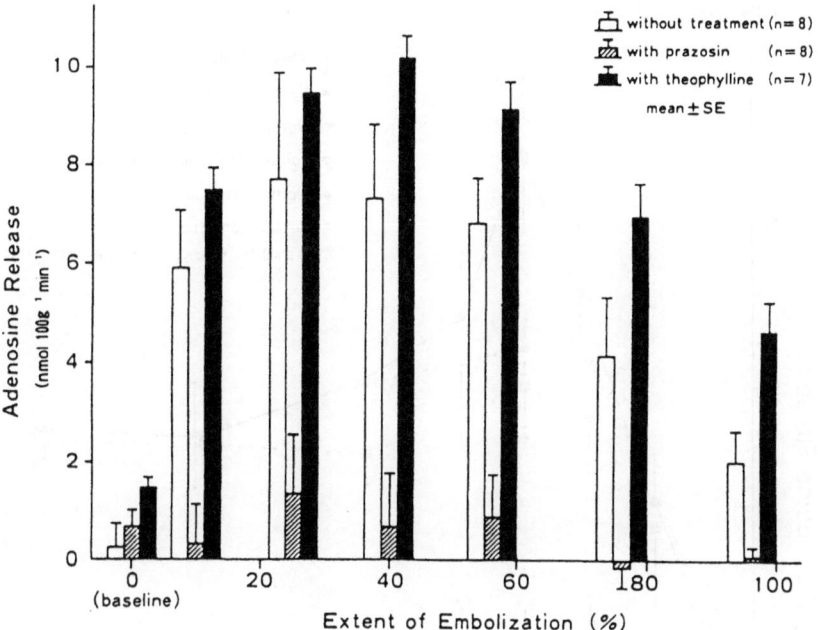

FIG. 3. Adenosine release during repetitive intracoronary injection of microspheres with and without treatment of prazosin and theophylline. The extent of embolization was subdivided into six ranges. Each column represents mean value from lumped data in each range. Adenosine release was significantly attenuated in the prazosin-treated group. (From [14] with permission)

release, although the peak release of adenosine (overshoot release) was significantly attenuated by propranolol. In contrast, with treatments of prazosin and phentolamine, adenosine release was markedly attenuated while contractile function and metabolic changes were not affected. These results strongly suggested that adenosine release during myocardial ischemia is mediated by alpha₁-adrenoceptor activity. It was further confirmed that withdrawal of prazosin restored the release of adenosine to the control level obtained at the untreated condition. Thus, alpha₁-adrenoceptor activity may regulate the release of adenosine directly, not by modification of the extent of ischemia.

What then, is the underlying mechanism by which adenosine release is regulated by alpha₁-adrenoceptor activity during ischemia? It is well known that adenosine is produced not only at the cardiomyocytes but also in the endothelial cells and vascular smooth muscle cells [29]. To clarify the cellular and subcellular mechanisms of alpha₁-adrenoceptor-mediated adenosine production, isolated cell preparations may be useful. For this purpose, cardiomyocytes were isolated from adult male Wistar rats and exposed to norepinephrine (10^{-9}–10^{-5} mol/l) while being treated with propranolol (beta-adrenoceptor blockade) and yohimbine (alpha₂-adrenoceptor blockade) [30]. Adenosine release was observed even without exposure of norepinephrine in a time-dependent manner; however, alpha₁-adreneceptor stimulation with norepinephrine or methoxamine significantly augmented the release of adenosine (Fig. 5). During hypoxic condition (incubation with 5% CO_2 and 95% N_2), the release of adenosine was further augmented in both untreated and alpha₁-adrenoceptor-stimulated conditions (Fig. 6). These results indicate that adenosine is produced in the cardiomyocytes and

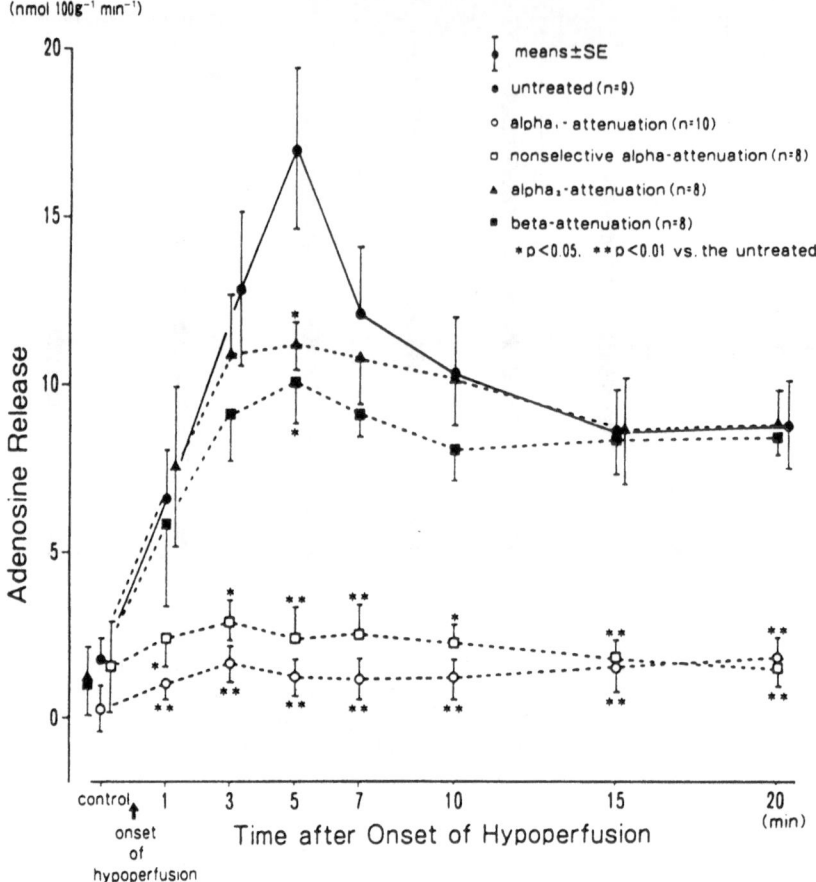

FIG. 4. Adenosine release during coronary hypoperfusion under administration of various agents that inhibit alpha- or beta-adrenoceptors. Alpha-adrenoceptor inhibition with phentolamine or prazosin markedly attenuated the release of adenosine during ischemia, but beta-adrenoceptor attenuation with propranolol or alpha$_2$-adrenoceptor inhibition with yohimbine minimally attenuated the release of adenosine. These results indicate that alpha$_1$-adrenoceptor activation is involved in adenosine release during myocardial ischemia. (From [8] with permission)

that alpha$_1$-adrenoceptor stimulation increases the release of adenosine in both normoxic and hypoxic conditions.

A major pathway of adenosine synthesis during ischemia and hypoxia is enzymatic dephosphorylation of 5'-AMP by 5'-nucleotidase. The synthesis pathway is switched from hydrolysis of S-adenosylhomocysteine (SAH) by SAH hydrolase to dephosphorylation of 5'-AMP during ishchemia or hypoxia [31]. 5'-Nucleotidase exists in two forms in the myocardium, ecto-5'-nucleotidase as a membrane-bound form and cytosolic 5'-nucleotidase as a free in the cytoplasm [32]. In our study, ecto-5'-nucleotidase activity was increased by norepinephrine and methoxamine during 30 min in a dose-dependent manner, but cytosolic 5'-nucleotidase was not activated [30]. Because alpha$_1$-adrenoceptors are coupled with phosphatidyl inositol hydrolysis, which activates protein kinase C through diacyl glycerol formation, increased activities of ecto-

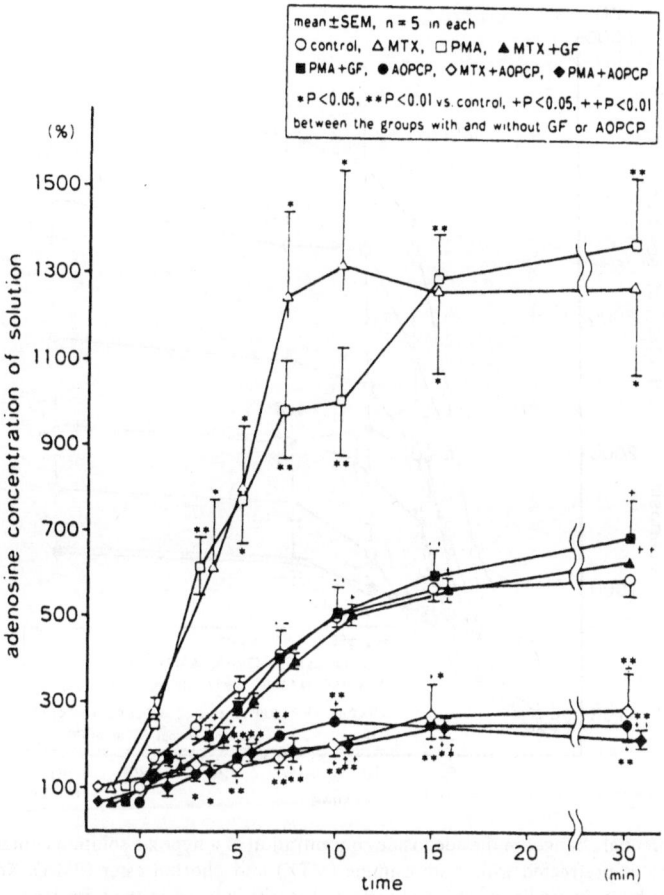

FIG. 5. Sequential changes in the adenosine concentration of a normoxic solution containing rat cardiomyocytes pretreated with methoxamine (MTX) and phorbol ester (PMA). Adenosine release was augmented in MTX- and PMA-treated cardiomyocytes more than in the untreated controls. Concomitant exposures to AOPCP (an inhibitor of 5′-nucleotidase) or GF 109203X (an inhibitor of protein kinase C) inhibited the increases in adenosine release from the myocytes, indicating that alpha-adrenoceptor stimulation augments the release of adenosine through activation of 5′-nucleotidase induced by protein kinase C activation. (From [30] with permission)

5′-nucleotidase by alpha$_1$-adrenoceptor stimulation may be attributable to activation of protein kinase C (Fig. 7). Indeed, increase in this enzyme activity by norepinephrine and methoxamine was inhibited by GF109203X, an inhibitor of protein kinase C in both normoxic and hypoxic conditions. Furthermore, enzyme activities were also increased by phorbol 12-myristate 13-acetate (PMA), an activator of protein kinase C. As expected, the increase in adenosine release was blunted by GF109203X and alpha,beta-methyleneadenosine 5′-diphosphate (AOPCP), an inhibitor of ecto-5′-nucleotidase. These results indicate that alpha$_1$-adrenoceptor stimulation enhances the 5′-nucleotidase activity through activation of protein kinase C.

Our results also indicate that ecto-5′-nucleotidase is more important for the pathway for increase of adenosine release in rat cardiomyocytes, because ecto-5′-nucleoti-

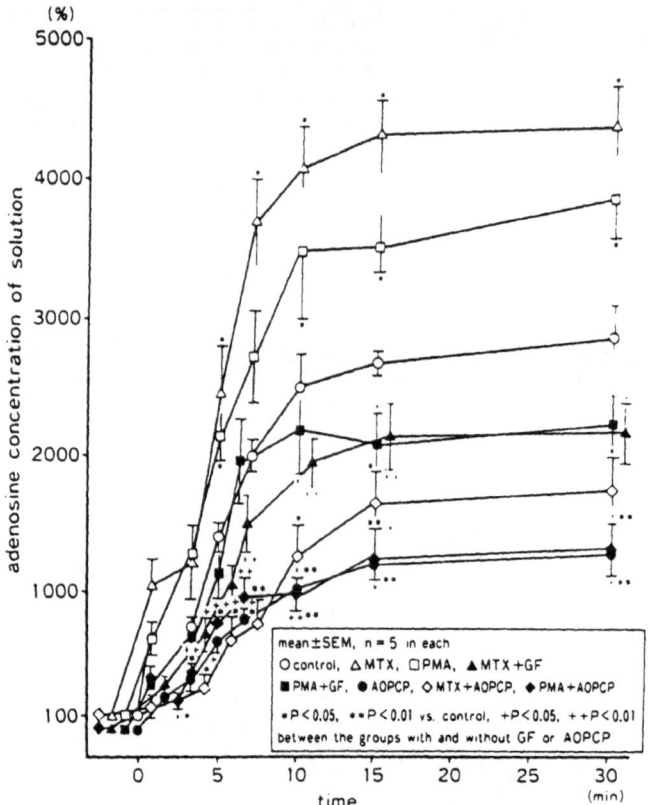

FIG. 6. Sequential changes in the adenosine concentration of a hypoxic solution containing rat cardiomyocytes pretreated with methoxamine (MTX) and phorbol ester (PMA). Adenosine release from hypoxic cardiomycytes was increased markedly even in the untreated condition. Adenosine release was augmented in MTX- and PMA-treated cardiomyocytes more than in the untreated controls. This augmentation was also inhibited by AOPCP or GF 109203X, as observed in the normoxic condition (see Fig. 5), indicating that alpha-adrenoceptor stimulation augments the release of adenosine from hypoxic cardiomyocytes. (From [30] with permission)

dase activity is predominantly increased by alpha$_1$-adrenoceptor stimulation and the release of adenosine is inhibited by AOPCP. Imai et al. [33] also postulated the importance of ecto-5'-nucleotidase in releasing adenosine in hypoxic cardiomyocytes. If this is the case, where is adenosine produced from 5'-AMP, outside the cardiomyocytes or inside the cells? We detected 5'-AMP in the medium in which the cardiomyocytes were suspended and observed that the amount of 5'-AMP is increased during hypoxic condition. It is reported that 5'-AMP can be released from cells and is converted to adenosine outside the cells [34]. Thus, adenosine synthesis is increased during hypoxia or ischemia because (1) the substrate of 5'-nucleotidase, 5'-AMP, is increased and (2) ecto-5'-nucleotidase activity is also increased.

During ischemia, norepinephrine is released and thereby alpha$_1$-adrenoceptors are activated, resulting an increase in ecto-5'-nucleotidase activity. This enzyme alteration could further increase the release of adenosine during ischemia. Because adenosine exerts cardioprotective effects, alpha$_1$- adrenoceptor stimulation during

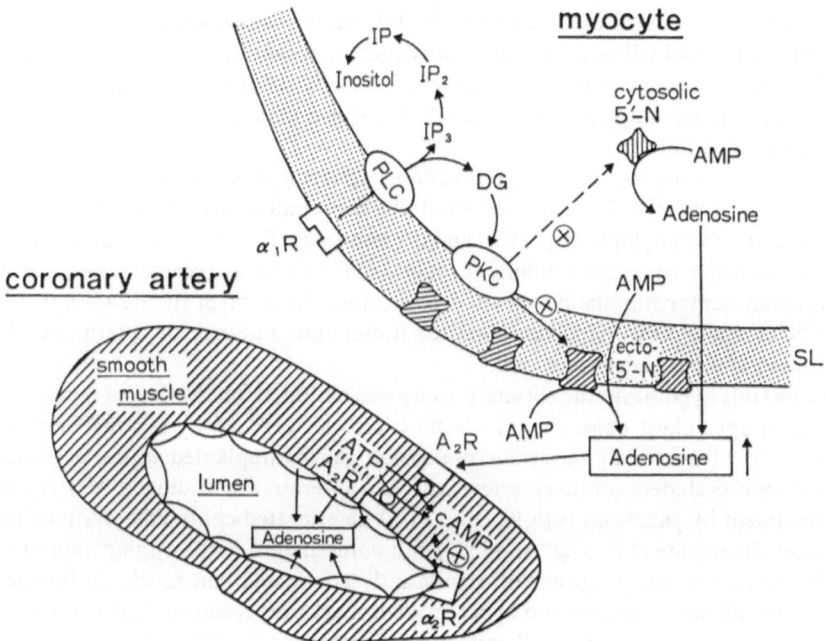

FIG. 7. Schemiatic diagram of possible actions of alpha-adrenergic stimulation on adenosine production and vascular effects of adenosine in ischemic hearts. (From [12] with permission)

ischemia may be beneficial for the heart [35,36], although excessive alpha-adrenoceptor stimulation causes coronary vasoconstriction and thereby increases ischemic injury.

Cardioprotective Effects of Alpha-Adrenoceptor Activity Against Ischemic Injury

It is well recognized that adenosine is cardioprotective against ischemic injury through (1) an increase in coronary blood flow, (2) inhibition of platelet activation and neutrophil activation, (3) attenuation of cardiac oxygen demand in beta-adrenoceptor-stimulated hearts, and (4) inhibition of Ca influx. If alpha-adrenoceptor stimulation activates 5'-nucleotidase, which synthesizes adenosine from 5'-AMP during ischemia, alpha-adrenoceptor stimulation may be beneficial because it augments adenosine release in the ischemic heart.

Thromboembolism in small coronary arteries is often observed in the ischemic heart [37], and this may sustain myocardial ischemia even during reperfusion. A previous report from our laboratory demonstrated that sustained hyperemic coronary flow response is observed in coronary microembolization because of a massive release of adenosine [13]. In the canine ischemic model in which the left anterior descending coronary artery is embolized with 15-μm microspheres, coronary blood flow increased to 170% ± 14% of the baseline flow at 16%–30% of maximal embolization. Intracoronary infusion of prazosin markedly attenuated adenosine release and hyperemic response, and regional contractile function and lactate

metabolism were significantly deteriorated [14]. These changes were compatible with
the effect of theophylline, an inhibitor of adenosine receptors. The salutary effect of
alpha-adrenoceptor activity was further confirmed by the improvement of ischemic
changes in the same dog after withdrawal of prazosin associated with an increase in
coronary blood flow.

Myocardial stunning, a sustained functional abnormality observed after transient
myocardial ischemia, is often observed in the clinical setting after coronary
recanalization by angioplasty (PTCA) and thrombolysis (PTCR). As discussed earlier,
adenosine could attenuate stunning through both A_1- and A_2-receptors. Because al-
pha$_1$-adrenoceptor stimulation enhances adenosine release, myocardial stunning may
also be attenuated by alpha$_1$-adrenoceptor stimulation and may be deteriorated by
inhibition of alpha$_1$-adrenoceptors.

To test this hypothesis, the coronary artery was occluded for 15 min and reperfused
for 3 h in open-chest dogs. Contractile function was assessed by regional segment
shortening, measured by ultrasonic dimension gauges implanted in the perfusion
area of the occluded coronary artery, the left anterior descending (LAD) artery.
Pretreatment by parazosin ($4 \mu g kg^{-1} min^{-1}$ i.c.) deteriorated contractile dysfunction,
while methoxamine ($1.0 \mu g kg^{-1} min^{-1}$ i.c.) and norepinephrine ($0.24 \mu g kg^{-1} min^{-1}$ i.c.)
with rauwolscine and propranolol, significantly attenuated contractile dysfunction
[24]. Both adenosine release and hyperemic coronary flow response during the early
reperfusion period were markedly attenuated by treatment with prazosin, and both
parameters were increased in alpha$_1$-adrenoceptor stimulation.

Thus, these results suggest that alpha$_1$-adrenoceptor stimulation is beneficial to
attenuate stunning because of the enhanced release of adenosine. This was further
confirmed by the fact that treatment of 8-phenyltheophylline completely abolished
the beneficial effect of norepinephrine and methoxamine. Furthermore, exogenous
administration of adenosine restored contractile function even with prazosin
treatment.

Recently, "ischemic preconditioning" has received much attention from both basic
and clinical points of view. Ischemic preconditioning is a phenomenon in which a
brief ischemia preceding lethal ischemia limits infarct size markedly. The limiting
effect on infarct size by ischemic preconditioning is remarkable, and thus the mechanism underlying this phenomenon has been extensively studied. Recently, Liu et al.
[38] demonstrated that adenosine A_1-receptor activation is responsible for the infarct
size-limiting effect. Several other investigators supported this idea, and recent reports
have also suggested that activation of protein kinase C plays an important role in the
subcellular mechanism of ischemic preconditioning [39]. A previous report by
Olafsson et al. [40] that intracoronary infusion of adenosine reduced infarct size by
75% in dogs has suggested the hypothesis that ischemic preconditioning augments
adenosine release on reperfusion. To test this idea, we measured adenosine release
after reperfusion following 40-min occlusion of the coronary artery in dogs preconditioned with four episodes of 5-min ischemia before the sustained ischemia [41].
Myocardial 5′-nucleotidase activity was also measured before and at 40 min of sustained ischemia with and without preconditioning. The adenosine concentration in
coronary venous blood during reperfusion was more than twofold higher in preconditioned hearts [41]. The significantly higher concentrations were observed until
30 min after reperfusion. Both ecto- and cytosolic 5′-nucleotidase activities were significantly increased in the preconditioned hearts [41]. Although the mechanisms of
activation of 5′-nucleotidase activity were not clarified in this study, increased 5′-

nucleotidase activities may be responsible for the enhanced adenosine release, and thereby infarct size was limited after reperfusion. If endogenous norepinephrine release in ischemia-preconditioned hearts is involved in activation of 5'-nucleotidase through alpha$_1$-adrenoceptor stimulation, administration of prazosin, an alpha$_1$-adrenoceptor antagonist, could attenuate the infarct size-limiting effect of preconditioning, and exogenous administration of alpha$_1$-adrenoceptor agonist may mimic the effect of preconditioning [42].

To test this hypothesis, prazosin ($4 \mu g kg^{-1} min^{-1}$) was constantly infused into the LAD coronary artery from 5 min before ischemic preconditioning to 60 min after reperfusion. The prazosin treatment significantly attenuated 5'-nucleotidase activities in both endocardium and epicardium, and blunted the infarct size-limiting effect of ischemic preconditioning [42] (Fig. 8). In contrast to prazosin, intermittent intracoronary administration of methoxamine ($40 \mu g kg^{-1} min^{-1}$) for four cycles for

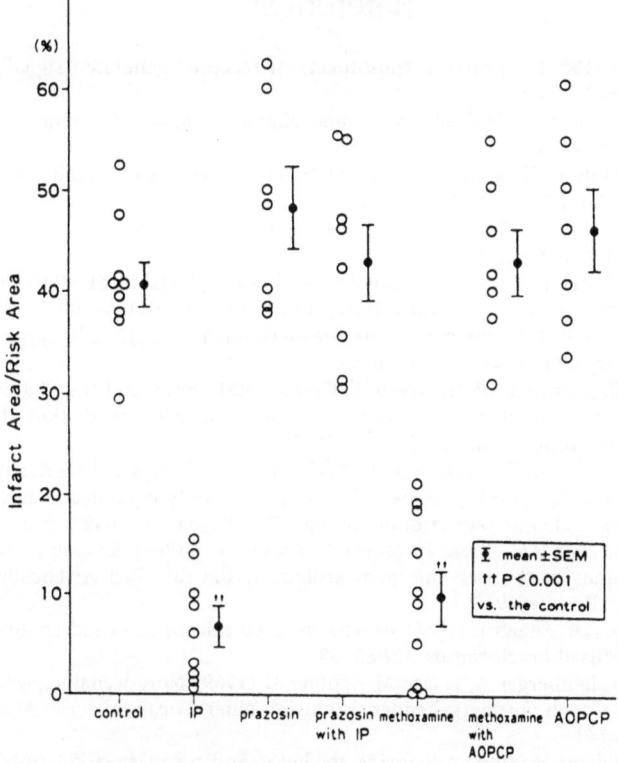

FIG. 8. Effects of ischemic preconditioning (IP), prazosin, and methoxamine on infarct size (infarct area/risk area) in dogs. Inositol phosphate (IP) was given to the heart during four cycles of 5-min occlusion of the left anterior descending coronary artery separated by 5 min reperfusion. IP markedly decreased the infarct size, but inhibition of alpha$_1$-adrenoceptors with prazosin completely blocked the infarct size-limiting effect of IP, indicating that alpha$_1$-adrenoceptor activation is important in the effect of IP. Pharmacological preconditioning with methoxamine mimicked the effect of IP, and this infarct size-limiting effect was abolished by concomitant treatment of AOPCP, an inhibitor of ecto-5'-nucleotidase. These results indicate that ischemic preconditioning increases the release of adenosine through activation of 5'-nucleotidase by intrinsic alpha$_1$-adrenoceptor stimulation. (From [42] with permission)

5 min at 5-min intervals increased 5'-nucleotidase activity, mimicking the ischemic preconditioning [42]. The infarct size was also attenuated by methoxamine as in ischemic preconditioning, and this beneficial effect was abolished by AOPCP, an inhibitor of ecto-5'-nucleotidase (Fig. 98).

Recent observations in our laboratory have demonstrated that the activation of 5'-nucleotidase is blunted by administration of the inhibitors of protein kinase C, polymixin B, and GF 109203X [43]. From these results, we conclude that ischemic preconditioning activates 5'-nucleotidase activities through activation of protein kinase C and increases adenosine release during ischemic preconditioning and reperfusion after sustained ischemia. In this signaling pathway, alpha-adrenoceptor activation plays a pivotal role in activation of this key enzyme, and exerts cardioprotective effects against ischemic and reperfusion injury through potentiation of adenosine release in ischemic hearts.

References

1. Gilman AG (1987) G proteins: transducers of receptor generated signals. Ann Rev Biochem 56:615–649
2. Homcy CJ, Graham RM (1985) Molecular characterization of adrenergic receptors. Circ Res 56:635–650
3. Vatner SF (1983) Alpha-adrenergic regulation of the coronary circulation in the conscious dog. Am J Cardiol 52:15A–21A
4. Angus JA, Cocks TM, Satoh K (1986) The α-adrenoceptors on endothelial cells (brief review). Fed Proc 45:2355–2359
5. Brady AJB, Warren JB, Poole-Wilson PA, Williams TJ, Harding SE (1993) Nitric oxide attenuates cardiac myocyte contraction. Am J Physiol 265:H176–H186
6. Cohen J, Eckstein L, Gutman Y (1980) The mechanism of alpha-adrenergic inhibition of catecholamine release. Br J Pharmacol 71:135–142
7. Camazine B, Shannon RP, Guerrero JL, Graham RM, Powell WJ Jr (1988) Neurogenic histaminergic vasodilation in canine skeletal nuscle: mediation by alpha$_2$-adrenoceptor stimulation. Circ Res 62:871–883
8. Kitakaze M, Hori M, Tamai J, Iwakura K, Koretsune Y, Kigiya T, Iwai K, Kitabatake A, Inoue M, Kamada T (1987) Alpha$_1$-adrenoceptor activity regulates release of adenosine from the ischemic myocardium in dogs. Circ Res 60:631–639
9. Schomig A, Dart AM, Dietz R, Mayer E, Kubler W (1984) Release of endogenous catecholamines in the ischemic myocardium of the rat. Part A: Locally mediated release. Circ Res 55:689–701
10. Wollenberger A, Shaab L (1965) Anoxia-induced release of noradrenaline from the isolated perfused heart. Nature 207:88–89
11. Shaab L, Wollenberger A, Haase M, Schiller U (1969) Noradrenalinaggabe aus dem Hundehezen nach vorubergehender Okklusion einer Koronararterie. Acta Biol Med Ger 22:135–143
12. Hori M, Kitakaze M (1991) Adenosine, the heart, and coronary circulation. Hypertension 18:565–574
13. Hori M, Inoue M, Kitakaze M, Koretsune Y, Iwai K, Tamain J, Ito H, Kitabatake A, Sato H, Kamada T (1986) Role of adenosine in hyperemic response of coronary blood flow in microembolization. Am J Physiol 250:H509–H518
14. Hori M, Tamai J, Kitakaze M, Iwakura K, Gotoh K, Iwai K, Koretsune Y, Kagiya T, Kitabatake A, Kamada T (1989) Adenosine-induced hyperemia attenuates myocardial ischemia in coronary microembolization in dogs. Am J Physiol 257:H244–H251
15. Kitakaze M, Hori M, Sato H, Takashima S, Inoue M, Kitabatake A, Kamada T (1991) Endogenous adenosine inhibits platelet aggregation during myocaridal ischemia in dogs. Circ Res 69:1402–1408

16. Cronstein BN, Levin RI, Belanoff J, Weissmann G, Hirchhorn R (1986) Adenosine: an endogenous inhibitor of neutrophil-mediated injury to endothelial cells. J Clin Invest 78:760–770

17. Cronstein BN, Kramer SB, Weissmann G, Hirschhorn R (1986) Adenosine : a physiological modulator of superoxide anion generation by human neutrophils. J Exp Med 158:1160–1177

18. Kitakaze M, Hori M, Takashima S, Sato H, Inoue M, Kamada T (1993) Ischemic preconditioning increases adenosine release and 5'-nucleotidase activity during myocardial ischemia and reperfusion in dogs. Implications for myocardial salvage. Circulation 87:208–215

19. Dobson JG Jr (1983) Mechanism of adenosine inhibition of catecholamine-induced responses in heart. Circ Res 52:151–160

20. Sato H, Hori M, Kitakaze M, Takashima S, Inoue M, Kitabatake A, Kamada T (1992) Endogenous adenosine blunts β-adrenoceptor-mediated inotropic response in hypoperfused canine myocardium. Circulation 85:1594–1603

21. Brauwald E, Kloner RA (1982) The stunned myocardium: prolonged postischemic ventricular dysfunction. Circulation 66:1146–1149

22. Karmazyn M (1988) Amiloride enhances postischemic ventricular recovery: possible role of Na^+-H^+ exchange. Am J Physiol 255:H608–H615

23. Brechler V, Pavoine C, Lotersztajin S, Garbarz E, Pecker F (1990) Activation of Na^+/Ca^{2+} exchange by adenosine in ewe heart sarcolemma is mediated by a pertussis toxin-sensitive G protein. J Biol Chem 265:16851–16855

24. Kitakaze M, Takashima S, Sato H (1990) Stimulation of adenosine A_1 and A_2 receptors prevents myocardial stunning (abstract). Circulation 82(suppl III):III-37

25. Bolli R, Patel BS, Jeroudi MO, Lai EK, McCay PB (1988) Demonstration of free radical generation in "stunned" myocaridium of intact dogs with the use of the spin trap alpha-phenyl N-tert-butyl-nitrone. J Clin Invest 82:476–485

26. Kitakaze M, Hori M, Takashima S, Iwai K, Sato H, Inoue M, Kitabatake A, Kamada T (1992) Superoxide dismutase enhances ischemia-indued reactive hyperemic flow and adenosine release in dogs. A role of 5'-nucleotidase activity. Circ Res 71:558–566

27. DeWitt DF, Wangler RD, Thompson CI, Sparkes HV Jr (1983) Phasic release of adenosine during steady-state metabolic stimulation in the isolated guinea pig heart. Circ Res 53:636–643

28. Hori M, Gotoh K, Kitakaze M, Iwai K, Iwakura K, Sato H, Koretsune Y, Inoue M, Kitabatake A, Kamada T (1991) Role of oxygen-derived free radicals in myocardial edema and ischemia in coronary microembolization 84:828–840

29. Schrader J, Borst M, Kelm M, Smolenski T, Deussen A (1991) Intra- and extracellular formation of adenosine by cardiac tissue. In: Imai S, Nagazawa M (eds) Role of adenosine and adenine nucleotides in the biological system. Elsevier, Amsterdam, pp 261–271

30. Kitakaze M, Hori M, Morioka T, Minamino T, Takashima S, Okazaki Y, Node K, Komamura K, Iwakura K, Itoh T, Inoue M, Kamada T (1995) α-Adrenoceptor activation increases ecto-5'-nucleotidase activity and adenosine release in rat cardiomyocytes by activating protein kinase C. Circulation 91:2226–2234

31. Lloyd HGE, Schrader J (1987) The importance of the transmethylation pathway for adenosine metabolism in the hearts. In: Gerlach E, Becker BF (eds) Topics and perspectives in adenosine research. Springer, Berlin Heidelberg New York, pp 199–207

32. Newby AC, Worku Y, Meghji P (1987) Critical evaluation of role of ecto- and cytosolic 5'-nucleotidase in adenosine formation. In: Gerlach E, Becker BF (eds) Topics and perspectives in adenosine research. Springer, Berlin Heidelberg New York, pp 155–168

33. Imai S, Nakazawa M, Imai H, Jin H (1987) 5'-Nucleotidase inhibitors and the myocardial reactive hyperemia and adenosine content. In: Gerlach E, Becker BF (eds) Topics and perspectives in adenosine research. Springer, Berlin Heidelberg New York, pp 416–424

34. Borst MM, Schrader J (1991) Adenine nucleotide release from isolated perfused guinea pig hearts and extracellular formation of adenosine. Circ Res 68:797–806

35. Hori M, Tamai J, Kitakaze M, Iwakura K, Gotoh K, Iwai K, Korestune Y, Kagiya T, Kitabatake A, Kamada T (1989) Adenosine-induced hyperemia attenuates myocardial ischemia in coronary microembolization in dogs. Am J Physiol 257:H244–H251

36. Kitakaze M, Hori M, Sato H, Iwakura K, Gotoh K, Inoue M, Kitabatake A, Kamada T (1991) Beneficial effects of alpha₁-adrenoceptor activity on myocardial stunning in dogs. Circ Res 68:1322–1339

37. Moschos CB, Lahiri K, Lyons M, Weisse AB, Oldwurted HA, Regan TJ (1973) Relation of microcirculatory thrombosis to thrombus in the proximal coronary artery: effect of aspirin, dipyridamole, and thrombolysis. Am Heart J 86:61–68

38. Liu GS, Thournton J, Van Winkle DM, Stanley AWH, Olsson RA, Downey JM (1991) Protection against infarction afforded by preconditioning is mediated by A_1 adenosine receptors in rabbit heart. Circulation 84:350–356

39. Speechly-Dick ME, Mocanu MM, Yellon DM (1994) Protein kinase C, its role in ischemic preconditioning in the rat. Circ Res 75:586–590

40. Olafsson B, Forman MB, Puett DW, Pou A, Cates CU, Friesinger GC, Virmani R (1987) Reduction of reperfusion injury in a canine preparation by intracoronary adenosine: importance of the endothelium and the no-reflow phenomenon. Circulation 76:1135–1145

41. Kitakaze M, Hori M, Takashima S, Sato H, Inoue M, Kamada T (1993) Ischemic preconditioning increase adenosine release and 5′-nucleotidase activity during myocardial ischemia and reperfusion in dogs. Implication for myocardial salvage. Circulation 87:208–215

42. Kitakaze M, Hori M, Morioka T, Minamino T, Takashima S, Sato H, Shinozaki Y, Chujo M, Mori H, Inoue M, Kamada T (1993) Alpha₁-adrenoceptor activation mediates the infarct size-limiting effect of ischemic preconditioning through augmentation of 5′-nucleotidase activity. J Clin Invest 93:2197–2205

43. Kitakaze M, Minamino T, Shinozaki Y, Sakamoto H, Mori H, Kurihara T, Hori M (1994) Activation of protein kinase C and subsequent activation of ectosolic 5′-nucleotidase; a major cause for the infarct size-limiting effect of ischemic precondtioning (abstract). Circulation 90(part 2):I–207

Immunomodulating Effects as New Aspects of a Positive Inotropic Agent

Shigetake Sasayama, Akira Matsumori, Sigeo Matsui,
Tetsuo Shioi, and Takehiko Yamada

Summary. Recently, a number of new inotropic agents have been developed to re-place or supplement digitalis glycosides. Though long-term treatment with most of these new agents was accompanied by an accelerated disease process and an adverse effect on survival, one quinorinone derivative, vesnarinone, has been confirmed to prolong the life of heart failure patients dramatically. We assessed the mechanism of action of this agent from the immunological point of view. Myocarditis and subse-quent heart failure were induced in mice by an encephalomyocarditis virus infection. Survival and myocardial damage were markedly improved by vesnarinone, although viral replication and virus-induced cell injury were not inhibited. The natural killer (NK) cell activity of the spleen cells obtained from infected mice was markedly elevated, but this specific cytotoxicity was substantially suppressed by treatment with vesnarinone. This effect appears to be related to the unique action of vesnarinone as a potassium-channel blocker which is capable of inhibiting T-cell activity. Vesnarinone also inhibited production of tumor necrosis factor (TNF)-α and several other cytokines. The observed benefits of vesnarinone on mortality may not be ex-plained solely by suppression of cytokine production because a similar effect was induced by amrinone, which had been shown to be deleterious to the clinical outcome of patients with heart failure. Nevertheless, the survival of mice subjected to lethal endotoxemia was significantly improved by vesnarinone through a reduction in TNF-α production. Cytokines exert depressant effects on myocyte function, and there appears to be a difference in cytokine regulation between normal subjects and heart failure patients. Therefore, we conclude that an inhibition of NK cell activity and suppression of cytokine production could mediate the beneficial effects of vesnarinone in the treatment of chronic heart failure.

Key words. Survival—Cytokine—Natural killer cell—Myocarditis—Heart failure

Introduction

Heart failure remains an obscure clinical entity and its definition has been disputed for many years. Cohn [1] has proposed that heart failure is defined as a syndrome in which cardiac dysfunction is associated with reduced exercise tolerance, a high

Department of Cardiovascular Medicine, Kyoto University, Sakyo-ku, Kyoto 606, Japan

incidence of ventricular arrhythmias, and shortened life expectancy. According to this concept, there can be only two goals in the management of heart failure: to relieve symptoms and improve the quality of life, and to prolong life.

New Orally Active Inotropic Agents

Depression of myocardial contractility plays an important role in the development of heart failure. However, in the early 1970s, the only drugs available to improve contractility of the failing myocardium were the digitalis glycosides. The role of digitalis in the management of heart failure has been disputed for many years [2]. Simple withdrawal of digitalis resulted in no clinical deterioration of many patients with mild to moderate heart failure [3], and the efficacy of chronic maintenance digoxin therapy was not evidenced in terms of exercise capacity on the basis of a placebo-controlled double-blind crossover study [4]. To replace or supplement digitalis in the management of heart failure, intensive interest and passion have been generated in the past few decades by the search for orally effective inotropic agents. Recently, a number of inotropic agents that are structurally unrelated to digitalis have been introduced [5].

The first exciting reports of amrinone, the synthetic phosphodiesterase (PDE) inhibitor which increases intracellular cyclic adenosine monophosphate (cAMP) by inhibiting its degradation, indicated that this agent could produce dramatic short-term hemodynamic benefits in patients with advanced left ventricular dysfunction [6]; however, important concerns were later expressed about an adverse reaction which accelerated disease progression during long-term treatment with this agent [7,8].

Subsequently, many oral PDE inhibitors were introduced, but again they were shown to induce short-term hemodynamic effects while no clinical improvement could be observed with sustained administration [9]. Even excess mortality was observed in patients who received active oral PDE inhibitors compared to placebo recipients [10]. Similarly, short-term therapy with β-receptor agonists produced marked hemodynamic benefits, but long-term treatment with these drugs was accompanied by an accelerated disease process and an adverse effect on survival [11,12].

There is substantial evidence that the failing heart is in an energy-depleted state. Administration of an inotropic agent to an energy-starved, failing heart would be expected to increase myocardial energy use and so could accelerate disease progression. A detrimental effect of positive inotropic drugs on survival of patients with chronic heart failure may also be explained by the exacerbation of ventricular tachyarrhythmias, which increases the probability of sudden death. An increase in the release of activator calcium into the cytosol by cardiotonic agents leads to the development of delayed afterdepolarizations [13]. Increased intracellular cAMP may also enhance automaticity and triggered responses.

A New Positive Inotrope with a Unique Mechanism of Action

Recently, another inotropic agent, vesnarinone, was synthesized in Japan. This compound is a quinolinone derivative and structurally unrelated to catecholamines, cardiac glycosides, or the xanthines. In addition to an increase in intracellular cAMP by inhibition of a specific isoform of PDE, the mechanism of action of this agent includes: (a) an increase in intracellular sodium ions, (b) an increase in the calcium-channel open frequency, and (c) prolongation of the action potential by inhibition of an outward potassium channel. Thus, vesnarinone appears to augment cardiac contractility via ion channels [14].

A preliminary study demonstrated that peak hemodynamic effects were observed 8 h after oral ingestion, when there was a significant rise in cardiac output with a concomitant decrease in diastolic pulmonary artery pressure. The heart rate remained unchanged throughout the study period and no marked increase in ventricular ectopy occurred with the agent [15].

The multicenter study conducted in Japan to evaluate the long-term clinical efficacy and safety of vesnarinone 60 mg given once daily demonstrated that 21% of patients in the placebo group were withdrawn from the trial due to death or worsening heart failure during 3 months of the study period, while only 2% of patients in the active-treated group were hospitalized because of increased congestive symptoms [16]. Subsequently, the survival study of this agent, which was carried out in the U.S., demonstrated a 62% reduction in mortality during 26 weeks of the study period in patients who received vesnarinone 60 mg once daily in addition to their usual therapeutic regimen [17]. We assessed the additional mechanisms of action of this agent, i.e., those other than PDE inhibition, using a murine model of myocarditis and heart failure. We assumed that the observed benefit might be related to the agent's effects on the immune system because treatment with vesnarinone was associated with a high incidence of reversible neutropenia [5,17].

Animal Model of Myocarditis and Heart Failure

It has long been postulated that dilated cardiomyopathy occurs as a "burned-out" stage of preceding viral myocarditis. A causal relationship between dilated cardiomyopathy and myocarditis is best characterized in murine models. We inoculated 4-week-old, male DBA/2 mice ($n = 60$) with encephalomyocarditis (EMC) virus. During the first 7 days, the virus invades the heart tissue and directly causes myocytolysis. Histopathological examination of the myocardium revealed that cellular infiltration and myocardial necrosis developed during this period. Congestive heart failure became apparent from 7 to 10 days post infection onwards, by which time most of the culturable virus had been eliminated, but the viral genome was detectable by polymerase chain reaction at the site of myocardial damage [18].

Survival of the Infected Mice

In the infected nontreated control group, 75% of the animals died during day 5 to day 8. When treatment with vesnarinone was started at the time of innoculation, the cumulative survival rate substantially improved in a dose-related manner [19]. In particular, all the animals treated with a higher dose had a delayed start of death and showed a threefold increase in survival on day 14. Treatment with equivalent molar doses of amrinone did not affect the survival (Fig. 1).

Histopathological Findings

The mice were killed 5 days after virus infection for histopathological examination. The heart weight to body weight ratio correlated closely with the congestive symp-

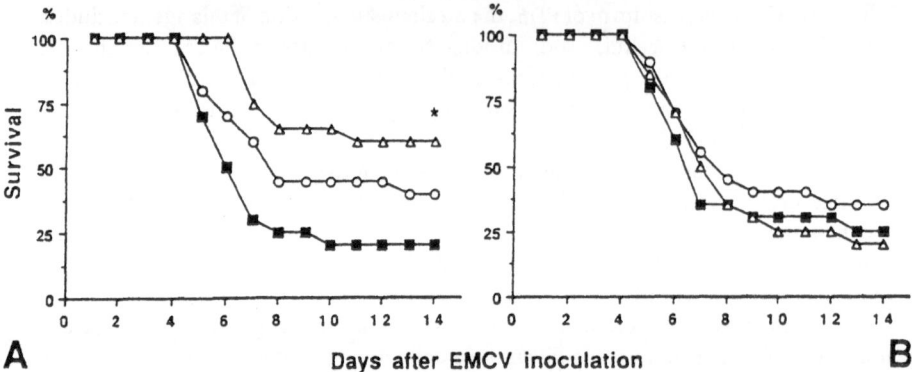

FIG. 1A,B. Cumulative survival curves of 4-week-old DBA/2 mice inoculated with encephalomyocarditis virus (*EMCV*). A Infected controls (*squares*), those treated with vesnarinone (VN) 10 mg/kg (*circles*), and with VN 50 mg/kg (*triangles*). B Infected controls (*squares*), those treated with amrinone (AM) 5 mg/kg (*circles*), and with AM 25 mg/kg (*triangles*). Survival of mice improved with vesnarinone in a dose-dependent manner, but was not affected by an equivalent molar dose of amrinone. (From [19] with permission)

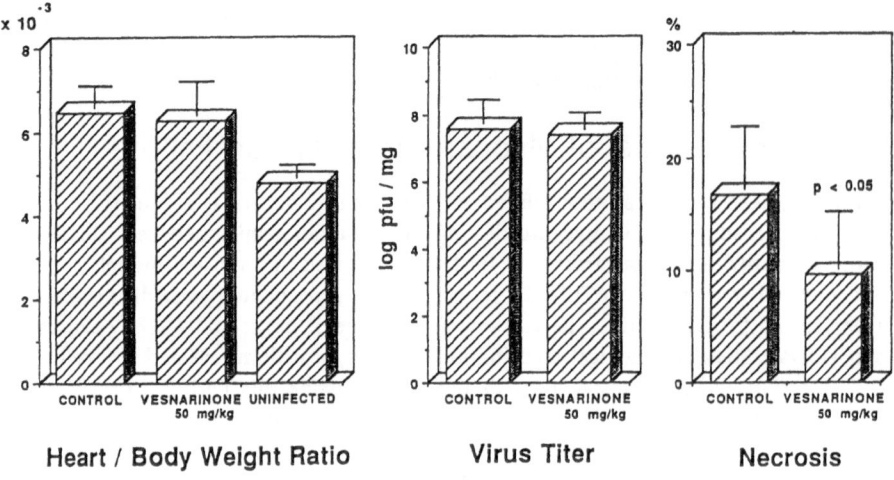

FIG. 2. Histopathologic findings and virus titer of the heart for the infected nontreated group (*control*) and for the infected vesnarinone-treated group. The data were obtained on day 5 of inoculation where severe heart failure had not yet developed. Heart weight had increased in both groups compared to the noninfected group. There were no differences in the myocardial virus titer between the two groups, whereas the percentage of necrosis area was significantly reduced in the treated group

toms but no appreciable differences were observed in group mean values between the infected control and the vesnarinone-treated groups. The virus titer determined by plaque-assay of the supernatants of homogenized myocardium was similar in the infected controls and the infected but vesnarinone-treated group. However, the percentage of myocardial necrosis was significantly reduced in the mice treated with vesnarinone (Fig. 2).

Virus Replication in Cultured Murine Myocytes

Myocytes of DDY murine neonates were cultured in 24-well plates and then infected with EMC virus. The plates were incubated for 24 h with or without various concentrations of vesnarinone, and then frozen and thawed for virus titration of the supernatants by plaque assay. The virus titer of the myocyte-free wells was 2.7 log pfu/ml and the virus yield in the infected control was 3.9 log pfu/ml. Treatment with vesnarinone did not affect virus yields regardless of concentration or preincubation with the drug before the virus infection.

Virus-Induced Cytopathic Effect

Murine myocytes were cultured on 96-well plates and labeled with ^{51}Cr, which is taken up by living cells and released only when cells die. The rate of ^{51}Cr release [100 × (sample cpm − spontaneous cpm)/(total cpm released after addition of Triton X − spontaneous cpm)] was 22% for control wells and 21% for wells treated with vesnarinone. Therefore, vesnarinone did not directly protect the myocytes from virus-induced cell injury.

Natural Killer (NK) Cell Activity

Then, we considered the contribution of immunological defense mechanisms to the observed beneficial effect of vesnarinone. The DBA/2 mice infected with EMC virus were killed on days 1, 3, and 5 and spleen cells were obtained. The ability of NK cells to kill their target was observed by incubating effector cells obtained from the spleen of the infected mice with ^{51}Cr-labeled target cells (YAC-1) and by measuring the amount of radioactivity released from the killed target. Incubation of the target cells with spleen cells was carried out at an effector-to target-cell ratio of 25:1, 50:1, and 100:1. The NK-cell activity of the spleen cells started to increase from the 2nd day after the virus infection, rising to 27% on day 5 from the initial value of 6.5% on day 1. These increases in specific cytotoxicity of NK cells were significantly suppressed by vesnarinone but not by an equal molar dose of amrinone (Fig. 3). In an additional experiment, we pretreated mice with antiasialo GM1 antibody before EMC virus infection. In these cases, cytotoxicity remained un-changed at any given level of effector-to target-cell ratio. Thus, the increase in specific cytotoxicity was due to an increase in the activity of asialo GM1-bearing NK cells, and the effects of vesnarinone could be attributed exclusively to inhibition of this activity.

This unique effect of vesnarinone appears to be related to its action on ion channels rather than its property as a PDE inhibitor. Lin and co-workers [20] have demonstrated that a blocker of small-conductance Ca^{2+}-ion activated potassium channels and voltage-gated potassium channels inhibits T-cell proliferation and lymphokine production when triggered through Ca^{2+}-associated signal transduction pathways. In particular, blockade of voltage-gated potassium channels leads to inhibition of the activation-induced rise in intracellular calcium through its role in setting the resting potential in T cells. Therefore, vesnarinone may exert immunosuppressive effects through this inhibition of the voltage-gated potassium channels involved in T-cell activation.

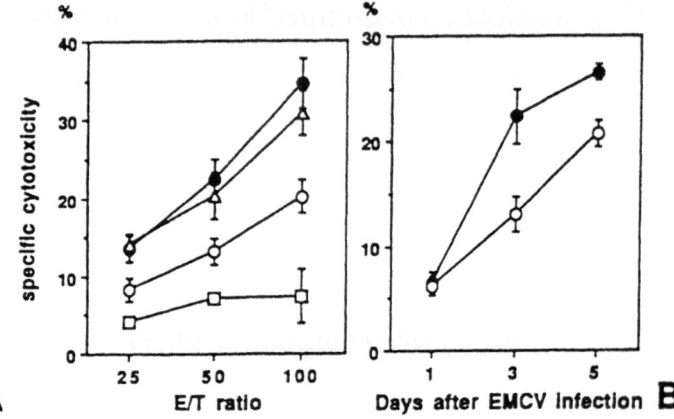

FIG. 3. **A** Natural Killer (NK) cell activity expressed as the rate of specific cytotoxicity measured at three different effector-to target-cell (E/T) ratios. The percentage of cytotoxicity of the NK cells obtained from the infected mice on day 3 was substantially elevated at each measurement (*solid circles*). NK cell activity was reduced by treatment with vesnarinone (*open circles*) but not to the levels of noninfected controls (*squares*). The effects of amrinone were not significant (*triangles*). **B** Time course of the percentage of specific cytotoxicity at an E/T ratio of 50:1. This value was 6.5% in both the nontreated (*solid circles*) and the vesnarinone-treated group (*open circles*) on day 1, but increased gradually thereafter. Treatment with vesnarinone suppressed these changes significantly. (From [19] with permission)

Cytokine Production

Recently, the intriguing possibility has been raised that some aspects of heart failure might be related to the biological effects of cytokines, most notably tumor necrosis factor (TNF)-α. TNF-α is mainly released from activated macrophages after viral infection, and the elaboration of TNF-α may potentially be cardioprotective by enhancing antiviral immune responses [21,22] or by inhibiting virus replication [23]. There is an increasing awareness that TNF-α may play a much broader pathophysiologic role in myocarditis and heart failure. In our murine model of myocarditis and heart failure, the plasma TNF-α concentration was elevated compared with noninfected mice on days 3, 5, and 7 after virus inoculation. Injection of recombinant human TNF-α increased the mortality of infected animals with greater histopathological changes and higher virus titer in the myocardium, while antimurine TNF-α antibody increased survival and caused an improvement in myocardial lesions [24].

PDE inhibitors which increase intracellular cAMP and modify protein kinase A suppress TNF-α gene expression at the transcriptional level. We cultured spleen cells obtained from the same DBA/2 mice in RPMI-FCS on microplates. Each well was incubated at 37°C in 5% CO_2 and stimulated with lipopolysaccharide (LPS) to produce TNF-α. Three different equal molar doses of vesnarinone and amrinone were added to the cell suspension. After 9 h of incubation, by which time TNF production reached a maximum, the TNF-α concentration in the supernatant of each well was assayed using enzyme-linkd immunosorbent assay (ELISA). Vesnarinone and amrinone similarly suppressed TNF-α production significantly in a dose-dependent manner (Fig. 4)

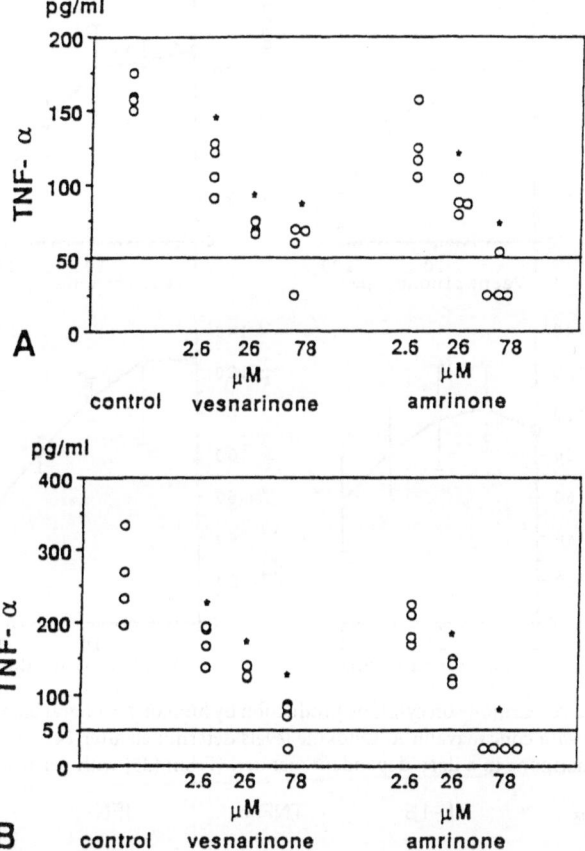

FIG. 4. The amount of tumor necrosis factor (*TNF*)-α produced in the cultured spleen cells stimulated with lipopolysaccharide (LPS) at 100 (A) and 1000 ng/ml (B). Addition of equivalent molar doses of vesnarinone and amrinone into the cell suspension similarly reduced TNF-α production in a dose-dependent manner. (From [19] with permission)

[19]. Vesnarinone also inhibited the production of interferon (IFN)-γ, interleukin (IL)-1β, and IL-2 as well as that of TNF-α by stimulated human peripheral lymphocytes, human T cell lines, and monocytic cell lines at concentrations similar to those found in the patients' plasma receiving vesnarinone treatment (Fig. 5) [25]. When the blood of 5 healthy male volunteers and 7 patients with heart failure was stimulated with 100 ng/ml of LPS, local cytokine production was more prominent in patients with heart failure. Vesnarinone inhibited the production of TNF-α and IFN-γ in both healthy and heart failure patients. Suppression of IL-1α and IL-1β was significant in healthy volunteers but not in patients with heart failure (Fig. 6) [26].

These productions of cytokines can be mediated through PDE inhibition, which leads to an increase in intracellular cAMP. Therefore, the reduced mortality associated with vesnarinone treatment may not be explained by its effect on cytokine production alone. However, a variety of cytokines have recently been shown to depress myocyte function either by a direct negative inotropic effect [27,28] or by a blunting of the effects of β -adrenergic stimulation [29,30]. In a murine model of lethal endotoxemia induced by intraperitoneal injection of LPS, we have shown that endog-

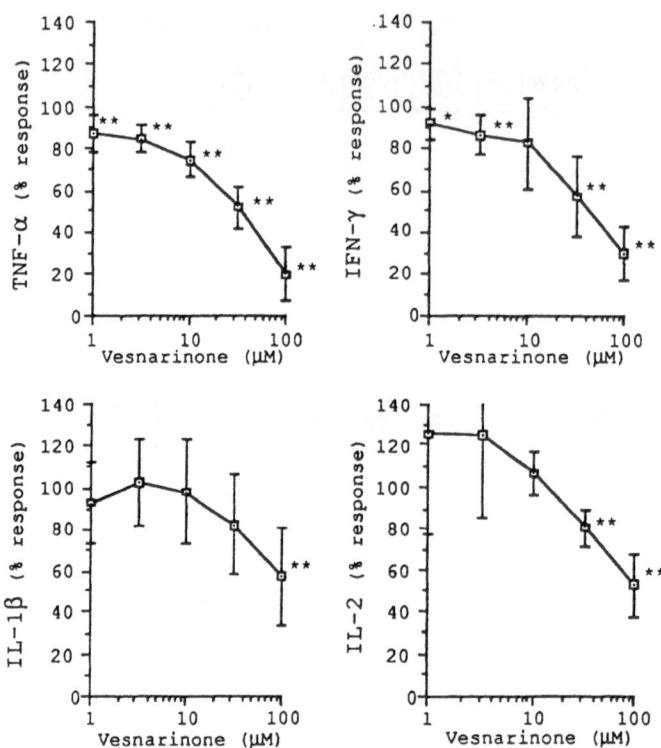

FIG. 5. Effects of vesnarinone on cytokine production by human peripheral blood mononuclear cells stimulated with concanavalin A. Cytokine levels determined after 24 h of incubation were reduced by vesnarinone in a dose-dependent manner. (From [25] with permission)

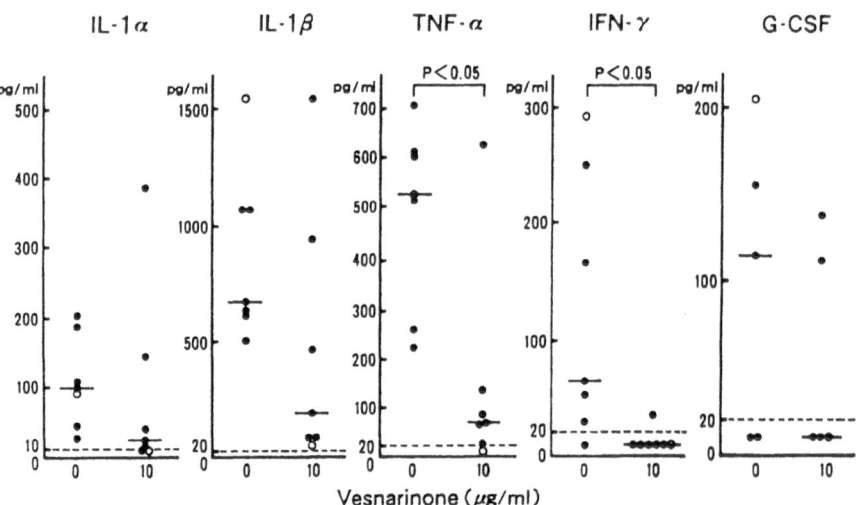

FIG. 6. Effects of vesnarinone on the production of cytokines in LPS-stimulated blood in patients with heart failure. A significant reduction in TNF-α and interferon (IFN)-γ was induced by vesnarinone 10 μg/ml. Suppression of interleukin (IL)-1α and IL-1β was significant in healthy volunteers but variable in heart failure patients. Marked depression of cytokines, most notably granulocyte colony-stimulating factor-(G-CSF) was observed in one patient who had developed neutropenia during vesnarinone treatment (open circle). (From [26] with permission)

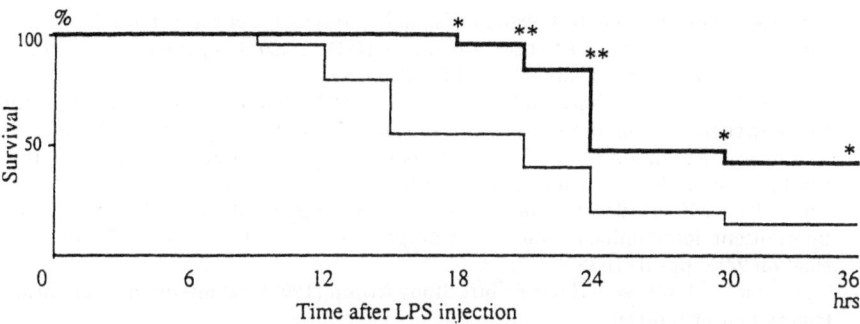

FIG. 7. Survival of 8-week-old female BALB/c mice with lethal endotoxemia induced by LPS injection. In the control group (*thin trace*), mice started to die 12 h after the injection of 300 µg LPS, but when treatment with vesnarinone (*thick trace*) 50 mg/kg po and 10 µg ip was started at the time of LPS injection, the mice survived the first 20 h, median survival time was prolonged, and lethality was reduced. The difference in mortality was most prominent at 24 h after LPS injection. (From [31] with permission)

enous proinflammatory cytokines play a pivotal role in mediating pathophysiological changes. Animals started to die 12 h after LPS injection with substantial elevation of plasma TNF-α, reaching a maximum level 1 h after LPS challenge. When vesnarinone was given by oral gavage together with simultaneous intraperitoneal injection with LPS, the median survival time was increased and lethality was significantly reduced (Fig. 7) [31]. These effects were associated with a significant reduction of the circulating TNF-α level at the maximal point.

Taken together, these findings suggest that cytokines certainly alter myocyte function, and that this cytokine-dependent cell damage can be related in part to clinical manifestation of heart failure. Therefore, the potent inhibitory effect of vesnarinone on cytokine production provides an additional modality for treatment of heart failure, as do its immunomodulating effects on NK-cell activation.

References

1. Cohn JN (1988) Current therapy of the failing heart. Circulation 78:1099–1107
2. Poole-Wilson PA, Robinson K (1989) Digoxin—A redundant drug in congestive cardiac failure. Cardiovasc Drugs Ther 2:733–741
3. Gheorghiade M, Beller GA (1983) Effects of discontinuing maintenance digoxin therapy in patients with ischemic heart disease and congestive heart failure in sinus rhythm. Am J Cardiol 51:1243–1250
4. Fleg JL, Gottlieb SH, Lakatta EG (1982) Is digoxin really important in treatment of compensated heart failure? A placebo-controlled crossover study in patients with sinus rhytum. Am J Med 73:244–250
5. Sasayama S (1992) What do the newer inotropic drugs have to offer? Cardiovasc Drugs Ther 6:15–18
6. Benotti JR, Grosman W, Braunwald E, Davolos DD, Alousi AA (1978) Hemodynamic assessment of amrinone: a new inotropic agent. N Engl J Med 299:1373–1377
7. Packer M, Leier CV (1987) Survival in congestive heart failure during treatment with drugs with positive inotropic actions. Circulation 75[Suppl IV]:IV-55-IV-63
8. Massie B, Bourassa M, DiBianco R, Hess M, Konstam M, Likoff M, Packer M, (for the Amrinone Multicenter Trial Group) (1985) Long-term oral administration of amrinone for congestive heart failure: lack of efficacy in a multicenter controlled trial. Circulation 71:963–971

9. Petein M, Levine B, Cohn JN (1986) Persistent hemodynamic effects without long-term clinical benefits in response to oral piroximone (MDL 19,205) in patients with congestive heart failure. Circulation 73[Suppl III]:230–236

10. Uretsky BF, Jessup M, Konstam MA, Dec W, Leier CV, Benotti J, Murali S, Herrmann HC, Dandberg JA (for the Enoximone Multicenter Trial Group) (1990) Multicenter trial of oral enoximone in patients with moderate to moderately severe congestive heart failure. Lack of benefit compared with placebo. Circulation 82:774–780

11. Dies F, Krell MJ, Whitlow P, Liang CS, Goldenberg I, Applefeld MM, Gilbert EM (1986) Intermittent dobutamine in ambulatory outpatients with chronic cardiac failure. Circulation 74[Suppl II]:II-38

12. The Xamoterol in Severe Heart Failure Study Group (1990) Xamoterol in severe heart failure. Lancet 336:1–6

13. Katz AM (1986) Potential deleterious effects of inotropic agents in the therapy of chronic heart failure. Circulation 73[Suppl III]:184–190

14. Iijima T, Taira N (1987) Membrane current changes responsible for the positive inotropic effect of OPC-8212, a new positive inotropic agent, in single ventricular cells of the guinea pig heart. J Pharmacol Exp Ther 240:657–662

15. Sasayama S, Inoue M, Asanoi H, Kodama K, Hori M, Sakurai T, Kawai C (1986) Acute hemodynamic effects of a new inotropic agent, OPC-8212, on severe congestive heart failure. Heart Vessels 2:23–28

16. Sasayama S (for the OPC-8212 Multicenter Research Group) (1990) A placebo-controlled, randomized, double-blind study of OPC-8212 in patients with mild chronic heart failure. Cardiovasc Drugs Ther 4:419–426

17. Feldman AM (for the Vesnarinone Study Group) (1993) Effects of vesnarinone of morbidity and mortality in patients with heart failure. N Engl J Med 329:149–155

18. Kyu BS, Matsumori A, Sato Y, Okada I, Chapman NM, Tracy S (1992) Cardiac persistence of cardioviral RNA detected by polymerase chain reaction in a murine model of dilated cardiomyopathy. Circulation 86:522–530

19. Matsui S, Matsumori A, Matoba Y, Uchida A, Sasayama S (1994) Treatment of virus-induced myocardial injury with a novel immunomodulating agent, vesnarinone. J Clin Invest 94:1212–1217

20. Lin CS, Boltz RC, Blake JT, Nguyen M, Talento A, Fischer PA, Springer MS, Sigal NH, Slaughter RS, Garcia ML, Kaczorowski GJ, Koo GC (1993) Voltage-gated potassium channels regulate calcium-dependent pathways involved in human T lymphocyte activation. J Exp Med 177:637–645

21. Henke A, Mohr C, Sprenger H, Graebner C, Stelzner A, Nain M, Gemsa D (1992) Coxsackievirus B$_3$-induced production of tumor necrosis factor-α, IL-1β, and IL-6 in human monocytes. J Immunol 148:2270–2277

22. Ostensen ME, Thiele DL, Lipsky PE (1987) Tumor necrosis factor-α enhances cytolytic activity of human natural killer cells. J Immunol 138:4185–4191

23. Jaattela M (1991) Biologic activities and mechanisms of action of tumor necrosis factor-α/cachectin. Lab Invest 64:724–742

24. Yamada T, Matsumori A, Sasayama S (1994) Therapeutic effect of anti-tumor necrosis factor-α antibody on the murine model of viral myocarditis induced by encephalomyocarditis virus. Circulation 89:846–851

25. Shioi T, Matsumori A, Matsui S, Sasayama S (1994) Inhibition of cytokine production by a new inotropic agent, vesnarinone, in human lymphocytes, T cell line, and monocytic cell line. Life Sciences 54:PL11–16

26. Matsumori A, Shioi T, Yamada T, Matsui S, Sasayama S (1994) Vesnarinone, a new inotropic agent, inhibits cytokine production by stimulated human blood from patients with heart failure. Circulation 89:955–958

27. Finkel MS, Oddis CV, Jacob TD, Watkins SC, Hattler BG, Simmons RL (1992) Negative inotropic effects of cytokines on the heart mediated by nitric oxide. Science 257:387–389

28. Yokoyama T, Vaca L, Rossen RD, Durante W, Hazarika P, Mann D (1993) Cellular basis for the negative inotropic effects of tumor necrosis factor-α in the adult mammalian heart. J Clin Invest 92:2303–2312

29. Gulick T, Pieper ST, Murphy MA, Lange LG, Schreiner GF (1991) A new method for assessment of cultured cardiac myocyte contractility detects immune factor-mediated inhibition of β-adrenergic responses. Circulation 84:313–321
30. Balligand JL, Ungureanu D, Kelly RA, Kobzik L, Pimental D, Michel T, Smith TW (1993) Abnormal contractile function due to induction of nitric oxide synthesis in rat cardiac myocytes follows exposure to activated macrophage conditioned medium. J Clin Invest 91:2314–2319
31. Matsui S, Matsumori A, Sasayama S (1994) Vesnarinone prolongs survival and reduces lethality in a murine model of lethal endotoxemia. Life Sci 55:1735–1741

Index